OESOPHAGOGASTRIC SURGERY

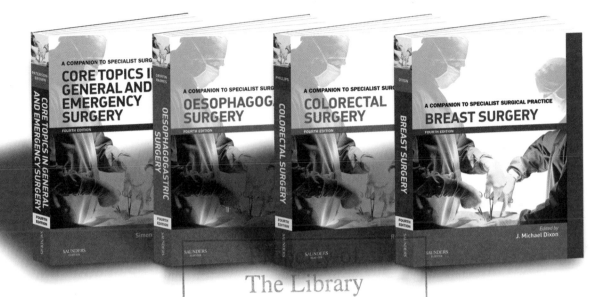

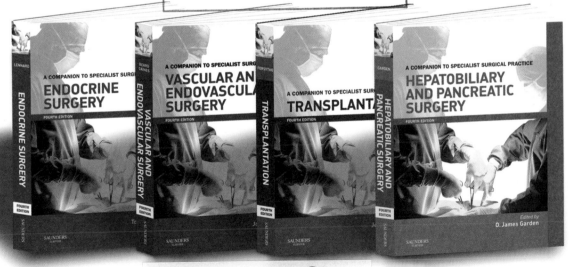

The Library
Prince Philip Hospital
Llanelli

A COMPANION TO SPECIALIST SURGICAL PRACTICE

A Companion to Specialist Surgical Practice

Series Editors
O. James Garden
Simon Paterson-Brown

OESOPHAGOGASTRIC SURGERY

FOURTH EDITION

Edited by

S. Michael Griffin
MD FRCS

Professor of Gastrointestinal Surgery
Northern Oesophago-gastric Unit
Royal Victoria Infirmary
Newcastle upon Tyne, UK

Simon A. Raimes
MD FRCS FRCS(Ed)

Consultant Upper Gastrointestinal Surgeon
Northern Oesophago-gastric Unit
Cumberland Infirmary
Carlisle, UK

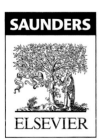

SAUNDERS

ELSEVIER

Edinburgh   London   New York   Oxford   Philadelphia   St Louis   Sydney   Toronto   2009

SAUNDERS
ELSEVIER

Fourth edition © 2009 Elsevier Limited. All rights reserved.

First edition 1997
Second edition 2001
Third edition 2005
Fourth edition 2009

ISBN 9780702030154

British Library Cataloguing in Publication Data
A catalogue record for this book is available from the British Library

Library of Congress Cataloging in Publication Data
A catalog record for this book is available from the Library of Congress

Notice

ELSEVIER your source for books, journals and multimedia in the health sciences
www.elsevierhealth.com

Working together to grow libraries in developing countries
www.elsevier.com | www.bookaid.org | www.sabre.org

ELSEVIER   BOOK AID International   Sabre Foundation

The Publisher's policy is to use paper manufactured from sustainable forests

Printed in China

Commissioning Editor: Laurence Hunter
Development Editor: Elisabeth Lawrence
Project Manager: Andrew Palfreyman
Text Design: Charlotte Murray
Cover Design: Kirsteen Wright
Illustration Manager: Gillian Richards
Illustrators: Martin Woodward and Richard Prime

Contents

Contents

Contributors

Derek Alderson, MB, BS, MD, FRCS
Barling Professor of Surgery
University of Birmingham
Birmingham, UK

William H. Allum, BSc, MD, FRCS
Consultant Surgical Oncologist
GI Surgery Unit
Royal Marsden NHS Foundation Trust
London, UK

Farzaneh Banki, MD
Assistant Professor of Surgery
Department of Surgery
Keck School of Medicine
University of Southern California
Los Angeles, CA, USA

Hugh Barr, MD, ChM, FRCS, FRCS(Ed), FHEA
Professor and Consultant Upper
Gastrointestinal Surgeon
Cranfield Postgraduate Medical School
Gloucestershire Royal Hospital
Gloucester, UK

Mark K. Bennett, MB, FRCPath
Consultant Histopathologist
Royal Victoria Infirmary
Newcastle upon Tyne, UK

Jane M. Blazeby, BSc, MD, FRCS(Gen Surg)
Professor of Surgery and Honorary
Consultant Surgeon
University of Bristol and University Hospitals
Bristol NHS Trust, Bristol, UK

Abraham J. Botha, MD, FRCS
Consultant Upper Gastrointestinal Surgeon
Department of Surgery
Guy's and St Thomas' NHS Foundation
London, UK

Geoffrey W.B. Clark, MB, ChB, MD, FRCS(Ed)
Consultant Oesophago-gastric Surgeon
Department of Surgery
University Hospital of Wales
Cardiff, UK

Adrian Crellin, MA, FRCP, FRCR
Consultant Clinical Oncologist
Leeds Cancer Centre
Cookridge Hospital
Leeds, UK

Christopher Deans, MB, ChB, MRCS, MRCS(Ed)
Specialist Registrar, General Surgery
University Department of Surgery
Edinburgh Royal Infirmary
Edinburgh, UK

Tom R. DeMeester, MD
Professor and Chairman
Department of Surgery
University of Southern California
Los Angeles, CA, USA

Simon Dexter, BSc, MB, BS, MRCS
Consultant Upper Gastrointestinal Surgeon
Department of Upper Gastrointestinal Surgery
St James's University Hospital
Leeds, UK

Richard S. Gillies, BSc, MB, BS, MRCS
Specialist Registrar, Oesophago-gastric Surgery
Oxford Oesophago-gastric Centre, Churchill Hospital
Oxford, UK

S. Michael Griffin, MD, FRCS
Professor of Gastrointestinal Surgery
Northern Oesophago-gastric Unit
Royal Victoria Infirmary
Newcastle upon Tyne, UK

Richard H. Hardwick, MD, FRCS
Consultant Upper Gastrointestinal Surgeon
Cambridge Oesophago-gastric Centre
Addenbrooke's Hospital
Cambridge, UK

John G. Hunter, MD
Professor and Chair of Surgery
Department of Surgery
Oregon Health and Science University
Portland, OR, USA

Contributors

Janusz Jankowski, MD, PhD, FRCP, FACG
Professor of Gastrointestinal Oncology
University of Oxford;
Digestive Disease Centre
Leicester Royal Infirmary
Leicester, UK

Simon Paterson-Brown, MB, BS, MPhil, MS, FRCS(Ed), FRCS
Honorary Senior Lecturer
Clinical and Surgical Sciences (Surgery)
University of Edinburgh;
Consultant General and Upper
Gastrointestinal Surgeon
Royal Infirmary of Edinburgh
Edinburgh, UK

Kyle A. Perry, MD
Minimally Invasive Surgery Fellow
Department of Surgery
Oregon Health and Science University
Portland, OR, USA

Simon A. Raimes, MD, FRCS, FRCS(Ed)
Consultant Upper Gastrointestinal Surgeon
Northern Oesophago-gastric Unit
Cumberland Infirmary
Carlisle, UK

Ian H. Shaw, BSc, PhD, MB, BChir, DA, FRCA
Consultant Anaesthetist
Department of Anaesthesia and Intensive Care
Newcastle General Hospital
Newcastle upon Tyne, UK

Jon Shenfine, MB, BS, FRCS
Specialist Registrar in Upper Gastrointestinal Surgery
Northern Oesophago-gastric Unit
Royal Victoria Infirmary
Newcastle upon Tyne, UK

Hubert J. Stein, MD
Professor of Surgery and Chairman
Department of Surgery
University Hospital of Salzburg
Salzburg, Austria

Rami R. Sweis, BSc, MRCP
Gastroenterology Specialist Registrar
Oesophageal Laboratory
Guy's and St Thomas' NHS Foundation
London, UK

Ashref Tawil, MB, BCH
Gastroenterology Specialist Registrar
Digestive Disease Centre
Leicester Royal Infirmary
Leicester, UK

Burkhard H.A. von Rahden, MD
Resident, General Surgery
Department of Surgery
University Hospital of Salzburg
Salzburg, Austria

David I. Watson, MB, BS, MD, FRACS
Professor of Surgery and
Head of Department of Surgery
Flinders University;
Senior Consultant Surgeon
Hepatobiliary and Oesophago-gastric Surgical Unit
Flinders Medical Centre
Bedford Park, Australia

John Wayman, MD, FRCS
Consultant Surgeon
Northern Oesophago-gastric Unit
Cumberland Infirmary
Carlisle, UK

Series preface

Since the publication of the first edition in 1997, the *Companion to Specialist Surgical Practice* series has aspired to meet the needs of surgeons in higher training and practising consultants who wish contemporary, evidence-based information on the subspecialist areas relevant to their general surgical practice. We have accepted that the series will not necessarily be as comprehensive as some of the larger reference surgical textbooks which, by their very size, may not always be completely up to date at the time of publication. This Fourth Edition aims to bring relevant state-of-the-art specialist information that we and the individual volume editors consider important for the practising subspecialist general surgeon. Where possible, all contributors have attempted to identify evidence-based references to support key recommendations within each chapter.

We remain grateful to the volume editors and all the contributors of this Fourth Edition. Their enthusiasm, commitment and hard work has ensured that a short turnover has been maintained between each of the editions, thereby ensuring as accurate and up-to-date content as possible. We remain grateful for the support and encouragement of Laurence Hunter and Elisabeth Lawrence at Elsevier Ltd. We trust that our aim of providing up-to-date and affordable surgical texts has been met and that all readers, whether in training or in consultant practice, will find this fourth edition an invaluable resource.

O. James Garden MB, ChB, MD, FRCS(Glas), FRCS(Ed), FRCP(Ed), FRACS(Hon), FRCSC(Hon)

Regius Professor of Clinical Surgery, Clinical and Surgical Sciences (Surgery), University of Edinburgh, and Honorary Consultant Surgeon, Royal Infirmary of Edinburgh

Simon Paterson-Brown MB, BS, MPhil, MS, FRCS(Ed), FRCS

Honorary Senior Lecturer, Clinical and Surgical Sciences (Surgery), University of Edinburgh, and Consultant General and Upper Gastrointestinal Surgeon, Royal Infirmary of Edinburgh

Editors' preface

We have aimed to thoroughly update this Fourth Edition of *Oesophagogastric Surgery* and to include the most recent expert opinion on some of the faster changing areas of this surgery. We have added two new chapters to the previous edition and have new authors for six of the original chapters. There is a new chapter on paraoesophageal hernia and gastric volvulus, and the previous chapter on early oesophageal and gastric cancer has been divided to deal with these separately and to incorporate descriptions of developing endoscopic and laparoscopic treatments. We have increased the international contribution to the book and are delighted to welcome Tom DeMeester, John Hunter and Hubert Stein as chapter authors. The authors who wrote the chapters for the Third Edition have been asked to update them and to focus on areas of changing practice. As previously, all the authors have been asked to incorporate the most recent references for their subject and to highlight the most important evidence-based ones. They have also included evidence-based text wherever possible. We have retained the use of the summary key points we introduced in the last edition as a résumé of the most important learning points at the end of each chapter. We would like to thank all our contributors for sharing their expertise and adhering to the criteria set for the series as a whole. We hope that this book presents the 'cutting edge' of the practice of oesophageal and gastric surgery that fulfils the need of both trainees and established specialists in our increasingly international readership.

S.Michael Griffin
Simon A.Raimes
Newcastle Upon Tyne
and Carlisle

Acknowledgements

Once again I am indebted to Theresa and our children for providing much needed support during the preparation of this new edition.

Simon A. Raimes
Carlisle

This new edition has greatly benefited from not only the many authors who have contributed to the volume from the first edition.

But also those new authors particularly from overseas who have provided an even greater breadth of experience.

I would acknowledge the tireless support and work of my secretary Alison Hood and my friend and co author Simon Raimes.

I dedicate this work to my family and in particular my mother and my inspirational late father.

S. Michael Griffin
Newcastle upon Tyne

Evidence-based practice in surgery

Critical appraisal for developing evidence-based practice can be obtained from a number of sources, the most reliable being randomised controlled clinical trials, systematic literature reviews, meta-analyses and observational studies. For practical purposes three grades of evidence can be used, analogous to the levels of 'proof' required in a court of law:

1. **Beyond all reasonable doubt.** Such evidence is likely to have arisen from high-quality randomised controlled trials, systematic reviews or high-quality synthesised evidence such as decision analysis, cost-effectiveness analysis or large observational datasets. The studies need to be directly applicable to the population of concern and have clear results. The grade is analogous to burden of proof within a criminal court and may be thought of as corresponding to the usual standard of 'proof' within the medical literature (i.e. $P < 0.05$).
2. **On the balance of probabilities.** In many cases a high-quality review of literature may fail to reach firm conclusions due to conflicting or inconclusive results, trials of poor methodological quality or the lack of evidence in the population to which the guidelines apply. In such cases it may still be possible to make a statement as to the best treatment on the 'balance of probabilities'. This is analogous to the decision in a civil court where all the available evidence will be weighed up and the verdict will depend upon the balance of probabilities.
3. **Not proven.** Insufficient evidence upon which to base a decision, or contradictory evidence.

Depending on the information available, three grades of recommendation can be used:

a. Strong recommendation, which should be followed unless there are compelling reasons to act otherwise.
b. A recommendation based on evidence of effectiveness, but where there may be other factors to take into account in decision-making, for example the user of the guidelines may be expected to take into account patient preferences, local facilities, local audit results or available resources.

c. A recommendation made where there is no adequate evidence as to the most effective practice, although there may be reasons for making a recommendation in order to minimise cost or reduce the chance of error through a locally agreed protocol.

Strong recommendation

Evidence where a conclusion can be reached 'beyond all reasonable doubt' and therefore where a **strong recommendation** can be given.
   This will normally be based on evidence levels:

- Ia. Meta-analysis of randomised controlled trials
- Ib. Evidence from at least one randomised controlled trial
- IIa. Evidence from at least one controlled study without randomisation
- IIb. Evidence from at least one other type of quasi-experimental study.

Expert opinion

Evidence where a conclusion might be reached 'on the balance of probabilities' and where there may be other factors involved which influence the recommendation given. This will normally be based on less conclusive evidence than that represented by scalpel icons:

- III. Evidence from non-experimental descriptive studies, such as comparative studies and case–control studies
- IV. Evidence from expert committee reports or opinions or clinical experience of respected authorities, or both.

Evidence in each chapter of this volume which is associated with either a strong recommendation or expert opinion is annotated in the text by either a **scalpel** or **pen-nib** icon as shown above. References associated with **scalpel** evidence will be highlighted in the reference lists, along with a short summary of the paper's conclusions where applicable.

Pathology of benign, malignant and premalignant oesophageal and gastric tumours

Mark K. Bennett

Introduction

Malignant tumours of the upper gastrointestinal tract appear as irregular mucosal ulcers, polypoid masses or diffuse thickening of the mucosa and wall. Dysplasia, the precursor for most cancers, is graded into a low- or high-grade form, in terms of cytological (individual cell) or architectural (glandular) atypia. Other mucosal changes, which predispose to the development of dysplasia, may be present. Investigations of the genetic/molecular changes in the mucosa confirm the stepwise progression from normal through dysplasia to cancer. This chapter describes the pathology of both benign and malignant tumours of the oesophagus and stomach. It also describes the pathological changes of dysplasia and premalignant lesions, and provides an insight into recent research into the molecular aspects of malignant transformation of normal epithelium.

Epithelial tumours of the oesophagus

Squamous carcinoma

The aetiology of these tumours is unknown, although there is a strong association between squamous cancer, alcohol intake and smoking in different parts of the world. Up to 80% of the male cases in the USA, Latin America and Japan have a history of either one or other factor, while in Iran and China these are not considered to be major causative agents.[1] Potential carcinogens (N-nitrosamines), which may be of environmental origin, have been found in areas where there is a high incidence of tumours. Similarly, diets lacking fresh fruit and vegetables and with an increased consumption of pickled foods are also found in these areas. This may reflect deficiencies in vitamins A, C and riboflavin and trace elements (zinc, molybdenum and selenium). There is evidence to suggest the human papillomavirus (HPV 16 and 18) may be important in some tumours.

Several predisposing factors have been reported (Box 1.1). Achalasia has a reported risk of cancer development of up to 33 times that of the normal population, with an incidence of 88 per 100 000 population.[2] The progression from a benign fibrous stricture as a result of chemically induced damage (e.g. lye ingestion)[3] to tumour has reportedly occurred in 0.8–7.2% of cases, with a latent period of up to 40 years. Tylosis, a rare autosomal dominant condition of abnormal keratinisation affecting the palms and soles of the feet, has been associated with oesophageal cancer. The tylosis-associated cancer susceptibility gene (TOC gene, tylosis oesophageal cancer gene) has recently been mapped to chromosome 17q25.[4,5] Postcricoid dysphagia with hypochromatic (iron deficiency) anaemia associated with mucosal webs is known as Plummer–Vinson or Paterson-Brown–Kelly syndrome. The webs consist of thin mucosal folds with some epithelial changes extending into the oral mucosa. These changes consist of epithelial atrophy or hyperkeratinisation and could account for the high incidence (up to 16%) of these patients having aerodigestive cancers.[6] The pharyngo-oesophageal (Zenker's) diverticulum found at the border of the cricopharyngeus and the inferior constrictor muscles has a reported incidence of cancer of between 0.3% and 0.8%.[7] The tumours tend to be at the apex of the diverticulum and by the time of diagnosis are usually in an advanced stage with extension through the wall. Barrett's oesophagus can occasionally be associated with a squamous carcinoma, though an adenocarcinoma is more usual.[8] There is a slightly increased incidence of squamous cancer in patients with coeliac disease though more frequently this condition has been complicated by small-bowel lymphoma.[9] The least frequent possible aetiology is that of irradiation treatment – only 13 cases have so far been reported.[10]

The tumours are found in the upper, middle and lower thirds in a ratio of approximately 1:5:2 respectively. They appear as fungating, ulcerating or infiltrating masses, though occasional verrucous (polypoid) or multifocal tumours are seen. Ulcerating lesions (**Fig. 1.1**) have raised rolled edges with necrotic centres while the stenosing variety show a diffuse full-circumferential infiltrating mass, often with a grey–white fibrous cut surface. The endoscopic appearances of early tumours, which may be better appreciated by use of the vital stains (toluidine blue or iodine), have been reported as showing a mosaic or hypervascular pattern or remain occult.[11] Improving endoscopic techniques, such as chromoendoscopy, narrowband imaging and laser confocal microendoscopy, may supersede this method. The pathological findings of these early tumours are similar to the advanced stages, with erosions, plaques or polypoid masses within the lumen.[12] The macroscopic appearances change with chemoradiation as a result of tumour shrinkage and scarring. A five-grade assessment of the effects of chemoradiation treatment has been suggested.[13]

Tumour infiltration and spread will depend on the site of the primary.[14] Approximately three-quarters of the tumours at presentation will extend through the submucosa and deep muscle layers into adventitial tissue. However, in Japan 40% are superficial (confined to the mucosa/submucosa).[15] Lymph node involvement increases with the depth of invasion; those confined to the mucosa/lamina propria (m1 and m2) show no metastatic spread while tumours extending to (but not through) the muscularis mucosa (m3) and the submucosal tumours (sm1) have <10% and 20% nodal involvement respectively. Because of the complexity of the mucosal lymphatic system approximately 40% of the upper-third tumours will spread to the abdominal nodes while similar numbers from the lower third will metastasise to the cervical lymph nodes. Metastatic tumour to visceral organs is a reflection of venous invasion,[16] most frequently to lung and liver, and has been demonstrated in 40–75%. There is an increase in second tumours within the aerodigestive tract as well as head and neck region, and in some this may be related to a family history or to the use of tobacco and alcohol. Depending on the degree of keratinisation, keratin whorl formation and the cytological atypia present, the histological appearances can be described as well, moderately or poorly differentiated (**Fig. 1.2**). Two variants of the squamous carcinoma are seen:

1. **Verrucous carcinoma** is similar to that found at other sites such as the head and neck. It has a predominantly exophytic papillary appearance and forms an intraluminal fungating mass.

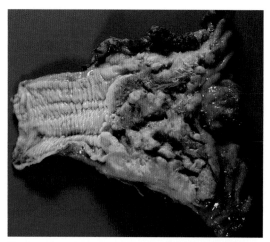

Figure 1.1 • Oesophageal carcinoma in the lower third, with a central ulceration and irregular margins.

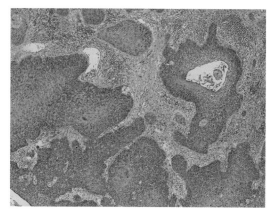

Figure 1.2 • Squamous carcinoma of the oesophagus. The tumour is formed from irregular islands of prickle cells with rudimentary keratin whorls.

Difficulties in histopathological interpretation of this tumour occur when superficial biopsies have been taken. The main differential diagnoses of this indolent malignant tumour are pseudoepitheliomatous hyperplasia, which is a benign reactive change, and the squamous papilloma, which is very uncommon in humans.

2. **Carcinosarcoma** (also known as sarcomatoid carcinoma and spindle cell carcinoma), which appears as an exophytic mass composed of a mixture of both squamous and spindle cells. The histogenesis of the spindle cells is unclear as they express cytokeratin, vimentin and smooth muscle actin, but a similar overexpression of the *p53* gene suggests a common origin for both the squamous and spindle elements.[17] Although the microscopic features are worrying, the tumour behaves in a less aggressive manner than the pure squamous carcinoma.

Molecular aspects

The multistep progression from normal mucosa to cancer shows that in up to half the cases of squamous carcinoma, the *p53* gene has been found to be abnormal. This gene is found on the short arm of chromosome 17 and normally acts as a brake on DNA replication and as a trigger for apoptosis (programmed cell death). As *p53* expression is found in normal and dysplastic epithelium, it has been suggested that abnormalities occur early in the pathway, leading to malignancy. Several defects are found, the most frequent being mutations of A:T base pairs, with a high prevalence of G to T transversions and/or loss of heterozygosity. *p53* can also be inactivated by methylation, which is mediated by the tumour suppressor gene *p14ARF*. Different mutations of *p53* are found in adenocarcinoma of the oesophagus.[18] The mutations allow abnormal cell growth and are associated with further damage to the genome, especially to the important tumour suppressor genes. This includes deletions or loss of heterozygosity (LOH) of the retinoblastoma gene (*Rb*, 48%), mutations in colorectal carcinoma (*MCC*, 63%) and adenomatous polyposis coli (*APC*, 67%) genes, and deletions in the colorectal cancer (*DCC*, 24%) gene. In nearly all cases one of these defective tumour suppressor genes is present, while nearly three-quarters of the squamous carcinomas have two abnormalities.

Continued cell growth will occur as a result of amplification and overexpression of growth factors and oncogenes. One of the most important is the protein kinase, epidermal growth factor receptor (EGFR), which shows amplification in 40–70% of squamous carcinomas. The ligands for EGFR, epidermal growth factor (EGF) and transforming growth factor-β (TGF-β), act on the receptor in an autocrine manner, further increasing the cellular proliferation. In addition to this important effect, EGF has at least one other effect on the tumour by phosphorylation of β-catenin.[19] This reduces the cellular adhesion and may account for more aggressive tumour behaviour. The *ras* oncogene family appears not to have an important role in the genesis of squamous carcinoma, unlike other gastrointestinal tract cancers.

Precancerous conditions: dysplasia

Dysplasia and carcinoma in situ are regarded as precancerous conditions of the oesophagus, and the atypia is similar to that found in other squamous epithelia such as the cervix or bronchial epithelium. There is irregular maturation of the keratinocytes with abnormally situated mitotic figures accompanied by nuclear enlargement and variation in size. When this dysplasia is full thickness it is referred to as non-invasive high-grade neoplasia (high-grade dysplasia or carcinoma in situ). The suggestion that these conditions are premalignant has come from the finding of dysplasia in up to 8% of the population in high-risk areas, with abnormalities of DNA, p53 and minichromosome maintenance (Mcm) proteins within the mucosa.[20,21] In screened high-risk populations the finding of dysplasia predates the development of carcinoma by approximately 5 years.

Non-invasive high-grade neoplasia can also be found at a distance from the primary tumour in up to 14% of resections. This is associated with the development of secondary oesophageal malignancy or other tumours in the aerodigestive tract. The precursor lesion for development of dysplasia is not well identified, although in areas of high risk there is an increased incidence of moderate to severe chronic oesophagitis, suggesting luminal damage may be in part responsible for this preneoplastic change.

Adenocarcinoma of the oesophagus

A significant rise in the incidence of adenocarcinoma of the oesophagus and gastric cardia has been reported. The tumours of the oesophagogastric junction share common epidemiological features; having a significant male predominance, they are more frequently associated with hiatus hernia, reflux and peptic strictures. Although smoking and alcohol are common factors they are less constant features than with squamous carcinoma. To improve epidemiological and demographic understanding, the following classification of these tumours has been suggested:[22,23]

- **Type I.** Adenocarcinoma of the distal oesophagus that usually arises from an area of specialised intestinal metaplasia of the oesophagus (Barrett's oesophagus) and which may infiltrate the oesophagogastric junction from above.

- **Type II.** True carcinoma of the cardia arising from the cardiac epithelium or short segments with intestinal metaplasia at the oesophagogastric junction; this entity is also referred to as 'junctional carcinoma'.
- **Type III.** Subcardial gastric carcinoma, which infiltrates the oesophagogastric junction and distal oesophagus from below.

Adenocarcinoma in Barrett's oesophagus (type I tumour)

First described in 1950,[24] Barrett's oesophagus is defined as the replacement of the squamous epithelium by a columnar-lined mucosa in the lower oesophagus (**Fig. 1.3**). Initially this was restricted to at least a 3-cm length but with time there has been recognition that short-segment (i.e. less than 3 cm) metaplastic change occurs. The metaplastic change develops as a consequence of chronic oesophagogastroduodenal reflux with the replacement of the squamous epithelium by the characteristic intestinal-type mucosa.[25] The differential diagnosis includes ciliated cell rests, tracheobronchial remnants and ectopic gastric mucosa. Further details of Barrett's oesophagus can be found in Chapter 15.

The incidence of malignancy in cases of Barrett's has been estimated to vary between 1 in 80 and 1 in 440 cases. From these figures it has been suggested that the risk of developing an adenocarcinoma is between 30 and 40 times that of the general population. This suggests that patients with Barrett's oesophagus may benefit from a surveillance programme, although the risk is questioned by others.[26,27] In particular, the area of involvement by the metaplasia and its duration appear insufficient to identify those patients at risk of developing malignancy.[28] The majority of the tumours are found in the lower third, though up to one-fifth are found in the middle third. Most appear as exophytic masses, ulcers or endophytic irregular masses. At presentation most are found to be at a late stage, with infiltration past the deep muscle layer in 70% of cases and lymph node metastases in up to three-quarters. Histologically the majority of these tumours show features similar to the intestinal type of gastric carcinoma.

Adenocarcinoma of the oesophagogastric junction (type II tumour)

These tumours form a distinct group from the more common subcardial tumours, occurring in slightly younger patients with a male predominance. As with type I tumours, symptoms related to hiatus hernia and reflux are common, as is a history of smoking and drinking alcohol. These tumours show an aggressive behaviour, with a worse prognosis than cancers in the rest of the stomach. There are several factors that might explain this, including large size (>5 cm) at presentation, early submucosal invasion, extension into the oesophagus and, because of their large size, the more frequent involvement of the serosa and lymph node metastases. Unlike the more distal tumours they are not associated with atrophic gastritis or intestinal metaplasia, suggesting that demographic and pathological features of these tumours are similar to the adenocarcinoma found in Barrett's oesophagus. The histological features of these tumours are similar to the other gastric adenocarcinomas. Multivariate analysis has shown that the staging of tumours is the most significant prognostic variable,[26] together with lymph node metastases. The majority of the nodal involvement is intra-abdominal, though metastatic spread to thoracic nodes was found in 7% of cases. Up to 80% of the tumours are aneuploid and have a shortened survival when compared with diploid tumours (10.6 vs. 20.4 months). A few studies have looked at the growth factors, their receptors and oncogenes in adenocarcinoma; EGFR is amplified and there is overexpression of TGF-β, h-*ras* and *erb*-B2. These factors are expressed in greater amounts with progression from normality to malignancy.

Other oesophageal tumours

In addition to squamous cell carcinoma and adenocarcinoma of the oesophagus, there are several other uncommon tumours to be considered in the differential diagnosis. Very uncommon tumours such as melanoma, choriocarcinoma, Paget's disease, squamous papilloma, cysts and also metastatic tumours to the oesophagus are not included in this discussion.

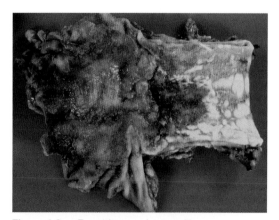

Figure 1.3 • Barrett's oesophagus with an adenocarcinoma: an irregular ulcerating tumour, which is encroaching upon the metaplastic mucosa. The residual squamous epithelium has been left as grey–white mucosal islands separated by the metaplastic mucosa.

Granular cell tumours

These are found in the skin, mouth and throughout the gastrointestinal tract, but most frequently in the oesophagus. They present with dysphagia or pain, the clinical symptoms possibly related to the size of the lesion (up to 4 cm in diameter). Nearly two-thirds of these tumours have been found in the lower third of the oesophagus and arise from the submucosa. The covering squamous epithelium is often thickened and the characteristic tumour cells fill the subjacent stroma. These are uniform plump cells with granular cytoplasm and stain with periodic acid–Schiff and S-100 protein. These benign tumours are thought to be derived from Schwann cells.

Basaloid carcinoma

Basaloid carcinoma (also known as adenoid cystic carcinoma and cylindroma) is an uncommon tumour usually found in males over 60 years. Most have been reported in small series and are thought to represent between 0.75% and 5% of oesophageal cancers. They are thought to arise from the ducts or acini of submucosal glands and present as ulcerating, infiltrating or fungating masses in the distal oesophagus. Microscopically they are similar to tumours found in the salivary gland and are composed of islands of basophilic cells with thickening of the basement membrane and microcystic structures. Most tumours show some differentiation towards squamous, glandular or even small-cell elements[29] and would indicate an origin from a multipotential stem cell. Similar neoplasms are reported in the trachea, breast, skin and cervix. They have a variable survival, though a recent study showed a 3-year survival rate of 51%. The expression of *p53*, *pRb* and *bcl*-2 was not related to the survival of the patients.

Mucoepidermoid carcinoma

This is an uncommon aggressive tumour found in males in the seventh decade. As the name implies, the tumour is composed of a mixture of glandular tissue, which forms cystic spaces and squamous elements.[30] They are most likely to have arisen from the submucosal glands (analogous to salivary gland tumours) and are found most frequently in the middle and lower thirds. There is extensive invasion, with lymph node metastases and a prognosis equivalent to the squamous carcinoma.[31]

Poorly differentiated endocrine carcinoma

This is an infrequent tumour representing 0.05–7.6% of all oesophageal cancers; approximately half of reported cases have come from Japan.[32] They present in the lower and middle thirds and are more usually found in males in the fifth to seventh decades. As with the equivalent lung lesion (oat cell carcinoma), ectopic hormone secretion

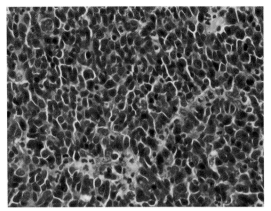

Figure 1.4 • Poorly differentiated endocrine (oat cell) carcinoma of the oesophagus, composed of sheets of undifferentiated cells with little cytoplasm. The appearances are similar to the more common bronchial oat cell carcinoma, from which they must be differentiated.

(adrenocorticotropic hormone, calcitonin, somatostatin or gastrin) has been reported. Macroscopically they appear as exophytic or ulcerative growths measuring on average 6 cm at presentation. Histologically these may appear as homogeneous tumours (**Fig. 1.4**) or as a mixture of squamous or mucoepidermoid elements. As a result of this heterogeneity it is unclear whether they arise from totipotential reserve cells at the base of the squamous epithelium or from oesophageal/tracheobronchial mucosa in the embryonic foregut. The possibility of metastatic or direct spread from the lung should also be considered. The prognosis is poor, with fewer than 14% of patients surviving 2 years.

Epithelial tumours of the stomach

Precursors of gastric carcinoma

The pathogenesis of gastric carcinoma is complex and multifactorial, with several potential precursor lesions (Box 1.2). Correa proposed a pathway from normal mucosa to cancer,[33] and this is discussed in detail in Chapter 2.

Box 1.2 • Precursors of gastric carcinoma

- Chronic gastritis
- Intestinal metaplasia of gastric mucosa
- Gastric polyps
- Gastric remnants (postgastrectomy state)
- Ménétrier's disease
- Chronic peptic ulcer
- Gastric epithelial dysplasia

Chronic atrophic gastritis and intestinal metaplasia

Inflammatory damage to the mucosa is the result of bacterial infection (*Helicobacter pylori*), chemical irritants (reflux of duodenal contents or ingested substances) or the consequence of an autoimmune process (pernicious anaemia). Continuation of the cellular destruction results in a chronic atrophic gastritis (**Fig. 1.5**) and intestinal metaplasia.

The most important of these insults in causing cell loss is *H. pylori* and is dependent on the bacterial strain as well as the host response. The bacteria survive within gastric mucus as a result of the effects of a urease in producing a pH-neutral internal and pericellular environment (**Fig. 1.6**). *Helicobacter pylori* also colonises the antrum, which has a higher pH than the corpus. Direct damage to the surface epithelium or more importantly to the proliferative zone is induced by several mechanisms, which include the production of acetaldehyde, a variety of toxins and mucolytic factors. In addition, *H. pylori* has a strong chemotactic effect for polymorphs and other inflammatory cells with activation of nuclear factor-κB and proinflammatory transcriptional targets on the adjacent epithelium. The polymorphs produce reactive oxygen metabolites, which cause further cellular damage resulting in an acute then chronic gastritis. Accumulation of lymphocytes results in lymphoid follicle formation, and this, together with the continuing cellular damage (which may be associated with antibody production to the bacteria), leads to an atrophic gastritis. Atrophy of the gastric mucosa may be seen as simple loss of the glands or as the replacement of the normal specialised glands by mucous neck cells with the resulting 'pyloric metaplasia'. In the past, environmental factors such as a high dietary intake of salt, or dried

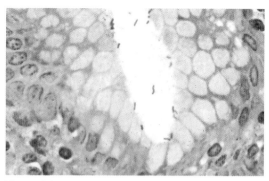

Figure 1.6 • *Helicobacter pylori*. The bacteria are found at the surface and in the mucus of the pits; in this silver stain they appear as black rods, often curved at the apex of the cell.

or pickled food were thought to enhance the development of the gastritis. The changes of an atrophic gastritis are a thinning of the mucosa, with loss of the specialised glands and a compensatory increase in turnover of cells in the proliferative zone.[34] The incidence of atrophic gastritis increases with age, being present in up to 40% of otherwise normal patients older than 60 years, indicating that further changes are required before malignant transformation can occur.

Eradication of *H. pylori* reduces the inflammatory reaction and halts the development of intestinal metaplasia. The linkage of *H. pylori* to gastric carcinogenesis has focused on strain differences (*cagA*, *vacA*, *iceA* and *babA*), but environmental and host genetic factors are important in the malignant transformation. In addition to the inflammatory damage, the cells of the pits may undergo metaplasia towards intestinal epithelium.[35,36] Intestinal metaplasia can be divided into three subtypes depending upon the altered cell phenotype most easily characterised by the type of mucin produced. The changes are a result of somatic mutations or epigenetic events in the stem cells. This includes hyperplasia of hTERT, DNA hypermethylation at the D17S5 locus, pS2 loss, RARβ loss, CD44 abnormalities and *p53* mutations:[37,38]

- **Type I (complete).** This is seen as a change from the production of neutral to acid mucins, a change in function from a secretory to an absorptive cell type, and the production of Paneth cells (which are usually found in the small bowel).
- **Type II.** The initial production of acid sialomucins is referred to as incomplete intestinal metaplasia (type II) and is found in association with Paneth cells and absorptive cells.
- **Type III.** With continuing damage, the pit cells change their morphology and produce an acid sulphamucin. This is more characteristic of

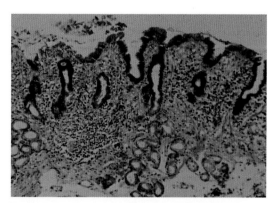

Figure 1.5 • Quiescent atrophic gastritis. The pyloric mucosa has an irregular surface with elongation of the pits and focal loss of the underlying glands in the lamina propria. There is a mild mononuclear cell inflammatory infiltrate.

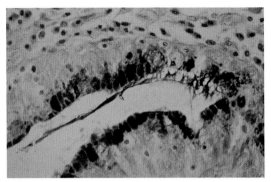

Figure 1.7 • Intestinal metaplasia (type III). The pits show both large solitary and multiple smaller secretory vacuoles within the apical portions of the cells. (Stained with alcian blue and High Iron Diamine HID.)

colonic mucosa and is accompanied by the loss of the Paneth cells, this appearance being known as incomplete intestinal metaplasia (type III) (**Fig. 1.7**).

These changes suggest selection pressure within the microenvironment of the pits, controlled by a complex hierarchy of transcription factors. In addition there are several genetic changes within the cells, which include telomere reduction, microsatellite instability and mutations of *p53*, *APC* and k-*ras*.

 There is continuing controversy as to the value of identifying this colonic-type mucin and its predictive value in identifying patients at risk of developing cancer.[39]

There is a significant difference in the expression of the sulphamucins between the intestinal and diffuse types of carcinoma (80% and 20% respectively), which has suggested differences in the underlying aetiology. It should be noted that intestinal metaplasia increases in prevalence and extent with age and is not infrequently associated with non-malignant disease, for example benign peptic ulceration. In these situations, as well as those associated with the cancers, there are abnormalities of the mucin genes and cell kinetics.[40,41]

Although it is possible to reverse the inflammatory and some of the intestinal metaplastic changes when associated with *H. pylori* infection, atrophy and the colonic-type intestinal metaplasia are regarded as irreversible. This may be because of the somatic mutations in the stem cells, or synergistic action between the inflammatory changes and such factors as bile reflux, high salt diet or alcohol. The mechanism by which damage to the nuclear DNA occurs is unclear, though several potential means are recognised. With the loss of the fundic glands, hypochlorhydria is found. In this changed environment

there exists the possibility for nitrosating bacteria to proliferate.[42] These bacteria are able to convert nitrates to nitrites, as well as creating N-nitroso compounds by catalysing reactions between amines and amides and the nitrites. Ascorbic acid, the reduced form of vitamin C, appears to protect against neoplasia, possibly by scavenging both nitrites and reactive oxygen metabolites. *Helicobacter pylori* blocks the secretion of ascorbic acid and hence would allow any carcinogen to exert an effect on the mucosa. A further potential mutagenic pathway is the production of potent N-nitrosating agents from nitric oxide by *H. pylori*. Both of these have been shown to cause mutations in *p53*, with its secondary effects on uncontrolled cell proliferation. The hyperproliferative state found in atrophic gastritis would perpetuate any damage to the genome. This could result in genomic instability[43] and together would initiate the steps required to convert the atrophic to a dysplastic mucosa.

Gastric mucosal polyps

Gastric polyps are found with increasing incidence with age; in some series they are present in up to 7% of patients over 80 years. The classification is important as it indicates whether or not they are premalignant or are just incidental and sometimes associated with tumours.[44,45] Gastric mucosal polyps fall into three main groups: the hyperplastic polyps; fundic gland polyps; and neoplastic polyps or adenomas.

Hyperplastic polyps are the most frequently found, usually with an equal sex distribution and occurring in later life, usually in the seventh decade. They represent between 80% and 85% of all gastric polyps, are found more often in the antrum than in the corpus, are often multiple and usually less than 1 cm in diameter. Histologically they are composed of disorganised and hyperplastic glandular elements, which are lined by regular epithelium and have an adjacent chronic gastritis. The risk of malignant transformation overall is approximately 0.5%, and with rare exceptions this occurs in those polyps greater than 2 cm in diameter.[46] The rate of detecting coexistent cancer in prospective studies varied from 4.5% to 13.5%.

Fundic gland polyps are present in up to 3% of endoscopies and form multiple sessile lesions confined to the body of the stomach. Originally described in association with familial adenomatous polyposis, they are found more frequently in a sporadic form.[47] They show alteration in mucin synthesis, increase in proliferation and expression of the sialyl-Tn epitope. There is no evidence that there is an increased risk of gastric cancer and they are regarded as hyperproliferative hamartomatous lesions.

Neoplastic polyps are also referred to as adenomas and histologically have a tubular configuration. They occur predominantly in the antrum, with no sex preference and more frequently in the elderly. They have been found in up to 0.23% of endoscopic studies; most are smaller than 2 cm. They are often associated with atrophic gastritis and intestinal metaplasia. Histologically the polypoid epithelium shows dysplastic features with hyperchromasia, irregularity of maturation and abnormally situated mitoses; there is no evidence to suggest infiltration through the basement membrane. Malignant transformation has been reported to occur in up to 40% of those adenomas greater than 2 cm. Although often found in isolation, co-existent cancers have been found in 3–25%, though the malignant change is generally reported in the range 5–10%.[48]

Gastroduodenal polyps are found with familial adenomatous polyposis, and are mainly fundic gland or hyperplastic types. These are often multiple and occur at an earlier age than the sporadic cases. Adenomas have been reported (35–100% of cases), are less frequent in the stomach than duodenum, and occur at a younger age (mean 37 years) than the sporadic adenoma. The lesions are usually small and multiple; with time they increase in number and exhibit frequent malignant transformation.[49] Except in Japan, the risk of gastric carcinoma is not increased in patients when compared with controls, though the relative risk of duodenal and periampullary carcinoma is markedly increased.

Flat adenomas similar to those found in the colon are another form of tubular adenoma with variable degrees of dysplasia.[50] Macroscopically, they appear as irregular impressions, being mistaken for a healing ulcer or depressed type of early gastric cancer. They occur in the distal two-thirds of the stomach, having similar demographic features to the more common polypoid adenomas. A larger percentage of the adenomas are described as having high-grade dysplasia, though the prevalence is unknown. In the Japanese literature, these lesions may represent up to 10% of all neoplastic polyps.

Gastric remnant

Following distal gastrectomy with gastroenteric anastomosis, a high incidence of carcinoma (2%) in the gastric remnant has been reported. Moreover, there has been a wide variation in the reported incidence, most likely related to the time factor. Those who are at most risk have been identified as patients who have undergone surgery before the age of 40 and who have had a postsurgery interval of between 15 and 20 years.[51] The type of gastrectomy and the nature of the preoperative disease are not factors. The risk of cancer is increased in countries with a high intrinsic rate of gastric cancer and is approximately twice that of the control population. There are a variety of benign histological changes associated with gastric remnants; these include a chronic gastritis and atrophy, fundic gland polyps, xanthomas, hyperplasia of the surface/foveolar epithelium and hyperplastic polyps with gastritis cystica profunda.

These cancers are termed 'stump cancers' and the majority are found at or close to the stoma site, rarely extend into the intestinal side of the anastomosis and show equal proportions of intestinal and diffuse histological types. Nearly 40% of cases have been restricted to the submucosa, in other words an early gastric cancer. It has been suggested that selective surveillance should be considered for patients who are symptomatic, who underwent surgery at a young age, who are 20 years or more after surgery, or who have high-grade dysplasia on endoscopy. In addition, cases of lymphoma of the stomach are now being described in the gastric stump.[52] A variety of non-gastric malignancies have been identified in follow-up series, and these have been predominantly lung, pancreatic ductal and colorectal cancers.

Ménétrier's disease (hypertrophic gastropathy)

This is a rare cause of rugal hypertrophy characterised by hyperplasia of the surface cells, hypochlorhydria and a protein-losing enteropathy. A review of the cases shows that approximately 10% are associated with cancer, diagnosed either simultaneously or within 12 months. However, follow-up in a total of 16 cases showed the risk of malignancy to be low or negligible.[53] A few cases have been associated with gastric dysplasia.

Chronic peptic ulcer disease

Chronic gastric ulcers were previously considered to be precancerous, but this is no longer supported by evidence as less than 1% of ulcers undergo malignant transformation.[54,55] The epidemiological evidence would suggest that ulcers do not have a significant role in gastric carcinogenesis. The natural history of early gastric carcinoma may explain why there was an initial over-reporting of the malignant change, since these tumours undergo episodes of mucosal ulceration followed by repair, some of which may be related to active medical therapy. It is essential, therefore, to ensure that any mucosal ulcer is adequately sampled before making a diagnosis of a benign ulcer.

Gastric epithelial dysplasia

Dysplasia may occur in an epithelium which shows intestinal metaplasia, and may be flat, depressed or polypoid. It has been previously classified in three grades: mild, moderate or severe.

There are several problems associated with histological interpretation, including interobservational variation, distinguishing regenerative atypia from true dysplasia, the ability to differentiate high-grade dysplasia from intramucosal carcinoma, and a lack of experience due to the rarity of dysplasia (especially in low incidence areas). This may be overcome with the recently published Vienna classification of gastric dysplasia (Box 1.3).[56]

The natural history of dysplasia is not relentless progression to cancer, as regression to normal mucosa occurs in mild and moderate dysplasia in 60% and 70% of cases respectively. Severe dysplasia can also regress, but this is less common; the majority of patients progress to carcinoma (50–80%).[57] Retrospective studies show that high-grade dysplasia is closely associated with gastric carcinoma in the adjacent mucosa; 40–100% of early gastric cancers and 5–80% of advanced tumours show dysplasia. In comparison, only 1–3% of gastric ulcers with an atrophic gastritis are associated with dysplasia. A diagnosis of severe dysplasia is a frequent marker of coexistent cancer when a gross endoscopic lesion such as an erosion, ulcer or polyp accompanies it. In this situation 50% of the tumours were diagnosed within 3–24 months of the initial finding of dysplasia on biopsy.

Early gastric cancer

This is defined as a malignant tumour limited to the mucosa or submucosa and is independent of any lymph node metastasis. The penetration of the muscularis mucosae allows subdivision of the tumours into those that are intramucosal or submucosal types.

 The Japanese Endoscopic Society introduced a macroscopic classification of these tumours (Fig. 1.8). This divides the lesions into predominantly protuberant (type I), a superficial type where there is minimal mucosal thickening (type II), or where there is a significant ulcerating lesion (type III).[58]

Type I protruding polypoid tumours appear as sessile, smooth, hemispherical nodules with a broad stalk, less than 3 cm in diameter and often paler than the adjacent mucosa. Type II tumours are subdivided into three subsets: the slightly elevated (IIa, in which the mucosal thickness is no greater than twice that of the adjacent mucosa); the flat

Box 1.3 • Vienna classification of epithelial neoplasias of the gastrointestinal tract

1. Negative for neoplasia
2. Indefinite for neoplasia
3. Non-invasive low-grade neoplasia
4. Non-invasive high-grade neoplasia:
   4.1. High-grade adenoma
   4.2. Non-invasive carcinoma
   4.3. Suspicious for invasive carcinoma
5. Invasive adenocarcinoma:
   5.1. Intramucosal carcinoma
   5.2. Submucosal carcinoma or beyond

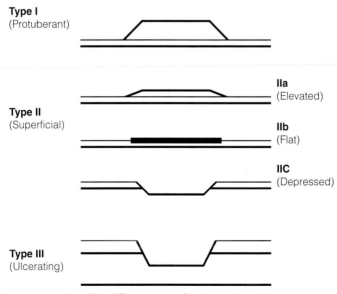

Figure 1.8 • Schematic representation of the different types of early gastric carcinoma.

(IIb, where no mucosal elevation or depression is seen); and the depressed group (IIc, in which there is mucosal erosion but no deep ulceration). More than one appearance can be found, especially if the tumours cover a large area. In this situation they are classified by the predominant type followed by the subsidiary type(s) – for example, IIa + IIc (**Fig. 1.9**). The appearances of these early gastric cancers was further studied by Kodama et al., who showed that the small tumours that penetrated the submucosa with an expanding margin (Pen A) tended to have more lymphatic and blood-borne metastases than the infiltrative type of tumour (Pen B).[59] The latter tumour had greater peritoneal recurrences.

Early gastric cancers are found predominantly within the lower two-thirds of the stomach and vary in size from 3–5 mm to more than 8 cm, although most are between 2 and 5 cm. Those lesions that are less than 5 mm in diameter are referred to as minute carcinomas. Mori et al.[60] have reported a small series of 21 patients with early carcinoma of the cardia. The ulcerating tumours (types III and IIc) are the most frequent, accounting for 64% of the neoplasms, followed by the exophytic lesions. The entirely flat IIb lesion is the least common and represents 14% of the tumours. Histologically the exophytic tumours tend to have a better differentiated intestinal type while the ulcerating tumours are more frequently associated with the signet ring or poorly differentiated histology. The flat lesions have a mixed histological pattern.

The prognosis for early gastric cancer is excellent, with a reported 5-year survival of 92%.[61] Long-term studies have shown that tumours confined to the mucosa have a 15-year survival of 87% and slightly less when there is infiltration into the submucosa (75%).[62] Despite this, reports from Japan indicate a recurrence rate of up to 2%, which is thought to be due either to residual tumour in the gastric remnant or haematogenous metastatic disease.[63] The features associated with haematogenous metastases are intestinal-type tumours, submucosal invasion and involvement of the epigastric lymph nodes. Intramucosal early gastric cancer rarely has perigastric nodal metastasis (less than 5%) due to the paucity of intramucosal lymphatics. Invasion of the submucosa is, however, associated with 10–20% nodal metastasis,[64] although reports from the UK have suggested even higher rates.[65] Interestingly, DNA analysis shows that aneuploid changes are more frequent in type I and IIa tumours, although the ploidy status and nodal metastasis have not been shown to be consistently correlated.[66]

Advanced gastric cancer

Approximately 90% of all malignant tumours of the stomach are adenocarcinomas. The majority of the remaining tumours are either malignant lymphoma or gastrointestinal stromal tumours. There are in addition a wide variety of other primary tumours arising from the stomach, which reflects the tissue present within the mucosa and deeper structures. These include squamous and oat cell carcinomas, carcinoid tumours, benign and malignant mesodermally derived tumours (i.e. those coming from blood vessels, fat cells and neural elements), and an assortment of rare tumours more often associated with extragastrointestinal sites such as the malignant fibrous histiocytoma, glomus tumours, teratoma and choriocarcinoma.

Advanced gastric cancer has shown significant changes over recent decades, with an overall decline in incidence, an increase in tumours of the cardia and oesophagogastric junction over the distal stomach, and finally an increase in the diffuse type (see below), which now represents up to 30% of all gastric neoplasms.[67]

Macroscopic features

The macroscopic appearances of an advanced gastric cancer have been divided into four types by Borrmann[68] (Box 1.4, **Figs 1.10** and **1.11**) and is now gaining acceptance throughout the English-speaking world. Approximately 50% of the tumours are confined to the antrum while a third are at the oesophagogastric junction. The tumours are large: more than a half are 6 cm in diameter with one in seven reaching 10 cm or more.

Histological features

The complexity of the histological features of gastric tumours is a reflection of the multiple cell types present. These include mucous and goblet cells, immature absorptive cells, pyloric gland cells, and Paneth, parietal and endocrine cells.

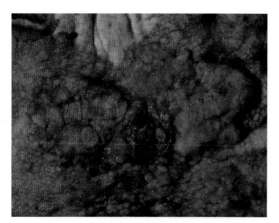

Figure 1.9 • An early gastric carcinoma of the fundus showing areas of both an elevated and superficially depressed tumour (type IIa + IIc).

Box 1.4 • Macroscopic appearances of advanced gastric carcinoma (Borrmann)

Type I (fungating): a polypoid protrusion with a broad base, often soft, red in colour and may be slightly ulcerated

Type II: an excavated carcinoma, which is dominated by the crater with slightly elevated margins. There is no definite infiltration of the adjacent mucosa

Type III: this is also ulcerative with mildly elevated margins and infiltrated

Type IV: a diffusely thickened (scirrhous type), also known as linitis plastica

The macroscopic appearances allow an assessment of similarities between types of tumour; it may also help in understanding the natural history of the tumours

This has led to a variety of classifications, the most widely accepted being that proposed by Lauren.[69] The tumours were divided into two main types: those forming glandular structures are known as intestinal (**Fig. 1.12**; 53%), while those with no structure that secrete mucin are referred to as diffuse carcinomas (**Fig. 1.13**; 33% – see Table 1.1).

The remaining 14% had a mixed appearance with elements from both types and were regarded as unclassified. The intestinal type of adenocarcinoma is associated with an increased incidence of chronic atrophic gastritis and gastric atrophy, while the diffuse cancers do not have this association.

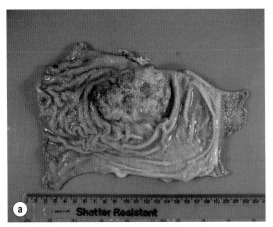

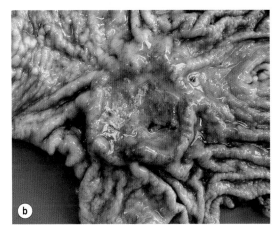

Figure 1.10 • The macroscopic appearances of advanced gastric cancer: **(a)** polypoid (Borrmann type I); **(b)** ulcerating (Borrmann type III).

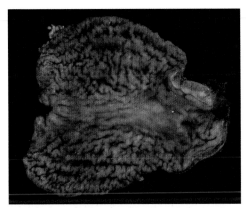

Figure 1.11 • A linitis plastica (Borrman type IV) in which there is diffuse infiltration of the wall of the stomach by tumour and apparent thickening of the rugal folds.

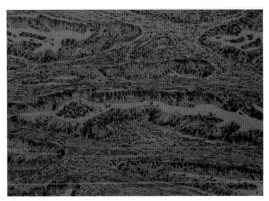

Figure 1.12 • An intestinal adenocarcinoma is composed of irregular glands, which are lined by attenuated cuboidal epithelium. In a well-differentiated tumour there is minimal nuclear pleomorphism or pseudostratification of the cells.

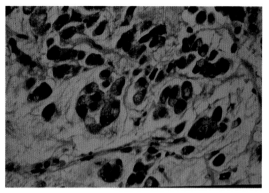

Figure 1.13 • A diffuse (signet-ring) adenocarcinoma in which the tumour cells are widely dispersed and separated by a variable amount of extracellular mucin. The nuclei of occasional cells are displaced by the intracytoplasmic secretory vacuoles, giving the typical signet-ring appearance.

The macroscopic appearance of these tumours depends on the relative proportions of stromal collagen and mucus produced. There are several other classification schemes proposed, including that of Ming, in which the tumours are split into expanding and infiltrating types,[70] and that of the World Health Organisation, where the tumours are organised into several different histological types (papillary, tubular, mucinous and signet ring cell adenocarcinomas).[71] Unfortunately these have not been conclusively shown to be independent factors in the prognosis of gastric cancer. In addition, Goseki et al. classified gastric carcinoma into four groups based on the degree of glandular differentiation and amount of intracytoplasmic mucin produced.[72] In the initial

studies they were able to show that liver metastases were more frequent in group 1 tumours (well-differentiated tubules with little mucin) while direct infiltration of peritoneum and lymph node metastases were seen in group IV tumours (little attempt at tubule formation with mucin-rich cells). A group of poorly differentiated tumours with a prominent lymphoid infiltrate, the lymphoepithelioma-like carcinomas, have been described.[73] In more than 80% of these tumours Epstein–Barr virus has been demonstrated within the tumour and adjacent mucosa, while it is found in only 9% of other adenocarcinomas. These tumours have a better prognosis, with 77% patients surviving 5 years

Prognostic pathological features

 Careful assessment of gastrectomy specimens has shown several prognostic features (TNM stage) in advanced gastric cancer,[74] the most important being the depth of tumour invasion (T stage).

Involvement of the resection margin by tumour, the presence of lymph node metastasis and recently the Goseki classification[75] has been shown to provide further prognostic information. Survival of patients with cancers of the cardia and upper third of the stomach is worse than that with cancers of the body and antrum (5-year survival of 15%, 25% and 30% respectively). Serosal involvement is an ominous feature with a 5-year survival of just 7%, while tumour infiltration restricted to the subserosa is associated with a 5-year survival of about 29%. Transcoelomic dissemination and direct infiltration

Table 1.1 • Comparative histological features of advanced gastric carcinoma

Features	Intestinal	Diffuse
Sex ratio M:F	2:1	Approximately 1:1
Mean age of detection (years)	55	48
Decreasing incidence in Western countries	Yes	No
5-year survival rate (all cases)	20%	Less than 10%
Major gross appearances	Intraluminal growth, fungating	Ulcerative, infiltrating
Microscopic features/differentiation	Well-differentiated, glandular, papillary, solid	Poorly differentiated, signet-ring cells
Growth pattern	Expansile	Non-cohesive diffuse
Mucin production	Confined to gland lumen	Extensive, often prominent in stroma around glands
Associated intestinal metaplasia	Almost 100%	Less frequent
Aetiological factors	Diet, environmental, *H. pylori*, associated with blood group A	Unknown, ? genetic factors, *H. pylori*

of adjacent structures may occur as a result of serosal involvement. Several authors have investigated the area of serosal involvement. Most have taken less than 2 cm in diameter as the limit that indicated a better prognosis. Abe et al.[76] showed that serosal involvement of less than 3 cm had a 5-year survival of 59.6% compared with 11.5% with tumours more than 3 cm. They have also suggested that if both the serosa and lymph nodes were involved then the diameter of serosal involvement is the more important factor in predicting ultimate survival. A significant underestimation of serosal involvement at surgery has been reported.[77] This tended to occur with large undifferentiated tumours and showed nearly 10% of cases had positive microscopic serosal involvement when the macroscopic appearances were thought to be tumour free.

The rate of lymph node metastases in early gastric cancer is related to tumour size, its growth pattern and the presence of ulceration. Survival is dependent upon the number of nodes involved,[78] the extension of metastasis through the capsule of nodes, involvement of the adjacent fibrovascular and fatty tissue, and whether or not the metastases were judged to be present microscopically.[79]

Involvement of the duodenum in tumours of the distal stomach has been reported in 9–69% of resections.[80,81] When present, it is regarded as a poor prognostic sign with a significant reduction in the 5-year survival rate to 8%, in comparison with those tumours restricted to the stomach. These tumours also show an increased involvement of the serosa, with evidence of lymphatic and vascular invasion. The suggestion that re-laparotomy should be undertaken to achieve a tumour-free resection line is controversial.

Other independent factors to show positive predictive value have included blood and lymphatic invasion,[82] intratumoral vessel count, patient age over 70, tumours with a diffuse infiltrating pattern, and tumours involving the entire stomach or that measure more than 10 cm in diameter. The only histological tumour type showing a worse prognosis is the adenosquamous carcinoma – this is an uncommon tumour composed of both glandular and squamous elements. Those tumours that macroscopically appear as early gastric carcinoma, but histologically are advanced cancers, have a prognosis that is intermediate between the two groups. Regression of tumour following chemotherapy is at present assessed by evaluating the degree of fibrosis, and any residual pools of mucin at the site of the primary tumour or within lymph nodes.[83]

Molecular aspects

As with most other tumours, a stepwise development of gastric cancer occurs and, as shown in **Fig. 1.14**, indicates that the underlying mechanisms may be different for the diffuse and intestinal types of tumour.[84] The development of gastric cancer requires that there is disruption of the genome and participation of many cancer-associated oncogenes, regulatory genes

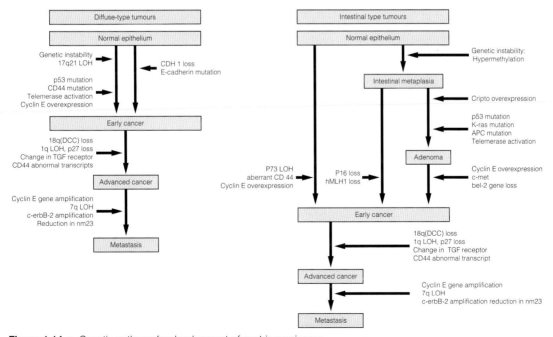

Figure 1.14 • Genetic pathway for development of gastric carcinoma.

and proteins to perpetuate the uncontrolled cell growth.[85] The consequence of these changes is the altered and aberrant expression of mucins, enzymes and hormones by the tumour epithelium.

Cytogenetic studies have failed to identify consistent chromosomal abnormalities, suggesting that many of the changes are non-specific or are secondary to the malignant transformation. Aneuploid tumours are common (60–70%), being more frequent in intestinal-type tumours. The most common abnormalities, apart from those mentioned below, are on chromosome 3 (rearrangement), chromosome 6 (deletions distal to 6q21), chromosome 8 (trisomy), chromosome 11 (aberration: 11p13–11p15), and on chromosome 13 (monosomy and translocations). The most consistent abnormality has been that of $p53$ in gastric cancer. Allelic loss and/or mutations of the $p53$ gene are found in intestinal metaplasia, adenomas and adenocarcinoma (14%, 33% and >60% respectively). Other tumour suppressor genes show LOH on chromosome 5p near the APC gene. Between 30% and 40% of tumours show this defect, and this suggests a possible further suppressor gene at this site. There is significant allelic loss (>60%) noted at the DCC gene locus on 18q.

Microsatellite instability has been found in a proportion of sporadic tumours from which there is the potential to establish multiple gene abnormalities. These changes are more frequently found in intestinal than diffuse-type tumours and in particular in subcardial intestinal tumours. There is a negative association with $p53$, suggesting this is a different pathway of accumulating genetic abnormalities. The target for the instability has been reported to be the TGF-β type II receptor. Oncogene expression appears early in tumour formation and may be the cause for increased cell division, though the significance of the genes and gene products is unclear at present. Two oncogenes, c-myc and $cripto$, show amplification and overexpression in intestinal metaplasia, some cases of dysplasia and advanced gastric cancer. C-met is amplified and present in 30% of intestinal cancers, especially the scirrhous tumours. This gene encodes the tyrosine kinase receptor for the hepatocyte growth factor but also interacts with EGF, TGF-β, interleukin-1α, amphiregulin, K-sam and others.[86] A member of the fibroblastic growth factor receptor family, K-sam is amplified in both diffuse and scirrhous carcinomas but not other types of tumours. The fibrosis seen in these tumours suggests interaction between receptors and oncogenes of the stromal and tumour cells. A strategy for the molecular–pathological diagnosis of gastric cancer using tissue samples has been suggested.[87]

Genetic abnormalities of the E-cadherin gene and reduced expression of the protein have been found in up to 90% of carcinomas, especially the diffuse type. E-cadherin is a transmembrane calcium-dependent cell adhesion molecule that is important in epithelial cell interactions. Loss of its binding properties could result in tumour infiltration and dissemination. Other molecules that have an anchoring function such as CD44 are also found to be defective.[88]

Familial clustering of cancers has uncommon (1–3%), occurring in patients with hereditary non-polyposis colorectal cancer (HNPCC) and familial gastric cancer. In HNPCC the patients are at risk not only of the colorectal tumours, but also of tumours in the stomach, endometrium, small bowel, ovary and ureter, and to a lesser extent kidney and hepatobiliary system.[89]

The criteria for the diagnosis of HNPCC are:

1. At least three affected relatives with verified colorectal cancer.
2. At least one of the above is a first-degree relative of the other two.
3. Familial adenomatous polyposis has been excluded.
4. At least two successive generations are affected.
5. One of the patients is younger than 50 years of age.

This is an autosomal dominant genetic disease due to a germ-line mutation in one of the DNA mismatch repair (MMR) genes. The most commonly mutated genes are hMSH2 and hMLH1 (60–70% of cases), but include hMSH6, PMS1 and PMS2. The tumours develop as a result of the loss of large relative segments of chromosomes, which are thought to include tumour suppressor genes. As a consequence the tissue becomes more liable to mutations and this accelerates carcinogenesis; the relative risk of developing gastric cancer is reported as 4.1 and the median age is 54 years.

Familial gastric cancer has now been recognised as encompassing three specific syndromes: hereditary diffuse gastric cancer (HDGC), familial diffuse gastric cancer and familial intestinal gastric cancer. The inclusion criteria for HDGC are:

1. Two or more documented cases of diffuse gastric cancer in first/second-degree relatives, with at lease one diagnosed before age 50.
2. Three or more cases of documented diffuse gastric cancer in first/second-degree relatives independent of age.

Those cases that do not fulfil these criteria are classified as familial diffuse gastric cancer. The genetic basis is an inactivating germ-line mutation in the E-cadherin gene (CDH-1)[90] in 30–40% of HDGC families. At present there have been up to 68 CDH-1 germ-line mutations identified. In cases where prophylactic gastrectomies have been performed the tumours have no site predilection, whereas gastrectomies for tumours which have come to light from surveillance programmes have been found in the antrum or antrum/transitional zone. The significance of this is unclear. In addition to the diffuse type of gastric cancer, lobular breast carcinoma and in some families colorectal cancer have been reported.

Mesenchymal tumours of the oesophagus and stomach

The stomach is the most frequent site for mesenchymal tumours within the gastrointestinal tract, accounting for 50–60%, with only 5% found in the oesophagus.[91] In the stomach they range in size from <1 cm, which are clinically asymptomatic, to bulky 20-cm masses. Multivariate analysis showed that the tumour location, size and mitotic index, and age were all independent prognostic factors. It is important to recognise that these tumours may be part of other clinical syndromes such as Carney's triad. This affects young women and consists of extra-adrenal paraganglioma together with pulmonary chondroma and stromal tumours of the stomach. The triad may be diagnosed if two of the three features are present. The stromal tumours and paragangliomas are often multiple.

Initially the tumours were thought to be leiomyomas or leiomyosarcomas as they were composed of spindle cells, with a variable amount of extracellular collagen. Electron microscopy shows heterogeneous features suggesting smooth muscle and/or neural differentiation, or no differentiation. This has led to problems with classification, which has now been clarified by immunocytochemisty. Variable expression of the markers of muscle (desmin and smooth muscle actin), nerve (S100, neurone-specific enolase and Protein Gene Product PGP 9.5) and interstitial cells of Cajal (CD117; also known as c-kit protein) has allowed classification into three major groups. Leiomyomas and leiomyosarcomas are positive for desmin and actin and negative for CD34. Neurofibroma and other neural tumours will be positive for S100 but negative for the other markers. The largest group of these tumours are positive for CD34 and CD117 and negative for the others, and are referred to as gastrointestinal stromal tumours (GISTs). The expression and the activation of c-kit protein is central to the histiogenesis of these tumours, and is the basis of the medical treatment with a tyrosine kinase inhibitor.

Predicting the clinical behaviour in GISTs is difficult, but malignant behaviour can be suggested if the tumours have a high cellularity with necrosis and there is mucosal invasion. It has been proposed that the relative risk of aggressive behaviour be assessed in terms of size and mitotic count, and that all tumours be assigned to one of four categories (very low, low, intermediate and high risk). Even so, up to 10% will behave in an unpredictable manner. This is further discussed in Chapter 11.

The inflammatory fibroid polyp is a benign lesion reported throughout the gastrointestinal tract with a predilection for the distal stomach and ileum. The gastric lesions typically present in the sixth decade, with slightly more males than females affected. The larger tumours cause outlet obstruction although most measure less than 3 cm in diameter. They present as polyps or expansile lesions in the submucosa, at or just proximal to the pyloric sphincter muscle. Plump spindle cells, numerous small blood vessels and a mixed inflammatory infiltrate, which includes eosinophils, are the cellular components of the tumour. The adjacent mucosa often shows features of atrophic gastritis. The underlying cause for the lesion is unknown. Ultrastructural features of the spindle cells shows them to be fibroblasts or myofibroblasts, suggesting that the tumours are reactive in nature – possibly an exuberant granulation tissue response.

In addition, small numbers of vascular tumours, glomus tumours, angiomas and Kaposi's sarcoma – the last associated with AIDS – have been reported.

Mucosa-associated lymphoid tissue (MALT) lymphoma

The stomach is the commonest site for gastrointestinal lymphomas, representing 3–6% of all gastric malignancies. The majority of the tumours are B-cell non-Hodgkin's lymphomas, the most common being the MALT lymphoma, with occasional T-cell lymphomas and Hodgkin's disease seen. These tumours arise from lymphoid tissue within the mucosa and are acquired as the result of *H. pylori* or *H. heilmannii* infection. The majority occur in patients over the age of 50 years, with equal sex distribution, who present clinically with symptoms suggesting a diagnosis of gastritis or peptic ulcer disease.[92] The tumours appear macroscopically as an ill-defined thickening of the mucosa with erosions, sometimes ulcerated (**Fig. 1.15**) and frequently multifocal. The gastric MALT lymphoma does not remain localised to the stomach, with spread occurring to the regional nodes though uncommonly to peripheral nodes. It is characteristic of these tumours that more remote spread is to other mucosal sites such as the small intestine, salivary gland and splenic marginal zone.

The lymphoma cells resemble follicle centre cells and are termed centrocyte-like, with other cells showing plasma cell differentiation and occasional blast cells. The characteristic lymphoepithelial lesion (**Fig. 1.16**) is composed of small to medium-sized tumour cells with irregular nuclei that infiltrate the pit epithelium. This lesion is not pathognomonic of a lymphoma as it can also be demonstrated in an *H. pylori*-associated gastritis, Sjögren's syndrome and Hashimoto's thyroiditis.

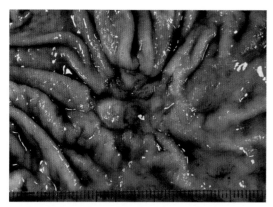

Figure 1.15 • Non-Hodgkin's lymphoma that shows superficial ulceration of the antrum with fibrous scarring of the adjacent mucosa.

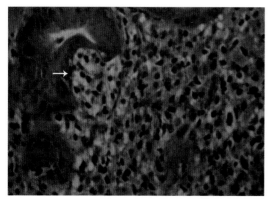

Figure 1.16 • Lymphoepithelial lesion – an intense mononuclear cell infiltrate is present within the mucosa extending into the pits. There is partial destruction of these (arrow).

Morphologically normal mucosa has been shown to have microlymphomatous lesions with widely scattered tumour cells detected by molecular analysis.

It is thought that the development of lymphoma is a multistage process, with the initiating phase being due to the interaction of the *H. pylori*, neutrophils, B cells and T cells within the mucosa. It is thought that the continuing B-cell proliferation, which is T-cell dependent (involving CD40 and CD40L), results from antigen (*H. pylori*) stimulation and may be bacterial strain specific. It has been postulated that in the presence of a mutator phenotype (from defective mismatch repair machinery) nuclear damage is caused by neutrophils generating oxygen radicals, resulting in genetic instability.

Cytogenetic studies show that three major translocations are seen in MALT lymphomas: t(11;18)(q21;q21)API2-MALT1 (30–40% of cases), t(14;18)(q32:q21)/IGH-MALT1 and t(1:14)(p22:q32)/IGH-BCL10. The first results in the fusion of the API2

gene product with the carboxy-terminus of the MALT1 gene product. The full protein product of API2 inhibits caspases 3, 7 and 9 and so is thought to inhibit apoptosis, while the function of MALT1 is unknown. When this translocation is present the MALT lymphoma is not responsive to *H. pylori* eradication. The other translocations account for less than 5%, and are associated with the juxtaposition of *BCL10* to the immunoglobulin gene with the resulting deregulation of the immunoglobulin. In addition there is loss or mutation of *p53* in 7% and 19% of low-grade cases, increasing to 29% and 33% of the transformed MALT lymphomas. Other chromosomal abnormalities include trisomy 3 (in up to 60% of cases), c-*myc* mutation, inactivation of *p15/p16* by hypermethylation and *Fas* gene mutation. This results in an abnormal clone, which undergoes clonal expansion and gives rise to a low-grade MALT lymphoma, the early phase of which is responsive to *H. pylori* eradication.[93,94]

Most low-grade MALT lymphomas are associated with disease confined to the gastric mucosa with slow dissemination. The favourable clinical behaviour may reflect the partial dependence on the *H. pylori* antigenic drive. In a minority of cases accumulation of further genetic abnormalities (such as inactivation of *p53* and *p16*) can be identified; however, in the majority the changes have not been recognised. The progression to the more common high-grade MALT lymphoma is thought to require the development of T-cell and *H. pylori* independence of the B-cell clone, together with further genetic abnormalities.[95] Overall 77% of patients with gastric MALT lymphoma show complete remission within 12 months of *H. pylori* eradication; however, in a few patients this can be prolonged up to 45 months. It should also be noted that tumour can be detected by polymerase chain reaction in the absence of histologically identifiable tumour. Less than 10% relapse and this could be due to reinfection with *H. pylori*; in the absence of reinfection the relapse is self-limiting. The use of *H. pylori* eradication treatment in transformed MALT lymphoma is controversial, although recently complete remission has been obtained in four of eight patients.[92]

Gastric MALT lymphoma with the t(11;18)(q21;q21) translocation should be treated with chemotherapy or radiation together, as *H. pylori* eradication alone is ineffective. It has also been found that these tumours show a worse response to some chemotherapy and have spread outside the gastric wall. The other lymphomas that are resistant to *H. pylori* eradication are those with abnormalities of the *BCL10* locus or ones associated with an autoimmune gastritis. These can be identified by strong nuclear staining with Bcl-10 in the former and in the latter by staining with the product of the *Fas* oncogene. These non-responsive lymphomas can be treated surgically or in combination with chemoradiotherapy. The 5-year survival for localised cases is 90–100% (stage Ig) and 82% (stage IIg). Continued follow-up of these patients is recommended as it is now recognised that synchronous and metachronous adenocarcinomas occur.[94]

Gastric neuroendocrine tumours

The gastric mucosa contains several types of endocrine cells, which contain, within membrane-bound vesicles, either a neurotransmitter, neuromodulator or neuropeptide hormone. These cells differ from neurones by having no axons or specialised terminals, and they contain marker proteins that include chromogranin and synaptophysin.[96] The neuroendocrine tumours (previously known as carcinoids) are derived from these cells, the most common arising from enterochromaffin-like (ECL) cells. Multistep progression from simple hyperplasia through nodule formation to dysplasia and tumour formation is thought to occur. These tumours will behave in a more malignant manner if they are single and are more than 2 cm in diameter. The histological features are increased numbers of mitoses or a high proliferative index, nuclear pleomorphism, accumulation of p53 within the nucleus and angioinvasion.[97,98] Gastric carcinoids represent only 0.54% of all malignant tumours.

Three subgroups of patients with gastric carcinoid tumours can be identified:

1. Multiple well-differentiated tumours affecting predominantly middle-aged females are associated with type A chronic atrophic gastritis and pernicious anaemia.[99] This group of patients is the most common and, where the tumours are invasive, they tend to be limited to the submucosa. Metastases are usually confined to the local lymph nodes (found in 7–12% of cases). No reported

deaths are associated with these tumours. The possibility of reversibility, by antrectomy (to reduce the hypergastrinaemia) or with octreotide, has demonstrated a reduction in the endocrine cell numbers at 1 month, although there tends to be a rebound phenomenon at 3 months after stopping treatment.

2. Carcinoid tumours associated with the Zollinger–Ellison syndrome or those patients with multiple endocrine neoplasia (MEN) type 1 have hypergastrinaemia and are also predominantly middle-aged females. The tumours tend to be multicentric with a minimal gastritis, but both hyperplasia and endocrine cell dysplasia are present. These tumours often extend into deep muscle, have lymph node metastases and have occasionally caused death. The loss of the *MEN1* gene locus is seen in the majority of these tumours, a defect also found in those tumours of the gut, pancreas and parathyroid associated with MEN-1.[100]

3. Solitary lesions that occur in middle-aged men tend to be larger (2 cm) and have a more aggressive behaviour. The adjacent mucosa shows a minimal non-specific gastritis, and only focal neuroendocrine hyperplasia and no dysplasia. Serosal infiltration with lymphatic and vascular invasion is more common. Liver metastasis with an accompanying carcinoid syndrome has been reported. Metastases are present in 52% of cases and approximately one-third of the patients will have died in a median interval of 51 months.

Recent guidelines from the British Society of Gastroenterology have incorporated the WHO classification of these tumours.[101] The likely prognosis is based on the depth of invasion, size and presence of any vascular invasion. The most aggressive tumours are similar to the small cell carcinoma (oat cell) and are regarded as high-grade malignancy.

Key points

- The multistep progression from normal mucosa to cancer shows that the *p53* gene has been found to be abnormal in up to half the cases of oesophageal squamous carcinoma. Different mutations of *p53* are found in adenocarcinoma of the oesophagus. The mutations allow abnormal cell growth and are associated with further damage to the genome, especially to the important tumour suppressor genes.
- Squamous dysplasia and carcinoma in situ are regarded as precancerous conditions of the oesophagus. In screened high-risk populations the finding of dysplasia predates the development of carcinoma by approximately 5 years.
- The precursor lesion for development of dysplasia is not well identified, although in areas of high risk there is an increased incidence of moderate to severe chronic oesophagitis, suggesting luminal damage may be in part responsible for this preneoplastic change.
- The pathogenesis of gastric carcinoma is complex and multifactorial with several potential precursor lesions (Box 1.2).
- Although it is possible to reverse the inflammatory and some of the intestinal metaplastic changes associated with *H. pylori* infection, atrophy and the colonic-type intestinal metaplasia (type III – incomplete metaplasia) are regarded as irreversible. There is continuing controversy as to the value of identifying the colonic-type mucin and its predictive value in identifying patients at risk of developing cancer.
- There are several problems associated with histological interpretation of grades of gastric dysplasia; these include interobservational variation, distinguishing regenerative atypia from true dysplasia, the ability to differentiate high-grade dysplasia from intramucosal carcinoma, and a lack of experience due to the rarity of dysplasia (especially in low incidence areas). This may be overcome with the recently published Vienna classification of gastric dysplasia (Box 1.3).
- There are a variety of classifications for gastric adenocarcinoma, the most widely accepted being that proposed by Lauren. The tumours are divided into two main types: those that form glandular structures are known as intestinal (53%), while those with no structure that secrete mucin are referred to as diffuse carcinomas (33%). The remaining 14% have a mixed appearance with elements from both types and are regarded as unclassified.
- There is a significant difference in the expression of the sulphamucins between the intestinal and diffuse types of gastric carcinoma (80% and 20% respectively), which has suggested differences in the underlying aetiology.
- Abnormalities of the E-cadherin gene and reduced expression of this protein have been found in up to 90% of carcinomas, especially the diffuse type, and is the defect in hereditary diffuse gastric cancer.
- The stomach is the commonest site for gastrointestinal lymphomas. The majority of the tumours are B-cell non-Hodgkin's lymphomas, the most common being the low-grade MALT lymphomas. It is thought that the development of lymphoma is a multistage process, with the initiating phase being due to the interaction of the *H. pylori*, neutrophils, B cells and T cells within the mucosa, and is associated with specific chromosomal translocations.
- Three subgroups of patients with carcinoid tumours can be identified. Most are benign and associated with overgrowth of the ECL cells. Solitary lesions frequently metastasise and can be highly malignant.

References

1. Munoz NC, Grassi A, Qiong S et al. Precursor lesions of oesophageal cancer in high-risk populations in Iran and China. Lancet 1982; 1:876–9.

2. Streitz J Jr, Ellis F Jr, Gibb SP et al. Achalasia and squamous cell carcinoma of the esophagus: analysis of 241 patients. Ann Thorac Surg 1995; 59(6):1604–9.

3. Applequist P, Salmo M. Lye corrosion carcinoma of the esophagus. A review of 63 cases. Cancer 1980; 45:2655–8.

4. O'Mahony MY, Ellis JP, Hellier M et al. Familial tylosis and carcinoma of the oesophagus. J R Soc Med 1984; 77:514–17.

5. Risk JM, Evans KE, Jones J et al. Characterization of a 500 kb region on 17q25 and the exclusion of candidate genes as the familial Tylosis Oesophageal Cancer (TOC) locus. Oncogene 2002; 21(41):6395–402.

6. Chisholm M. The association between webs iron and post-cricoid carcinoma. Postgrad Med J 1974; 50:215.

7. Huang BS, Unni KK, Payne WS. Long term survival following diverticulectomy for cancer in pharyngooesophageal (Zenker's) diverticulum. Ann Thorac Surg 1984; 38:207–10.

8. Tamura H, Schulman SA. Barrett-type esophagus associated with squamous carcinoma. Chest 1971; 59:330–3.

9. Swinson CM, Slavin G, Coles EC et al. Coeliac disease and malignancy. Lancet 1983; i:111–15.

10. Sherrill DG, Grishkin BA, Galal FS et al. Radiation induced associated malignancies of the oesophagus. Cancer 1984; 54:726–8.

11. Contini S, Consigli GF, Di Lecee F et al. Vital staining of oesophagus in patients with head and neck cancer: still a worthwhile procedure. Ital J Gastroenterol 1991; 23:5–8.

12. Bogomoletz WV, Molas G, Gayet B et al. Superficial squamous cell carcinoma of the esophagus. A report of 76 cases and review of the literature. Am J Surg Pathol 1989; 13:535–46.

13. Mandard AM, Dalibard F, Mandard JC et al. Pathologic assessment of tumor regression after preoperative chemoradiotherapy of esophageal carcinoma: clinicopathologic correlations. Cancer 1994; 73:2680–6.

14. Jaskiewicz K, Banach L, Mafungo V et al. Oesophageal mucosa in a population at risk of oesophageal cancer: postmortem 72 studies. Int J Cancer 1992; 50:32–5.

15. Takubo K, Aida J, Sawabe M et al. Early squamous cell carcinoma of the oesophagus: the Japanese viewpoint. Histopathology 2007; 51:733–42.

16. Sarbia M, Porschen R, Borchard F et al. Incidence and prognostic significance of vascular and neural invasion in squamous cell carcinomas of the esophagus. Int J Cancer 1995; 61(3):333–6.

17. Handra Luca A, Terris B, Couvelard A et al. Spindle cell squamous carcinoma of the oesophagus: an analysis of 17 cases, with new immunohistochemical evidence for a clonal origin. Histopathology 2001; 39(2):125–32.

18. Montesano R, Hainaut P. Molecular precursor lesions in oesophageal cancer. Cancer Surv 1998; 32:53–68.

19. Shiozaki H, Kadowaki T, Doki Y et al. Effect of epidermal growth factor on cadherin-mediated adhesion in a human oesophageal cancer cell line. Br J Cancer 1995; 71(2):250–8.

20. Going JJ, Keith WN, Neilson L et al. Aberrant expression of minichromosome maintenance proteins 2 and 5, and Ki-67 in dysplastic squamous oesophageal epithelium and Barrett's mucosa. Gut 2002; 50(3):373–7.

21. Matsuura H, Kuwano H, Morita M et al. Predicting recurrence time of esophageal carcinoma through assessment of histologic factors and DNA ploidy. Cancer 1991; 67:1406–11.

22. Ruol A, Merigliano S, Baldan N et al. Prevalence, management and outcome of early adenocarcinoma (pT1) of the esophago-gastric junction. Comparison between early cancer in Barrett's esophagus (type I) and early cancer of the cardia (type II). Dis Esoph 1997; 10(3):190–5.

23. Siewert JR, Stein H. Classification of adenocarcinoma of the oesophagogastric junction. Br J Surg 1998; 85:1457–9.

24. Barrett N. Chronic peptic ulcer of the oesophagus and 'oesophagitis'. Br J Surg 1950; 38:175–82.

25. Womack C, Harvey L. Columnar epithelial lined oesophagus (CELO) or Barrett's oesophagus: mucin histochemistry, dysplasia, and invasive adenocarcinoma [letter]. J Clin Pathol 1985; 38(4):477–8.

26. Thomas P, Doddoli C, Lienne P et al. Changing patterns and surgical results in adenocarcinoma of the oesophagus. Br J Surg 1997; 84(1):119–25.

27. van der Burgh ADJ, Hop WCJ, van Blankenstein M. Oesophageal cancer is an uncommon cause of death in patients with Barrett's oesophagus. Gut 1996; 39:5–8.

28. Iftikhar SY, Steele RJ, Watson S et al. Assessment of proliferation of squamous, Barrett's and gastric mucosa in patients with columnar lined Barrett's oesophagus [see comments]. Gut 1992; 33(6):733–7.

29. Cho KJ, Jang JJ, Lee SS et al. Basaloid squamous carcinoma of the oesophagus: a distinct neoplasm with multipotential differentiation. Histopathology 2000; 36(4):331–40.

30. Matsuki A, Nishimaki T, Suzuki T et al. Esophageal mucoepidermoid carcinoma containing signet-ring

cells: three case reports and a literature review. J Surg Oncol 1999; 71(1):54–7.

31. Mafune K, Takubo K, Tanaka Y et al. Sclerosing mucoepidermoid carcinoma of the esophagus with intraepithelial carcinoma or dysplastic epithelium. J Surg Oncol 1995; 58(3):184–90.

32. Takubo K, Nakamura K, Sawabe M et al. Primary undifferentiated small cell carcinoma of the esophagus. Hum Pathol 1999; 30(2):216–21.

33. Correa P, Chen VW. Gastric cancer. Cancer Surv 1994; 20:55–76.

34. Xia HH, Talley NJ. Apoptosis in gastric epithelium induced by *Helicobacter pylori* infection: implications in gastric carcinogenesis. Am J Gastroenterol 2001; 96(1):16–26.

35. Silva S, Filipe M. Intestinal metaplasia and its variants in the gastric mucosa of Portuguese subjects. A comparative analysis of biopsy and gastrectomy material. Hum Pathol 1986; 17:988–95.

36. Sipponen P, Kimura K. Intestinal metaplasia, atrophic gastritis and stomach cancer: trends over time. Eur J Gastroenterol Hepatol 1994; 6(1):S79–83.

37. Dixon MF. Prospects of intervention in gastric carcinogenesis: reversibility of gastric atrophy and intestinal metaplasia. Gut 2001; 49:2–4.

38. Smith MG, Hold GL, Tahara E et al. Cellular and molecular aspects of gastric cancer. World J Gastroenterol 2006; 12(19):2979–90.

39. Stemmermann GN. Intestinal metaplasia of the stomach. A status report. Cancer 1994; 74(2):556–64.

40. Ho SB, Shekels LL, Toribara NW et al. Mucin gene expression in normal, preneoplastic, and neoplastic human gastric epithelium. Cancer Res 1995; 55(12):2681–90.

41. Saegusa M, Takano Y, Okayasu I. Bcl-2 expression and its association with cell kinetics in human gastric carcinomas and intestinal metaplasia. J Cancer Res Clin Oncol 1995; 121(6):357–63.

42. Yamaguchi N, Kakizoe T. Synergistic interaction between *Helicobacter pylori* gastritis and diet in gastric cancer. Lancet Oncol 2001; 2(2):88–94.

43. Correa P, Fox J, Fontham E et al. *Helicobacter pylori* and gastric carcinoma: serum antibody prevalence in populations with contrasting cancer risks. Cancer 1990; 66:2569–74.

44. Ming S-C. Malignant potential of epithelial polyps of the stomach. In: Ming S-C (ed.) Precursors of gastric cancer. New York: Praeger, 1984; pp. 219–31.

45. Nakamura T, Nakano G. Histopathological classification, and malignant change in gastric polyps. J Clin Pathol 1985; 38:754–64.

46. Hattori T. Morphological range of hyperplastic polyps and carcinomas arising in hyperplastic polyps of the stomach. J Clin Pathol 1985; 38:622–30.

47. Lida M, Yao T, Watanabe H et al. Fundic gland polyposis in patients without familial adenomatosis coli: its incidence and clinical features. Gastroenterology 1984; 86:1437–42.

48. Kolodziejczyk P, Yao T, Oya M et al. Long-term follow-up study of patients with gastric adenomas with malignant transformation. An immunohistochemical and histochemical analysis. Cancer 1994; 74(11):2896–907.

49. Sarre R, Frost A, Jagelman D et al. Gastric and duodenal polyps in familial adenomatous polyposis. A prospective study of the nature and prevalence of upper gastrointestinal polyps. Gut 1987; 28:306–14.

50. Xaun Z, Ambe K, Enjoji M. Depressed adenoma of the stomach revisited: histologic, histochemical and immunohistochemical profiles. Cancer 1991; 67:2382–9.

51. Fujiwara T, Hirose S, Hamazaki K et al. Clinicopathological features of gastric cancer in the remnant stomach. Hepato-Gastroenterology 1996; 43(8): 416–19.

52. Sebagh M, Flejou JF, Potet F. Lymphoma of the gastric stump. Report of two cases and review of the literature. J Clin Gastroenterol 1995; 20(2):147–50.

53. Johnson MI, Spark JI, Ambrose NS et al. Early gastric cancer in a patient with Ménétrier's disease, lymphocytic gastritis and *Helicobacter pylori*. Eur J Gastroenterol Hepatol 1995; 7(2):187–90.

54. Morson BC, Sobin LH, Grundmann E et al. Precancerous conditions and epithelial dysplasia in the stomach. J Clin Pathol 1980; 33:711–21.

55. Lee SI, Iida M, Yao T et al. Long-term follow-up of 2529 patients reveals gastric ulcers rarely become malignant. Dig Dis Sci 1990; 35:763–8.

56. Schlemper RJ, Riddell RH, Kato Y et al. The Vienna classification of gastrointestinal epithelial neoplasms. Gut 2000; 47:251–5.

57. You WZ, Zhao L, Chang YS et al. Progression of precancerous gastric lesions. Lancet 1995; 345:866.

58. Murakami T. Pathomorphological diagnosis. Definition and gross classification of early gastric cancer. GANN Monogr 1971; 11:53–5.

59. Kodama YI, Inokuchi K, Soejima K et al. Growth patterns and prognosis in early gastric carcinoma. Superficial spreading and penetrating growth types. Cancer 1983; 51:320–6.

60. Mori M, Sakaguchi H, Akazawa K et al. Correlation between metastatic site, histological type, and serum tumor markers of gastric carcinoma. Hum Pathol 1995; 26(5):504–8.

61. Saragoni L, Gaudio M, Vio A et al. Early gastric cancer in the province of Forli: follow-up of 337 patients in a high risk region for gastric cancer. Oncol Rep 1998; 5(4):945–8.

62. Tsuchiya A, Kikuchi Y, Ando Y et al. Lymph node metastases in gastric cancer invading the submucosal layer. Eur J Surg Oncol 1995; 21(3):248–50.

63. Kitamura K, Yamaguchi T, Okamoto K et al. Total gastrectomy for early gastric cancer. J Surg Oncol 1995; 60(2):83–8.

64. Kim JP, Hur YS, Yang HK. Lymph node metastasis as a significant prognostic factor in early gastric

cancer: analysis of 1136 early gastric cancers. Ann Surg Oncol 1995; 2(4):308–13.

65. Hayes N, Karat D, Scott D et al. Radical lymphadenectomy for early gastric carcinoma. Br J Surg 1996; 83:1421–3.

66. Brito MJ, Filipe MI, Williams GT et al. DNA ploidy in early gastric carcinoma (T1). A flow cytometric study of 100 European cases. Gut 1993; 34:230–4.

67. Ikeda Y, Mori M, Kamakura T et al. Improvements in diagnosis have changed the incidence of histological types in advanced gastric cancer. Br J Cancer 1995; 72(2):424–6.

68. Borrmann R. Makroskopische Formen des vorgeschrittenen Magenkrebses. In: Henke F, Lubarach O (eds) Handbuch der speziellen pathologischen Anatomie und Histologie. Berlin: Springer, 1926; Vol. 4/1.

69. Lauren P. The two histological main types of gastric carcinoma: diffuse and so called intestinal-type carcinoma. Acta Pathol Microbiol Scand 1965; 64:31–49.

70. Ming S-C. Gastric carcinoma. A pathobiological classification. Cancer 1977; 39:2475–85.

71. Hamilton SR, Aaltonen LA. WHO histological classification of gastric tumours. In: World Health Organization of tumours: pathology and genetics of tumours of the digestive system. Lyon: IARC Press, 2000; pp. 38–67.

72. Goseki N, Maruyama M, Takizawa T et al. Morphological changes in gastric carcinoma with progression. J Gastroenterol 1995; 30(3):287–94.

73. Matsunou H, Konishi F, Hori H et al. Characteristics of Epstein–Barr virus-associated gastric carcinoma with lymphoid stroma in Japan. Cancer 1996; 77(10):1998–2004.

74. Boku T, Nakane Y, Minoura T et al. Prognostic significance of serosal invasion and free intraperitoneal cancer cells in gastric cancer. Br J Surg 1990; 77(4):436–9.

75. Songun I, van de Velde CJ, Arends JW et al. Classification of gastric carcinoma using the Goseki system provides prognostic information additional to TNM staging. Cancer 1999; 85(10):2114–18.

76. Abe S, Shiraishi M, Nagaoka S et al. Serosal invasion as the single prognostic indicator in stage IIIA (T3N1M0) gastric cancer. Surgery 1991; 109(5):582–8.

77. Ichiyoshi Y, Maehara Y, Tomisaki S et al. Macroscopic intraoperative diagnosis of serosal invasion and clinical outcome of gastric cancer: risk of underestimation. J Surg Oncol 1995; 59(4):255–60.

78. Noda N, Sasako M, Yamaguchi N et al. Ignoring small lymph nodes can be a major cause of staging error in gastric cancer. Br J Surg 1998; 85(6):831–4.

79. Di Giorgio A, Botti C, Sammartino P et al. Extracapsular lymph node metastases in the staging and prognosis of gastric cancer. Int Surg 1991; 76(4):218–21.

80. Nakamura K, Ueyama T, Yao T et al. Pathology and prognosis of gastric carcinoma. Findings in 10,000 patients who underwent primary gastrectomy. Cancer 1992; 70(5):1030–7.

81. Kakeji Y, Korenaga D, Baba H et al. Surgical treatment of patients with gastric carcinoma and duodenal invasion. J Surg Oncol 1995; 59(4):215–19.

82. Setala LP, Kosma VM, Marin S et al. Prognostic factors in gastric cancer: the value of vascular invasion, mitotic rate and lymphoplasmacytic infiltration. Br J Cancer 1996; 74:766–72.

83. Becker K, Mueller JD, Schulmacher C et al. Histomorphology and grading of regression in gastric carcinoma treated with neoadjuvant chemotherapy. Cancer 2003; 98:1521–30.

84. Correa P. Human gastric carcinogenesis: a multistep and multifactorial process. First American Cancer Society Award Lecture on Cancer Epidemiology and Prevention. Cancer Res 1992; 52(24):6735–40.

85. Tahara E. Genetic alterations in human gastrointestinal cancers. The application to molecular diagnosis. Cancer 1995; 75(6, Suppl):1410–17.

86. Stemmermann G, Heffelfinger SC, Noffsinger A et al. The molecular biology of esophageal and gastric cancer and their precursors: oncogenes, tumor suppressor genes, and growth factors. Hum Pathol 1994; 25(10):968–81.

87. Yasui W, Oue N, Aung PP et al. Molecular–pathological prognostic factors of gastric cancer: a review. Gastric Cancer 2005; 8:86–94.

88. Harn HJ, Ho LI, Chang JY et al. Differential expression of the human metastasis adhesion molecule CD44V in normal and carcinomatous stomach mucosa of Chinese subjects. Cancer 1995; 75(5):1065–71.

89. Aarnio M, Salovaara R, Aaltonen LA et al. Features of gastric cancer in hereditary non-polyposis colorectal cancer syndrome. Int J Cancer 1997; 74(5):551–5.

90. Carneiro F, Oliveira C, Suriano G et al. Molecular pathology of familial gastric cancer, with an emphasis on hereditary diffuse gastric cancer. J Clin Pathol 2008; 61:25–30.

91. Fletcher CD, Berman JJ, Corless C et al. Diagnosis of gastrointestinal stromal tumors: a consensus approach. Hum Pathol 2002; 33(5):459–65.

92. Wotherspoon AD, Doglioni C, Diss TC et al. Regression of primary low-grade B-cell gastric lymphoma of mucosa associated lymphoid tissue type after eradication of *Helicobacter pylori*. Lancet 1993; 342:575–7.

93. Zucca E, Bertoni F, Roggero E et al. Molecular analysis of the progression from *Helicobacter pylori*-associated chronic gastritis to mucosa-associated lymphoid-tissue lymphoma of the stomach. N Engl J Med 1998; 338(12):804–10.

94. Bacon CM, Du Ming-Q, Dogan A. Mucosa-associated lymphoid tissue (MALT) lymphoma: a practical guide for pathologists. J Clin Pathol 2007; 60:361–72.

95. Du Ming Q, Isaccson PG. Gastric MALT lymphoma: from aetiology to treatment. Lancet Oncol 2002; 3(2):97–104.

96. Fahrenkamp AG, Wibbeke C, Winde G et al. Immunohistochemical distribution of chromogranins A and B and secretogranin II in neuroendocrine tumours of the gastrointestinal tract. Virchows Arch 1995; 426(4):361–7.

97. Modlin IM, Sandor A, Tang LH et al. A 40-year analysis of 265 gastric carcinoids. Am J Gastroenterol 1997; 92(4):633–8.

98. Solcia E, Rindi G, Paolotti D et al. Natural history, clinicopathologic classification and prognosis of gastric ECL cell tumors. Yale J Biol Med 1998; 71(3–4):285–90.

99. Sculco D, Bilgrami S. Pernicious anemia and gastric carcinoid tumor: case report and review. Am J Gastroenterol 1997; 92(8):1378–80.

100. Debelenko LV, Emmert-Buck MR, Zhuang Z et al. The multiple endocrine neoplasia type I gene locus is involved in the pathogenesis of type II gastric carcinoids. Gastroenterology 1997; 113(3):773–81.

101. Ramage JK, Davies AHG, Ardill J et al. Guidelines for the management of gastroenteropancreatic neuroendocrine (including carcinoid) tumours. Gut 2005; 54:1–16.

2

Epidemiology, genetics and screening for oesophageal and gastric cancer

William H. Allum

Introduction

Approximately 25 years ago the outline of oesophageal and gastric cancer appeared well defined. Oesophageal cancer was essentially squamous cell in origin and a disease of low socio-economic populations reflecting high intake of tobacco and alcohol. Gastric cancer similarly affected lower socio-economic groups. It tended to be found in the distal stomach and histopathologically comprised the intestinal type described by Lauren. Correa had postulated a progressive process from atrophic gastritis through intestinal metaplasia and dysplasia to intestinal-type adenocarcinoma. Evidence accumulated to support a key role for *Helicobacter pylori* as an instigator of this progression. The majority view amongst epidemiologists proposed that health strategies to reduce smoking and alcohol as well as eradicating *Helicobacter* would significantly reduce the incidence of both diseases.

However, cancer registries began to report increases in the incidence of adenocarcinoma of the oesophagus. During the early 1990s it became obvious that this was a general problem and oesophageal adenocarcinoma became the most rapidly increasing cancer in Western countries. Concurrently there was an increase in cardia cancer of the stomach with a parallel reduction in more distal lesions in the West.

There are now three main types of oesophageal and gastric cancer: squamous cell carcinoma of the oesophagus (SCC), non-cardia cancer of the stomach, and adenocarcinoma of the oesophagogastric junction including the cardia (ACA). Each presents a major health problem in different parts of the world, and much effort has been directed at improving our understanding of aetiology and detecting disease at an early and treatable stage. Preventative strategies have been studied with varying degrees of success. More recently, as understanding of cancer genetics has evolved, there has been considerable interest in evaluating genetic mutations within gastric cancer families and patients who develop gastric cancer at an early age.

The overall poor results of treatment have reflected the advanced stage of most cases at presentation. Those parts of the world with high incidence have developed and pursued active mass screening programmes. These have certainly identified precursor lesions and premalignant conditions. Indeed, application of these programmes has produced a significant improvement in survival rates for gastric cancer, particularly in Japan. Knowledge of these changes and underlying conditions has enabled areas of lower incidence to pursue examination of those assessed to be at high risk and as a result to increase the number of cancers diagnosed at an early stage.

Definitions

The change in site of cancers of the oesophagus and stomach with concentration around the oesophagogastric junction has created differences in opinion with regard to classification. This partly reflects differences in the pathological behaviour of tumours arising at different sites, and consequently indications for specific treatments. In epidemiology it is important to ensure a clear classification in order to understand differences in incidence and to appreciate aetiological evidence for the observed changes in these cancers.

For the purposes of the following discussion, carcinoma of the oesophagus will include cancers of the thoracic and abdominal oesophagus but will exclude the cervical oesophagus. Non-cardia gastric cancer will include all cancers of the fundus, body and pyloric antrum. Oesophagogastric junctional cancers will be considered according to the Siewert and Stein classification:[1]

- **Type I** is adenocarcinoma of the distal oesophagus, which usually arises from an area of Barrett's metaplasia and which may infiltrate the oesophagogastric junction from above.
- **Type II** is true carcinoma of the cardia arising from the cardiac epithelium or short segments with intestinal metaplasia at the oesophagogastric junction, often referred to as 'junctional carcinoma'.
- **Type III** is subcardial gastric carcinoma that infiltrates the oesophagogastric junction and distal oesophagus from below.

Although this classification has some limitations, including lack of consensus over pathological behaviour, approach to treatment and ability to site endoscopically, it has become accepted as a practical system.

Epidemiology

Incidence

Cancer epidemiology studies are often limited by the nature of data collection, frequently being retrospective and by necessity incomplete and not standardised. An apparent increase in disease incidence may be influenced by improvements in registration efficiency, an effect of the increasing age of the population and an overall increase in the incidence of the disease itself. Changes in incidence and the actual burden of new cases over time are the result of changes in the size and composition of population and in the actual risk for a specific cancer. Cancer registration may be based upon clinical details only without histological confirmation or on histology of cancer rather than specific reference to squamous cell or adenocarcinoma. These approaches will cause bias to incidence data, although more thorough standardised approaches have latterly reduced these influences.

Oesophageal cancer

Carcinoma of the oesophagus (ICD code 150) was the eighth commonest cancer in 2000.[2] Worldwide there were 412 000 new cases representing 4.1% of the total cases of cancer. Mortality was high, with 338 000 deaths or 82% of all registered cases. Incidence varies across the world, with the highest risk in the so-called Asian 'oesophageal cancer belt', which extends from Northern Iran through Central Asia to North Central China, where incidence is

up to 200 per 100 000. There are also high rates in East and South-East Africa, east South America and parts of France and Switzerland. Overall the male to female ratio is 2.1:1, although there are variations. There is a majority of cases in women in India, and in parts of France males are more frequently affected. SCC predominates in the less developed countries, where 83% of all cases occur. The incidence rates have remained stable. In more developed countries the incidence of SCC has declined. In the USA, SCC in black males has decreased from 17.9 per 100 000 in 1973 to 10.4 per 100 000 in 2002.[3]

Oesophagogastric junctional cancer

The migration of cancer of the oesophagus and stomach towards the oesophagogastric junction has been progressing over the past 50 years. Although the increase has included both histological subtypes, the rate of increase has been greatest for ACA[4,5] (**Fig. 2.1**). In the more developed countries (North America, Europe, Australia, New Zealand and Japan) the increased incidence has been predominantly in males. In the USA the incidence of ACA in white males has increased from 1.0 per 100 000 to 4.8 per 100 000 between 1973 and 2002. In parts of Australia and the UK incidence in white males is 8–12 per 100 000. Over the past 20 years the annual increase in incidence has been approximately 10% per year. Demographically the peak age group affected is between 50 and 60 years of age, and the male to female ratio varies between 2:1 and 12:1. There have been parallel increases in ACA of the gastric cardia.[6] In the USA and the UK cardia cancer accounts for approximately 50% of all gastric cancers. The age group affected and the sex incidence are similar to ACA of the lower oesophagus, suggesting a similar aetiology.

Gastric cancer

Gastric cancer (ICD code 151) is the fourth most frequent cancer worldwide. In 2000 there were 876 000 new cases with 647 000 deaths. This represents 8.7% of all new cases of malignancy and 10.4% of all cancer deaths. The majority of cases (62%) occur in less developed countries, where the male to female ratio is 1.8:1. This contrasts with a ratio of 1.6:1 in more developed countries. Highest incidence rates are found in Japan (male 69.2 per 100 000 and female 28.6 per 100 000). Other countries with high incidence include East Asia, Eastern Europe, and Central and South America. In most countries the rates of incidence continue to decline, with rates 11% lower in 2000 compared with 1990. Although distal cancers still predominate in countries with highest incidence, proximal migration is steadily increasing, particularly in Japan and Korea.

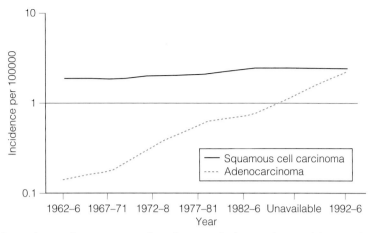

Figure 2.1 • Incidence changes for squamous cell carcinoma and adenocarcinoma of the oesophagus, 1962–1996. Reproduced from Powell J, McConkey CC, Gillison EW et al. Continuing rising trend in oesophageal adenocarcinoma. Int J Cancer 2002; 102:422–7. Copyright 2002 John Wiley & Sons, Inc. Reprinted with permission of John Wiley & Sons, Inc.

Inter-country variations are well known between the Far East and the West. There are, however, significant intra-country variations. These largely reflect a north to south gradient, which is particularly apparent in the northern hemisphere. In both Japan and China mortality rates in the northern provinces are almost double those in the south. Similar differences are observed in the UK, with higher standardised mortality rates in north and northwestern regions. In the southern hemisphere, however, the gradient is reversed. Indeed, the higher geographical latitudes in both hemispheres are more temperate or colder and have a higher risk of gastric cancer, thus implicating environmental and particularly dietary factors in aetiology.

Aetiology

Squamous cell carcinoma of the oesophagus

Smoking and alcohol

Smoking and alcohol are established risk factors for SCC, particularly in the West. Smokers have a five-fold higher risk than non-smokers, which doubles in heavy smokers. There is a positive dose–response effect for both duration and intensity of smoking, although long-term use of tobacco appears to be the stronger influence. The risk reduces after stopping. In the USA tobacco consumption decreased between the 1960s and 1990s, and this is reflected in the decrease in disease incidence. However, the reduction in smoking was less apparent in the black population, in which SCC rates have remained high.

The effect of alcohol is similar to smoking, although the amount consumed appears to be the greater risk factor. Several studies have demonstrated relative risks ranging from 2.9 to 7.4 for heavy drinkers. As with smoking, abstention from alcohol does appear to decrease the risk. Alcohol and smoking seem to have synergistic and independent effects. The mechanism of action for the damaging effect of alcohol is unclear. It may directly damage the oesophageal mucosa or increase its susceptibility to other carcinogens, or may have its effect via the secondarily associated dietary deficiencies.

Socio-economic and dietary influences

Areas of highest incidence are those countries of low socio-economic status where poverty and malnutrition predominate and this is reflected in dietary habits and customs. Hot drinks, coarse foods and a low intake of fresh fruit and vegetables have all been implicated in aetiological studies. The development of SCC appears to be related to a type of chronic oesophagitis which is different from that found in the West and is often complicated by atrophy and dysplasia (see Chapter 1). It is not usually associated with gastro-oesophageal reflux and is often asymptomatic. It may be induced directly by mechanical irritation, thermal injury or vitamin deficiencies. Alternatively the inflammatory injury producing oesophagitis increases the sensitivity of the oesophageal mucosa to carcinogens and hence malignant transformation.

In a case–control analysis of 15- to 26-year-olds in a high-risk area, Chang-Claude et al.[7] compared a series of factors in those with mild and moderate oesophagitis with those with very mild oesophagitis and with normal subjects. Significant changes were associated with ingestion of very hot beverages, a family history of oesophageal cancer, prevalence of oesophagitis among siblings, and a low intake of fresh fruits and wheat flour products. Cigarette smoking and the use of cottonseed oil for cooking were usually observed in those with oesophagitis but there was no striking difference according to level of risk. The lack of any effect with smoking and alcohol may have reflected the rural nature of the population with low socio-economic status and hence low use of both tobacco and alcohol.

Other similar studies have identified riboflavin deficiency and vitamin A and C deficiency[8] as risk factors that are particularly important at a young age. Conversely vitamin C intake confers a protective benefit; Hu et al.,[9] in a case–control study, found that 100 mg of vitamin C per day decreased risk by 39%. Overall, those with a nutritionally deficient diet have a higher incidence of oesophageal cancer in the high-risk areas.[10]

Corrosive injury
SCC is also associated with a variety of uncommon conditions that relate to some form of inflammatory injury. Oesophageal strictures developing after ingestion of corrosive agents, particularly in childhood, are associated with a 1000-fold increase in the risk of carcinoma. There is a time delay of 20–40 years after ingestion of the corrosive, and as a result tumours are seen at a younger age than normal.

Achalasia
Achalasia is associated with SCC, but the magnitude of the risk is unclear. Brucher et al.[11] report from their single institution series that the risk of developing a carcinoma in long-standing achalasia is increased 140-fold when compared with the general population. The risk appears to relate to retention oesophagitis secondary to stasis and exposure to possible carcinogens in fermenting food residue. There is a lead time of approximately 15–20 years and these cases probably warrant long-term surveillance. Treatment of the achalasia does not seem to reduce the risk.

Associated syndromes and familial risk
The Plummer–Vinson syndrome of dysplasia, iron-deficiency anaemia, koilonychia and oropharyngeal mucosal atrophy is associated with an increased risk of cervical oesophageal cancer.

Finally, there is a familial tendency suggesting a genetic predisposition. Tylosis palmarum is a rare inherited autosomal dominant condition in which there is a very high incidence of SCC. Perhaps of greater significance is the finding of the increased risk in low-risk areas for offspring of parents with oesophageal cancer.[12] There are numerical and structural chromosomal aberrations in patients with a family history not seen in those without a family history (see below).

Adenocarcinoma of the oesophagus and junctional cancers

Gastro-oesophageal reflux disease (GORD)
Gastro-oesophageal reflux is now the most common symptomatic presentation of all conditions affecting the upper gastrointestinal tract. Estimates suggest that 4–9% of all adults experience daily heartburn and up to 20% experience symptoms on a weekly basis.[13] Many are self-treated and do not attend for further investigation. The relationship of GORD and oesophageal ACA has been evaluated in case–control studies. Chow et al.[14] found a relationship between oesophageal and cardia cancer associated with a past history of oesophageal reflux, hiatus hernia, oesophagitis or dysphagia, with an odds ratio of between 2 and 5. The individual cancer risk is small because of the high frequency of GORD. In the USA hospital activity data confirm parallel trends in incidence of reflux disease and ACA. However, population-based studies have not shown a definite increase in the prevalence of reflux. Furthermore the annual incidence of ACA in patients over 50 years of age with reflux is 65 per 100 000, yet 40% of patients developing cancer do not have a background of chronic reflux.[14] Lagergen et al.[15] have estimated the risk of developing ACA of the oesophagus by scoring symptoms of heartburn and regurgitation (alone or in combination), timing of symptoms (particularly at night) and frequency of symptoms. Among those with recurrent symptoms of reflux, the odds ratio of developing cancer was 7.7 in comparison with those without symptoms. More frequent, more severe and longer-lasting symptoms of reflux were associated with a much greater risk (odds ratio 44). The risk associated with GORD is related to the development of Barrett's metaplasia. Approximately 12% undergoing endoscopy for symptomatic GORD have Barrett's. Further detailed discussion of the role of Barrett's in the aetiology of ACA is presented in Chapter 15.

Obesity and dietary factors
Evidence is accumulating to implicate obesity as an independent risk factor for oesophagogastric junctional cancer. In the last 20 years the incidence of junctional cancer has increased in parallel with the epidemic of obesity. There is a three- to sixfold excess risk among overweight individuals.[16] Obesity predisposes to hiatus hernia and reflux, and hence contributes mechanically to increase risk. However, data from a number of studies demonstrate an effect independent of reflux. Lindblad et al.[17] have reported a 67% increase in the risk of oesophageal

ACA in patients with a body mass index (BMI) greater than 25, and this increases with increasing BMI. This effect was noted irrespective of the presence of reflux symptoms.

There appears to be a sex difference in that the effect was only found in women with a BMI greater than 30, whereas in men it was observed in both overweight and obese individuals. Recently this effect in women has been confirmed, with 50% of cases of oesophageal adenocarcinoma in postmenopausal women in the Million Women study being attributed to obesity.[18] Vaughan et al.[19] have examined the potential relationship between a series of biological markers of progression from metaplasia to cancer in obese and overweight patients. There was little evidence of change in the biomarkers in association with increasing obesity. However, abnormalities in the biomarkers were observed in individuals with high anthropometric measures of abdominal fat. The study concluded that increased BMI contributed to reflux and development of metaplasia but it was the 'male pattern' of abdominal obesity that was actually associated with malignant transformation. Further evidence is accumulating to support different types of obesity. The distribution of abdominal fat tends to be central and retroperitoneal. This acts as a potent source of growth factors, hormones and regulators of the cell cycle. Such individuals develop the metabolic syndrome, which is linked to raised serum cholesterol and triglycerides, hypertension and hyperglycaemia. In the general population the metabolic syndrome occurs in 10–20%. Power and colleagues[20] have recently demonstrated that 46% of those with Barrett's oesophagus and 36% of those with GORD have features of the metabolic syndrome. The factors released by centrally deposited fat may have an effect on the process of metaplasia transforming to dysplasia.

The effect of diet on the risk of junctional cancer is probably a reflection of BMI. High intake of calories, fat and animal protein with a low intake of dietary fibre have all been implicated as risk factors. Consumption of red meat as opposed to white meat (poultry) appears to have an effect, although studies only show a trend rather than a significant risk.

Helicobacter pylori

The role of *Helicobacter pylori* infection in the aetiology of junctional cancer is unclear but appears to be evolving. Gastric infection with *H. pylori* is characterised by gastric atrophy and hypochlorhydria. It has been suggested that this reduction in acid production could, in association with ammonia production from urea by the bacteria, protect the lower oesophagus by changing the content of the refluxing gastric juice. In countries with an increase in junctional cancer, there has been a corresponding decrease in incidence of *H. pylori* infection.

Furthermore community-based approaches to eradicate *H. pylori* infection in the treatment of ulcer and non-ulcer dyspepsia may be inadvertently contributing to the increase in these cancers.

Increases in incidence in true cardia (type II) and type III junctional cancers have paralleled the increase in type I cancers and the natural history appears to be similar. Guanrei et al.[21] reported on a group of patients with early oesophageal SCC and early ACA of the cardia who refused any treatment. Progression to advanced disease was similar at 4–5 years. Survival from diagnosis was also similar, with a median of 74 months. However, the pathological features, the outcome and surgical approaches are more akin to gastric cancer than oesophageal cancer. Some consider the inflammation and metaplasia associated with cardia cancer to be caused by *H. pylori* infection despite many cases presenting with reflux. Recently Hansen et al.[22] have proposed that cardia cancer has two distinct aetiologies. In a nested case–control study, serum from a defined population cohort followed for the development of gastric cancer was tested for *H. pylori* antibodies and for evidence of atrophic gastritis, using as surrogate markers gastrin levels and the pepsinogen I to pepsinogen II ratio. *Helicobacter pylori* seropositivity and gastric atrophy were associated with the risk of non-cardia gastric cancer. In cardia cancer there were two distinct groups. In one serology for *H. pylori* was negative and there was no evidence of gastric atrophy, and in the other *H. pylori* was positive and there was evidence of atrophy. The authors concluded that the former group behaved like non-cardia cancer and were more likely to be diffuse type and the latter like oesophageal ACA and likely to be intestinal type. Further support for this hypothesis is reflected in differences at the molecular level. Differences in the pattern of cell surface cytokeratins have been reported: the cytokeratin 7 and 20 pattern is essentially restricted to Barrett's metaplasia but is absent or rare in intestinal metaplasia of the gastric cardia.[23] Such different characteristics would imply a different carcinogenic process at the two sites.

Socio-economic factors

Lifestyle has an effect on the risk for junctional cancers. There is an association with lower socio-economic class but this is not as strong as for SCC. Powell and McConkey[4] demonstrated that the increase of ACA of the lower third of the oesophagus and the cardia was mainly in social classes I and II – that is, in professional and managerial occupations. In addition in a large surgical series, Siewert and Ott[24] reported that patients with ACA were more frequently from an educated background, a characteristic which was not present in the population with SCC. However, the effect of socio-economic class may not be independent as, when adjusted for GORD, BMI and smoking, Jansson et al.[25] found the effect to be less apparent.

Gastric cancer

The Correa hypothesis[26] (**Fig. 2.2**) describes the steps in the process of malignant transformation for gastric cancer. It highlights where environmental factors stimulate changes, particularly in the development of intestinal-type gastric cancer (see Chapter 1). These include socio-economic and dietary influences, as well as exposure to carcinogens.

Socio-economic influences

Gastric cancer is a disease of lower socio-economic groups. The incidence of tobacco smoking tends to be higher in these groups and there is a 1.6-fold risk of developing stomach cancer for smokers in comparison to non-smokers.

An excess risk has been linked to certain occupations. Coalmining in the UK and the USA is associated, as is the pottery industry in the north Midlands of

the UK. The proposed mechanism involves swallowing dust-contaminated mucus cleared from the lungs and nasal passages. Evidence for such a relationship is circumstantial, and as certain occupations reflect social background the risk may equally reflect lifestyle, particularly dietary habits, rather than actual occupational risk.

Exposure to potentially carcinogenic agents at an early age is clearly crucial to the risk of developing both precursor lesions and subsequently gastric cancer. Evidence for this risk is available from migrant studies. Initial evidence from Japanese migrants to the USA showed that the high risk of Japanese ethnicity was retained despite the lower incidence of the disease in the USA. The longer the migrant lives in the area of lower incidence, the more likely it is that the risk of gastric cancer reduces; however, it does not reach that of the host environment. For example, the US-born offspring of migrants show a similar risk to their country of birth. This would suggest that it is an environmental influence that is important rather than a genetic one. Interestingly, Correa et al.[27] have subsequently demonstrated that

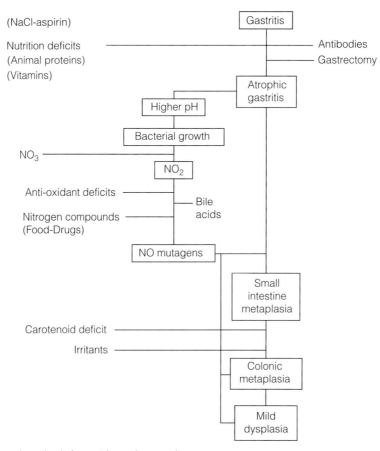

Figure 2.2 • Correa hypothesis for gastric carcinogenesis.

migrants developing gastric cancer are more likely to develop the diffuse type, consistent with their new host country, further suggesting a relationship of the intestinal type to environmental influences.

Diet

The prevalence of gastric cancer in poor communities reflects both malnutrition and intake of a poor-quality diet. Foodstuffs that are cheap prevail, as well as low-cost methods of food preservation and preparation. High carbohydrate intake has been implicated. Case–control studies have demonstrated consumption of cooked cereals, rice and starch to be higher in gastric cancer patients than controls. Other studies have shown no difference. It may, however, be an effect of the balance of carbohydrate in proportion to protein and fat. Areas with a high dietary carbohydrate content have a low protein intake. Protein deficiency will impair gastric mucosal repair and indeed high carbohydrate/low protein may impair defence mechanisms against injurious agents.

Salt preservation of food was common during the early years of the 20th century throughout the world; in some landlocked parts of the world this still occurs. In such areas and in those still using salt preservation there have been high rates of gastric cancer. The consumption of salted and pickled fish is high in Japanese and Colombians and correlates with their disease incidence. On the basis that salt induces injury to the gastric mucosa it may act like high carbohydrate intake, as an initiator to allow access for more potent carcinogens. By contrast the rapid and widespread adoption of refrigerators in the 1950s and 1960s has significantly affected the preservation of fresh foods. The reduction in mortality observed in Japan shows an inverse relationship with the increase in ownership of domestic refrigerators.[28]

Fresh vegetables and fruit theoretically act to protect against gastric carcinogenesis. Vitamin C inhibits intragastric formation of nitrosamines from nitrite and amino precursors. Both vitamins A and E act as antioxidants within cells, as well as regulating cell differentiation and protecting the gastric mucosal barrier. However, dietary studies have failed to confirm these proposed effects. An intercountry variation in fruit and vegetable intake has not paralleled differences in gastric cancer incidence. It is possible, however, that prolonged exposure is more relevant, again supporting the philosophy of a balanced diet rather than one supplemented with a potentially beneficial foodstuff.

Helicobacter pylori

In 1994 the International Agency for Research on Cancer designated *H. pylori* to be a type I carcinogen.[29] The initial effect of *H. pylori* is acute inflammation. Since the infection does not resolve spontaneously, an effect is likely to persist and may proceed to chronic gastritis and associated mucosal atrophy and intestinal metaplasia, dysplasia and eventually cancer. The evidence for its role is from a number of sources. Areas of high cancer incidence have a high rate of *H. pylori* infection. In a prospective population-based study in Japan, 2.9% of those infected developed gastric cancer compared with none from the uninfected population; 4.7% of those infected who had non-ulcer dyspepsia progressed to cancer.[30] The decline in prevalence of *H. pylori*, particularly in developed countries, parallels the decrease in gastric cancer incidence. *Helicobacter pylori* infection tends to occur early in life but varies later in life, which appears to be a cohort effect. In the USA and Japan less than 20% of the population are infected at 20 years of age; however, by 50 years 50% are infected in the USA compared with 80% in Japan. The early rates of infection are linked to low income, poor education, poor sanitation and overcrowding. Epidemiology studies using serology have demonstrated that seropositive populations representing previous infection have a 2.1–16.7-fold greater risk of developing gastric cancer than corresponding seronegative populations.

Although the evidence for *H. pylori* inducing gastric cancer is convincing, not all those infected develop the disease. The risk of malignant transformation appears to be enhanced by bacterial virulence and host factors (see below). *Helicobacter pylori* with cytotoxin-associated gene A (*cagA*) appears to be associated with the greatest risk.[31] In the West, 60% of *H. pylori* infections are *cagA* positive compared with 100% in Japan.[32,33] It is likely that *H. pylori* induces an environment which is susceptible to malignant transformation. It induces tissue monocytes to produce reactive oxygen intermediates, which are potent carcinogens. Infection is associated with a significant reduction in gastric juice ascorbic acid,[34] which acts to scavenge and suppress *N*-nitroso compounds and oxygen free radicals. It also facilitates the proliferation of nitrosating bacteria, which promote the development of *N*-nitroso compounds.

Prevention of oesophageal and gastric cancer

Prevention strategies are either primary or secondary. Primary approaches aim to prevent cancer developing, whereas secondary prevention is intended to identify precancerous processes and conditions and to intervene to prevent progression to cancer.

In oesophageal and gastric cancer primary prevention approaches are currently limited to population education to alter social habits (such as decreasing or stopping tobacco or alcohol consumption) and dietary habits (such as maintaining a diet containing fresh fruit and vegetables with a low or minimal salt intake). In addition the need to prevent obesity is now well established. The role of *H. pylori* eradication is important but programmes of eradication should only be considered according to the level of risk for oesophageal or gastric cancer in the population. In populations with a high risk of gastric cancer, eradication is indicated; however, in populations in which oesophageal ACA is common, eradication may have an adverse effect. The overall benefit of these approaches would be greatly enhanced if specific markers of risk could be identified to focus prevention strategies. Current understanding of such markers is limited but identification of molecular biomarkers, for example, may be advantageous (see below).

Secondary prevention depends upon understanding the natural history and detection of premalignant conditions. In SCC there is limited evidence that secondary measures could be effective because of lack of understanding of the histological changes leading to cancer. In oesophageal ACA surveillance of Barrett's metaplasia to identify progression to dysplasia is theoretically a positive approach (see Chapter 15). Identification of p53 expression and aneuploidy in biopsies of Barrett's has been shown to predict the risk of progression.[35] In both gastric and oesophageal cancer there is a potential role for chemoprevention. Increasing levels of cyclo-oxygenase-2 (COX-2) are present in the progression of atrophic gastritis to intestinal metaplasia and gastric cancer.[36] Smoking, acid and *H. pylori* are all associated with COX-2 expression. Aspirin and other non-steroidal agents inhibit COX-2 and their use may act as a chemopreventive for gastric cancer. Aspirin also seems to have an effect in Barrett's metaplasia and in combination with acid suppression may minimise progression to dysplasia. The ASPECT trial in the UK is assessing whether such a strategy can have a secondary preventive effect.[37]

Genetics of oesophageal and gastric cancer

The majority of the available evidence for the aetiology of oesophageal and gastric cancer implicates environmental factors. In oesophageal adenocarcinoma this is consistent with the sequence of Barrett's metaplasia to dysplasia and on to cancer, and in gastric cancer with the Correa hypothesis of atrophic gastritis, intestinal metaplasia, dysplasia and cancer. There is, however, an increasing body of evidence supporting a genetic predisposition. In oesophageal cancer there is some evidence of genetic effects from study of rare coexistent conditions such as tylosis palmaris. Epidemiology studies have shown a familial clustering in approximately 10% of gastric cancers,

with 1–3% related to a hereditary gastric cancer precancer syndrome (hereditary diffuse gastric cancer). Gastric cancer is also one of the cancers in hereditary tumour syndromes. In addition certain genes have been implicated with a greater risk for oesophageal and gastric carcinogenesis from environmental factors, suggesting a link between host genetic make-up and established aetiological agents.

Oesophageal cancer

Evidence for an inherited type of oesophageal cancer is limited. However, the rare skin condition of tylosis palmarum and familial clustering for Barrett's cancer raise the possibility of an hereditary risk. The relationship of tylosis palmaris with SCC had been recognised from epidemiological studies. Investigation of a group of families in Liverpool including several generations has identified a specific tylosis oesophageal cancer gene.[38] Subsequent studies have detected this gene in 69% of cases of sporadic SCC. Recently more specific proteins coded by this gene have been reported to be related to poorly differentiated SCC and potentially predict for those with a poorer prognosis.[39]

There have been a number of reports of families with Barrett's metaplasia who have developed adenocarcinoma. In these families the frequency of Barrett's was more than 20% and the frequency of GORD was approximately 40%. In a case–control study, 24% of those with Barrett's, oesophageal or junctional ACA had a family history compared to 5% in the control group.[40] Multivariate analysis confirmed that family history was an independent risk factor with equal weighting to age, male gender, obesity and alcohol consumption. Further analysis of similar families is required to evaluate possible genetic linkages.

Gastric cancer

Hereditary diffuse gastric carcinoma (HDGC)

The first description of a germ-line mutation was in 1998 in three New Zealand Maori families. Mutations in the CDH1 tumour suppressor gene (the E-cadherin gene) has since been described in several families of different ethnic backgrounds. The CDH1 mutation occurs along the gene in these families as opposed to clustering in one site as observed in sporadic cases. In order to develop a common approach for HDGC, the International Gastric Cancer Linkage Consortium defined HDGC as including families with more than two pathologically proven diffuse gastric cancers in individuals under 50 and families with more than three close relatives with pathologically proven diffuse gastric cancer at any age.[41]

HDGC is an autosomal dominantly inherited syndrome. Carriers of the CDH1 mutation have in excess of 70% lifetime risk of developing diffuse gastric cancer. Female carriers have an additional risk of lobular breast cancer in about 40% of patients. Screening for CDH1 mutations in the research setting has shown its presence in 40% of families with multiple gastric cancers and at least one diffuse gastric cancer in a member under 50. The criteria for potential screening have been extended to include a number of other combinations of presentation (Box 2.1).

The proportion of HDGC families which have the CDH1 germ-line mutation, however, is only approximately 30%. In the remaining two-thirds either the detection methods to identify the mutation have been insensitive or there are other, as yet unidentified, HDGC susceptibility genes. A number of genes have been proposed, including those coding for other cell adhesion molecules such as β-catenin and γ-catenin and those involved in other hereditary cancer syndromes. Although some data support a role, this remains investigational.

The clinical issues raised for these families is their optimal management. In view of the 70% or more chance of developing diffuse gastric cancer with its attendant poor long-term survival, the options

Box 2.1 • Criteria for screening for CDH1 in HDGC

Three or more cases of gastric cancer at any age with at least one case of diffuse gastric cancer

Isolated individual with diagnosis of diffuse gastric cancer <40

Isolated individual with both diffuse gastric cancer and lobular breast cancer

One family member with diffuse gastric cancer and another with lobular breast cancer

One family member with diffuse gastric cancer and another with signet-ring colon cancer

are either prophylactic total gastrectomy or endoscopic surveillance. There have been a number of reports of the pathology of resected stomachs after prophylactic gastrectomy. In clinically, endoscopically 'normal' stomachs, supported by biopsy, diffuse multifocal intramucosal disease was identified in all specimens.[42,43] Some studies have shown concentration of disease in the distal third, whereas others have more widespread involvement.[44] The question arises, however, as to the appropriateness of total gastrectomy in essentially a young population for whom the nutritional sequelae will be lifelong. Furthermore the morbidity and mortality of such a procedure must be minimal. Therefore the role for endoscopy must be explored. Standard surveillance is limited but the distribution of disease from the pathology studies indicates where biopsies should be concentrated. Advances in endoscopy, which include endoscopic autofluorescence spectroscopy and chromoendoscopy, have the potential to enhance accuracy. A further point is that 20–30% of CDH1 germ-line mutations do not progress to clinically diffuse gastric cancer. There are some data to suggest intramucosal disease may not progress and be of biological rather than clinical importance analogous to prostatic cancer in elderly men. Thus counselling of individuals from HDGC families produces very difficult questions, particularly as knowledge is incomplete as to risk, most appropriate management and the role of genetic intervention, as well as the sequelae of life following total gastrectomy.

Hereditary cancer syndromes

The development of molecular genetics has allowed confirmation of primary genetic aetiology for a spectrum of cancers which epidemiology studies had suggested were inherited (Table 2.1). Gastric cancer has been found to be coexistent in these syndromes, further supporting a genetic basis for

Table 2.1 • Hereditary cancer syndromes

Syndrome	Main tumours	Associated tumours
Lynch syndrome (hereditary non-polyposis colorectal cancer)	Colon carcinoma	Endometrial, gastric, small bowel and urothelial cancer
Li–Fraumeni syndrome	Breast cancer, osteosarcoma, brain tumours, soft tissue sarcoma	Gastric and colon cancer, adrenocortical carcinoma, haematological and gynaecological
Familial adenomatous polyposis coli	Colon cancer	Gastric cancer, papillary thyroid cancer, desmoid tumours, medulloblastoma and hepatoblastoma
Peutz–Jeghers syndrome	Hamartomatous polyps of the small bowel, colon and stomach	Gastrointestinal carcinomas, breast, testicular and ovarian cancers
Juvenile polyposis	Hamartomatous polyps of the colon and occasionally stomach and small bowel	Gastrointestinal cancer

its development.[45] There are differences across the world, consistent with evidence that the gene pool varies within different populations. In patients with familial adenomatous polyposis (FAP) there is an excess of gastric cancer in Japanese families which is not observed in US non-oriental families. Similarly in the Lynch syndrome, gastric cancer is more common in China and Korea yet rare in Caucasians. Thus screening surveillance in such populations should be directed accordingly. Unless there is gastric cancer in the family then upper gastrointestinal endoscopy is not routinely required in those with the Lynch syndrome.

Moderate cancer risk

Worldwide studies have shown that approximately 5–10% of patients with gastric cancer have a family history but without other features to suggest an inherited aetiology. However, it is possible that in this population there is some hereditary predisposition to increased susceptibility to environmental factors such that their risk is increased. Studies have shown increased rates of *H. pylori* infection with atrophic gastritis and hypochlorhydria in first-degree relatives of gastric cancer patients compared with normal controls. This could of course be purely due to environmental factors. Alternatively normal variations in the genetic coding sequence of multiple genes (polymorphisms) which are inheritable may lead to differential inflammatory responses to agents such as *H. pylori* or tobacco. Thus the combined effect of inflammation promoting host genetic polymorphisms and different microbiological genotypes such as CagA *H. pylori* may increase the risk in a particular population. Specific studies including p53 have shown certain polymorphisms to be associated with the production of variant proteins.[46] These have been identified more frequently in patients with diffuse gastric cancer than in matched controls. DNA polymorphism in the interleukin-1 gene cluster has been associated with a response to *H. pylori* infection. It is postulated that the polymorphism increases the production of interleukin-1β, a proinflammatory cytokine, which inhibits gastric acid secretion and hence achlorhydria and gastric atrophy.

There is similar evidence for oesophageal adenocarcinoma. As previously described, GORD, diet, obesity and tobacco are all environmental aetiological factors for oesophageal ACA. However, although 12% of patients with GORD have Barrett's metaplasia, not all progress to cancer and Barrett's metaplasia can occur without a history of GORD. It is likely that there are host polymorphisms which interact with the environmental factors to promote progression to malignant transformation. The largest evidence supports a role for p53 and aneuploidy as markers of risk. These, however, remain investigational and await larger patient cohort studies to

ensure validity. As in gastric cancer the progression of change to cancer is non-linear, multifactorial and variable between populations.

Molecular genetics of oesophageal and gastric cancer

The development and progression of oesophageal and gastric cancer has been clearly demonstrated in numerous studies to have a genetic basis. Alterations in tumour suppressor genes and oncogenes have been identified in both cancers. Specifically genes which have roles in diverse functions such as cell adhesion, signal transduction, differentiation, development, gene transcription or DNA repair have been demonstrated in both oesophageal and gastric cancer. **Figure 2.3** shows some of the changes described in oesophageal cancer arising in Barrett's metaplasia, and **Fig. 2.4** shows the changes in gastric cancer and highlights different mechanisms for the intestinal and diffuse types. Studies of cDNA microarrays

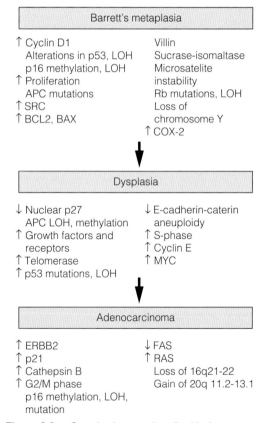

Figure 2.3 • Genetic changes described in the progression from Barrett's metaplasia to oesophageal adenocarcinoma. Reproduced from Lin J, Beer DG. Molecular biology of upper gastrointestinal malignancies. Semin Oncol 2004; 31:476–86. With permission from Elsevier.

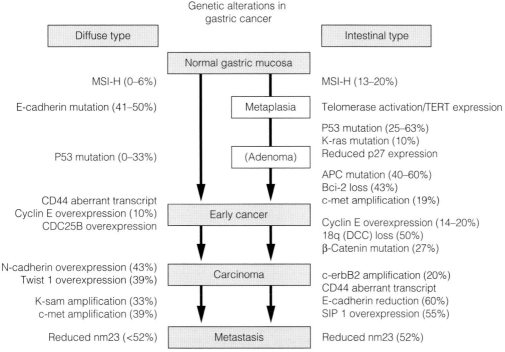

Figure 2.4 • Genetic alterations described in gastric cancer. Abbreviations: *APC*, adenomatous polyposis coli; Bcl-2, B-cell CLL/lymphoma 2; CD44, CD44 antigen; CDC25B, cell division cycle 25B; c-*erbB2*, v-*erb*-B2 erythroblastic leukaemia viral oncogene homologue 2; c-*met*, met proto-oncogene (hepatocyte growth factor receptor); *DCC*, deleted in colon cancer; K-*ras*, v-Ki-*ras* 2 Kirsten rat sarcoma viral oncogene homologue; K-*sam*, encodes fibroblast growth factor receptor 2; MSI-H, microsatellite instability – high; nm23, non-metastatic cells 1 (protein, NM23, expressed in); p53, tumour protein p53 (Li–Fraumeni syndrome); SIP-1, SMAD-interacting protein 1; TERT, telomerase reverse transcriptase; TWIST 1, twist homologue 1. Reproduced from Keller G, Hofler H, Becker K-F. Molecular medicine of gastric adenocarcinomas. Expert Rev Molec Med 2005; 7:1–13. With permission from Cambridge University Press.

for gastric cancer have reported characteristic patterns of gene expression in chronic gastritis, intestinal metaplasia, and intestinal and diffuse gastric cancer. These raise opportunities for identification of molecular markers and gene profiling in cancer progression and for the prediction of prognosis and treatment sensitivity.[45,47]

Screening for oesophageal and gastric cancer

Screening programmes for any disease are dependent on a number of criteria. Firstly, the disease must be common in the target population. Secondly, a reliable and accurate test that is as sensitive and specific as possible is required, and the test should be acceptable to the screened population. There should be an effective treatment for the screened abnormality with minimum morbidity and mortality. Finally, not only does the treatment need to show an improvement in results, but implementation of the screening programme should also result in an overall benefit for the screened population.

The worldwide differences in incidence of oesophageal and gastric cancer allow the implementation of screening programmes for asymptomatic populations only in those areas where the incidence is high. However, lessons from these programmes have increased knowledge of natural history and have allowed high-risk groups to be targeted in low-risk areas in order to detect disease at an earlier stage.

Asymptomatic screening

Oesophageal cancer

Evaluation of asymptomatic screening for carcinomas of the oesophagus has centred on those parts of China with the highest incidence. The screening test involves swallowing a small deflated balloon, which is then inflated at the lower end of the oesophagus. The balloon surface is covered with a fine mesh; on withdrawal from the oesophagus, this scrapes the mucosa to collect cells. A cytological smear is then made from the scrapings for microscopic examination. Those individuals found to have abnormalities are then subjected to endoscopy and appropriate biopsy. Radiology has very little place. In 132 subjects with early oesophageal cancer detected in this way, 26% had normal radiological appearances.[48]

The efficiency of this technique has had varying reports. Reviewing data based on 500 000 examinations, Shu[49] suggested an accuracy for the differentiation of benign from malignant of 90%. Mass surveys have shown that 73.8% of detected cancers were either in situ or minimally invasive. In a provincial review, Huang[50] reported on 17 000 examinations screened during a 1-year period. Abnormalities were found in 68% of the population, with low-grade dysplasia in 37%, high-grade in 26% and in situ cancer in 2%. A group with high-grade dysplasia were followed for up to 8 years. Regression to normal or low-grade change was observed in 40%, 20% remained as high grade, 20% fluctuated between high and low grade, and 20% developed cancer. In the absence of dysplasia, 0.12% developed cancer. Progression from dysplasia to in situ cancer occurred over 3–12 years and from in situ to invasive cancer over 3–7 years. Tumour risk was consistent, with a known distribution of middle-third chronic oesophagitis in 76%. It would seem that the duration of severe dysplasia is the greatest risk for malignant transformation. Follow-up by endoscopy is therefore important and in order to ensure biopsy of the same site vital stains have been used. Huang[51] reported that staining with toluidine blue was effective for identifying neoplastic epithelium; 84% of cancers were identified in positively staining areas.

The problem associated with this approach is the management of dysplasia. Oesophageal dysplasia is a dynamic process with both spontaneous regression and progression. Furthermore, even if in situ cancer develops, progress to advanced disease is often prolonged and may be associated with prolonged survival. In one series of 23 untreated patients, 11 developed late-stage disease at a mean of 55 months. In the remainder there was no change for over 6 years and the 5-year survival of the group was 78%.[52] Five-year survival needs to be considered with caution as detection of asymptomatic slowly progressive disease introduces lead-time bias and this can falsely give the impression that treatment results for screen-detected cases are better.

As a result an International Union Against Cancer (UICC) recommendation has been to limit oesophageal cancer screening to areas of high risk.[53] The aim is to identify the natural history of dysplasia more completely. Common standards are required for the classification of dysplasia to identify those changes with greatest risk. Once the assessment is more reliable, control studies should be developed to determine whether screening intervention could reduce mortality for oesophageal cancer.

In areas of low risk, asymptomatic screening is not justifiable. Endoscopic screening is, however, useful for those individuals who have coexisting conditions that are associated with a high risk for oesophageal or gastric cancer. Thus for tylosis, achalasia and corrosive stricture, regular endoscopies are recommended. This should start 10 years after diagnosis for achalasia and ingestion of the corrosive agent.

Gastric cancer

The prominence of gastric cancer as a public health problem in Japan led to the development during the 1960s of a mass screening programme for all men over the age of 40 years. The programme has been based on double-contrast radiology with endoscopy assessment of any abnormalities.[54] Members of the public are invited to undergo radiology in mobile units at which seven films are taken after the ingestion of an effervescent contrast agent. Screening is undertaken annually or biannually depending on the area of Japan and the associated risk of disease. Government recommendations set a target of 30% for the annual examination rate. Despite the recognition of gastric cancer as a public health problem, attendance for screening is low. In 1985 over 5 million were examined, representing 13% of the at-risk population. Therein lies one of the problems with any screening programme, namely the cooperation of the public.

Approximately half the cases diagnosed are limited to the mucosa or submucosa (early gastric cancer). Half of those detected are symptomatic and an alternative approach could be envisaged. In keeping with the criteria for a screening programme there has been a highly significant decrease in mortality. However, as already discussed, there may be other reasons for the decline in mortality.

Oshima et al.[55] compared screened and unscreened populations to determine whether screening was important over and above the other influences on the decrease in mortality. In a case-controlled study they found that the risk of dying from gastric cancer among screened cases was at least 50% less than that for non-screened cases. Other Japanese groups have reported similar results. However, the actual effect on mortality remains to be proven as none of the studies have been randomised or controlled. As a result the UICC recommended that studies should be continued in Japan to resolve the problem, but screening in this way should not be adopted as public health programmes in other parts of the world.[53] As with oesophageal cancer, screening an asymptomatic population in low-risk areas is not worthwhile, although there are groups for whom surveillance endoscopy should be considered (see below).

Symptomatic screening and early detection

Symptomatic presentation is an unreliable predictor of significant pathology as the cardinal upper gastrointestinal symptoms of reflux and dyspepsia are very common and can be associated with a wide range of conditions from normal to malignancy. However, since half of the early gastric cancers detected in Japan through screening had symptoms, a variety of approaches have been investigated in order to increase early detection and by implication improve outcome. These can be considered as either methods of selecting symptomatic patients for early investigation or the development of surveillance programmes for those with high-risk conditions.

Early diagnostic endoscopy

The rate of dyspepsia and reflux in the general population is too high to justify endoscopic assessment for all newly presenting patients. Studies have therefore evaluated methods of selecting those potentially at higher risk of having a significant diagnosis.

Symptom profiling has been evaluated based on symptomatic presentation of patients with oesophageal and gastric cancer. Dyspepsia has been classified as uncomplicated or complicated by alarm symptoms including weight loss, anorexia, vomiting, dysphagia and signs of anaemia or an abdominal mass. Further classification according to age has also been studied as early gastric cancer tends to present approximately 10 years younger than advanced disease.[56] Although such studies have increased rates of detection of early gastric cancer to approximately 15–20%, many patients with uncomplicated dyspepsia have undergone normal examinations. In a series of 25 patients under 55 years with gastric cancer, 24 had complicated dyspepsia.[57] Furthermore, in a population database of 3293 oesophageal and gastric cancers, 290 were under 50 and 21 (7%) had uncomplicated dyspepsia.[58] The simple conclusion of this evidence is to restrict endoscopy for those under 55 years to complicated dyspepsia. However, the alarm symptoms used to define complicated dyspepsia are those of established locally advanced disease with the expected poor prognosis. This has been confirmed in a large case series of open access endoscopy from Newcastle upon Tyne.[59] It could be argued that the low index of suspicion for the significance of simple dyspepsia in younger patients had led to a delay in investigation until they developed more significant or alarm symptoms. The failure to diagnose earlier cancers in younger patients may be a result of a failure to initiate investigations until the cancer is advanced and raising the age threshold to 55 for uncomplicated dyspeptics would decrease the rate of diagnosis of upper gastrointestinal cancer. Indeed, the effect of early intervention in unselected dyspepsia not only increases the rate of earlier diagnoses of cancer, but this is also translated into a survival advantage (**Fig. 2.5**).[60]

Much effort has been made to refine the indications for endoscopy based on symptoms and it may be that all that can be achieved has been by this approach. However, symptomatic presentation is the most practical route for selection for endoscopy and it is therefore essential that any service can assess patients in the most efficient manner. In the UK a pragmatic approach has been adopted.[61] Urgent specialist referral or endoscopic investigation (within 2 weeks) is indicated for people with dyspepsia of any age when presenting with chronic gastrointestinal bleeding, progressive unintentional weight loss, iron-deficiency anaemia, progressive dysphagia, persistent vomiting, epigastric

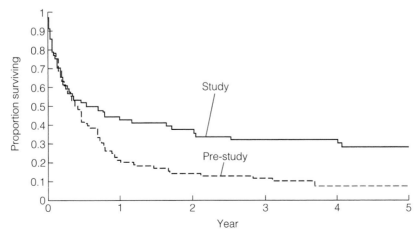

Figure 2.5 • Survival after early detection of gastric cancer (study population) compared with historical control population (pre-study population).

mass or suspicious barium meal. In addition to these alarm symptoms similar referral is required for a dyspeptic patient over 55 years with onset of symptoms within the last year and/or continuous symptoms since onset. The advantage of referral within 2 weeks is largely procedural and has only limited support from the literature. Gastric cancers limited to the mucosa and submucosa have a doubling time of 1.5–10 years, whereas advanced disease has a doubling time of between 2 months and 1 year.[62,63] Reducing symptomatic delay is unlikely to significantly alter outcome for early disease, but may render more advanced disease amenable to resection. In a comparative audit of 2-week referrals (TWRs) with conventional presentations, Radbourne et al.[64] have found that although the TWR produced more cancers, the stage of disease was equivalent at diagnosis and survival was comparable between the two groups.

High-risk groups

Helicobacter pylori

The role of *H. pylori* as a marker for endoscopy has received considerable attention. Both serological estimation and breath tests depending on exhalation of urea have been investigated. Serology has been assessed for concordance with the underlying histological presence of *H. pylori*. Farinati et al.[65] found 82% agreement between a measurable antibody response and histological evidence of *H. pylori* infection. Urea breath tests are in routine use in *Helicobacter* eradication programmes for duodenal ulceration. Again, the problem is one of specificity and sensitivity.

Helicobacter pylori seropositivity does not necessarily imply active infection. Equally seropositivity is a common finding and may not be specific for the at-risk population. It increases with age and to a certain extent parallels gastric atrophy, which is equally an age-related phenomenon and in the majority does not progress to cancer. There is also evidence that seroreversion may occur with seropositivity frequently seen in early gastric cancer and seronegativity in more advanced disease.[66] However, evidence of infection at an early age does identify a group at risk and therefore worthy of consideration for endoscopic follow-up. Whiting et al.[67] reported a retrospective analysis of *H. pylori* seropositivity in cancer patients compared with a group of undiagnosed dyspeptics. Although the cancer patients were significantly more likely to be seropositive, this was very much site related. In this study cardia cancers were not usually seropositive. Thus any screening programme based on *H. pylori* serology could miss the proximal tumours, which are currently the more common cancers. Further investigation is required and longitudinal studies may resolve the issue of whether patients with *H. pylori* seropositivity warrant close endoscopic follow-up.

Precancerous conditions

Pernicious anaemia imposes a three- to fourfold increased risk of gastric cancer compared with the normal population. However, screening of such individuals may be of limited value, as in one survey of gastric cancer only 1.3% had pernicious anaemia. Patients who have undergone gastric resection for benign disease have been considered to have a greater risk, possibly because of increased alkaline reflux. However, again this group provides only a small proportion of gastric cancers detected in a screening programme.

In parallel with the increased risk for patients with pernicious anaemia who have associated chronic atrophic gastritis, those found at endoscopic biopsy to have gastric atrophy and columnar-type gastric intestinal metaplasia may form a risk group. Whiting et al.[68] have followed a group of patients by annual endoscopy who were found to have chronic atrophic gastritis and intestinal metaplasia at diagnostic endoscopy for dyspepsia. This group was reported to have an 11% risk of developing gastric cancer and the authors suggest that such patients should be considered a high-risk group.

Summary and future

Our understanding of oesophageal and gastric cancer has undergone a radical change in the last 30 years. The traditional view that oesophageal cancer was commonly squamous cell and associated with heavy smoking and alcohol and, like gastric cancer, was a disease of deprived socio-economic populations has been overturned by the dramatic increase in tumours close to the oesophagogastric junction. The reason for this change remains to be fully explained. There are a number of indicators, but evidence is inconsistent and confusing. Developments in molecular biology with greater understanding of the genetics of oesophageal and gastric cancer look promising and have the potential to improve rates of detection of premalignant lesions so that earlier intervention can prevent malignant transformation occurring.

The poor end results of the past remain as potent influences on the philosophy towards treatment of gastro-oesophageal cancer. Greater appreciation of the curability of early disease by both medical and public education must become a priority.

Key points

- The incidence of adenocarcinoma of the oesophagogastric junction is increasing rapidly, while that of gastric cancer is decreasing in most Western countries.
- The incidence of oesophageal squamous cell cancer has decreased slightly in recent years in Western countries.
- Proximal gastric cancer is now more common than distal cancer in Western countries – in the USA, cancer of the cardia accounts for more than half of all cases of gastric cancer.
- The epidemiology of gastric cardia cancer may be flawed by the inconsistency in the definition of this cancer, as this has led to imprecise subsite reporting. The apparent rise in incidence of this cancer may have other explanations.
- The aetiology of squamous cancer of the oesophagus is linked to chronic oesophagitis and strongly influenced by diet, smoking and the ingestion of nitrosamines.
- The link between gastro-oesophageal reflux disease (GORD), Barrett's oesophagus and adenocarcinoma of the oesophagus is now proven. This poses a major health problem in Western and developed countries.
- The risk of adenocarcinoma of the oesophagus is eight times higher in men than women. The predisposing factors for adenocarcinoma include GORD and obesity.
- Adenocarcinoma of cardia of the stomach may have two aetiologies, one similar to non-cardia gastric cancer and the other similar to oesophageal ACA.
- The intestinal type of gastric cancer is strongly linked to environmental factors, in particular to diet (especially nitrate ingestion).
- The International Agency for Cancer Research has classified *Helicobacter pylori* as a group I carcinogen for gastric cancer.
- Genetic studies confirm that oesophageal and gastric cancer can be inherited either as the sole cancer or as part of hereditary cancer syndromes.
- Sporadic oesophageal and gastric cancer may be caused by interactions between genetic polymorphisms, increasing risks from environmental factors.
- Asymptomatic screening for oesophageal squamous cell cancer is only justified in high-risk populations and in those with conditions known to predispose to this cancer, such as achalasia.
- Asymptomatic screening for gastric cancer is only justified in high-risk populations. There is evidence that the mortality in the screened population is less than 50% of that in a matched unscreened population (though not from controlled studies).
- Screening of dyspeptic patients remains controversial, as the number of malignancies detected is small. This requires further research in countries that do not have asymptomatic screening programmes, so that an 'at-risk' population can be better defined.
- The role of *H. pylori* screening as a means to identify those at most risk of developing gastric cancer requires further research. At present it is not specific enough to be of clinical use.

References

1. Siewert JR, Stein HJ. Classification of adenocarci-noma of the oesophago-gastric junction. Br J Surg 1998; 85:1457–9.

2. Parkin DM. Global cancer statistics in the year 2000. Lancet Oncol 2001; 2:533–43.

3. Holmes RJ, Vaughan TL. Epidemiology and patho-genesis of oesophageal cancer. Semin Radiat Oncol 2006; 17:2–9.

4. Powell J, McConkey CC. The rising trend in oesophageal adenocarcinoma and gastric cardia. Eur J Cancer Prevent 1992; 1:265–9.

5. Powell J, McConkey CC, Gillison EW et al. Continuing rising trend in oesophageal adenocarci-noma. Int J Cancer 2002; 102:422–7.

6. Allum WH, Powell DJ, McConkey CC et al. Gastric cancer: a 25-year review. Br J Surg 1989; 76:535–40.

7. Chang-Claude JC, Wahrendorf J, Liang QS et al. An epidemiological study of precursor lesions of oesophageal cancer among young persons in a high risk population in Huixian, China. Cancer Res 1990; 50:2268–74.

8. Iran – IARC Study Group. Oesophageal cancer studies in the Caspian Littoral of Iran: results of population studies. A prodrome. J Natl Cancer Inst 1979; 59:1127–38.

9. Hu J, Nyren O, Wolk A et al. Risk factors for oesophageal cancer in northeast China. Int J Cancer 1994; 57:38–46.

10. Yang CS. Research on oesophageal cancer in China: a review. Cancer Res 1980; 40:2633–44.

11. Brucher BL, Stein HJ, Bartels H et al. Achalasia and oesophageal cancer: incidence, prevalence and prognosis. World J Surg 2001; 25:745–9.

12. Li JY, Ershaw AG, Chen ZJ et al. A case–control study of cancer of the oesophagus and gastric cardia in Linxian. Int J Cancer 1989; 43:755–61.

13. Cameron AJ. Epidemiology of columnar-lined oesophagus and adenocarcinoma. Gastroenterol Clin North Am 1997; 26:487–94.

14. Chow WH, Finkle WD, McLaughlin JK et al. The relation of gastro-oesophageal reflux disease and its treatment to adenocarcinomas of the oesophagus and gastric cardia. JAMA 1995; 274:474–7.

15. Lagergen J, Bergstrom R, Londgren A et al. Symptomatic gastro-oesophageal reflux as a risk factor for oesophageal adenocarcinoma. N Engl J Med 1999; 340:825–31.

16. Cheng KK, Sharp L, McKinney PA et al. A case–control study of oesophageal adenocarcinoma in women: a preventable disease. Br J Cancer 2000; 83:127–32.

17. Lindblad M, Rodriguez LA, Lagergen J. Body mass, tobacco and alcohol and risk of oesophageal, gastric cardia and gastric non-cardia adenocarcinoma among men and women in a nested case control study. Cancer Causes Control 2005; 16:285–94.

18. Reeves GK, Pirie K, Beral V et al. Cancer incidence and mortality in relation to body mass index in the Million Women Study; cohort stuffy. Br Med J 2007; 335:1134–9.

19. Vaughan TL, Kristal AR, Blount PL et al. Non steroidal anti-inflammatory drug use, body mass index and anthropometry in relation to genetic and flow cytometric abnormalities in Barrett's oesophagus. Cancer Epidemiol Biomark Prev 2002; 11:745–52.

20. Power DG, Ryan AM, Healy LA et al. Barrett's oesophagus: prevalence of central adiposity, metabolic syndrome and a pro-inflammatory state. Proceedings of Gastrointestinal Cancer Symposium, American Society for Clinical Oncology, 2008; 70.

21. Guanrei Y, Songliang Q, He H et al. Natural history of early oesophageal squamous carcinoma and early adenocarcinoma of the gastric cardia in the People's Republic of China. Endoscopy 1988; 20:95–8.

22. Hansen S, Vollset SE, Derakhshan MH et al. Two distinct aetiologies of cardia cancer; evidence from premorbid serological markers of gastric atrophy and Helicobacter pylori status. Gut 2007; 56:918–25.

23. Orsmby AH, Vaezi MF, Richter JE et al. Cytokeratin immunoreactivity patterns in the diagnosis of short-segment Barrett's oesophagus. Gastroenterology 2000; 119:683–90.

24. Siewert JR, Ott K. Are squamous and adenocarcinoma of the oesophagus the same disease? Semin Radiat Oncol 2006; 17:38–44.

25. Jansson C, Johansson AL, Nyren O et al. Socioeconomic factors and risk of oesophageal adenocarcinoma within the European Prospective Investigation into Cancer and Nutrition (EPIC). J Natl Cancer Inst 2006; 98:345–54.

26. Correa P. A human model of gastric carcinogenesis. Cancer Res 1988; 48:3554–60.

27. Correa P, Sasano N, Stemmerman N et al. Pathology of gastric carcinoma in Japanese populations: comparisons between Miyagi prefecture, Japan, and Hawaii. J Natl Cancer Inst 1973; 51:1449–59.

28. Hirayama T. Actions suggested by gastric cancer epidemiological studies in Japan. In: Reed PI, Hill MJ (eds) Gastric carcinogenesis. Amsterdam: Excerpta Medica, 1988; pp. 209–28.

29. International Agency for Research on Cancer Working Group on the Evaluation of Carcinogenic risks to Humans. Schistosomes, liver flukes and Helicobacter pylori. Luon: International Agency for Research on Cancer, 1994; pp. 177–240.

30. Uemara N, Okamoto S, Yamamoto S et al. Helicobacter pylori infection and the development of gastric cancer. N Engl J Med 2001; 345:784–9.

31. Tomb JF, White O, Kerlavage AR et al. The complete genome sequence of the gastric pathogen Helicobacter pylori. Nature 1997; 388:539–47.

32. Vicari JJ, Peek RM, Falk GW et al. The seroprevalence of cagA-positive Helicobacter pylori: strains in the spectrum of gastro-oesophageal reflux disease. Gastroenterology 1998; 115:50–7.

33. Ito Y, Azuma T, Ito S et al. Analysis and typing of the vacA gene from cagA-positive strains of Helicobacter pylori isolated in Japan. J Clin Microbiol 1997; 35:1710–14.

34. Sobala GM, Schorah CJ, Shires S. Gastric ascorbic acid concentration and acute Helicobacter pylori infection. Rev Esp Enf Digest 1990; 78(Suppl 1):63.

35. Fitzgerald RC Molecular basis of Barrett's oesophagus and oesophageal adenocarcinoma. Gut 2006; 55:1810–18.

36. Ristimaki A, Houkanen N, Jankala H et al. Expression of cyclo-oxygenase-2 in human gastric carcinoma. Cancer Res 1997; 57:1276–80.

37. Jankowski J, Barr H. Improving surveillance for Barrett's oesophagus: AspECT and BOSS trials provide an evidence base. Br Med J 2006; 332:1512.

38. von Brevern M, Hollstein MC, Risk JM et al. Loss of heterozygosity in sporadic oesophageal tumours in the tylosis oesophageal cancer gene region of chromosome 17q. Oncogene 1998; 17:2101–5.

39. Moodley R, Reddi A, Chetty R et al. Abnormalities of chromosome 17 in oesophageal cancer. J Clin Pathol 2007; 60:990–4.

40. Chak A, Lee T, Kinnard MF et al. Familial aggregation of Barrett's oesophagus, oesophageal adenocarcinoma, and oesophago-gastric junctional adenocarcinoma in Caucasian adults. Gut 2002; 51:323–8.

41. Lynch HT, Grady W, Suriano G et al. Gastric cancer: new genetic developments. J Surg Oncol Semin 2005; 90:114–33.

42. Huntsman DG, Carneiro F, Lewis FR et al. Early gastric cancer in young asymptomatic carriers of germline E cadherin mutation. N Engl J Med 2001; 344:1904–9.

43. Chun YS, Linder NM, Smyrk TC et al. Germline E-cadherin germ mutations. Is prophylactic total gastrectomy indicated. Cancer 2001; 92:181–7.

44. Charlton A, Blair V, Shaw D et al. Hereditary diffuse gastric cancer: predominance of multiple foci of signet ring cell carcinoma in distal stomach and transitional zone. Gut 2004; 53:814–20.

45. Keller G, Hofler H, Becker KF. Molecular mechanisms of gastric adenocarcinoma. Expert Rev Molec Med 2005; 7:1–13.

46. Hiyama T, Tanaka S, Kitadai Y et al. p53 codon 72 polymorphism in gastric cancer susceptibility in patients with *Helicobacter pylori* associated chronic gastritis. Int J Cancer 2002; 100:304–8.

47. Lin J, Beer DG. Molecular biology of upper gastrointestinal malignancies. Semin Oncol 2004; 31:476–86.

48. Wang G-Q. Endoscopic diagnosis of early oesophageal carcinoma. J R Soc Med 1981; 74:502–3.

49. Shu Y-J. Cytopathology of the oesophagus. Acta Cytol 1983; 27:7–16.

50. Huang G-J. Recognition and treatment of the early lesion. In: Delarae NC, Wilkins EW, Wong J (eds) Oesophageal cancer. International trends: general thoracic surgery, 4th edn. St Louis: Mosby, 1988; pp. 149–52.

51. Huang GJ. Early detection and surgical treatment of oesophageal carcinoma. Jpn J Surg 1981; 11:399–405.

52. Yanjun M, Li G, Xianzhil G et al. Detection and natural progression of early oesophageal carcinoma – preliminary communication. J R Soc Med 1981; 74:884–6.

53. Chamberlain J, Day NE, Hakama M et al. UICC workshop of the project on evaluation of screening programmes for gastrointestinal cancer. Int J Cancer 1986; 37:329–34.

54. Hisamichi S. Screening for gastric cancer. World J Surg 1989; 13:31–7.

55. Oshima A, Hirata N, Ubakata T et al. Evaluation of a mass screening programme for stomach cancer with a case–control study design. Int J Cancer 1986; 38:829–34.

56. Fielding JWL, Ellis DJ, Jones BG et al. Natural history of 'early' gastric cancer: results of a 10-year regional survey. Br Med J 1980; 281:965–7.

57. Christie J, Shepherd NA, Codling BW et al. Gastric cancer below the age of 55: implications for screening patients with uncomplicated dyspepsia. Gut 1997; 41:513–17.

58. Salmon CA, Park KGM, Rapson T et al. Age threshold for endoscopy and risk of missing upper GI malignancy: data from the Scottish Audit of Gastric and Oesophageal Cancer. Gut 2003; 52:A26.

59. Bowrey DJ, Griffin SM, Wayman J et al. Using alarm symptoms to select dyspeptics for endoscopy which result in patients with curable oesophago-gastric cancer being overlooked. Surg Endosc 2006; 20:1725–8.

60. Hallissey MT, Jewkes AJ, Allum WH et al. The impact of the dyspepsia study on deaths from gastric cancer. In: Nishi M, Sugano H, Takahashi T (eds) International gastric cancer congress, Bologna: Monduzzi Editore-International Proceedings Division, 1995; Vol. 1, p. 264.

61. NHS Executive. Referral guidelines for suspected cancer. London: HMSO, 2000.

62. Martin IG, Young S, Sue-Ling H et al. Delays in the diagnosis of oesophago-gastric cancer: a consecutive case series. Br Med J 1997; 314:467–71.

63. Kohli Y, Kawai K, Fujita S. Analytical studies on growth of human gastric cancer. J Clin Gastroenterol 1981; 3:129–33.

64 Radbourne D, Walker G, Joshi D et al. The 2 week standard for suspected upper GI cancers: its impact on staging. GUT 2008; 52:A116.

65. Farinati F, Valiante F, Germania B et al. Prevalence of *Helicobacter pylori* infection in patients with precancerous changes and gastric cancer. Eur J Cancer Prevent 1993; 2:321–6.

66. Kikuchi S. Epidemiology of *Helicobacter pylori* and gastric cancer. Gastric Cancer 2002; 5:6–15.

67. Whiting JL, Hallissey MT, Fielding JWL et al. Screening for gastric cancer by *Helicobacter pylori* serology: a retrospective study. Br J Surg 1998; 85:408–11.

68. Whiting JL, Sigurdsson A, Rowlands DC et al. The long term results of endoscopic surveillance of premalignant gastric lesions. Gut 2002; 50:378–81.

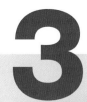

3

Staging of oesophageal and gastric cancer

Christopher Deans
Simon Paterson-Brown

Introduction

Accurate staging of patients with oesophageal and gastric cancer is essential in order to determine the most appropriate management option for each patient. This has become particularly important with the recent introduction of alternative potentially curative treatments for early tumours, such as endoscopic resection and photodynamic therapy, and the recognition that surgical resection is no longer considered the best form of palliation for the majority of patients with gastro-oesophageal cancer who cannot be cured by resection.[1,2] Furthermore, as new therapeutic and neoadjuvant regimens are designed and tested, accurate staging is an essential requirement, not only in terms of patient selection but also in assessing outcome.

This chapter will describe the main staging classifications currently in use for gastric and oesophageal cancer and will propose a staging algorithm for patients following histological confirmation of cancer. The various modalities available for preoperative staging will be discussed, along with their limitations. Techniques involved in surgical (intraoperative) staging will also be outlined and the important role of the multidisciplinary team will be highlighted. Finally, possible prognostic factors that might influence the future staging of gastro-oesophageal cancer will be discussed.

Principles of staging

The purpose of all cancer staging is to determine the extent of disease burden in the patient. Stage takes into account the primary tumour and aims to determine whether the tumour has spread to adjacent tissues and distant organs. Complete staging relies on a combination of clinical staging, surgical staging and ultimately final pathological staging with microscopic analysis of the resected specimen.

Clinical staging

Clinical staging depends on the anatomical extent of the tumour that can be determined before treatment. Assessment includes physical examination, endoscopic biopsies, laboratory studies and imaging. The location of the tumour, depth of invasion, and evidence of nodal and distant spread needs to be determined as fully as possible.

Surgical (intraoperative) staging

This is based on the macroscopic findings at surgical exploration and the assessment of tumour resectability.

Histopathological staging

This involves histological examination of the resected specimen with en bloc structures and other tissue biopsies. Extension of the tumour into adjacent structures and evidence of distant spread should be carefully documented.

Staging classifications

In 1986 a single TNM ('tumour–node–metastasis') staging classification was agreed between the American Joint Committee on Cancer (AJCC), the Japanese Joint Committee (JJC) and the International Union Against Cancer (UICC). This collaboration has resulted in a common staging language that aims to reduce confusion and facilitate the exchange of information between treatment centres. This classification system is now strongly recommended by the majority of centres in Europe and North America and it is this system that will be used throughout this chapter.[3]

This system was approved by the UICC and AJCC in 1985 and in Japan in 1986. Table 3.1 illustrates the 2003 update of the unified TNM staging system for gastric cancer. Use of this system is strongly recommended.

Internationally unified staging system (TNM)

The TNM system is based on an anatomical classification of disease involvement, where T represents the extent of the primary tumour, N the absence or presence and extent of regional lymph node metastases, and M the absence or presence of distant metastases. The addition of numbers to these groups indicates the progression of the disease (Table 3.2). Subdivisions of some of these categories enable increased specificity where required and allow tighter prognostic grouping. In all cases microscopic proof of malignancy is required before a final TNM stage can be assigned.

The TNM staging can be based on either clinical or pathological information. The clinical classification is designated with a 'c' prefix (cTNM) and represents the pretreatment stage of disease. This may be derived from physical examination, imaging and other relevant investigations. The pathological classification (pTNM) incorporates all the information from the clinical classification and the additional evidence provided from histopathological analysis. Other prefixes may be used to give additional information on the timing of the staging; an example in modern practice is the addition of 'y' for those patients who have undergone multimodal therapy, such as preoperative chemotherapy then surgery, as in ypTNM.

Once a TNM category has been decided, a stage grouping is assigned (Table 3.1). This simplifies the staging analysis, allowing easier comparison of outcomes. The groupings are chosen to ensure that each group is similar in terms of prognosis, while at the same time maintaining the differences between TNM categories.

Gastric cancer staging

The unified TNM system for gastric cancer

The current 6th edition of the 'TNM Classification of Malignant Tumours'[3] for gastric cancer is shown in Table 3.2. In terms of nodal assessment in gastric cancer, regional lymph nodes are defined as the

Table 3.1 • Internationally unified TNM stage groupings for gastric cancer

Stage grouping	T	N	M
Stage 0	Tis	N0	M0
Stage Ia	T1	N0	M0
Stage Ib	T1	N1	M0
	T2A or B	N0	M0
Stage II	T1	N2	M0
	T2A or B	N1	M0
	T3	N0	M0
Stage IIIa	T2A or B	N2	M0
	T3	N1	M0
	T4	N0	M0
Stage IIIb	T3	N2	M0
Stage IV	T4	N1, N2, N3	M0
	T1, T2, T3	N3	M0
	Any T	Any N	M1

Table 3.2 • Internationally unified TNM staging system for gastric cancer

T factor

Tx	Primary tumour cannot be assessed
T0	No evidence of primary tumour
Tis	Carcinoma in situ: intraepithelial tumour without invasion of the lamina propria
T1	Tumour invades lamina propria or submucosa
T2A	Tumour invades muscularis propria
T2B	Tumour invades the subserosa
T3	Tumour penetrates serosa (visceral peritoneum) without invasion of adjacent structures
T4	Tumour invades adjacent structures

N factor

Nx	Regional lymph nodes cannot be assessed
N0	No regional lymph node metastasis
N1	Metastasis in 1–6 regional lymph nodes
N2	Metastasis in 7–15 regional lymph nodes
N3	Metastasis in more than 15 regional lymph nodes

M factor

Mx	Distant metastasis cannot be assessed
M0	No distant metastasis
M1	Distant metastasis

perigastric nodes along the greater and lesser curvatures, the nodes along the left gastric, common hepatic, splenic and coeliac arteries, and the left hepatoduodenal nodes. Involvement of other intra-abdominal lymph nodes, such as the para-aortic and mesenteric nodes, are classified as distant metastases (M1).

A requirement for complete N staging of gastric cancer is that a minumum of 15 lymph nodes must be included for histological analysis. Although some studies suggest that as few as 10 nodes are sufficient to accurately assess pN stage,[4,5] a large series from Japan examining 926 patients with gastric cancer found that, stage for stage, patients with 20–30 examined nodes that were negative for metastatic disease had a better prognosis compared to those with 10–19 examined negative nodes.[6] Not surprisingly, these authors went on to recommend that at least 30 nodes must be examined for accurate N staging. However, many reports do not reach these numbers and only 31% of gastric resections in a recent UK-based study included 15 or more lymph nodes for histological analysis.[7] More recent studies, however, have examined the prognostic significance

of the ratio between metastatic and dissected lymph nodes (n ratio) in gastric cancer patients.[8,9] One such study, involving nearly 800 patients, identified the n ratio, but not the total number of lymph node metastases, as an independent prognostic indicator on multivariate analysis.[8] Therefore, in all cases of potentially curative gastrectomy, an attempt should be made to maximise the total number of lymph nodes removed at the time of resection and to record the ratio of metastatic versus the total number of harvested lymph nodes in order to optimise the staging accuracy (see also Chapter 7).

AJCC and WCC modifications of the TNM system

These two systems are modifications of Kennedy's original description of the TNM system.[10] The American Joint Committee on Cancer Staging Systems and the UICC staging systems were widely adopted in the USA and Europe.[11,12] The AJCC system has gained more popularity in the UK and is outlined in Table 3.3. In this system R is used to indicate whether there is evidence of residual cancer after the resection: R0 indicates complete resection, R1 microscopic evidence of residual cancer and R2 macroscopic residual cancer. This R factor should not be confused with the previous Japanese use of R for the level of nodal resection, which has now been changed to D to avoid confusion.

Oesophageal cancer staging

As with gastric cancer there are multiple staging systems currently in use. The Japanese PHNS system

Table 3.3 • Clinical staging of gastric cancer (AJCC)

T factor

T_1	Confined to the mucosa and submucosa
T_2	Involving the muscularis propria and the subserosa
T_3	Spread to involve the serosa
T_4	Spread to contiguous structures

N factor

N_0	No nodal metastases
N_1	Perigastric nodes within 3 cm of primary tumour
N_2	Nodes greater than 3 cm from tumour involved
N_3	Non-excised nodes involved

M factor

M_0	Absence of metastatic disease
M_1	Presence of metastatic disease

is again the most meticulous, but is not widely used outside Japan. Use of the TNM system is strongly recommended and is shown in Table 3.4.

The unified TNM system for oesophageal cancer

The TNM classification of oesophageal cancer is shown in Table 3.4. Oesophageal tumours are staged according to the anatomical site of the primary tumour within the oesophagus and then classified with respect to the primary tumour, nodal spread and distant metastases (TNM) as for gastric cancer (Table 3.4). The anatomical location of the tumour is based on a variation of the original description by the Japanese Society for Esophageal Diseases.[13]

Table 3.4 • Internationally unified TNM staging system for oesophageal cancer and stage groupings

T factor			
Tx	Primary tumour cannot be assessed		
T0	No evidence of primary tumour		
Tis	Carcinoma in situ		
T1	Tumour invades lamina propria or submucosa		
T2	Tumour invades muscularis propria		
T3	Tumour invades adventitia		
T4	Tumour invades adjacent structures		
N factor			
Nx	Regional lymph nodes cannot be assessed		
N0	No regional lymph node metastasis		
N1	Regional lymph node metastasis		
M factor			
Mx	Distant metastasis cannot be assessed		
M0	No distant metastasis		
M1	Distant metastasis		
For tumours of the lower thoracic oesophagus:			
M1a	Metastasis in coeliac lymph nodes		
M1b	Other distant metastasis		
For tumours of the upper thoracic oesophagus:			
M1a	Metastasis in cervical lymph nodes		
M1b	Other distant metastasis		
For tumours of the mid-thoracic oesophagus:			
M1a	Not applicable		
M1b	Non-regional lymph node or other distant metastasis		
Stage grouping: oesophageal cancer			
Stage 0	Tis	N0	M0
Stage I	T1	N0	M0
Stage IIA	T2, T3	N0	M0
Stage IIB	T1, T2	N1	M0
Stage III	T3	N1	M0
	T4	Any N	M0
Stage IV	Any T	Any N	M1
Stage IVA	Any T	Any N	M1a
Stage IVB	Any T	Any N	M1b

Anatomical description of the primary tumour

This system divides the oesophagus into four parts:

1. **Cervical oesophagus.** From the lower border of the cricoid cartilage to the thoracic inlet at the suprasternal notch, approximately 18 cm from the upper incisor teeth.
2. **Intrathoracic oesophagus.**
   (a) **Upper thoracic portion.** From the thoracic inlet to the level of the tracheal bifurcation, approximately 24 cm from the upper incisor teeth.
   (b) **Mid-thoracic portion.** The proximal half of the oesophagus between the tracheal bifurcation and the oesophagogastric junction. The lower level is approximately 32 cm from the upper incisor teeth.
   (c) **Lower thoracic portion.** The distal half of the oesophagus between the tracheal bifurcation and the oesophagogastric junction. The lower level is approximately 40 cm from the upper incisor teeth. This portion is approximately 8 cm in length and includes the abdominal oesophagus.

Regional lymph nodes (N stage)

The regional lymph nodes are defined according to the anatomical location of the primary tumour within the oesophagus:

- **Cervical oesophagus** – scalene, internal jugular, upper and lower cervical, paraoesophageal and supraclavicular.
- **Intrathoracic oesophagus** – internal jugular, tracheobronchial, superior mediastinal, paratracheal, perigastric (excluding coeliac), carinal, pulmonary hilar, perioesophageal, left gastric, paracardial, nodes of the lesser curve of the stomach and posterior mediastinal nodes.

Tumour involvement of any node outwith those described above are classified as metastatic disease (M1a). The TNM classification recommends that at least six lymph nodes are assessed as part of the histopathological staging of oesophageal tumours, although some authors have claimed a minimum of 18 lymph nodes are required for accurate staging.[14]

Distant metastases: M stage

This is subdivided into M0, where no distant metastases are detected, and M1, where there is evidence of distant metastases. Metastatic involvement may be further subclassified into M1a or M1b according to which structures are involved (Table 3.4). Again, definitions vary depending on the site of the primary tumour within the oesophagus. Distant metastases may occur at any site; however, the most commonly affected sites are the liver, lungs, pleura and, less frequently, the kidneys and brain. Tumour may also extend directly into mediastinal structures before distant spread is evident.

Oesophagogastric junctional (OGJ) tumours

These tumours are rapidly increasing in incidence and are defined as those that are centred within 5 cm proximal or distal of the anatomical cardia. They may arise in one of three ways:

- from metaplastic columnar epithelium in the lower oesophagus;
- from glandular epithelium of the cardia of the stomach;
- from the fundus of the stomach with proximal spread.

The International Society for Diseases of the Oesophagus has endorsed a classification of junctional tumours that is based on the likely origin of the tumour.[15] Type I represents adenocarcinoma of the distal oesophagus with the centre of the tumour lying 2–5 cm above the anatomical cardia. Type III cancer is a gastric carcinoma with its centre 2–5 cm below the anatomical cardia. Type II lesions are true junctional tumours with centres 2 cm above or below the anatomical cardia.

Adenocarcinomas arising in the region of the oesophagogastric junction pose a problem for staging, with the main difficulty lying in the identification of regional lymph nodes. Due to their anatomical location, these tumours may metastasise to lymph nodes above or below the diaphragm. Involvement of these nodes may therefore be classified as regional nodal involvement (N) or metastatic (M), both of which may have significant implications for management decisions and prognosis. At the present time, type I tumours are staged as oesophageal cancers and type III lesions are staged as gastric tumours, but debate still exists as to the best staging system for type II tumours, and some authors have proposed the need for a separate staging system in order to address these particular problems.[16,17] One pragmatic solution at the present time would be to follow the procedure performed, with gastric staging used for a total gastrectomy and oesophageal staging for an oesophagogastrectomy.

Chapter 3

Preoperative staging

 The decision-making algorithm demonstrated in **Fig. 3.1** takes the reader through the investigation pathway of a patient with histological confirmation of either oesophageal or gastric cancer for whom surgical intervention with curative intent is the primary objective. This is based on a review of the current data from multiple prospective and retrospective series comparing accuracy with final stage.

Clinical assessment

In the age of technological advances and novel investigations it is easy to forget the importance of a careful history, examination and simple investigations in the assessment of patients with cancer of the oesophagus and stomach. Clinical evidence of disseminated disease early in a patient's staging process will prevent further unnecessary, expensive, invasive and distressing investigations. In addition, identifying patients' symptoms and signs may help direct specific investigations for individual patients to aid the detection of metastatic disease – for example, back pain may represent vertebral metastases and suggest further investigation by bone scan. Palpable supraclavicular nodes may indicate disseminated disease and again, if metastatic tumour is confirmed on needle aspiration cytology, curative resection will not be possible.

 In June 2006 the Scottish Intercollegiate Guidelines Network (SIGN) published guidelines on the management and staging of patients with oesophageal and gastric cancer based on a review of the current evidence.[18] The staging process outlined in this chapter reflects these recommendations.

Contrast radiography

Endoscopy has largely replaced the use of contrast swallows/meals as the investigation of choice for investigation of suspected upper gastrointestinal malignancy. However, contrast studies may be of use in selected patients, for example in the investigation of a suspected oesophagotracheal fistula.

Endoscopy

Endoscopic fibreoptic examination of the upper gastrointestinal tract (with biopsies) is the most important investigation in the diagnosis of oesophageal and gastric carcinoma and should be performed on any patient in whom the disease is suspected. In addition to providing definitive diagnostic information, endoscopy also provides important staging and prognostic information. The position, size and morphology of the cancer may be assessed as well as, interestingly, depth of tumour invasion. A blinded study that prospectively staged 117 patients with gastric or oesophageal cancer found that the macroscopic appearance at endoscopy was more accurate than computed tomography (CT) for assessing T stage (67% vs. 33%) and comparable for assessing local nodal metastatic involvement (68% vs. 67%).[19] Surprisingly, endoscopic macroscopic appearance and endoscopic ultrasonography (EUS) also appear comparable as techniques for estimating depth of tumour invasion.[20]

It is routine practice in many surgical units for patients to undergo a repeat endoscopy by a member of the surgical team before surgical resection, not only to plan the proposed procedure, but also to confirm the exact position of the tumour, recheck its measurements and dimensions and to note the presence of any associated lesions, such as Barrett's change or satellite nodules.

Computed tomography (CT)

Following diagnostic endoscopy and histological confirmation of cancer, CT is often the initial staging investigation undertaken (Fig. 3.1). The main role of CT is in the detection of metastatic disease which, if present, precludes the patient from curative treatments and further staging investigations become unnecessary, allowing more appropriate resources to be directed towards palliation. The initial value of CT in the locoregional assessment of oesophageal and gastric tumours has been disappointing. Early studies utilised older generation scanners and the data comparing CT staging with other techniques, such as endoscopic ultrasonography and laparoscopic ultrasonography, were poor. The introduction and increased availability of new multislice spiral scanners has renewed interest in the role of CT in the local assessment of gastro-oesophageal tumours and more recent studies have suggested improved staging accuracy (see below). In addition, advances in computing software, coupled with better quality images, now allow three-dimensional reconstruction of the upper gastrointestinal tract to be performed, resulting in the development of novel techniques such as virtual endoscopy. These techniques may assist in operative planning in the future.

Oesophagus

Previous studies found poor correlation between the local assessment of oesophageal tumours on CT and findings at surgery and autopsy. More recent studies involving newer generation spiral CT machines have shown improved accuracy for locoregional

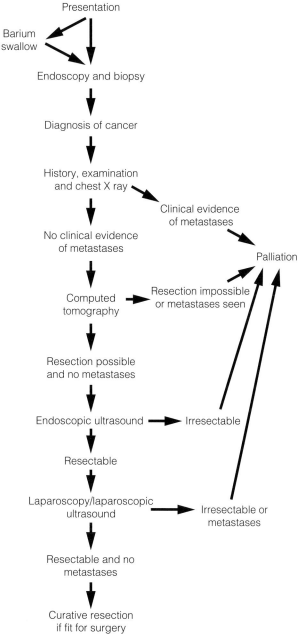

Figure 3.1 • Algorithm for the investigation of patients with oesophagogastric carcinoma.

(T and N stage) assessment of oesophageal tumours (**Fig. 3.2**). When compared with histopathological stage of resected specimens, T stage accuracies have been reported in the region of 43–92% for oesophageal cancer, and accuracies ranging between 27% and 86% have been published for N stage (sensitivity 48–68% with a specificity of 90–95%) (Table 3.5).[21–25] Increased accuracies have been

reported through the use of novel techniques such as virtual endoscopy.[22,23] Following detailed multidimensional scanning the computer software allows the radiologist to generate a three-dimensional reconstruction of the upper gastrointestinal tract from the endoluminal perspective. The radiologist is then able to perform a 'virtual endoscopy' with hopes of better local tumour assessment. Currently,

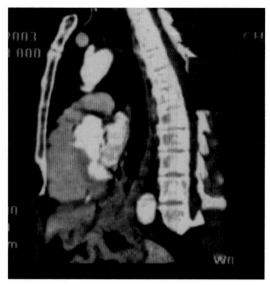

Figure 3.2 • Sagittal CT reconstruction of a distal oesophageal tumour. This example shows a T3 malignant stricture above the oesophagogastric junction.

difficulties in maintaining adequate oesophageal insufflation have limited the usefulness of this technique for assessing oesophageal T stage.

One of the main limitations of CT is correctly identifying malignant lymph nodes. It remains impossible to differentiate abnormally enlarged nodes that contain tumour from those that are enlarged as a result of benign reactive hyperplasia. The size of the lymph node that different authors regard as a criterion for malignant involvement varies from 5 to 15 mm.[26] Lymph nodes of more than 1 cm in diameter can, however, be seen within the mediastinum in healthy people,[27] and nodes of normal size may contain metastatic deposits. One study which retrospectively reviewed the histology of more than 23 000 lymph nodes from gastric cancer resections[28] demonstrated that the mean diameter of a metastatic node was 7.8 mm, and if 5 mm was used as a cut-off, 38% of metastatic nodes would still be missed. Improved image quality associated with modern scanners allows the identification of even smaller regional lymph nodes, but the pathological significance of these smaller lymph nodes remains unknown.

Malignant cervical or supraclavicular lymphadenopathy occurs in about 60% of patients with upper-third carcinomas. A recent study comparing ultrasonography with CT detection of supraclavicular nodes confirmed that ultrasonography is the more sensitive modality. It should be performed in addition to CT and combined with fine-needle aspiration of abnormal nodes greater than 5 mm in diameter along the short axis.[29]

The ability to accurately predict resectability is of key importance to the surgeon and CT continues to play an important role. One particular area of controversy is the loss of the perioesophageal fat plane. When present, invasion is highly unlikely but when absent, even in well-nourished patients, it cannot be taken as absolute evidence of invasion. This may account for the overestimation of tracheal, bronchial, aortic and cardiac invasion in many studies. Extraoesophageal tumour extension, in particular to the tracheobronchial tree, aorta and heart, can be determined using the following signs:

- the presence of an intraluminal bud;
- obvious displacement and deformation of the tracheobronchial tree, aorta or pericardium;
- increased thickness of the membranous trachea, bronchus, wall of the aorta or left atrium;
- growth extending beyond the posterior wall of the trachea at the level of the aortic arch.

Invasion of the aorta is more difficult to ascertain and although it occurs very infrequently, its presence is of great importance to the surgeon. It has been suggested that aortic invasion is considered indeterminate with contact of 45–90% between the aorta and tumour, and that invasion can only be predicted with accuracy if there is more than 90% contact; however, this is not universally accepted.[26,30] A recently introduced criterion for aortic invasion is based on the loss of the paravertebral fat space present in the triangle formed by the aorta, oesophagus and vertebral body.[30]

Table 3.5 • Reported accuracy of new generation spiral CT for T and N stages for oesophageal cancer compared with final histopathology

Authors	Number of patients	T stage accuracy (%)	N stage accuracy (%)
Kim et al.[21]	23	43	86
Panebianco et al.[22]	39	88	69
Onbas et al.[23]	44	92	83
Moorjani et al.[24]	50	–	62
Pfau et al.[25]	56	–	27

The true value of CT, however, is in the detection of distant metastases, and several studies have demonstrated the overall accuracy in detecting liver metastases to range between 86% and 98%.[31–33] Advances in technique and the evolution of newer CT scanners have brought the size of lesions easily seen to less than 1 cm. Pulmonary metastases are shown more frequently on CT than on simple chest radiography and small lesions are more readily identified. In the assessment of peritoneal disease, small-volume ascites is clearly identified and omental or mesenteric thickening may be detected; however, small-volume peritoneal disease may still go undetected. Therefore, even in the era of modern scanners, laparoscopy maintains a valuable role in the preoperative assessment of tumours below the diaphragm (see later section on staging laparoscopy).

Gastro-oesophageal junction

Owing to the variability of the normal anatomy at the gastro-oesophageal junction, the CT findings in patients with carcinoma of the gastro-oesophageal junction should be interpreted with caution.[31,32] A coexisting hiatus hernia may mimic or obscure both oesophageal and gastric invasion of the crura. However, diaphragmatic invasion in itself is unlikely to influence surgical resection as adjacent diaphragm can be excised en bloc with the tumour.

Stomach

Early hopes that conventional CT would provide accurate staging for gastric carcinoma were disappointing. The CT appearances of gastric carcinoma are variable and usually present with focal or diffuse wall thickening, frequently projecting into the lumen of the stomach with or without ulceration. Assessment of extension into adjacent organs is unreliable unless a large bulk of tumour is present within the involved structure. However, technical improvements with high-resolution dynamic two-phase CT with intravenous contrast and oral ingestion of water to distend the stomach and spasmolytics to inhibit peristalsis have certainly improved the diagnostic accuracy in assessing the primary tumour.[34,35] The overall accuracy of dynamic CT in determining the T stage is now in the region of 77–89% (Table 3.6).[33,36–39] The greatest accuracies have been reported, once again, by combining conventional high-definition CT with virtual endoscopy. This technique has proved more useful in the assessment of gastric malignancies than oesophageal tumours due to better success at maintaining adequate insufflation. Patients swallow bubble-making granules which produce a gas-filled stomach and this improves picture quality. In a study of 63 patients with gastric lesions noted at conventional gastroscopy, virtual endoscopy detected the same lesions with a sensitivity of 93% and a specificity of 91%.[40] This technique has also been associated with increased rates of detection of early gastric cancer by CT.[41]

The ability of CT to detect organ invasion by the primary tumour remains disappointing even with modern scanners. A study from Japan that assessed high-resolution CT and adjacent organ invasion showed that an absence of fat plane or an irregularity of the border between the tumour and the adjacent organ was not significantly related to invasion.[42] However, when the mean densities at the region of interest were measured they were found to be significantly greater at invasion sites than at non-invasion sites. Although this allowed invasion of the pancreas, liver and colon to be assessed with an accuracy of 75%, 61% and 78% respectively, these authors still found that CT had a limited value in differentiating inflammatory adhesions with fibrosis or oedema from true invasion.

Modest improvements in the detection of metastatic regional lymph nodes have also been reported with the use of newer scanners. Accuracies ranging between 63% and 80% have been reported for N staging by CT when compared with histological staging of the resected specimen (sensitivity 74%, specificity 65%).[34,36–40] Limitations to CT nodal staging relate to the detection of involved perigastric nodes close to the primary tumour. These lymph

Table 3.6 • Reported accuracy of new generation spiral CT for T and N stages for gastric cancer compared with final histopathology

Authors	Number of patients	T stage accuracy (%)	N stage accuracy (%)
Kim et al.[33]	106	84	64
Yang et al.[37]	44	88	80
Chen et al.[38]	55	89	78
Hur et al.[39]	84	77	67
Kim et al.[36]	63	84	63

nodes often appear confluent with the primary tumour and therefore CT will continue to struggle for accurate nodal staging for some gastric cancers.

As for oesophageal cancer, the main use of CT is in the detection of distant metastases and accuracy figures are similar to those seen for oesophageal malignancy. Despite the increasing accuracy of dynamic spiral CT, assessment of the primary tumour remains disappointing and currently cannot be used to plan surgery.

Further improvements in the accuracy of CT staging may be achieved through establishment of radiologists with a special interest. One report demonstrated improved levels of sensitivity and specificity among radiologists who regularly stage patients with gastric cancer,[43] with an associated reduction in the open and closed laparotomy rate. Such findings provide additional support for the formation of specialist multidisciplinary teams for the management of gastro-oesophageal cancer (see later in chapter).

Ultrasonography

The modern role of ultrasonography in the staging of oesophagogastric cancer is mainly complementary to CT and is largely in the assessment of metastatic disease, such as the further delineation of liver lesions. However, some authors have advocated the routine use of ultrasonography in the evaluation of cervical lymph nodes. It has been estimated that 10–28% of patients with upper/middle oesophageal tumours have metastatic involvement of neck lymph nodes.[44–46] Recent studies have compared the accuracies of CT and ultrasonography for the detection of malignant cervical lymph nodes that were otherwise not clinically palpable. The sensitivity of CT alone was 25–28%, ultrasonography alone 75–85% and CT/ultrasonography combined 80%, and the specificities were 99% for CT, 91% for ultrasonography and 91% for CT/ultrasonography combined.[47,48] In one study, CT failed to identify malignant cervical lymphadenopathy in 36 of 65 patients, whereas ultrasonography only missed 4 of 65 patients.[47] Unsurprisingly, these authors have promoted the use of neck ultrasonography in the routine staging of patients with oesophageal cancer in conjunction with CT. Conversely, another group failed to demonstrate any additional staging benefit to performing routine neck ultrasonography in patients with oesophageal cancer; however, in that study patients with stage T3/4 and/or N1 disease also underwent further staging by positron emission tomography (PET), which also detected cervical lymphadenopathy (see later in chapter).[49] Cytological analysis should be performed on all suspicious neck lymph nodes detected by ultrasonography to confirm metastatic disease.

Endoscopic ultrasonography (EUS)

If metastatic disease is excluded by CT (and ultrasonography if appropriate) the next staging investigation undertaken is often EUS. This is more accurate at staging depth of tumour invasion (T stage) and lymph node metastasis (N stage) than CT and, consequently, EUS has become an established tool for the local assessment of oesophageal and gastric carcinoma.[19,50,51]

EUS of the primary tumour

Using 7.5–12 MHz frequency, the wall of the oesophagus and stomach can be seen as five layers of alternating bright (hyperechoic) and dark (hypoechoic) bands (**Fig. 3.3**). From inside to out these layers correspond to: the wall of the balloon, the mucosa, the submucosa, the muscularis propria and finally the adventitia (oesophagus) or serosa (stomach). The presence of thickening through these layers as caused by a carcinoma can clearly be seen (**Fig. 3.4**).

EUS of lymph nodes

Unlike CT, which can only assess lymph node size, EUS provides additional information regarding shape, border demarcation, echo intensity and echo texture. As already stated lymph node size is an unreliable guide for determining metastatic involvement and other criteria are now used. In general it is thought that rounded, sharply demarcated, homogeneous, hypoechoic features indicate

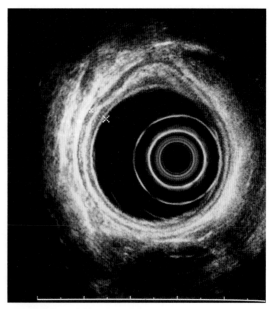

Figure 3.3 • EUS of oesophagus showing the five different layers. Note the small T1 tumour at 12 o'clock. With thanks to Dr John Plevris, Royal Infirmary, Edinburgh.

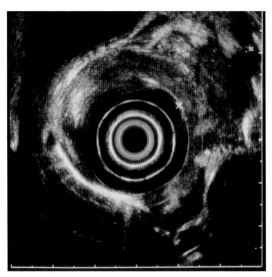

Figure 3.4 • EUS of oesophagus showing a T4 tumour with extension into the mediastinum and aortic fascia (seen at 4 o'clock). With thanks to Dr John Plevris, Royal Infirmary, Edinburgh.

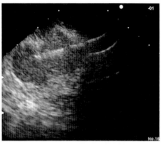

Figure 3.5 • EUS-guided fine-needle aspirate of a mediastinal lymph node in a patient with oesophageal malignancy. The 22G FNA needle is visible within the node. The subsequent cytology confirmed malignancy. With thanks to Dr Ian Penman, Western General Hospital, Edinburgh.

malignancy, whereas elongated, heterogeneous, hyperechoic lymph nodes with indistinct borders are more likely to be benign/inflammatory. However, these endosonographic features may not be evident in cases of micrometastases and evaluation of these features is subjective and may vary between different observers, possibly even between the same observer on different occasions. In a study of 100 patients with oesophageal carcinoma, one study found an overall sensitivity of 89% for the detection of malignant lymph nodes.[52] When EUS identified any lymph nodes the likelihood of N1 disease was 86%, whereas when lymph nodes were not seen the chance of N0 disease was 79%. When at least one of the predictive features of malignancy was present, specificity increased from 75% to 92%, and when all four features were present, metastases were found histologically in 100%. The features most sensitive for discriminating benign from malignant lymph nodes appear to be the central echo pattern followed, in order, by border, shape and size.

EUS can be also used to perform fine-needle aspiration (FNA) of mediastinal masses or lymph nodes (**Fig. 3.5**), although care should be taken not to traverse the primary tumour with the needle. In one study, the additional benefit of performing FNA cytology in addition to EUS alone on N stage accuracy and influence on treatment decisions was analysed.[53] These authors identified 3 out of 35 (9%) patients who were staged as N0 by EUS alone and who were later found to have metastatic lymph node involvement following FNA and cytological analysis.

Although tumour involvement of local lymph nodes is not in itself a contraindication to resection, it does allow the surgeon to discuss more accurately the risks and benefits of resection with the patient, particularly if the node in question is some distance from the primary tumour. Depending on local protocols, it may also help identify patients for neoadjuvant therapy.

EUS is also a valuable tool in the identification of coeliac lymph nodes, with one study demonstrating that it was possible to perform routine FNA cytology of the coeliac nodes in 95% of patients with oesophageal cancer.[54] The authors found positive cytology for metastatic disease in 79% of nodes that were greater than 5 mm in diameter. However, seven patients had subsequent histological proof of metastatic involvement of the coeliac nodes despite a negative FNA examination and the nodes being smaller than 5 mm. In the future the introduction of molecular techniques, such as polymerase chain reaction (PCR) and in situ hybridisation, could assist in the identification of malignant cytology that may be missed by conventional staining methods.

EUS-guided FNA has also been used to evaluate response to neoadjuvant treatment and to distinguish postoperative/postradiotherapy fibrosis from disease recurrence. However, the staging accuracy of EUS following preoperative chemo/radiotherapy is poor compared to that undertaken at the time of diagnosis due to difficulty in the ability to distinguish tumour from inflammatory change.[55] Similarly, EUS has proved disappointing in evaluating treatment response to neoadjuvant therapy. Although a reduction in the thickness of the primary tumour is associated with downstaging, the accuracy of identifying residual nodal disease is poor.[56] The addition of FNA may improve the diagnostic accuracy in future studies.

Performing FNA cytological analysis in conjunction with EUS is safe and is associated with improvements in local staging accuracy and may improve accuracies in detecting response to preoperative therapies and detecting disease recurrence.

EUS for metastatic disease

Although the main use of EUS is in the locoregional (T and N) assessment of tumours, ascitic fluid and lesions within the left lobe of the liver can also be detected.[57]

EUS staging of oesophageal carcinoma

The transducer is introduced into the stomach and then withdrawn at 1-cm intervals through the oesophagus. The clinician should determine the extent of maximal tumour penetration and the relationship of the tumour to surrounding structures. Lymph nodes should be classified as described above and the layers of the oesophagus examined (T and N staging).

The accuracy of EUS in staging oesophageal cancer is shown in Table 3.7.[58–61] The overall accuracy for T stage determined by EUS compared with pathological stage from resected specimens is in the region of 61–78%.[62–64] A recent systematic review of EUS accuracy in staging both oesophageal and gastric cancer concluded that EUS was highly effective at discriminating stages T1/2 from T3/4.[65] This has clear clinical relevance in assisting in the process of selecting patients for neoadjuvant therapies. Extension of tumour outside the wall of the oesophagus and possible extension into heart, aorta, vertebrae and pulmonary vessels can be readily assessed (**Fig. 3.6**), although invasion of the airways is more difficult due to the artefact produced by air.

EUS has reported accuracies between 65% and 75% for the assessment of nodal disease.[58–61] Further improvements in N staging accuracy can be achieved by performing FNA of suspicious lymph nodes identified at the time of EUS examination. Overall accuracies between 83% and 97% have been described for the identification of malignant lymph nodes following EUS with cytological analysis.[66,67] One study has reported even better accuracies by performing simultaneous trucut biopsy at the same time as FNA.[68] In that study, accuracy of positively identifying malignant lymph nodes was 76% by FNA alone, 76% by trucut biopsy alone and increased to 95% following combination of FNA and trucut biopsy.

The main problem with EUS is failure to pass through the stricture, leading to an incomplete assessment of the tumour, which in the series from Bristol occurred in 1 in 5 patients.[69] However, this same group went on to demonstrate that adequate information can still be provided by these incomplete examinations in relation to surgical decision-making.[70] This problem can be circumvented by using the non-viewing smaller probe, which is passed over a guidewire under gastroscopic and/or fluoroscopic vision. Accuracies of 90% for T stage and 78% for N stage have been reported with this method.[71] Another alternative is to pass the smaller catheter miniature echo probe, and several small trials have shown that this has a similar sensitivity and specificity for staging oesophageal cancer to standard EUS examination.[72]

EUS staging of gastric carcinoma

Although the results of EUS in assessing T stage of gastric tumours is not quite as good as for the oesophagus due to the distensibility of the stomach, accuracies of 83% in T1, 61% in T2, 87% in T3 and 76% in T4 have been reported in one large series of 403 patients, with an overall accuracy of 81%.[73] These results confirm those of previous studies (Table 3.8).[59,60,74,75] In the light of recent developments in endoscopic treatment for early gastric cancer, accurate staging is essential and figures from several studies suggest that EUS has an overall accuracy for staging early gastric cancer of around 77%.[73,76]

In using EUS it is important to recognise the problems in interpretation of any findings in the presence

Table 3.7 • Accuracy of EUS in oesophageal carcinoma (T + N stage) (%)

| | Reference | | | |
Histology	Catalano et al.[58]	Rosch et al.[59]	Grimm et al.[60]	Dittler and Siewert[61]
T1	33	50	90	81
T2	75	78	86	77
T3	82	91	93	89
T4	89	80	83	88
N0	94	42	85	70
N1	89	89	88	74

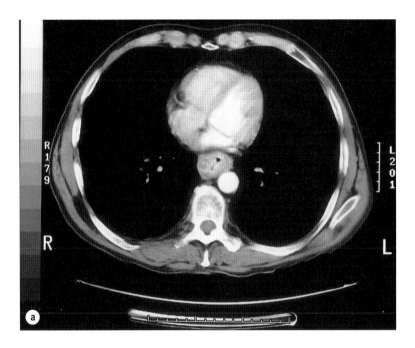

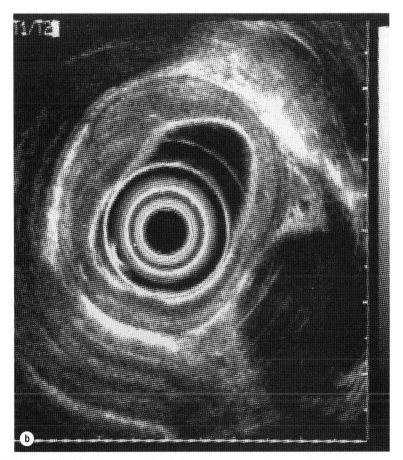

Figure 3.6 • CT **(a)** and EUS **(b)** of the same patient with a T3 N1 tumour in the mid-oesophagus.

Table 3.8 • Accuracy of EUS in gastric carcinoma (T + N stage) (%)

	Reference			
Histology	Rosch et al.[59]	Grimm et al.[60]	Dittler and Siewert[74]	Ziegler et al.[75]
T1	71	90	81	91
T2	64	79	71	81
T3	83	62	87	86
T4	64	89	79	89
N0	75	85	93	88
N1	86	50	65	64

of peptic ulceration due to distortion of the normal layers of the stomach wall.[77] Furthermore, fibrous proliferation in reaction to benign peptic ulcer disease is often indistinguishable from the fibrotic reaction induced by malignant invasion.[78] The ultrasonographic appearances of oedema around a tumour are similar to those of the tumour itself and can lead to overstaging, whereas microinfiltration of tumour cannot be visualised with EUS, resulting in understaging. Reports of the detection of malignant lymph nodes in gastric cancer vary from 55% to 87%, with accuracy highest for the perigastric nodes of the lesser curve.[74,79] EUS assessment of nodes in other locations is significantly less accurate.

Future developments in probe design and technology, including the introduction of three-dimensional EUS which provides a 3-D computer-generated reconstruction of the region under examination, are emerging and may provide improvements in staging accuracy and allow better operative planning.[80] Increasing experience and expertise in the use of EUS, along with adopting a policy of performing FNA on suspicious lymph nodes, should ensure that EUS continues to be the most accurate modality for the local assessment of upper gastrointestinal cancers.

Laparoscopy

Despite improved resolution with new multislice scanners, the detection of low-volume peritoneal disease by CT remains disappointing. Previously, sensitivities for the detection of peritoneal disease by CT alone have been in the region of 58% for oesophageal cancer and 33% for gastric cancer.[81] It is in the detection of peritoneal metastatic disease that staging laparoscopy is of particular value, but assessment of serosal involvement may also be determined as well as assessment of invasion of adjacent tissues and detection of low-volume ascites (**Fig. 3.7**). Several studies, old and current, have consistently shown laparoscopy to be significantly more sensitive at demonstrating these modes of metastasis than either CT or percutaneous ultrasonography for lower oesophageal and gastric cancer.[32] In one

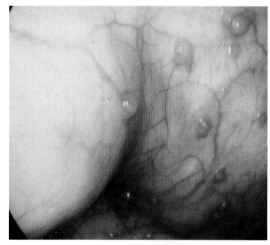

Figure 3.7 • Laparoscopic view of peritoneal tumour deposits identified at staging laparoscopy in a patient with gastric cancer. These nodules were not detected on CT.

study of more than 500 patients with oesophageal cancer, staging by laparoscopy changed management decisions for 20% of patients and the sensitivity of laparoscopy for determining resectability was 88%.[82] Several studies have shown that, as a result of preoperative assessment by laparoscopy, 10–20% of patients avoid unnecessary surgery.[83–85] Unsurprisingly, a recent systematic review has recommended the use of laparoscopy for the staging of patients with oesophagogastric cancer.[86]

Laparoscopic ultrasonography (lapUS)

This technique was introduced as an adjunct to staging laparoscopy. In addition to providing visual information regarding overt peritoneal, serosal and liver metastases obtained by conventional laparoscopy, lapUS also demonstrates tumour depth (**Fig. 3.8**), associated lymphadenopathy (**Fig. 3.9**), small metastases deep within the liver parenchyma (**Fig. 3.10**) and assessment of invasion of adjacent organs (**Fig. 3.11**). Early reports suggested that lapUS

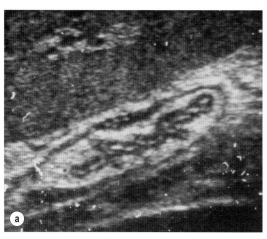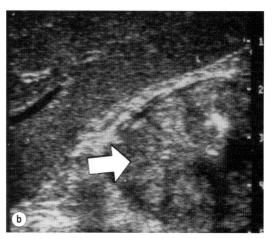

Figure 3.8 • Laparoscopic ultrasound examination of the lower (intra-abdominal) oesophagus in a normal patient **(a)** and a patient with a T3 carcinoma of the lower oesophagus extending across the oesophagogastric junction **(b)**.

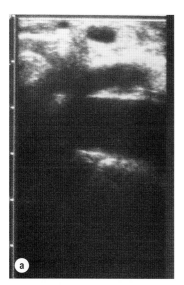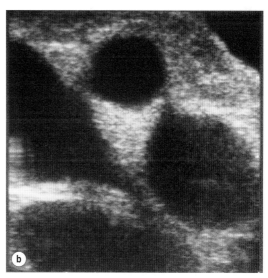

Figure 3.9 • Laparoscopic ultrasound examination of the coeliac axis in two patients with lower oesophageal carcinoma showing an enlarged left gastric lymph node in one patient (N1 disease) **(a)** and malignant lymphadenopathy around the coeliac axis in the other (M1 disease) **(b)**.

was more accurate at staging gastric and oesophageal cancer than CT or laparoscopy alone, with accuracies quoted between 80% and 90%.[87,88] However, recent improvements in the quality of CT imaging have resulted in the increased detection of smaller liver lesions and enlarged lymph nodes. As such the additional benefit of performing lapUS over and above conventional laparoscopy is now less clear.

Peritoneal cytology

The increased application of laparoscopy in the routine staging of gastric and lower oesophageal cancers

has allowed easy access to the abdominal cavity for cytological assessment of tumour spread. The presence of malignant ascites would represent metastatic disease and assign a patient irresectable. However, the significance of free intraperitoneal cancer cells in the absence of ascites was less clear and has undergone extensive research. Cancer cells within peritoneal washings without macroscopic evidence of disease have been identified in 8–42% of patients with gastric cancer (**Fig. 3.12**).[89–91] Positive cytology has been identified as an independent adverse prognostic indicator for gastric cancer and its presence results in a stage-matched reduction in survival.[91–93]

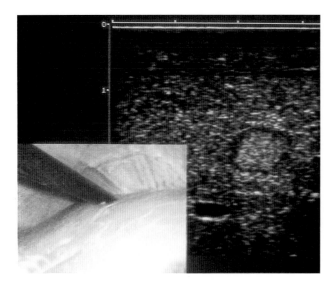

Figure 3.10 • Laparoscopic ultrasonography of a patient with gastric carcinoma showing a 6-mm liver metastasis deep within the right lobe of the liver.

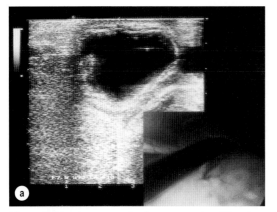

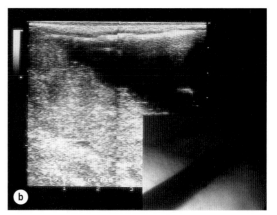

Figure 3.11 • Laparoscopic ultrasonography of the stomach showing a small T2 carcinoma **(a)** and an extensive T4 tumour with invasion of the pancreas **(b)**. Note the disrupted plane between the posterior surface of the tumour and the anterior surface of the pancreas.

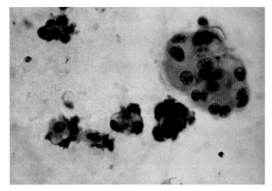

Figure 3.12 • Malignant cells identified in peritoneal washings taken from a patient with gastric cancer.

In one study, the median survival for patients with positive peritoneal washings was 11 months compared with more than 72 months for stage-matched controls, and all patients who had positive cytology subsequently developed peritoneal recurrence.[94] Newer techniques for the analysis of peritoneal fluid include measurement of carcinoembryonic antigen (CEA) concentration and determination of CEA mRNA expression by PCR.[95] The authors here noted that these techniques increased the sensitivity of positive identification of cancer cells in their series from 31% to 77% above cytological analysis alone. An elevated peritoneal fluid CEA mRNA concentration has also been associated with reduced survival duration among patients with gastric cancer who underwent 'curative' R0 resection.[96]

The routine cytological analysis of peritoneal washings (or ascitic fluid) during laparoscopy provides valuable additional information for the staging accuracy of patients with gastric and oesophageal cancer and may help identify those patients likely to develop peritoneal recurrence.

Positron emission tomography (PET)

PET differs from other imaging techniques such as CT and magnetic resonance imaging (MRI) in that it measures biological/physiological function rather than the anatomical detail of tissues.[97] The technique is based on the detection of radioactivity emitted after an intravenous injection of a radioactive tracer. The tracer is typically labelled with fluorine-18 or carbon-11 and the total radioactive dose is similar to that used in CT. PET therefore offers quantitative analysis, allowing relative changes over time to be monitored, for example in response to therapy. Whole-body scans may be performed to stage a cancer within 10–40 minutes and can be undertaken with the patient fully clothed. A common method used in cancer staging is to measure the rate of consumption of a radiolabelled glucose analogue, 18-fluorodeoxyglucose (FDG). This is based on the premise that malignant tumours consume glucose at a faster rate than benign tissues and this differential rate is detected by the scanner (**Fig. 3.13**).[98] Modern scanners allow images generated by PET to be fused with CT images (CT-PET) to enable better anatomical localisation of areas of increased uptake and improve spatial resolution (**Fig. 3.14**). One of the potential advantages of PET is in overcoming the difficulties in interpreting the significance of non-specifically enlarged lymph nodes encountered by CT. This is particularly true of new generation CT scanners where better resolution results in the identification of more 'indeterminate' lesions. PET also has the advantage of detecting metastatic involvement

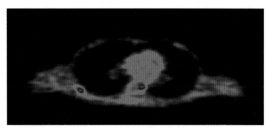

Figure 3.13 • PET scan of a patient illustrating adenocarcinoma of the distal oesophagus with adjacent lymphadenopathy and right rib metastases (red 'hot spots').

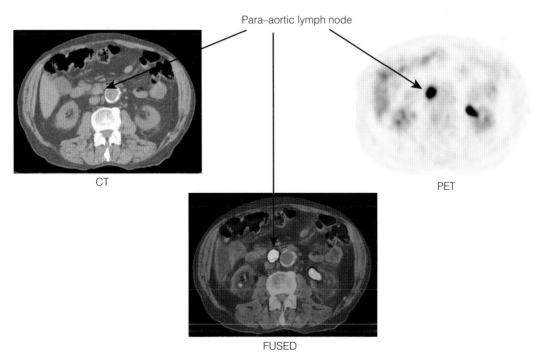

Para–aortic lymph node

CT

PET

FUSED

Figure 3.14 • This para-aortic lymph node with metastatic involvement was initially overlooked on the CT scan but subsequently identified on PET scanning. The two images may be superimposed to help in the anatomical localisation of disease. With thanks to Daren Francis, University College Hospital, London.

in lymph nodes that are not pathologically enlarged. In most instances, metastatic involvement at sites of increased tracer uptake identified by PET should be confirmed histologically.

The role of PET in the preoperative staging of patients with oesophagogastric cancer and its role in assessing response to neoadjuvant therapies has been extensively investigated. Several studies have investigated the accuracy of PET in the initial staging of gastro-oesophageal cancer and although some suggested it was useful in the identification of the primary tumour, it is poor for the accurate assessment of T stage.[99,100] PET has also been used in the locoregional assessment of lymph node metastases, with variable results.[101] Overall accuracy rates for nodal assessment range between 48% and 90% (sensitivity 43–78% and specificity 86–100%) depending on the criteria used for the detection of metastatic lymph nodes.[101–103] The relatively disappointing diagnostic accuracy of PET in the assessment of regional lymph nodes is probably due to the fact that lymph node metastases in oesophageal cancer are frequently located close to the primary tumour. The limited spatial resolution of PET (in the region of 5–8 mm for modern machines) makes interpretation of increased uptake due to regional lymph nodes or the primary tumour difficult to decipher.

The main staging role of PET is in the detection of distant nodal and metastatic disease. A recent review of CT-PET found an overall sensitivity of 67% and specificity of 97% for the identification of distant metastases in oesophageal cancer.[101] In several studies PET has demonstrated significantly better specificity than CT, even when combined with endoscopic ultrasonography, for the identification of both nodal and distant metastasis.[103–105] The accuracy of PET in the identification of metastatic disease was 82% in a prospective study of patients with oesophageal cancer compared with an accuracy of 64% for CT and EUS combined.[104] Several recent studies have consistently shown that PET leads to a change in UICC stage in up to 20% of patients who were staged by CT and EUS alone.[106,107] However, a meta-analysis of several small studies concluded that PET offered little improvement in the overall staging accuracy for oesophageal cancer.[108] A more recent study of 199 patients with oesophageal cancer investigated the value of CT-PET in addition to optimum staging by CT and EUS.[109] In this study, hot spots were identified by PET in 30 of 199 patients. In eight patients, these hot spots were subsequently confirmed as metastases and non-curative surgery was avoided. However, in seven patients the areas of increased uptake were due to benign lesions, such as colonic polyps, and in the remaining 15 patients the findings were due to false positives. As a result,

these patients underwent additional unnecessary investigations with delay in the initiation of treatment. At the present time, and as a consequence of these few studies, current guidelines do not recommend the routine use of CT-PET in the initial staging of patients with upper gastrointestinal cancer.[18] However, CT-PET does have an important role in the further assessment of 'indeterminate' lesions identified by CT where the positive identification of metastatic disease would significantly alter management decisions.

Another potential role of PET is in the assessment of response to preoperative chemo/radiotherapy. Conventional imaging modalities cannot easily distinguish viable tumour from necrotic or fibrotic tissue following neoadjuvant treatment, whereas PET can measure changes in metabolic activity within the tissues and this may identify residual disease. This has been supported in a recent systematic review of the accuracy of different staging modalities in assessing tumour response to preoperative therapy.[110] PET was significantly better than CT at predicting tumour response and, in addition, the response detected by PET was also seen to correlate with long-term survival. Residual tracer uptake after completion of preoperative treatment appears to be a marker for viable residual tumour and poor prognosis. In the future, PET may be used to identify patients who are not responding to neoadjuvant therapy early in the treatment process to avoid further potentially toxic treatment without overall benefit or may lead to a change in the chemotherapy agents used.[101] Attempts using PET to prospectively predict which patients are likely to be responders to preoperative therapy have been disappointing.[111]

Although not routinely indicated in the staging of oesophageal and gastric cancer, selected use of CT-PET is valuable in the further assessment of 'indeterminate' lesions identified by other staging modalities where the positive identification of metastatic disease would significantly alter management decisions. PET may also have a potential role in assessing response to neoadjuvant therapies.

A recent meta-analysis of staging modalities for oesophageal cancer concluded, for the detection of regional lymph node metastases, that EUS was superior in terms of sensitivity and specificity when compared with CT and PET. For the identification of distant metastases PET was the best single modality; however, the authors advocated a combined approach involving both PET and CT for the optimum assessment of distant disease.[112]

Magnetic resonance imaging (MRI)

MRI is an alternative to CT and many studies have compared the accuracies of the two techniques.[111,113,114] Overall accuracies for the locoregional assessment of gastric and oesophageal tumours are comparable to those for CT and pooled accuracy values are of the order of 78% for T stage and 59% for N stage. However, when compared with EUS, MRI was significantly worse at assessing accuracy of T stage (60% vs. 84%) for oesophageal cancer.[114] MRI fares better in the local assessment of gastric tumours. A recent systematic review comparing local staging accuracy of MRI, EUS and spiral CT for stomach cancer found overall T stage accuracies for EUS of 65–92%, for CT of 77–89% and for MRI of 71–83%.[115] One study reported MRI to be superior to EUS in the assessment of gastric wall infiltration (accuracy 53% vs. 35%).[116] Of recent interest, a novel lymphotrophic contrast agent (ferumoxtran-10) has been trialled during MRI staging. This contrast agent is accumulated within lymphatic tissue with hopes of improving accuracy rates in the assessment of nodal disease. A recent study reported a sensitivity of 100%, specificity of 93% and an accuracy rate of 95% for the preoperative identification of regional lymph node metastases among patients with gastric cancer using this technique.[117] Another new development in MRI staging of oesophagogastric cancer is endoscopic MRI. This technique involves an endoscope with a radiofrequency receiver coil incorporated into its tip. Accuracies of T and N staging of gastric and oesophageal cancers by this technique are similar to EUS.[118] However, as with conventional MRI, movement artefact remains a problem and in the above series up to 38% of the examinations had to be repeated due to inadequate views. At present this technique is limited to research.

As with modern CT, the real value of MRI is the detection of distant metastatic disease and to assist in the prediction of resectability. The accuracy of CT and MRI in the detection of mediastinal invasion, for example tracheal or bronchial invasion, is similar between CT and MRI and is in the region of 90%.[31,113] However, there are drawbacks to the use of MRI that, when combined with its more limited availability and higher cost, make CT the preferred investigation for staging of both oesophageal and gastric tumours at the present time. MRI is limited in its ability to examine more than one organ system or one area of the body during a single examination. It is not as good as CT for evaluation of pulmonary metastases, and a high-quality study of the entire mediastinum and the upper abdomen in one sitting is difficult to obtain due to movement artefacts. Currently, MRI is reserved as a complementary staging modality, and is most often used when additional information is required on particular abnormalities identified by CT, for example liver lesions or adrenal gland abnormalities.

Bronchoscopy

Rigid bronchoscopy used to be considered essential for all patients with upper- and middle-third oesophageal carcinomas to assess invasion of the tracheobronchial tree. With the improvements in other staging modalities already discussed, this is no longer necessary. However, if EUS or CT demonstrates a bulky tumour in the upper/middle third of the oesophagus that extends outside the adventitial layer and a good view of the interface between tumour and airway cannot be seen, then flexible bronchoscopy, perhaps with ultrasonography (see below), is indicated.

Endobronchial ultrasonography (EBUS)

EBUS is a technique that enables ultrasound examination of the endobronchial tree using a modified bronchoscope, similar in principle to EUS examination of the upper gastrointestinal tract. Several studies have reported improved accuracy rates compared with CT assessment in cases where endobronchial invasion by the tumour is suspected. Accuracy rates in the region of 90–95% have been reported for EBUS (sensitivity values around 90%, specificity 80–100%), whereas the reported accuracy of CT in distinguishing endobronchial invasion from compression by the tumour is much lower, at around 50–60%.[119–121] EBUS may also be used to examine carinal and mediastinal lymph nodes and EBUS-directed FNA can also be performed on any suspicious nodes noted at the time of examination.

Thoracoscopy

As indicated previously, lymph node size is a poor indicator of metastatic involvement and this has limited the accuracy of CT in detecting mediastinal disease in oesophageal cancer. This is particularly true of patients who may have lymphadenopathy due to concomitant lung disease or smoking. The main uses of video-assisted thoracoscopy (VATS) are in the assessment of local tumour invasion (T4 disease), lymph node sampling for histological analysis, and in identifying metastatic disease within the chest cavity. Most of the studies relating to thoracoscopy in the staging of oesophageal cancer have come from North America and have shown the accuracy of VATS at around 94% for N staging (sensitivity 63% and specificity 100%).[122,123] In one study, thoracoscopy detected mediastinal lymph node metastases in an additional 5% of patients that had not been detected by CT and EUS staging.[124] There is little doubt that thoracoscopy has an important role in the assessment of thoracic disease in those patients with locally advanced but still potentially resectable disease in whom other staging investigations have been inconclusive.

Other investigations

Further investigations in patients with oesophageal and gastric cancer should be carried out if there are any other suggestions of potential metastatic disease, following clinical assessment and the results of other investigations. These might include isotope bone scanning, CT of the brain and echocardiography to assess the possibility of pericardial invasion in bulky middle and lower oesophageal tumours.

The multidisciplinary team (MDT)

The results of each staging investigation should be discussed at regular multidisciplinary team meetings where a consensus opinion on the overall clinical stage of individual patients can be agreed. Involvement of MDTs that include surgeons, interventional endoscopists, radiologists, radiation oncologists, pathologists and palliative care physicians greatly enhance this process of patient assessment and allow the most appropriate management to be provided for each patient. The improved accuracy of CT staging with the involvement of specialist radiologists within the MDT setting has already been discussed.[43] Furthermore, it has now been shown that involvement of the MDT improves overall clinical staging accuracy and is associated with improved outcomes after surgery for gastro-oesophageal cancer.[64,125]

Re-staging following neoadjuvant therapy

On completion of neoadjuvant therapy it is necessary to re-stage patients to evaluate response to treatment and detect any disease progression during the treatment period before embarking on surgical resection. Current methods to evaluate response are based upon changes in symptoms, endoscopic appearance and radiological assessment.

Patients with tumours responding to preoperative therapy often describe improvements in swallowing ability; however, symptomatic improvement in dysphagia alone is not a good indicator of response.[126] The accuracy of endoscopy at predicting pathological response is reported between 21% and 59% and patients predicted endoscopically to have a response have significantly better prognosis than those who do not.[127] However, a high false-negative rate (27%) was also reported in the same study, which may have a detrimental effect for those patients proceeding to resection. When a 50% reduction in tumour diameter is used as the definition of tumour response, then the positive predictive value of EUS for detecting pathological response is around 75%.[128] The assessment of

nodal disease following preoperative chemo/radiotherapy by EUS is disappointing. Difficulties lie in the ability to distinguish tumour from inflammatory change.[55,56]

The value of CT in predicting response to chemotherapy also remains disappointing.[129] One study of patients with oesophageal cancer who underwent CT before and after preoperative chemotherapy found that 93% of patients had a reduction in tumour volume following chemotherapy; however, this showed no correlation to histological evidence of tumour response or to survival.[130] Studies evaluating tumour response with PET have been much more encouraging, where changes in rates of tracer uptake relate to the volume of residual tumour cells (see section above on PET).

On completion of preoperative therapy, each patient should therefore be re-staged to reassess disease burden before proceeding to surgical resection. Additional investigations such as EUS or PET may be undertaken should further doubt remain as to potential resectability.

Intraoperative assessment and staging

With the current preoperative staging techniques already discussed, there should not be unexpected findings at operation, and thus it should be possible to undertake surgery with a clear plan on type of procedure and extent of resection. However, occasionally surprises do occur and before embarking on resection careful operative staging of the cancer must be carried out. This has two objectives: firstly, to confirm preoperative staging and in particular ensure that the cancer has not been understaged; secondly, to reassess whether the planned operative procedure remains appropriate in the light of any revised findings.

The extent of the primary tumour and in particular the proximal and distal palpable margins must be carefully examined. The lateral margins must also be evaluated to stage the depth of invasion and the presence of fixity to adjacent structures. It is also important to decide whether adherence to another organ is inflammatory or neoplastic, although this is often difficult to determine with certainty and without a full trial dissection.

The extent of lymph node involvement may also alter the surgical procedure. If enlarged nodes are within the planned extent of the en bloc resection then it is not vital to decide whether they are malignant. However, enlarged nodes that either cannot be safely resected or lie outside the margins of the resection should be regarded as distant metastases and sampled for frozen section analysis. If positive for metastases, the surgical decision can be altered as appropriate.

One study has compared accuracy of surgical TNM staging with final pathological TNM stage.[131] The presence of liver metastases was correct in 92%, T stage was correct in 60% and nodal involvement in 61%. Although all three were correct in only 21%, none of the 78 patients who was undergoing laparotomy for gastric carcinoma underwent inadequate resection.

Sentinel nodes

The concept of sentinel node sampling has been introduced with some success in planning the extent of lymphadenectomy for patients with breast cancer and malignant melanoma. Studies exploring the value of sentinel node sampling in patients with gastric and oesophageal cancer is less clear. One large study from Newcastle examined over 1600 lymph nodes resected from patients with distal oesophageal or gastro-oesophageal junction tumours and found sentinel lymph node biopsies to be 96% accurate at determining lymph node metastatic disease.[132] However, another study of 143 patients treated by oesophagectomy and two-field lymphadenectomy identified skip lesions in 55% of resected specimens, suggesting that the sentinel node concept is not reliable for patients with oesophageal cancer.[133] Certainly the lymph node drainage of the upper digestive tract is complicated with variable lymphatic drainage patterns, variable patterns of lymphatic spread by the tumour (above or below the diaphragm) and relatively high rates of skip lesions.[134] Future hopes of using the sentinel node concept to tailor the extent of lymphadenectomy in patients with oesophagogastric cancer will have to await the outcome of two large-scale prospective multicentre trials currently ongoing in Japan.

Final histopathological staging

The final staging of oesophageal and gastric cancer is important for a number of reasons: firstly, it allows an accurate prediction of prognosis and may indicate the need for adjuvant therapy; secondly, when results are compared with preoperative and intraoperative staging it provides ongoing quality control and educational feedback; and thirdly, it allows the results from different centres to be compared.

Histological features that may, in addition to the pTNM stage, influence prognosis can also be identified on microscopic analysis of the resected specimen. Tumour cell invasion of blood vessels and lymphatics are established as poor prognostic indicators independent of stage for gastric cancer.[135,136] The grading of the cancer represents the degree of differentiation of the tumour expressed as how much it resembles the tissue at the site of origin (Table 3.9). Less differentiation of the tumour is associated with poorer outcome as is the presence of a signet-ring morphology of the cancer cells.[137] A recent Medical Research Council randomised trial for gastric cancer identified the presence of eosinophils within the resection specimen as a favourable prognostic indicator.[138]

Lymph node micrometastases

Malignant cells are often found in normal-looking lymph nodes resected at surgery that retain their normal macroscopic and microscopic architecture. These malignant cells may be missed by conventional haematoxylin/eosin staining and often require specialist techniques, such as immunohistochemistry, to aid their detection. Although the prognostic significance of these lymph node micrometastases remains debatable, one small study that used immunohistochemistry methods detected micrometastases in 32% of regional nodes resected following gastrectomy that were staged pN0 by conventional histological analysis,[139] and this was associated with a significantly poorer 5-year survival (66% vs. 95%). Although this survival difference in the presence of micrometastases has been supported by other studies,[140,141] this has not been universal and especially for early gastric cancer.[142,143] It is presumably one of the mechanisms behind locoregional recurrence following potentially curative surgery.

Potential future novel staging modalities

This chapter has focused on current conventional staging modalities that determine the anatomical stage of disease. Recent interest in staging has investigated novel staging techniques that address the biological behaviour of tumours, which aim to predict tumour behaviour, including metastatic potential, likelihood of response to chemo/radiotherapy,

Table 3.9 • UICC classification of tumour grading

Histological grade (G)	
Gx	Grade cannot be assessed
G1	Well differentiated
G2	Moderately differentiated
G3	Poorly differentiated
G4	Undifferentiated

and risk of recurrence. To date many prognostic indicators have been investigated, including tumour markers, acute-phase proteins and cytokines, heat-shock proteins, adhesion molecules and proto-oncogenes. Many more novel markers are reported regularly in the literature but most of these require further validation in future studies.

The presence of systemic inflammation (elevated serum C-reactive protein concentration) has been established as an independent prognostic indicator for most epithelial cancers, including gastro-oesophageal cancer.[144-146] Other acute-phase proteins such as fibrinogen have also been shown to correlate with stage of disease in oesophageal cancer.[147] The presence of systemic inflammation may be used, in addition to TNM stage (and degree of weight loss), to improve accuracy in estimating prognosis and likely survival duration following surgery.[148] Recent work has suggested that interleukin-10 may be useful as a predictor of recurrence for gastric cancer;[149] there is also some evidence that allelic polymorphisms in cytokines, such as tumour necrosis factor, provide prognostic information in oesophageal cancer.[150] This suggests that the patient's immunological/inflammatory response to oesophageal cancer may influence survival and appears to be genetically predetermined rather than secondary to tumour phenotype. Although measuring markers of systemic inflammation does not provide direct information on anatomical tumour stage (TNM), such variables may provide additional information on tumour behaviour which can improve accuracy for estimations of prognosis and assist in patient selection for neo/adjuvant therapy.

Other researchers have developed complex computer models to predict outcome based on established prognostic variables, such as nodal involvement. Some of these have led to the development of nomograms to estimate prognosis following oesophagectomy.[151] Artifical neural networks, which utilise computer-generated equations, have also been used to improve prognostic accuracy following surgical resection.[152] However, both of these systems include pathological variables in their calculations and so cannot be used prospectively to aid management decision-making.

Many other prognostic factors have been proposed and these are beyond the scope of this chapter, but may prove their worth in the future. Clearly, not only the anatomical stage of disease is important for estimating prognosis and determining outcome, but also tumour biological behaviour. Currently the decision to proceed to curative resection is determined by the fitness of the patient for surgery and how far the disease has spread (anatomical stage). In the future additional independent prognostic indicators such as those described above may enable clinicians to stratify their patients more accurately and reduce the number of failed curative resections.

Key points

- The appropriate management of patients with oesophageal and gastric cancer depends on accurate staging of the disease from the preoperative work-up, through surgery (if indicated), to final detailed histological analysis.
- The use of the unified TNM system is strongly recommended for the staging of both gastric and oesophageal cancer.
- More recently, some authors have also proposed a separate additional staging method for tumours arising from the gastro-oesophageal junction. There is now an agreed system that classifies these tumours into types I (lower oesophageal), II (true junctional cancers) and III (proximal gastric).
- Accurate preoperative staging is essential to avoid futile attempts at radical treatment of incurable disease and to guide the use of the different available treatment modalities. The decision-making algorithm is demonstrated in Fig. 3.1. This is based on a review of the current data from multiple prospective and retrospective series comparing accuracy with final stage.
- Endoscopic ultrasonography is the most accurate staging modality for locoregional (T and N) staging of oesophageal cancer. It is not as accurate for gastric cancer, but is still the most sensitive test for T and N staging. Performing EUS-guided FNA of suspicious lymph nodes further improves local staging accuracy.
- In lower oesophageal and gastric cancer information on peritoneal metastases can often only be obtained from laparoscopy. This can prevent unnecessary laparotomy by

identifying patients with advanced disease, not detected by other diagnostic modalities, who will not benefit from surgery.

• Positive peritoneal cytology has been identified as an independent prognostic indicator for gastric cancer and its presence results in a stage-matched reduction in survival. The routine cytological analysis of peritoneal washings during laparoscopy is likely to add to the staging accuracy of patients with gastric cancer and help identify those patients likely to develop peritoneal recurrence.

• Recent improvements in CT, MRI and PET may help further improve the accuracy of the staging process and identification of metastatic disease.

• Recently, more research interest has focused on staging techniques that address the biological behaviour of tumours, which is important in determining the pattern of spread, progression of disease, response to chemoradiotherapy and likelihood of recurrence. This is a potentially exciting area for future research.

• Every patient with oesophageal and gastric cancer has a right to expect the most accurate staging available throughout their care and this can only be provided by the clinicians within the MDTs incorporating many of the investigative techniques described here into their routine practice.

Acknowledgements

The previous editions of this chapter have been written/contributed to by John Anderson and Jonathan Ferguson. Some of the original background data from their text remains and we wish to acknowledge their contributions.

References

1. Blazeby JM, Alderson D, Farndon JR. Quality of life in patients with oesophageal cancer. In: Lange J, Siewert JR (eds) Recent results in cancer research – esophageal carcinoma, Vol. 55. Berlin: Springer-Verlag, 2000; pp. 193–204.

2. Avery KNL, Metcalfe C, Barham CP et al. Quality of life during potentially curative treatment for locally advanced oesophageal cancer. Br J Surg 2007; 94:1369–76.

3. Sobin LH, Wittekind CH. TNM classification of malignant tumours, 6th edn. New York: John Wiley, 2003.

   This system was approved by the UICC and AJCC in 1985 and in Japan in 1986. **Table 3.1** illustrates the 2003 update of the unified TNM staging system for gastric cancer. Use of this system is strongly recommended.

4. Bruno L, Nesi G, Montinaro F et al. Clinicopathologic characteristics and outcome indicators in node-negative gastric cancer. J Surg Oncol 2000; 74:30–2.

5. Bouvier AM, Haas O, Piard F et al. How many nodes must be examined to accurately stage gastric carcinomas? Results from a population based study. Cancer 2002; 94:2862–6.

6. Ichikura T, Ogawa T, Chochi K et al. Minimum number of lymph nodes that should be examined for the International Union Against Cancer/American Joint Committee on Cancer TNM classification of gastric carcinoma. World J Surg 2003; 27:330–3.

7. Mullaney PJ, Wadley MS, Hyde C et al. Appraisal of compliance with the UICC/AJCC staging system in the staging of gastric cancer. Union Internacional Contra la Cancrum/American Joint Committee on Cancer. Br J Surg 2002; 89:1405–8.

8. Saito H, Fukumoto Y, Osaki T et al. Prognostic significance of level and number of lymph node metastases in patients with gastric cancer. Ann Surg Oncol 2007; 14(5):1688–93.

9. Kunisaki C, Shimada H, Nomura M et al. Clinical impact of metastatic lymph node ratio in advanced gastric cancer. Anticancer Res 2005; 25(2B):1369–75.

10. Kennedy BJ. TNM classification for stomach cancer. Cancer 1970; 26:971–83.

11. Beahrs OH, Henson DE, Hunter RVP et al. Manual of staging of cancer. Philadelphia: JB Lippincott, 1992.

12. Hermanek P, Sobin LH (eds) UICC:TNM classification of malignant tumours, 5th edn. Berlin: Springer-Verlag, 1996.

13. Japanese Society for Esophageal Diseases. Guide for the clinical and pathological studies on carcinoma of the esophagus. Jpn J Surg 1976; 6:69–78.

14. Rizk N, Venkatramen E, Park B et al. The prognostic importance of the number of involved lymph nodes in esophageal cancer: implications for revisions of the American Joint Committee on Cancer

staging system. J Thorac Cardiovasc Surg 2006; 132(6):1374–81.

15. Siewert JR, Stein HJ. Classification of adenocarcinoma of the oesophagogastric junction. Br J Surg 1998; 85:1457–9.

16. Hardwick RH, Williams GT. Staging of oesophageal adenocarcinoma. Br J Surg 2002; 89:1076–7.

17. Wijnhoven BPL, Siersema PD, Hop WCJ et al. Adenocarcinomas of the distal oesophagus and gastric cardia are one clinical entity. Br J Surg 1999; 86:529–35.

18. http:www.sign.ac.uk

19. Kienle P, Buhl K, Kuntz C et al. Prospective comparison of endoscopy, endosonography and computed tomography for staging of tumours of the oesophagus and gastric cardia. Digestion 2002; 66:230–6.

20. Yanai H, Noguchi T, Mizumachi S et al. A blind comparison of the effectiveness of endoscopic ultrasonography and endoscopy in staging early gastric cancer. Gut 1999; 44:361–5.

21. Kim SH, Lee JM, Han JK et al. Three-dimensional MDCT imaging and CT esophagography for evaluation of esophageal tumors: preliminary study. Eur Radiol 2006; 16(11):2418–26.

22. Panebianco V, Grazhdani H, Iafrate F et al. 3D CT protocol in the assessment of the esophageal neoplastic lesions: can it improve TNM staging?. Eur Radiol 2006; 16(2):414–21.

23. Onbas O, Eroglu A, Kantarci M et al. Preoperative staging of esophageal carcinoma with multidetector CT and virtual endoscopy. Eur J Radiol 2006; 57(1):90–5.

24. Moorjani N, Junemann-Ramirez M, Judd O et al. Endoscopic ultrasound in oesophageal carcinoma: comparison with multislice computed tomography and importance in the clinical decision making process. Minerva Chir 2007; 62(4):217–23.

25. Pfau PR, Perlman SB, Stanko P et al. The role and clinical value of EUS in a multimodality esophageal carcinoma staging program with CT and positron emission tomography. Gastrointest Endosc 2007; 65(3):377–84.

26. Fekete F, Gayet B, Frija J. CT scanning in the diagnosis of oesophageal disease. In: Jamieson GG (ed.) Surgery of the oesophagus. Edinburgh: Churchill Livingstone, 1988; pp. 85–9.

27. Schnyder PA, Gamsu G. CT of the pretracheal retrocaval space. Am J Roentgenol 1981; 136:303–8.

28. Noda N, Sasako M, Yamaguchi N et al. Ignoring small lymph nodes can be a major cause of staging error in gastric cancer. Br J Surg 1998; 85:831–4.

29. Overhagen IT, Lameris JS, Berger MY et al. Improved assessment of supraclavicular and abdominal metastases in oesophageal and gastrooesophageal carcinoma with the combination of ultrasound and computed tomography. Br J Radiol 1993; 66:203–8.

30. Halvorsen RA, Thompson WM. Gastrointestinal cancer, diagnosis staging and the follow-up role of imaging. Semin Ultrasound, CT, MRI 1989; 10:467–80.

31. Thompson WM, Halverson RA. Staging esophageal carcinoma II: CT and MRI. Semin Oncol 1994; 21:447–52.

32. Watt I, Stewart I, Anderson D et al. Laparoscopy, ultrasound and computed tomography in cancer of the oesophagus and cardia: a prospective comparison for detecting intra-abdominal metastases. Br J Surg 1989; 76:1036–9.

33. Kim HJ, Kim AY, Oh ST et al. Gastric cancer staging at multi-detector row CT gastrography: comparison of transverse and volumetric CT scanning. Radiology 2005; 236(3):879–85.

34. Cho JS, Kim JK, Rho SM et al Pre-operative assessment of gastric carcinoma: value of two-phase dynamic CT with mechanical i.v. injection of contrast material. Am J Roentgenol 1994; 163:69–75.

35. Mani NB, Suri S, Gupta S et al. Two-phase dynamic contrast-enhanced computed tomography with water-filling method for staging of gastric carcinoma. Clin Imaging 2001; 25:38–43.

36. Kim AY, Kim HJ, Ha HK. Gastric cancer by multidetector row CT: preoperative staging. Abdom Imaging 2005; 30(4):465–72.

37. Yang DM, Kim HC, Jin W et al. 64 multidetector-row computed tomography for preoperative evaluation of gastric cancer: histological correlation. J Comput Assist Tomogr 2007; 31(1):98–103.

38. Chen CY, Hsu JS, Wu DC et al. Gastric cancer: preoperative local staging with 3D multi-detector row CT – correlation with surgical and histopathologic results. Radiology 2007; 242(2):472–82.

39. Hur J, Park MS, Lee JH et al. Diagnostic accuracy of multidetector row computed tomography in T and N staging of gastric cancer with histopathologic correlation. J Comput Assist Tomogr 2006; 30(3):372–7.

40. Inamoto K, Kouzai K, Ueeda T et al. CT virtual endoscopy of the stomach: comparison study with gastric fiberscopy. Abdom Imaging 2005; 30(4):473–9.

41. Shin KS, Kim SH, Han JK et al. Three-dimensional MDCT gastrography compared with axial CT for the detection of early gastric cancer. J Comput Assist Tomogr 2007; 31(5):741–9.

42. Tsubnraya A, Naguchi Y, Matsumoto A et al. A preoperative assessment of adjacent organ invasion by stomach carcinoma with high resolution computed tomography. Jpn J Surg 1994; 24:299–304.

43. Barry JD, Edwards P, Lewis WG et al. Special interest radiology improves the perceived preoperative stage of gastric cancer. Clin Radiol 2002; 57:984–8.

44. Bressani Doldi S, Lattuada E, Zappa MA et al. Ultrasonographic evaluation of the cervical lymph nodes in preoperative staging of eosphageal neoplasms. Abdom Imaging 1998; 23:275–7.

45. Van Overhagen H, Lameris JS, Zonderland HM et al. Ultrasound and ultrasound-guided fine needle aspiration biopsy of supraclavicular lymph nodes in patients with esophageal carcinoma. Cancer 1991; 67:585–7.

46. Bonvalot S, Bouvard N, Lothaire P et al. Contribution of cervical ultrasound and ultrasound fine-needle aspiration biopsy to the staging of thoracic oesophageal carcinoma. Eur J Cancer 1996; 32A:893–5.

47. Van Vliet EP, van der Lugt A, Kuipers EJ et al. Ultrasound, computed tomography, or the combination for the detection of supraclavicular lymph nodes in patients with esophageal or gastric cardia cancer: a comparative study. J Surg Oncol 2007; 96(3):200–6.

48. Van Vliet EP, Steyerberg EW, Eijkemans MJ et al. Detection of distant metastases in patients with oesophageal or gastric cardia cancer: a diagnostic decision analysis. Br J Cancer 2007; 97(7):868–76.

49. Schreurs LM, Verhoef CC, van der Jagt EJ et al. Current relevance of cervical ultrasonography in staging cancer of the esophagus and gastroesophageal junction. Eur J Radiol 2008; 67(1):105–11.

50. Terada M, Tsukaya T, Saito Y. Technical advances and future developments in endoscopic ultrasonography. Endoscopy 1998; 30(Suppl 1):a3–7.

51. Botet JF, Lightdale CJ, Zaiber AG et al. Preoperative staging of gastric cancer: comparison of endoscopic US and dynamic CT. Radiology 1991; 181:426–32.

52. Catalano MF, Sivak MV, Rice T et al. Endosonographic features, predictive of lymph node metastasis. Gastrointest Endosc 1994; 40:442–6.

53. Marsman WA, Brink MA, Bergman JJ et al. Potential impact of EUS-FNA staging of proximal lymph nodes in patients with distal esophageal carcinoma. Endoscopy 2006; 38(8):825–9.

54. Reed CE, Mishra G, Sahai AV et al. Esophageal cancer staging: improved accuracy by endoscopic ultrasound of celiac lymph nodes. Ann Thorac Surg 1999; 67:319–22.

55. Kalha I, Kaw M, Fukami N et al. The accuracy of endoscopic ultrasound for restaging esophageal carcinoma after chemoradiation therapy. Cancer 2004; 101(5):940–7.

56. Rabeiro A, Franceschi D, Parra J et al. Endoscopic ultrasound restaging after neoadjuvant chemotherapy in esophageal cancer. Am J Gastroenterol 2006; 101(6):1216–21.

57. Chen CH, Yang CC, Yeh YH. Preoperative staging of gastric cancer by endoscopic ultrasound: the prognostic usefulness of ascites detected by endoscopic ultrasound. J Clin Gastroenterol 2002; 35:321–7.

58. Catalano MF, Van Dam J, Sivak MV. Malignant esophageal strictures: staging accuracy of endoscopic ultrasonography. Gastrointest Endosc 1995; 541:535–9.

59. Rosch T, Lorenz R, Zehker K et al. Local staging and assessment of resectability in carcinoma of the esophagus, stomach and duodenum by endoscopic ultrasonography. Gastrointest Endosc 1992; 38:460–7.

60. Grimm H, Binmoeller KF, Hamper K et al. Endosonography for preoperative locoregional staging of esophageal and gastric cancer. Endoscopy 1993; 25:224–30.

61. Dittler HI, Siewert JR. Role of endoscopic ultrasonography in esophageal carcinoma. Endoscopy 1993; 25:156–61.

62. Barbour AP, Rizk NP, Gerdes H et al. Endoscopic ultrasound predicts outcomes for patients with adenocarcinoma of the gastroesophageal junction. J Am Coll Surg 2007; 205(4):593–601.

63. Kutup A, Link BC, Schurr PG et al. Quality control of endoscopic ultrasound in preoperative staging of esophageal cancer. Endoscopy 2007; 39(8):715–19.

64. Davies AR, Deans DAC, Penman I et al. The multidisciplinary team meeting improves staging accuracy and treatment selection for gastro-esophageal cancer. Dis Esophagus 2006; 19(6):496–503.

65. Kelly S, Harris KM, Berry E et al. A systematic review of the staging performance of endoscopic ultrasound in gastro-oesophageal carcinoma. Gut 2001; 49:534–9.

EUS, combined with FNA of suspicious lymph nodes, is currently the most accurate staging modality for T and N staging of oesophageal cancer.

66. Murata Y, Ohta M, Hayashi K et al. Preoperative evaluation of lymph node metastasis in esophageal cancer. Ann Thorac Cardiovasc Surg 2003; 9(2):88–92.

67. Chang KJ, Soetikno RM, Bastas D et al. Impact of endoscopic ultrasound combined with fine-needle aspiration biopsy in the management of esophageal cancer. Endoscopy 2003; 35(11):962–6.

68. Storch I, Jorda M, Thurer R et al. Advantage of EUS Trucut biopsy combined with fine-needle aspiration without immediate on-site cytopathologic examination. Gastrointest Endosc 2006; 64(4):505–11.

69. Vickers J, Alderson D. Influence of luminal obstruction on oesophageal cancer staging using endoscopic ultrasonography. Br J Surg 1998; 85:999–1001.

70. Vickers J, Alderson D. Oesophageal cancer staging using endoscopic ultrasonography. Br J Surg 1998; 85:994–8.

71. Hunerbein M, Ghadimi BM, Haensch W et al. Transendoscopic ultrasound of esophageal and gastric cancer using miniaturized ultrasound catheter probes. Gastrointest Endosc 1998; 48:371–5.

72. Akahoshi K, Chijiiwa Y, Sasaki I et al. Preoperative TN staging of gastric cancer using a 15 MHz ultrasound miniprobe. Br J Radiol 1997; 70:703–7.

73. Shim CS. Role of endoscopic ultrasonography for gastric lesions. Endoscopy 1998; 30(Suppl 1):A55–9.

74. Dittler HJ, Siewert JR. Role of endosonography in gastric carcinoma. Endoscopy 1993; 25:162–6.

75. Ziegler K, Sanft C, Zimmer T et al. Comparison of computed tomography, endosonography, and

intra-operative assessment in the TN staging of gastric carcinoma. Gut 1993; 34:604–10.

76. Abe S, Lightdale CJ, Brennan MF. The Japanese experience with endoscopic ultrasonography in the staging of gastric cancer. Gastrointest Endosc 1993; 39:586–91.

77. Shimizu S, Tada M, Kawai K. Endoscopic ultrasonography for early gastric cancer. Endoscopy 1994; 26:767–8.

78. Ohashi S, Nakazawa S, Yoshino J. Endoscopic ultrasonography in the assessment of invasive gastric cancer. Scand J Gastroenterol 1989; 24:1039–48.

79. Grimm H. EUS in gastric carcinoma. 10th Int Symp Endosc Ultrasonogr 1995; pp. 109–11.

80. Hunerbein M, Ghadimi BM, Gretschel S et al. Three-dimensional endoluminal ultrasound: a new method for the evaluation of gastrointestinal tumors. Abdom Imaging 1999; 24:445–8.

81. Lightdale CJ. Endoscopic ultrasonography in the diagnosis, staging and follow-up of esophageal and gastric cancer. Endoscopy 1992; 24:297–303.

82. De Graaf GW, Ayantunde AA, Parsons SL et al. The role of staging laparoscopy in oesophagogastric cancers. Eur J Surg Oncol 2007; 33(8):988–92.

83. Yau KK, Siu WT, Cheung HY et al. Immediate pre-operative laparoscopic staging for squamous cell carcinoma of the esophagus. Surg Endosc 2006; 20(2):307–10.

84. Smith A, Finch MD, John TG et al. Role of laparoscopic ultrasonography in the management of patients with oesophagogastric cancer. Br J Surg 1999; 86:1083–7.

85. Molloy RG, McCourtney JS, Anderson JR. Laparoscopy in the management of patients with cancer of the gastric cardia and oesophagus. Br J Surg 1995; 82:352–4.

86. Rao B, Hunerbein M. Diagnostic laparoscopy: indications and benefits. Langenbeck's Arch Surg 2005; 390(3):187–96.

    A systematic review which recommends the use of laparoscopy for the staging of patients with oesophago-gastric cancer.

87. Finch MD, John TG, Garden OJ et al. Laparoscopic ultrasonography for staging gastroesophageal cancer. Surgery 1997; 121:10–17.

88. Anderson DN, Campbell S, Park KG. Accuracy of laparoscopic ultrasonography in the staging of upper gastrointestinal malignancy. Br J Surg 1997; 84:580.

89. Suzuki T, Ochiai T, Hayashi H et al. Importance of positive peritoneal lavage cytology findings in the stage grouping of gastric cancer. Surg Today 1999; 29:111–15.

90. Ribeiro U, Gama-Rodrigues JJ, Safatle-Ribeiro AV et al. Prognostic significance of intraperitoneal free cancer cells obtained by laparoscopic peritoneal lavage in patients with gastric cancer. J Gastrointest Surg 1998; 2:24.

91. Bryan RT, Cruickshank NR, Needham SJ et al. Laparoscopic peritoneal lavage in staging gastric and oesophageal cancer. Eur J Surg Oncol 2001; 27:291–7.

92. Kodera Y, Yamamura Y, Shimizu Y et al. Peritoneal washing cytology: prognostic value of positive findings in patients with gastric carcinoma undergoing a potentially curative resection. J Surg Oncol 1999; 72:60–5.

93. Suzuki T, Ochiai T, Hayashi H et al. Peritoneal lavage cytology findings as prognostic factor for gastric cancer. Semin Surg Oncol 1999; 17:103–7.

94. Nekarda H, Gess C, Stark M et al. Immunocytochemically detected free peritoneal tumour cells (FPTC) are a strong prognostic factor in gastric carcinoma. Br J Cancer 1999; 79:611–19.

95. Kodera Y, Nakanishi H, Ito S et al. Quantitative detection of disseminated cancer cells in the greater omentum of gastric carcinoma patients with real-time RT–PCR: a comparison with peritoneal lavage cytology. Gastric Cancer 2002; 5:114–17.

96. Katsuragi K, Yashiro M, Sawada T et al. Prognostic impact of PCR-based identification of isolated tumour cells in the peritoneal lavage fluid of gastric cancer patients who underwent a curative R0 resection. Br J Cancer 2007; 97(4):550–6.

97. Berger A. Positron emission tomography. How does it work? Br Med J 2003; 326:1449.

98. Valk PE, Bailey DL, Townsend DW. Positron emission tomography: principles and practice. London: Springer-Verlag, 2002.

99. McAteer D, Wallis F, Couper G et al. Evaluation of 18F-FDG positron emission tomography in gastric and oesophageal carcinoma. Br J Radiol 1999; 72:525–9.

100. Kole AC, Plukker JT, Nieweg OE et al. Positron emission tomography for staging of oesophageal and gastro oesophageal malignancy. Br J Cancer 1998; 78:521–7.

101. Ott K, Weber W, Siewert JR. The importance of PET in the diagnosis and response evaluation of esophageal cancer. Dis Esophagus 2006; 19:433–42.

102. Kato H, Kuwano H, Nakajima M et al. Comparison between positron emission tomography and computed tomography in the use of the assessment of esophageal carcinoma. Cancer 2002; 94:921–8.

103. Lerut T, Flamen P, Ectors N et al. Histopathologic validation of lymph node staging with FDG-PET scan in cancer of the esophagus and gastroesophageal junction: a prospective study based on primary surgery with extensive lymphadenectomy. Ann Surg 2000; 232:743–52.

104. Flamen P, Lerut A, Van Cutsem E et al. Utility of positron emission tomography for the staging of patients with potentially operable esophageal carcinoma. J Clin Oncol 2000; 18:3202–10.

105. Luketich JD, Friedman DM, Weigel TL et al. Evaluation of distant metastases in esophageal cancer:

100 consecutive positron emission tomography scans. Ann Thorac Surg 1999; 68:1133–7.

106. Kato H, Miyazaki T, Nakajima M et al. The incremental effect of positron emission tomography on diagnostic accuracy in the initial staging of oesophageal carcinoma. Cancer 2005; 103:148–56.

107. Stahl A, Stollfuss J, Ott K et al. FDG PET and CT in locally advanced adenocarcinomas of the distal oesophagus. Clinical relevance of discordant PET findings. Nuklearmedizin 2005; 44:249–55.

108. Van Westreenen HL, Westerterp M, Bossuyt PM et al. Systematic review of the staging performance of 18-FG positron emission tomography in esophageal cancer. J Clin Oncol 2004; 22(18):3805–12.

109. Van Westreenen HL, Westerterp M, Sloof GW et al. Limited additional value of positron emission tomography in staging oesophageal cancer. Br J Surg 2007; 94(12):1515–20.

110. Westerterp M, van Westreenen HL, Reitsma JB et al. Esophageal cancer: CT, endoscopic ultrasound, and FDG PET for assessment of response to neoadjuvant therapy – systematic review. Radiology 2005; 236:841–51.

111. Swisher SG, Erasmus J, Maish M et al. 2-Fluoro-2-deoxy-d-glucose positron emission tomography imaging is predictive of pathologic response and survival after preoperative chemoradiation in patients with esophageal carcinoma. Cancer 2004; 101:1776–85.

112. Van Vliet EPM, Heijenbrok-Kal MH, Hunink MGM et al. Staging investigations for oesophageal cancer – a meta-analysis. Br J Cancer 2008; 98:547–57.

A meta-analysis of staging modalities for oesophageal cancer which concluded that, for the detection of regional lymph node metastases, EUS was superior in terms of sensitivity and specificity when compared with CT and PET. For the identification of distant metastases PET was the best modality; however, the authors advocated a combined approach involving both PET and CT for the optimum assessment of distant disease.

113. Takashima S, Takeuchi N, Shiozaki H et al. Carcinoma of the esophagus: CT vs MR imaging in determining resectability. Am J Roentgenol 1991; 156:297–302.

114. Wu LF, Wang BZ, Feng JL et al. Preoperative TN staging of esophageal cancer: comparison of miniprobe ultrasonography, spiral CT and MRI. World J Gastroenterol 2003; 9:219–24.

115. Kwee RM, Kwee TC. Imaging in local staging of gastric cancer: a systematic review. J Clin Oncol 2007; 25(15):2107–16.

116. Arocena MG, Barturen A, Bujanda L et al. MRI and endoscopic ultrasonography in the staging of gastric cancer. Rev Esp Enferm Dig 2006; 98(8):582–90.

117. Tatsumi Y, Tanigawa N, Nishimura H et al. Preoperative diagnosis of lymph node metastases in gastric cancer by magnetic resonance imaging with ferumoxtran-10. Gastric Cancer 2006; 9(2):120–8.

118. Kulling D, Feldman DR, Kay CL et al. Local staging of esophageal cancer using endoscopic magnetic resonance imaging: prospective comparison with endoscopic ultrasound. Endoscopy 1998; 30:745–9.

119. Herth F, Ernst A, Schulz M et al. Endobronchial ultrasound reliably differentiates between airway infiltration and compression by tumor. Chest 2003; 123(2):458–62.

120. Osugi H, Nishimura Y, Takemura M et al. Bronchoscopic ultrasonography for staging supracarinal esophageal squamous cell carcinoma: impact on outcome. World J Surg 2003; 27(5):590–4.

121. Wakamatsu T, Tsushima K, Yasuo M et al. Usefulness of preoperative endobronchial ultrasound for airway invasion around the trachea: esophageal cancer and thyroid cancer. Respiration 2006; 73(5):651–7.

122. Krasna MJ, Mao YS, Sonett J et al. The role of thoracoscopic staging of esophageal cancer patients. Eur J Cardiothorac Surg 1999; 16:S31–3.

123. Krasna MJ. Advances in staging of esophageal carcinoma. Chest 1998; 113:107S–111S.

124. Krasna MJ, Jiao X, Mao YS et al. Thoracoscopy/laparoscopy in the staging of esophageal cancer: Maryland experience. Surg Laparosc Endosc Percutan Tech 2002; 12:213–18.

125. Stephens MR, Lewis WG, Brewster AE et al. Multidisciplinary team management is associated with improved outcomes after surgery for oesophageal cancer. Dis Esophagus 2006; 19:164–71.

126. Geh JI, Crellin AM, Glynne-Jones R. Preoperative chemoradiotherapy in oesophageal cancer. Br J Surg 2001; 88:338–56.

127. Brown WA, Thomas J, Gotley D et al. Use of oesophagogastroscopy to assess the response of oesophageal carcinoma to neoadjuvant therapy. Br J Surg 2004; 91:199–204.

128. Willis J, Cooper GS, Isenberg G et al. Correlation of EUS measurement with pathologic assessment of neoadjuvant therapy response in esophageal carcinoma. Gastrointest Endosc 2002; 55:655–61.

129. Jones DR, Parker LA, Detterbeck FC et al. Inadequacy of computed tomography in assessing patients with esophageal carcinoma after induction chemoradiotherapy. Cancer 1999; 85:1026–32.

130. Griffith JF, Chan AC, Chow LT et al. Assessing chemotherapy response of squamous cell oesophageal carcinoma with spiral CT. Br J Radiol 1999; 72:678–84.

131. Madden MV, Price SK, Learmonth GM et al. Surgical staging of gastric carcinoma: sources and consequences of error. Br J Surg 1987; 74:119–21.

132. Lamb PJ, Griffin SM, Burt AD et al. Sentinel node biopsy to evaluate the metastatic dissemination of oesophageal adenocarcinoma. Br J Surg 2005; 92:60–7.

133. Schroeder W, Prenzel K, Baldus SE et al Localization of isolated lymph node metastases in esophageal cancer – does it influence the sentinel node concept? Hepatogastroenterology 2007; 54(76):1116–20.

134. Tangoku A, Seike J, Nakano K et al. Current status of sentinel lymph node navigation surgery in breast and gastrointestinal tract. J Med Invest 2007; 54(1–2):1–18.

135. Kooby DA, Suriawinata A, Klimstra DS et al. Biologic predictors of survival in node-negative gastric cancer. Ann Surg 2003; 237:828–35.

136. Dhar DK, Kubota H, Tachibana M et al. Long-term survival of transmural advanced gastric carcinoma following curative resection: multivariate analysis of prognostic factors. World J Surg 2000; 24:588–93.

137. Kim J, Kim S, Yang H. Prognostic significance of signet ring cell carcinoma of the stomach. Surg Oncol 1994; 3:221–7.

138. Cuschieri A, Talbot IC, Weeden S. Influence of pathological tumour variables on long-term survival in resectable gastric cancer. Br J Cancer 2002; 86:674–9.

139. Yasuda K, Adachi Y, Shiraishi N et al. Prognostic effect of lymph node micrometastasis in patients with histologically node-negative gastric cancer. Ann Surg Oncol 2002; 9:771–4.

140. Lee E, Chae Y, Kim I et al. Prognostic relevance of immunohistochemically detected lymph node micrometastasis in patients with gastric carcinoma. Cancer 2002; 94:2867–73.

141. Okada Y, Fujiwara Y, Yamamoto H et al. Genetic detection of lymph node micrometastases in patients with gastric carcinoma by multiple-marker reverse transcriptase–polymerase chain reaction assay. Cancer 2001; 92:2056–64.

142. Choi HJ, Kim YK, Kim YH et al. Occurrence and prognostic implications of micrometastases in lymph nodes from patients with submucosal gastric carcinoma. Ann Surg Oncol 2002; 9:13–19.

143. Morgagni P, Saragoni L, Folli S et al. Lymph node micrometastases in patients with early gastric cancer: experience with 139 patients. Ann Surg Oncol 2001; 8:170–4.

144. Nozoe T, Saeki H, Sugimachi K. Significance of preoperative elevation of CRP as an indicator of prognosis in oesophageal carcinoma. Am J Surg 2001; 182:197–201.

145. Crumley ABC, McMillan DC, McKernan M et al. Evaluation of an inflammation-based prognostic score in patients with inoperable gastro-oesophageal cancer. Br J Cancer 2006; 94(5):637–41.

146. Ikeda M, Natsugoe S, Ueno S et al. Significant host and tumour-related factors for predicting prognosis in patients with esophageal carcinoma. Ann Surg 2003; 238(2):197–202.

147. Wayman J, O'Hanlon D, Hayes N et al. Fibrinogen levels correlate with stage of disease in patients with oesophageal cancer. Br J Surg 1997; 84:185–8.

148. Deans DAC, Wigmore SJ, de Beaux A et al. A clinical prognostic scoring system to aid management decision-making for gastro-oesophageal cancer. Br J Surg 2007; 94(12):1501–8.

149. Galizia G, Lieto E, De Vita F et al. Circulating levels of interleukin-10 and interleukin-6 in gastric and colon cancer patients before and after surgery: relationship with radicality and outcome. J Interferon Cytokine Res 2002; 22:473–82.

150. Deans DAC, Rose-Zerilli M, Wigmore S et al. Host cytokine genotype is related to adverse prognosis and systemic inflammation in gastro-oesophageal cancer. Ann Surg Oncol 2007; 14(2):329–39.

151. Lagarde SM, Reitsma JB, de Castro SMM et al. Prognostic nomogram for patients undergoing oesophagectomy for adenocarcinoma of the oesophagus or gastro-oesophageal junction. Br J Surg 2007; 94(11):1361–84.

152. Mofidi R, Deans DAC, Duff MD et al. Prediction of survival from carcinoma of the oesophagus and oesophago-gastric junction following surgery with curative intent using an artificial neural network. Eur J Surg Oncol 2006; 32(5):533–9.

4

Preoperative assessment and perioperative management in oesophageal and gastric surgery

Ian H. Shaw

Introduction

All of the evidence suggests that the quality of perioperative anaesthetic care is an important determinant in the outcome of patients undergoing oesophageal or gastric resection. As preoperative assessment and optimisation is invariably a multidisciplinary process, early communication and dialogue between the surgical, anaesthetic and critical care teams is essential to identify and minimise potential problems. The benefit derived from a particular therapy will depend not only on the stage of the gastric or oesophageal disease, but also on the fitness of the patient to withstand potentially prolonged anaesthesia and surgery, as well as a protracted and physiologically challenging postoperative period.

The preoperative physiological status of the patient has a significant impact on operative mortality and morbidity. Decreased functional status has consistently been identified as a predictor of poor postoperative outcome.[1–5] Operability in oesophageal and gastric disease is therefore determined by a combination of surgical resectability and the preoperative physiological status of the patient.

Upper gastrointestinal surgery and anaesthesia is a major undertaking that significantly impinges on the patient's cardiorespiratory system. The perioperative management necessitates strict vigilance and close monitoring of the patient's cardiorespiratory status and prompt intervention instituted as the situation demands. A thorough preoperative assessment of the patient is mandatory before assigning the patient to a particular therapeutic option. The time facilitated by the preoperative staging period

should be utilised efficiently to render the patient optimally fit. The provision of a high-quality service throughout the perioperative period is essential for a successful outcome.

Preoperative assessment

Role of the multidisciplinary team (MDT)

All decisions about management and standards for potentially curative therapy follow a documented clinical policy that has been agreed throughout each cancer network. All members of the specialist team are involved in discussions on policy decisions and in particular auditing the adherence to them. Audit of outcomes, participation in national clinical trials and data collection systems are all part of the multidisciplinary process. The specialist oesophagogastric cancer team includes a designated lead clinician who is most commonly a surgeon, together with specialist oesophagogastric surgeons from the team, a medical gastroenterologist, a consultant intensivist and anaesthetist, both clinical and medical oncologists, an interventional radiologist and a cross-sectional imager together with a dietician, a clinical nurse specialist and a palliative care specialist. A histopathologist and a cytopathologist are also part of the MDT.

Since the publication of the Improving Outcomes Guidance document from the Department of Health on upper gastrointestinal (GI) cancers, there has been a significant improvement in trial recruitment and

Chapter 4

patient outcomes.[6] The role in preoperative assessment is well established. All physical assessments described in the following section are discussed for each individual patient in the multidisciplinary setting, including a full appraisal of the patient and family's physical and mental circumstance and expectations of therapy. The clinical nurse specialist is key to this process. All potential options of curative therapy are considered in the context of objective and subjective fitness assessment and the opinions of the team documented. More than one option is often presented to the patient and family as the patient and family's wishes are paramount and may be at variance with the views of the MDT.

Patients who are managed by an MDT are more likely to be offered appropriate treatment and to receive continuity of care through all the stages of their disease. Increasing specialisation has offered valuable opportunities for improving specialist clinical training as well as research opportunities, recruitment into clinical trials, and in particular perioperative and overall patient outcome.

Patient selection and risk stratification

The aim of preoperative assessment is to optimise the patient's physiological status and so make an objective evaluation as to the likelihood of a successful surgical outcome. Thoracic and upper gastrointestinal surgery carries the greatest risk of postoperative pulmonary complications.[5,7–9] In consequence, much attention continues to be devoted to identifying reliable preoperative clinical risk predictors that will improve patient selection and facilitate appropriate preoperative physiological optimisation. Despite a number of risk predictors being identified (Box 4.1), there is still no consensus on the selection criteria for patients undergoing gastric and oesophageal resection for cancer. The reliability of many of the risk predictors remains contentious. The situation is further complicated by differing predictor risk factors between patients with oesophageal squamous carcinoma as compared to adenocarcinoma.[21]

 Although predicting postoperative outcome remains an inexact science, the evidence does suggest a poorer outcome in patients with increasing complexity of comorbidity.[22] Comorbidity, particularly cardiorespiratory impairment, is common in patients presenting for upper GI surgery.[5,7,23] Advancing age is repeatedly identified as one of a number of perioperative risk factors that correlate with an increased risk of postoperative complications following oesophagectomy.[7,10,11,24]

Box 4.1 • Preoperative clinical risk predictors that have been reported as associated with an increase in postoperative morbidity and mortality following oesophagectomy*

Increasing age[2,5,10–15]
Impaired functional status[2–5,14,16]
Impaired cardiac function[3,15]
Impaired pulmonary function[3,13–15]
Low P_aO_2[3,10,17]
Cigarette smoking[18]
Surgical approach[19]
Diabetes mellitus[5,15]
Impaired hepatic function[15,16]
Raised alkaline phosphatase[5]
Raised urea or impaired renal function[5,15]
Low serum cholesterol[12]
Low serum albumin[5,17]
Low BMI[18]
Preoperative chemotherapy†[11,15]

*Many patients will exhibit more than one risk factor. Pulmonary complications are a notably major cause of postoperative mortality.
†Although not substantiated in other studies.[12,20]

Old age per se is not a contraindication to upper GI surgery, but coexisting medical conditions and organ dysfunction increase with age. The need for vasoactive support in patients over 80 years of age admitted to intensive care after surgery correlates strongly with hospital mortality. Provided patients are selected with care and perioperative management is intensive, advanced age alone is not a contraindication to successful oesophageal resection.[3]

In an attempt to categorise surgical risk the Physiological and Operative Severity Score for the enUmeration of Mortality and morbidity (POSSUM) scoring system was proposed. POSSUM amalgamates a physiological score with an operative severity score to give an estimation of the risk of mortality and morbidity. The value of such a system is that it acknowledges the significance of both the patient's physiological parameters and the magnitude of surgical intervention to surgical outcome. Despite this POSSUM has a poor predictive accuracy for both morbidity and mortality following oesophagectomy.[25] As a result of the general over-prediction of mortality in low-risk groups, a modified system, P-POSSUM, was proposed.[26] P-POSSUM, although slightly more reliable in predicting outcome after gastrointestinal surgery, was not specific to gastric and oesophageal surgery. Therefore O-POSSUM, a risk-adjusted surgically specific model for predicting outcome after upper GI surgery, was developed.[27] O-POSSUM accurately predicted mortality after gastrectomy but was found to be lacking in accurately predicting outcome after oesophagectomy.[28] In a study of 545 patients undergoing transthoracic oesophagectomy, P-POSSUM was found to be superior to O-POSSUM,[29] the latter over-predicting mortality in low-risk and elderly patients.[30] Concerns have been raised as to the comparability of the patients, their tumour status, the failure to acknowledge transfused blood, a factor known to correlate with poor outcome, and the operations used to formulate O-POSSUM scores. The more reliable predictability of O-POSSUM following gastrectomy when compared to oesophagectomy may reflect that the two operations do not share the same risk factors.[30]

An alternative specific composite scoring system that facilitates the prediction of mortality following oesophagectomy for cancer based on objective preoperative physiological parameters has been proposed.[7,15] By considering the patient's general status, tumour stage, and selected measurable aspects of pulmonary, hepatic, renal, cardiac and endocrine function, the authors claim to have developed a system for refining patient selection.

In more general terms, the most familiar and simple classification of preoperative physical status and risk is that of the American Society of Anesthesiologists (ASA) (Table 4.1). Although the correlation of ASA grade with perioperative risk has limitations, it does provide a useful global assessment tool and its use is universal and familiar.

As might be expected, perioperative morbidity and mortality increase with increasing ASA score, including after oesophagectomy.[22] Oesophageal resection performed on ASA 3 patients via the transhiatal route had a better outcome when compared to the transthoracic route. The appropriateness of undertaking major surgery in ASA 4 patients requires very careful multidisciplinary consideration as surgery in this group is associated with a very high morbidity and mortality.[22]

Table 4.1 • The American Society of Anesthesiologists' assessment of physical status

Grade	Definition
ASA 1	Normal healthy patient
ASA 2	Patient with mild systemic disease
ASA 3	Patient with a severe systemic disease that limits activity but is not incapacitating
ASA 4	Patient with incapacitating disease that is a constant threat to life
ASA 5	Moribund patient not expected to survive 24 hours with or without surgery

Coexisting cardiovascular disease

Ischaemic heart disease has repeatedly been identified as a major perioperative risk factor[31,32] in upper GI surgery. Up to 10% of patients who have undergone an oesophagectomy will have cardiovascular complications.[8] Patients presenting with active cardiovascular risk factors (Box 4.2)[31,32] should be evaluated and treated as directed by the current American College of Cardiology/American Heart Association (ACA/AHA) joint guidelines on perioperative cardiovascular evaluation and care.[33] The need to investigate asymptomatic patients with identifiable risk factors will depend on the magnitude of the proposed surgery (**Fig. 4.1**) and the functional capacity of the patient. Between 5% and 10% of asymptomatic patients have an abnormal electrocardiogram (ECG) of significance to anaesthesia. Silent myocardial ischaemia, which can be associated with significant decreases in coronary blood flow, is recognised as a frequent and potentially serious marker of morbidity. A myocardial infarction within 6 months of any proposed surgery represents an appreciable increased operative risk, the risk of reinfarction and death being greatest within the first 3 months.

Patients who have had a recent coronary artery bypass graft or angioplasty do not appear to be at an increased risk provided they have good residual ventricular function, remain asymptomatic and have no other cardiac risk factors.[31,32]

Mild hypertension is not an independent risk factor for perioperative cardiovascular complications but poorly controlled hypertension may be associated with an increased perioperative morbidity.[31,32] Exaggerated responses to surgical stimulation and manipulation, changes in posture, hypovolaemia and anaesthetic agents can occur in hypertensive patients.

Congestive heart failure has repeatedly been identified as being associated with a poorer postoperative outcome.[31,32]

Patients presenting with a significant degree of ventricular impairment, as reflected by a low ejection fraction, need extremely careful assessment as they may not be suitable candidates for major upper GI surgery. Heart failure precipitated by hypertension may carry a different perioperative risk compared with heart failure secondary to ischaemic heart disease.

There is little evidence that the routine evaluation of left ventricular function in asymptomatic patients is of any benefit. However, patients with prior heart failure, worsening dyspnoea and dyspnoea of unknown origin should have their left ventricular function evaluated preoperatively.[33,34]

For a full and detailed discussion of perioperative cardiovascular evaluation prior to non-cardiac surgery, the reader should consult the literature.[31–33,35]

Box 4.2 • Clinical predictors of increased perioperative risk of myocardial infarction, heart failure and death during non-cardiac surgery*

Major clinical risk predictors

- Unstable coronary syndromes
- Acute or recent myocardial infarction with evidence of important ischaemic risk by clinical symptoms or non-invasive study
- Unstable or severe angina (Canadian class III and IV)
- Decompensated heart failure
- Significant arrhythmias
- High-grade atrioventricular block
- Symptomatic ventricular arrhythmias in the presence of underlying heart disease
- Supraventricular arrhythmias with uncontrolled ventricular rate
- Severe valvular disease

Intermediate clinical risk predictors

- Mild angina pectoris (Canadian class I and II)
- Previous myocardial infarction by history or pathological Q waves
- Compensated or prior heart failure
- Diabetes mellitus (particularly insulin dependent)
- Renal insufficiency

Minor clinical risk predictors

- Advanced age
- Abnormal ECG (left ventricular hypertrophy, left bundle branch block, ST-T abnormalities)
- Rhythm other than sinus (e.g. atrial fibrillation)
- Low functional capacity (e.g. inability to climb one flight of stairs carrying groceries)
- History of stroke
- Uncontrolled systemic hypertension

*Patients presenting for upper gastrointestinal surgery who have any of these conditions should undergo careful evaluation and treatment before elective surgery.[34]
Reproduced with the permission of the American College of Cardiology and Elsevier Science Publications.

Coexisting respiratory disease

Patients over the age of 65 years with operable oesophageal cancer are known to be at a higher risk of postoperative complications. Much of the evidence correlating preoperative pulmonary function to postoperative outcome after thoracotomy concerns pulmonary surgery involving a reduction in lung volume. The collapse of the non-dependent lung during oesophageal surgery is temporary in order to facilitate surgical access. Although this does not involve any permanent reduction in lung volume, transient pulmonary impairment during the immediate postoperative period is a common finding.[18] As one might expect, significantly impaired preoperative pulmonary function results in difficulties in maintaining adequate oxygenation during one-lung anaesthesia (OLA) and in the postoperative period.

The aetiology of postoperative pulmonary complications is multifactorial and cannot reliably be predicted by pulmonary function tests alone.[3,7,18] Impaired peak expiratory flow rate and forced vital capacity have been identified as reliable risk predictors following oesophagectomy, the latter particularly when associated with a lower than normal arterial oxygen tension.[3,17]

Attempts to develop a preoperative predictive scoring system for pulmonary complications following oesophagectomy have met with limited success.[7] Increasing age over 50, diminished performance status and a progressively falling forced expiratory volume in 1 second (FEV_1) <90% of predicted appeared to correlate with increasing pulmonary complications, the accuracy of prediction being 65%. Unfortunately the surgical procedures were not entirely comparable. Regardless, patients with an FEV_1 of <65% predicted value were at a greater risk of postoperative pulmonary complications following oesophagectomy.[7,11] Although there appears to be insufficient evidence to support preoperative spirometry as a tool to stratify pulmonary risk for non-cardiothoracic surgery, it would still be prudent to implement appropriate risk-reduction strategies prior to surgery (Box 4.3)[36] when the results of pulmonary function testing suggest suboptimal function, particularly when the patient is symptomatic.

A low preoperative oxygen saturation is known to correlate with persistent postoperative hypoxaemia following thoracotomy for non-pulmonary surgery and a higher incidence of pulmonary complications and mortality after oesophagectomy.[3,10]

Anaesthetic considerations

All studies agree that coexisting medical conditions, major abdominal or thoracic surgery and increasing age increase the risk of perioperative morbidity and mortality.[24,31,32] Although the literature fails to identify a single specific preoperative risk factor that reliably predicts surgical outcome following upper GI surgery, the data do strongly support the view that patients with a reduced cardiorespiratory reserve tolerate upper abdominal and thoracic surgery poorly.[2,3,7,10]

A careful assessment of patient's preoperative functional cardiorespiratory reserve should be undertaken and the efficacy of any prescribed medication evaluated. Suboptimal treatment of cardiorespiratory disease can add appreciably to the perioperative risks in a patient undergoing thoracic or upper abdominal surgery.

Two conditions merit special mention when considering a patient for upper GI surgery: diabetes mellitus and tobacco abuse. An increase in mortality and morbidity has been observed in diabetic patients following oesophageal surgery,[5,7] although this was not confirmed in an earlier study.[3] Diabetes mellitus,

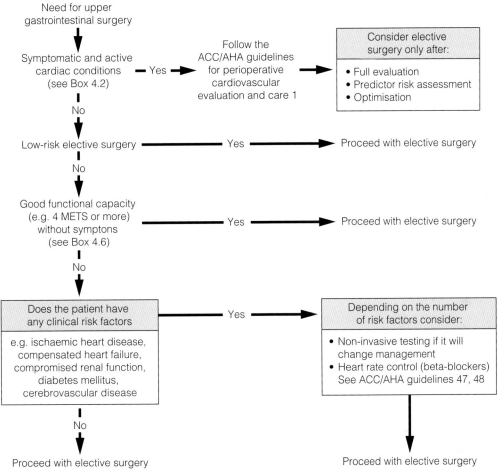

Figure 4.1 • Cardiovascular evaluation and care aligorithm for patients over 50 years of age being considered for elective upper gastrointestinal surgery. For a critical appraisal of the best current practice on the preoperative cardiovascular evaluation for patients undergoing non-cardiac surgery, the reader should consult the American College of Cardiology/American Heart Association (AHA/ACC) joint 2006 and 2007 guidelines.[33,34]

Box 4.3 • Preoperative pulmonary risk-reduction strategies for patients undergoing upper gastrointestinal surgery

- Cessation of cigarette smoking for a minimum of 8 weeks
- Aggressively treat airflow obstruction in patients with COPD or asthma under the direction of a respiratory physician
- Optimise haemoglobin concentration
- Treat any respiratory tract infection with antibiotics having first cultured the sputum
- Begin patient education regarding adequate exercise and lung expansion techniques with the assistance of a physiotherapist if necessary
- Encourage patient to lose weight if appropriate
- Nutritional support for patients considered to be significantly undernourished

particularly if control has been erratic, is associated with end-organ dysfunction and has a strong association with cardiovascular, cerebrovascular and renal dysfunction and hypertension, factors known to increase perioperative risk. Long-standing diabetic patients can develop cardiovascular instability secondary to autonomic dysfunction as well as experiencing silent myocardial infarctions.

Smoking has long been regarded as a major aetiological factor in perioperative morbidity. Smoking is a predisposing factor in the aetiology of postoperative myocardial infarction and adult respiratory distress syndrome following oesophagectomy.[7,18] Smoking and a high alcohol consumption have been identified as particular risk factors in patients presenting with oesophageal squamous carcinoma.[21] A sixfold increase in postoperative pulmonary complications has been observed in patients who continue to smoke. Smoking years positively correlate with late postoperative hypoxaemia and complications after upper abdominal surgery even in patients with no apparent preoperative cardiorespiratory dysfunction. Smoking cessation and encouraging the patients to exercise preoperatively is known to improve measured exercise tolerance.[16] Previous thoracic surgery and a history of industrial inflammatory lung disease may impede the collapse of the non-dependent lung during a thoracotomy as a result of adhesions. In patients who have undergone lung reduction surgery of the dependent lung, OLA will be precluded, thereby limiting the surgical options.

Preoperative investigations

Although specific preoperative tests are of limited value in predicting risk following gastric and oesophageal surgery, they can be helpful with regards perioperative care. Firstly, they provide a reference baseline for the anaesthetic and postoperative management of these often complex patients. The interference with normal oxygenation and ventilation, the potential for haemodynamic instability and the appreciable operative and postoperative fluid requirements make gastric and oesophageal surgery a major insult on the body's normal physiological processes. Maintaining homeostasis with reference to preoperative values is essential. Secondly, preoperative investigations aim to identify any remediable abnormality and facilitate optimisation of the patient's physical status within the limits of any coexisting disease.

The majority of patients undergoing upper GI surgery require only basic preoperative investigations (Box 4.4). Elaborate preoperative investigation and testing should be limited to circumstances in which the results will affect patient treatment and outcome.

Preoperative pulmonary function test results setting strict criteria as regards acceptable pulmonary function should be avoided as this may deny the patient's only chance of curative surgery. For example, hypercarbia alone, although suggestive of ventilatory compromise, is not a good predictor of postoperative morbidity in the absence of impaired exercise tolerance.[12]

Pulmonary function test results must be considered in relation to the clinical findings and the arterial blood gas analysis, particularly the P_aO_2. In selected patients, where oxygenation during OLA is regarded as borderline, any imbalance of pulmonary ventilation and perfusion may be predicted by V/Q scanning, indicating which, if any, is the dominant lung. Where further investigation is deemed necessary this should be conducted under the supervision of a chest physician.

Almost a third of the patients presenting for oesophagectomy showed some macroscopic abnormality of the trachea and main bronchi. The anaesthetist will need to know of any anatomical or pathological factors that may impede endotracheal intubation.

Box 4.4 • Minimum routine preoperative investigations for a patient presenting for upper gastrointestinal surgery

Haematological
- Haemoglobin
- Full blood count
- Coagulation screen
- Blood cross-match (2–4 units) or Group and Save as appropriate

Biochemical
- Urea and electrolytes
- Blood glucose
- Liver function tests
- Arterial blood gases on air

Electrocardiogram
- Resting 12-lead

Pulmonary function tests
- Before and after bronchodilation
- Saturation on room air

Radiology
- Chest radiology
- Computed tomography (CT) scan

Exercise test
- Stair climb
- Saturation on room air before and after exercise

Supplementary
- Bronchoscopy
- Echocardiography
- Lung diffusion capacity

Even minor degrees of abnormality can be especially problematic. Endobronchial intubation is not a benign technique and life-threatening injuries to the airway have been reported. Evidence of bronchial involvement of oesophageal carcinoma must be carefully evaluated. It has been advocated that all patients with potentially operable oesophageal tumours extending above the carina should have routine bronchoscopy.

Oral and dental hygiene should be addressed as this can be a source of chronic sepsis that could disseminate infection to the tracheobronchial tree during intubation.

Assessment of patient's preoperative functional cardiorespiratory reserve

Whilst the preoperative assessment of organ function as a predictor of postoperative morbidity and mortality following gastric and oesophageal surgery remains a contentious issue, the view

that suboptimal preoperative cardiorespiratory function is associated with a higher incidence of complications is undisputed.[3,11,13,17,21,23]

Upper GI surgery places substantial metabolic demands on patients, particularly in the immediate postoperative period. Patients with impaired oxygen delivery present an increased operative risk. In this regard there is growing interest in the predictive value of preoperative exercise testing. Poor exercise tolerance correlates with an increased risk of perioperative complications that are independent of age and all other patient characteristics. In recognition of this observation, the incorporation of an objective assessment of functional reserve into new standards of preoperative evaluation has been proposed. Whilst of great interest and potential, the true value of preoperative exercise testing currently remains debatable and is probably of minimal value in asymptomatic healthy individuals.

Exercise testing

Although the patient's exercise capacity is a subjective estimation it can be a useful measure of the patient's functional cardiorespiratory reserve. Any patient who remains asymptomatic after climbing several flights of stairs, walking up a steep hill, running a short distance, cycling, swimming or performing heavy physical activity should tolerate the rigours of upper GI surgery. However, it is important to appreciate that an apparent ability to perform these activities does not exclude cardiorespiratory disease[37] and, indeed, this is a major criticism of exercise testing performed in the absence of cardiopulmonary monitoring. Malnourished patients, not untypical in upper GI surgery, will also exhibit a reduced exercise tolerance.

Metabolic equivalents

A simple measure of a patient's cardiorespiratory reserve can be made at the bedside by expressing functional capacity in terms of metabolic equivalents (METs). METs are a measure of aerobic demands for common daily activities and pastimes (Box 4.5). One metabolic equivalent equals 3.5 mL/kg/min of oxygen uptake in a 70-kg 40-year-old man at rest. Functional capacity is classified as excellent if the METs are >7, moderate if 4–7 and poor if <4. Perioperative cardiac and long-term risk is increased in patients unable to meet a 4-MET demand during normal daily activities, particularly in patients under 65 years of age.[31,32]

Stair climbing

Patients with poor exercise tolerance, defined as an inability to climb two flights of stairs, have more comorbidity, higher ASA scores and postoperative complications. Although a subjective assessment, a patient unable to climb two flights of stairs has

Box 4.5 • Estimate of energy requirements for some daily activities expressed as metabolic equivalents (METs)

1 MET
- Self-care, eating, dressing, using the toilet
- Walking indoors around the house
- Gentle walk on level ground
- Light work, housework

4 METs
- Climbing a single flight of stairs or walking up an incline
- Walking briskly on level ground
- Running a short distance
- Heavy housework such as lifting, scrubbing, gardening, moving furniture
- Leisurely cycling
- Moderate recreational activities like golf, bowling, dancing

>10 METs
- Strenuous sports like swimming, tennis, football, jogging, skipping
- As the intensity of the exercise can vary with the activity, this should be considered when making any assessment

almost a 90% chance of developing postoperative cardiorespiratory complications.[38] Oncological surgery involving a thoracotomy and anaesthesia of over 8 hours duration has been noted as of particular risk in exercise-limited patients. Conversely, unlimited exercise tolerance was associated with fewer serious complications.

Desaturation during exercise equivalent to climbing three flights of stairs, suggesting an inability to meet the increased metabolic demands of exercise, appears to have some predictive power as regards postoperative complications in patients undergoing lung reduction surgery. Exercise-induced hypotension, possibly indicating ventricular impairment secondary to coronary artery disease,[37] is an ominous sign and must be investigated.

Cardiopulmonary exercise testing

Surgery precipitates an increase in oxygen demand that extends well into the postoperative period.[39] Patients whose cardiorespiratory systems are unable to meet this increased oxygen demand have a worse prognosis after major surgery.[1] Cardiopulmonary exercise testing (CPX) is a dynamic non-invasive objective test that evaluates the ability of a patient's cardiorespiratory system to adapt to a sudden increase in oxygen demand. The ramped exercise test is performed on a cycle ergometer with ECG monitoring and analysis of expired carbon dioxide and oxygen consumption, the latter being directly related to oxygen delivery and a linear function of cardiac output when exercising.[40] A 24% incidence of previously undetected and 'silent' ischaemic heart disease has been reported during CPX testing.[40]

With increasing exercise, oxygen consumption will eventually exceed oxygen delivery. Aerobic metabolism becomes inadequate to meet the metabolic demands and blood lactate rises reflecting supplementary anaerobic metabolism. The value for oxygen consumption at this point is known as the anaerobic threshold (AT), expressed as mL/kg/min. A greater mortality has been reported in patients with an AT below 11 mL/kg/min undergoing major abdominal surgery,[41] the risk being compounded by the presence of ischaemic heart disease.[40]

Advocates of CPX claim the results can be used to stratify operative risk, identify those who will most benefit from preoptimisation, and facilitates anaesthetic and postoperative care, so allowing the efficient use of limited resources. Where CPX testing may have a role is in evaluating the patients in the intermediate-risk group of the ACC/AHA preoperative cardiac evaluation guidelines (see Box 4.2). Making a valued reliable preoperative assessment of risk is crucial in this group but can be fraught with difficulties.[41]

Patients who have undergone neoadjuvant therapy for oesophageal cancer have been reported as having impaired pulmonary diffusion capacity and cardiopulmonary exercise performance.[42] Despite this observation the literature does not fully support the view that this increases the risk of postoperative morbidity and mortality.

In a study of 91 patients who had undergone transthoracic oesophagectomy, maximum oxygen uptake during exercise correlated well with postoperative cardiopulmonary complications.[4] The authors concluded that transthoracic oesophagectomy can safely be performed on patients with a maximum oxygen uptake of at least 800 mL/min/m^2. This conclusion has been disputed in a recent study of 78 consecutive patients who had CPX prior to oesophagectomy, where CPX testing was found to be only of limited value in predicting postoperative cardiopulmonary morbidity.[43]

Shuttle walk test

It is both impractical and unnecessary to CPX all patients presenting for upper GI surgery. CPX testing is expensive, elaborate and not widely accessible. A simpler and more viable alternative to CPX testing is incremental and progressive shuttle walk testing (SWT).[44] SWT endurance appears to correlate well with oxygen utilisation seen in CPX testing. In a study of 51 patients undergoing oesophageal resection, preoperative SWT was a sensitive indicator of 30-day operative mortality. Although the cause of death or complications were not recorded, no patient who walked more than 350 m on SWT died.[16] The authors suggest that the inability to maintain adequate oxygen delivery, as reflected by an exercise tolerance of <350 m at SWT, may impair wound healing and facilitate anastomotic failure.

Patients with musculoskeletal disease and morbid obesity may be unable to complete any form of dynamic exercise testing. In such circumstances upper limb ergometry, pharmacologically induced myocardial stress testing monitored by thallium imaging or echo cardiography may be an alternative. However, their reliability has been questioned. For a comprehensive review of exercise testing, the reader should consult Fletcher et al.[37] and Older et al.[41]

Meticulous history taking, clinical examination, baseline investigations and exercise testing will help identify those patients who need further non-invasive or invasive investigation such as echocardiography, myocardial stress testing, imaging and angiography.[33] Specialist multidisciplinary involvement should be sought. Only after thorough assessment can the appropriateness of the planned anaesthesia and surgery be determined.

Perioperative optimisation

The literature supports the view that appropriately directed perioperative care is associated with an improved surgical outcome in those patients with recognised risk predictors. However, there remains no clear consensus as to how this can best be brought about. Prior to any interventional preoptimisation it is important to establish that current treatment for coexisting cardiorespiratory disease is optimal. Optimisation may be a multidisciplinary process and specialist advice should be sought as early as the situation demands.

Beta-blockade

Coronary artery disease significantly increases mortality and myocardial infarction is more likely to be fatal in high-risk procedures such as thoracoabdominal surgery. There has been much interest in adrenergic beta-blockade prior to major surgery as a means of improving ischaemic ventricular dysfunction.[31] The best approach on how to pharmacologically protect selected high-risk patients with identifiable perioperative clinical predictors from perioperative cardiovascular complications remains to be fully elucidated. Patients who have been on long-term beta-blockade can exhibit adrenergic hypersensitivity if the therapy is withdrawn suddenly. Current practice states that patients taking chronic beta-blockers should therefore continue their medication throughout the perioperative period as sudden withdrawal may be associated with an increase in mortality. The cardioprotective effect of beta-blockers has been reported as persisting for up to 6 months into the postoperative period, even after cessation of therapy.[34]

Myocardial ischaemia correlates closely with postoperative cardiac events.[34] Maintaining a perioperative heart rate of <80 beats per minute to reduce perioperative ischaemia and the risk of myocardial infarction and death in high-risk patients has been proposed.[32] In patients with no clinical risk predictors, perioperative beta-blockade is probably of little value. However, identifying those patients who will benefit from perioperative beta-blockade remains debatable. Current ACC/AHA guidelines suggest beta-blockers should be considered in all patients with an identifiable cardiac risk as defined by the presence of more than one clinical risk factors.[33,34] For the therapy to be efficacious patients should be optimally beta-blocked in the weeks preceding elective surgery and continued throughout the immediate postoperative period. Although no particular beta-blocker has been identified as preferable, long-acting beta-blockers initiated before surgery were thought to be superior to shorter-acting drugs.[34]

The protective mechanism of beta-blockers is unclear, the control of heart rate being only part of the explanation. By contrast, recent critical expert re-evaluation of perioperative beta-blockage has questioned the validity of some of the evidence that beta-blockers are indeed cardioprotective.[45] Adverse effects can be associated with beta-blockade, especially the non-selective beta-blockers. Vagal responses to surgery and anaesthesia can be exacerbated by concomitant beta-blockade and responses to sympathomimetic inotropes may be altered. For more information, the reader should consult Auerbach and Goldman[46] and Beckman et al.[34]

Statins

There is growing interest in statins as a pre-emptive intervention therapy in the preoperative period in patients with ischaemic heart disease or hypercholesterolaemia. A meta-analysis of postoperative outcome following cardiac, vascular and non-cardiac surgery demonstrated a significant reduction in early postoperative mortality in patients taking long-term statins.[47] The effects on postoperative cardiovascular morbidity were less obvious due to insufficient and unreliable data. An alternative review, however, felt the evidence for the routine perioperative use of statins to reduce cardiovascular risk was currently lacking.[48] To date no specific studies evaluating perioperative statin therapy and postoperative outcome following gastric or oesophageal surgery have been reported. Current ACC/AHA guidelines on perioperative cardiovascular care recommends that patients should continue statin therapy throughout the operative period.[33] Until further prospective studies can clarify the true value of statins in the perioperative period, continuing statins throughout the perioperative period may remain at the personal judgement of the attending clinician.

Goal-directed haemodynamic preoptimisation

Surgery is associated with an increased metabolic demand, which continues well into the postoperative period. The normal physiological response is to increase oxygen delivery by an increase in cardiac output. Shoemaker et al.[1] showed that those patients who incurred an oxygen debt as a consequence of limited cardiorespiratory reserve incurred more postoperative morbidity and mortality. Nonsurvivors tended to have the greatest and most persistent oxygen debt. In an attempt to address this issue goal-directed therapy, within 12 hours of major high-risk surgery, has been proposed. Goal-directed optimisation aims to attain predetermined target physiological parameters that are known to correlate with a favourable outcome. With the aid of invasive monitoring, using crystalloid, colloid, blood, inotropes and oxygen, four physiological variables are amenable to manipulation. They are heart rate, stroke volume, haemoglobin and oxygen saturation. By increasing oxygen delivery to supranormal levels (>600 mL/min/m^2) it was hoped to reduce morbidity and mortality.

Not all patients are suitable for goal-directed therapy. It has been advocated that only those patients undergoing surgery for which mortality exceeds 20% and those identified as high risk during risk stratification should be considered.

During a period of preoptimisation, Wilson et al.[49] ensured an adequate circulating haemoglobin concentration, and administered various regimens of fluids and inotropes to patients in an attempt to enhance oxygen delivery. Reductions in mortality and length of hospital stay were reported. Preoperative fluid loading was regarded as the most important factor. A subsequent evidence-based review supported the view that fluid alone improved morbidity but not mortality after major surgery.[50] This finding contradicts studies that demonstrated a positive effect on surgical outcome after oesophagectomy with judicious fluid administration.[51] The reported administration of bolus doses of perioperative vasopressor drugs as required further complicates the interpretation of many of the goal-directed studies.[52]

When fluid loading alone fails to attain the predetermined physiological targets, inotropes such as dopexamine, dobutamine and epinephrine have all been used. In one study dopexamine appeared to be superior in reducing morbidity and hospital stay.[49] The pathogenesis of postoperative morbidity is ill-understood but the GI tract, as a source of potent inflammatory triggers, may be pivotal. In addition to improving oxygen delivery, inotropes appear to modulate the cytokine response and this may account for some of the beneficial effects reported.[53]

The use of inotropes is not without consequence. They can alter regional blood flow, cause tissue hypoxia and increase myocardial oxygen demand, provoking ischaemia. An adequate cardiac output is not necessarily synonymous with good regional or anastomotic blood flow. The data as regards the use of goal-directed therapy with fluids and inotropes are often conflicting when postoperative morbidity is considered, with many reports being regarded as underpowered to come to a definitive conclusion.[50]

Whilst few studies are not without criticism, goal-directed preoptimisation may be beneficial in appropriately selected high-risk patients. Despite the perceived advantages of preoptimisation it is still not widely practised on account of limited resources and concerns over the need for potentially hazardous invasive monitoring such as pulmonary artery catheters. The increasing availability of less invasive cardiac output monitors such as LiDCO and PiCCO may partly resolve this situation. Further details on the role and methodology of goal-directed preoptimisation can be found in the literature.[53]

Nutritional status

Both malnutrition and weight loss are associated with alterations in cellular physiology and organ function, which can compromise the upper GI patient in the postoperative period. Patients who receive neoadjuvant therapy prior to oesophageal surgery are more likely to be nutritionally compromised. A consensus group of clinicians[54] have defined malnutrition as a body mass index (BMI) of <18.5 kg/m^2, weight loss within the preceding 2 months of greater than 5% of usual body weight, and a serum albumin of <35 g/L. Along with diabetics, smokers, the elderly and the persistently hypoxic, malnourished patients are more prone to infection, pulmonary complications and delayed wound healing.[36,54]

A falling BMI, particularly if <20 kg/m^2,[7] and serum protein are associated with an increased risk of postoperative complications after oesophagectomy,[11,17] including acute respiratory distress syndrome (ARDS).[18] Marked weight loss may reflect advanced disease and requires careful evaluation of nutritional status. After a retrospective analysis of published data, the European Society for Clinical Nutrition and Metabolism (ESPEN) have proposed a nutritional risk screening system for patients undergoing major abdominal surgery. Assessment is based on the identifiable nutritional risk factors of a weight loss of >5% in the preceding 3 months, a BMI of <20.5 kg/m^2 and a food intake of <75% of normal requirements in the preceding week.[55]

Specialist oesophagogastric cancer units with a dedicated dietician are more likely to perform routine preoperative nutritional assessment, although this is far from universal.[56] Routine preoperative nutritional support for malnourished patients in the form of parenteral nutrition, nasogastric feeding, sip feeds and food snacks was provided in only 17% of specialist units. Early postoperative nutritional support under dietetic guidance was more common, low-residue whole-protein jejunal feeding being the most popular.

The published evidence suggests perioperative nutritional supplementation is associated with less postoperative infections, although this was not supported by one meta-analysis.[36] The same study did, however, find that patients fed with enhanced immunonutrition enteral formulations had a reduced incidence of postoperative pneumonia. Surgery, and possibly anaesthesia, is associated with immune suppression. Providing those malnourished patients with an early immunonutritional dietary source containing arginine, ribonucleic acid and omega-3 fatty acids has been reported as reducing infections, hospital stay and ventilatory requirements. A recent randomised controlled study of immunonutrition in patients undergoing resection for oesophageal and gastric cancer has failed to demonstrate clinical benefit when compared with standard enteral feeds.[57] Nutritional supplementation has been shown to improve SWT endurance.[11]

In a study of 104 patients, 50% of the patients with oesophageal adenocarcinoma were overweight.[21] Obesity (BMI >30 kg/m^2) has been associated with increased operative risk, and there is some evidence that patients at their ideal body weight do better after surgery. Obese patients have a higher incidence of coexisting cardiovascular disease, are prone to hypoventilation syndromes, postoperative airway obstruction and diabetes, a known risk predictor in upper gastrointestinal surgery. Chronic obstructive pulmonary disease (COPD) patients who smoke and are obese appear to be more prone to postoperative pulmonary complications.

Operative anaesthetic management

With a few exceptions, such as angiotensin-converting enzyme inhibitors and oral hypoglycaemics, the patient's current medication should be given right up until and including the day of surgery. To reduce the incidence of thromboembolism prophylactic low-dose heparin together with antithromboembolism stockings (TED) should be provided perioperatively. Pneumatic calf compression should be applied preoperatively and care taken in positioning the patient during surgery. Where postoperative extradural analgesia is being proposed unfractionated heparin and low-molecular-weight heparins should be discontinued 6 and 12 hours respectively before the insertion of the epidural catheter.

Non-steroidal anti-inflammatory drugs (NSAIDs) and low-dose aspirin are not a contraindication to neuroaxial blockade and opinion supports the latter's continuation throughout the surgical period. Increasingly, patients are presenting for surgery with drug-eluting coronary stents. They present a difficult dilemma when the planned surgery could involve major blood loss. Stents are highly thrombogenic and especially prone to thrombosis in the postoperative hypercoagulable state, a situation exacerbated by multiple stents, diabetes, renal impairment and other thromboembolic triggers. Stent thrombosis is associated with a high mortality. Although well-controlled clinical trials are lacking, opinion is moving away from uniformly stopping all antiplatelet medication in the perioperative period, the rationale being that the risks of serious ischaemia exceed that of haemorrhage. The exception is cranial, spinal and ophthalmic surgery, where the risk of haemorrhage into a closed cavity is high. Non-cardiac surgery on patients with coronary stents maintained on antithrombotic therapy throughout the operative period has been conducted without major morbidity from bleeding.[58] Stopping an individual patient's antiplatelet medication 7–14 days before elective surgery should only be done after consideration of the balance between haemorrhage and thrombotic risk and in consultation with haemotologists and the patient's cardiologist. Antiplatelet medication should only be restarted when the risk of postoperative bleeding has passed and any indwelling catheters have been removed. Continuing antiplatelet medication or medication given within 7–14 days of surgery will, however, preclude the use of epidural analgesia.[58]

Optimisation of the preoperative haemoglobin will help avoid the need for preoperative blood transfusion but unnecessary transfusion must be avoided.[51] Patients who have a low haemoglobin prior to upper abdominal surgery are more likely to receive a blood transfusion.

There is good evidence that the prophylactic administration of antibiotics can decrease morbidity, shorten hospital stay and reduce infection-related costs in general surgical operations. Broad-spectrum antibiotic prophylaxis against respiratory and wound infections should be administered immediately preoperatively or on induction of anaesthesia in accordance with locally agreed antibiotic policies.

During oesophageal resection, most of the difficulties for the anaesthetist arise from the need for OLA during the second stage of the procedure. Surgical manipulation of the hiatus and mediastinum is often associated with sudden cardiovascular instability. Excessive peritoneal traction can cause an increase in vagal tone manifest as a profound bradycardia. Manipulation of the heart can precipitate unstable dysrhythmias. A misplaced retractor, hand or surgical pack can result in a sudden reduction in venous return and a fall in cardiac output and blood pressure. Delivering the stomach through the hiatus into the chest is especially hazardous in this respect. If cardiovascular instability is associated with a period of relative hypoxia during OLA the situation can become potentially life-threatening if uncorrected. Consequently, the peroperative monitoring of patients undergoing oesophageal and gastric surgery should be comprehensive, taking into consideration the patient's medical status (Box 4.6). Good communication between the surgeon and the anaesthetist is essential.

Lung isolation techniques in oesophageal surgery

Transthoracic oesophageal resection invariably involves the temporary deflation of the non-dependent lung to aid surgical access. The anaesthetist has available two techniques to bring this about, endobronchial intubation and endobronchial occlusion.

Endobronchial intubation

Anaesthesia for oesophageal surgery should only be undertaken by anaesthetists familiar with the complexities of one-lung ventilation. Both gastric and oesophageal surgery can be performed in a patient intubated with a standard endotracheal tube. To facilitate the peroperative collapse of the right lung, as during a two-stage transthoracic oesophagectomy, a left-sided double-lumen endobronchial tube is used (**Fig. 4.2**). The upper lobe bronchus is very susceptible to occlusion during endobronchial intubation owing to its close proximity to the carina. Failure to recognise inadvertent upper lobe occlusion will make adequate oxygenation during OLA impossible. Correct placement of the double-lumen endobronchial tube is confirmed by auscultation of the chest and confirmatory fibreoptic bronchoscopy. Fibreoptic examination may not always be possible, particularly when smaller diameter double-lumen

Box 4.6 • Minimum perioperative monitoring of a patient during upper gastrointestinal surgery

Vital functions
- Electrocardiogram
- Blood pressure: non-invasive or invasive
- Central venous pressure as clinically indicated
- Hourly urine output
- Oximetry
- Core temperature

Ventilation
- Clinical observation
- End tidal carbon dioxide
- Inspired oxygen concentration
- Airway pressure

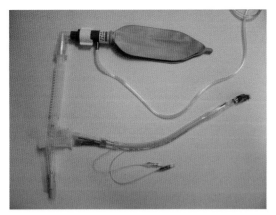

Figure 4.2 • A disposable polyvinyl chloride Broncho-Cath double-lumen endobronchial tube with a continuous positive airway pressure (CPAP) circuit attached. A positive pressure of 5–10 cm H_2O can be applied to the collapsed non-dependent lung to aid oxygenation (see text) during the thoracic stage of an oesophagectomy. Reproduced from Fleisher, LA, Beckman JA, Brown KA et al. ACC/AHA 2006 guideline update on perioperative cardiovascular evaluation for non-cardiac surgery; focused update on perioperative beta-blocker therapy. J Am Coll Cardiol 2006; 47:2345-55. With kind permission from the American College of Cardiology/Elsevier.

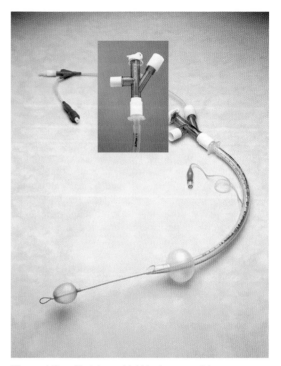

Figure 4.3 • Endobronchial blockers provide an alternative technique to isolate the non-dependent lung during the thoracic stage of an oesophagectomy when placement of a double-lumen endobronchial tube is impossible (see text). The endobronchial blocker is passed through a single-lumen endotracheal tube and optimally positioned in the appropriate main bronchus under direct fibreoptic guidance. Photograph reproduced by courtesy of Cook Medical, Bloomingtom, IN.

tubes have been used. Intraoperative displacement of the endobrochial tube during surgical manipulation of mediastinal structures can lead to precipitous desaturation during one-lung ventilation.

Endobronchial blockers

When presented with a patient who is difficult to intubate, double-lumen tubes can be unforgiving owing to their size and bulk. Tracheal intubation with a double-lumen endobronchial tube can be problematic or impossible in the presence of prominent or irregular dentition, limited neck or temporomandibular joint movement, factors which make normal laryngoscopy difficult. An alternative technique is to isolate the non-dependent lung with an endobronchial blocker (**Fig. 4.3**) passed fibreoptically through a single-lumen endotracheal tube.

Endobronchial blockers have been used successfully for routine oesophageal resection in preference to endobronchial intubation.[59] One limiting factor is the tendency of blockers to be more prone to displacement with mediastinal manipulation, either dropping proximally out of the bronchus into the trachea resulting in the sudden reinflation of the non-dependent lung, or migrating distal to the upper lobe bronchus with reinflation of the upper lobe. Full non-dependent lung deflation can take up to 20 minutes or more owing to the small internal lumen of the blocker, but may be accelerated by prior preoxygenation or manual deflation. Despite this, endobronchial blockers provide a very valuable alternative when double-lumen endobronchial

intubation is not possible, such as in a patient with a pre-existing tracheostomy. Endobronchial blockers are associated with a lower incidence of airway injuries and postoperative hoarseness when compared to a double-lumen tube.

Management of one-lung anaesthesia (OLA) during oesophageal surgery

During the thoracic stage of a two-stage oesophagectomy, the patient is placed in the left lateral position and the dependent lung preferentially ventilated through the longer endobronchial limb. To facilitate surgical access the non-dependent lung is collapsed by occluding the gas flow through the tracheal limb and opening the lumen to the atmosphere. Adequate ventilation must now be delivered to the dependent lung to avoid hypoxaemia.

Collapsing the non-dependent lung substantially reduces the area available for respiratory exchange. Fortuitously, in adopting the lateral position gravity allows the dependent lung to be preferentially perfused. Blood perfusing the collapsed lung is no longer oxygenated and will mix with oxygenated blood from the ventilated lung in the heart, causing venous admixture and a fall in arterial oxygen tension.

The aetiology of hypoxia during one-lung anaesthesia is complex, multifactorial and not exclusively due to the collapse of one lung (Box 4.7).

Hypoxia during OLA for non-pulmonary surgery can be of a greater magnitude than during lung-reduction surgery. Diseased lung is often poorly perfused and the ensuing hypoxia activates the hypoxic pulmonary vasoconstrictor response, an important homeostatic mechanism that serves to direct blood flow to better oxygenated parts of the lungs. In a patient undergoing an oesophagectomy a healthy lung is suddenly deflated and a substantial imbalance of ventilation and perfusion occurs. Pulmonary hypoxic vasoconstriction counteracts the effects of non-ventilated alveoli on gas exchange by the redistribution of capillary blood towards oxygenated lung.

During oesophagectomy the ventilated lung is subjected to compressive forces that can result in a degree of pulmonary atelectasis. Surgical manipulation, the effects of gravity on mediastinal structures, the weight of the abdominal contents acting through a paralysed diaphragm, plus the weight of the patient lying on the dependent lung all contribute in this respect. Patchy atelectasis within the dependent lung is a common finding on a postoperative chest radiograph.

OLA during an oesophagectomy elicits a marked inflammatory response that is known to increase the risk of postoperative ARDS.[18,60] The response is exacerbated if the OLA time is prolonged and associated with cardiovascular instability.

Using protective ventilatory strategies with tidal volumes as low as 5 mL/kg and 5 cm positive end-expiratory pressure (PEEP) during oesophageal

surgery appears to reduce inflammatory mediator release and improve oxygen exchange.[61] Low-level pressure-controlled ventilation with PEEP, in contrast to the more commonly used volume-controlled ventilation, has also been reported as improving oxygenation with the added benefit of concomitant lower airway pressures.

Provided the endobronchial tube is correctly positioned and cardiac output maintained, adequate oxygenation can usually be achieved simply by increasing the fractional inspired oxygen concentration. Patients vary in their ability to maintain arterial oxygen tension during OLA, and a few are very intolerant of this major physiological insult. Up to 10% of patients develop severe hypoxia during OLA, possibly due to persistent perfusion of the non-dependent lung. Attempts to predict which patients may be intolerant to OLA have met with only limited success. A haematocrit >0.45 and increasing age were associated with impaired oxygenation during OLA, the latter probably reflecting the observation that P_aO_2 decreases with increasing age. If hypoxia develops the anaesthetist has several options available, not all of which have been fully substantiated as totally beneficial (Box 4.8).

The application of continuous positive airway pressure (CPAP) to the collapsed lung may improve oxygenation (Fig. 4.2), although excessive CPAP can result in reinflation of the collapsed lung interfering with surgical access. Alternatively, PEEP applied to the dependent lung may increase the functional residual capacity by recruiting collapsed alveoli, so reducing any shunt. PEEP is potentially harmful as it increases the pulmonary vascular resistance within

Box 4.7 • Aetiology of perioperative hypoxia during one-lung anaesthesia for oesophageal surgery

- One-lung anaesthesia in a patient with healthy lungs
- Pre-existing disease in the dependent ventilated lung
- Displaced endobronchial tube or endobronchial blocker
- Partly occluded endobronchial tube
- Low cardiac output due to:
  - hypovolaemia
  - mediastinal manipulation
  - compression of the inferior vena cava
  - compression of the right atria
- Perioperative deterioration of the dependent lung
- Exaggerated intrapulmonary shunting secondary to a high thoracic epidural block
- Massive blood transfusion

Box 4.8 • Manoeuvres to minimise hypoxia and pulmonary trauma during the thoracic stage of an oesophagectomy

Dependent lung ventilation
- Increasing the inspired oxygen concentration
- Positive end-expiratory pressure (PEEP)
- Recruitment manoeuvres at start of one-lung ventilation
- Low-volume-controlled ventilation with PEEP
- Pressure-controlled ventilation with PEEP

Non-dependent deflated lung
- Oxygen insufflation
- Continuous positive airway pressure (CPAP)

Both lungs
- Intermittent two-lung ventilation
- Continuous two-lung ventilation with lung retraction

Circulation
- Maintenance of an adequate cardiac output
- Temporary interruption of arterial blood flow to non-dependent lung

the ventilated lung and can redirect blood through the non-ventilated lung. The risk of barotrauma is ever present. OLA, and surgical manipulation of the lung, is associated with the release of inflammatory mediators.[60,61] Combined CPAP and PEEP has also been postulated. In practice, however, this combined manoeuvre is often associated with a significant reduction in cardiac output.

Surgical behaviour is an important factor in the well-being of the patient. Inadvertent surgical compression of the inferior vena cava or the right atrium can precipitate a sudden reduction in cardiac output with deleterious effects on oxygenation and organ perfusion. Supraventricular and ventricular ectopics are common during mediastinal manipulation. Where an appreciable shunt already exists (>30%) a fall in cardiac output will markedly exacerbate any systemic hypoxia. A linear relationship between operative hypotension and surgical manipulation of the mediastinum has been reported.

Although oesophagectomy performed under two-lung ventilation is associated with less pulmonary shunting, surgical access is suboptimal, making radical lymphadenectomy unlikely. Re-identifying the surgical plane after repeated lung inflation and deflation can be difficult (S.M. Griffin, personal communication). Temporary occlusion of the pulmonary artery supplying the non-ventilated lung has been advocated in the past where the hypoxia is persistent and unresponsive to the above measures. In practice this is almost never necessary and, besides, it is not a manoeuvre that can be executed quickly.

On completion of the surgery the collapsed lung is reinflated under direct vision. Failure to reinflate the lung fully can be a major cause of postoperative hypoxia. Difficulty in reinflation, although uncommon, may be encountered if endobronchial secretions are especially tenacious; suction bronchoscopy is then indicated.

Fluid therapy and blood transfusion during upper gastrointestinal surgery

Patients who have received blood transfusions during oesophagectomy for carcinoma have a less favourable outcome.[5,10,12,62,63] Although Craig et al.[64] found long-term survival unaffected, short-term survival was decreased. Where massive blood transfusion is required the association between volume and poor outcome may reflect the circumstances necessitating such large transfusions. Transfused patients have a higher incidence of prominent ulcerative tumours, blood vessel invasion, longer operation times[62] and preoperative chemoradiotherapy, particularly in the elderly.

Anaesthesia, surgery and transfused blood are all immunosuppressant, the latter effect being volume related. Transfused patients are more prone to infection. Operation-induced immunosuppression is maximal in the first 48 hours after surgery. One study reported a deleterious effect in oesophageal surgery after only 3 units.[63]

Indications for blood transfusion should be based entirely on the need for oxygen delivery and haemodynamics rather than an arbitrary haemoglobin level. In a randomised controlled trial in critically ill patients, haemoglobin in the range 7–9 g/dL did not adversely affect mortality when compared with the more liberal use of blood transfusion.[65] Provided the patient is kept normovolaemic and pulmonary gas exchange is unimpeded a degree of postoperative haemodilution will be tolerated by most patients. The exception to this may be patients with known coronary artery disease. Consideration must also be given to the viability of any GI anastomosis. Adequate tissue oxygenation can be maintained at a haematocrit of 25–30%.

Perioperative fluid therapy in relation to surgical outcome remains controversial and the literature often contradictory. Much of current practice is unsupported by sound evidence-based data.[52] Fluid overload as reflected in an increase in postoperative body weight can impair pulmonary gas exchange and GI function, and be deleterious to surgical outcome after abdominal surgery. Sources of excess perioperative fluids, which cause haemodilution, include fluid challenges given to counteract the cardiovascular effects of general anaesthesia and neuroaxil analgesia, the latter of doubtful efficacy and probably unnecessary.[52] Replacing blood lost during surgery with crystalloid or colloid, so avoiding transfusion, necessitates administering fluid volumes several times in excess of the blood volume lost. Fluid retention secondary to the surgical stress response and estimations of evaporative losses from the surgical site are notoriously difficult to assess. Conversely, hypovolaemia is also detrimental to tissue and anastomotic perfusion.[52]

Consensus does prevail in that perioperative fluid losses from preoperative starvation, insensible and nasogastric sources, wound exudation and urine output should be replaced. Hourly evaporative fluid losses from the abdominal and chest cavities during a two-stage oesophagectomy can be well in excess of 32 g/h. Endocrine-mediated water and salt retention during surgery leads to a fall in urine output during upper GI surgery. Provided the patient is normovolaemic and does not have pre-existing renal disease, a lower than normal hourly urine output is usually well tolerated.

Significant reductions in oesophagectomy-related pulmonary morbidity can be achieved by a regime of perioperative fluid restriction. Kita et al.[66]

maintained a central venous pressure of <5 mmHg and an adequate urine output with intraoperative fluids given at 4–5 mL/kg/h, and reported less postoperative respiratory complications after oesophagectomy.

Goal-directed fluid therapy that avoids immediate postoperative weight gain has been shown to be beneficial in lower GI surgery.[52]

Postoperative care

Timing of extubation following gastric and oesophageal surgery

All patients who have undergone an uncomplicated gastrectomy are usually extubated in theatre and then nursed in a ward or high-dependency unit. In the past a short period of overnight elective ventilation was popular following oesophageal resection,[43] but current consensus supports early extubation, either in theatre or in the intensive care unit (ICU)[67] shortly afterwards, as both feasible and desirable leading to shorter critical care stays.[44,67,68] The prerequisite to successful extubation is satisfactory pain control.[67] Michelet et al.,[69] using an OLA ventilatory strategy that reduced inflammatory mediator release, were able to demonstrate an improvement in lung function that resulted in earlier extubation. Prolonged periods of postoperative ventilation put patients at increased risk. Elderly patients admitted to ICU after major surgery, ventilation beyond 24 hours and the need for vasoactive drugs are known to be associated with increased mortality. Successful extubation is dependent on several variables (Box 4.9).

Postoperative analgesia

Pain after upper abdominal and thoracic surgery can be considerable and elicits a marked neurohumoral metabolic response. It has been postulated that attenuation of this stress response will improve surgical outcome. In practice very high concentrations

Box 4.9 • Criteria for successful extubation following gastrointestinal surgery

- Stable cardiovascular system
- Less than 50 mL/h blood loss from the surgical drains
- Absence of hypercarbia
- Adequate oxygen saturation/P_aO_2 on an F_iO_2 of <0.4 whilst breathing spontaneously
- Active cough and gag reflex
- Ability to respond to commands
- Absence of distressing pain and confusion
- Absence of surgical complications

Neoadjuvant therapy was not predictive of extubation failure.[67]

of opiates are required necessitating postoperative ventilatory support or an intense neuraxial block at a high dermatome level. The literature still remains divided as to the long-term value of suppressing the stress response.

Pain after gastrectomy or oesophagectomy inhibits movement and coughing, leading to sputum retention, atelectasis and pulmonary complications. Vital capacity, residual volume and functional residual capacity are all compromised.

 Effective postoperative analgesia following upper GI surgery has been shown to correlate with a reduction in postoperative cardiopulmonary complications.

Pain exacerbates GI ileus. Although the main source of pain will be the surgical site, discomfort can arise from elsewhere. Inability to move around freely in the immediate postoperative period, shoulder pain arising from an unfamiliar posture during thoracotomy, difficulties with micturition, GI distension and hypothermia can all exacerbate existing pain.

Most studies acknowledge that good pain relief following upper GI surgery, however delivered, is crucial to a favourable outcome but the literature remains contradictory as to whether long-term surgical outcome is improved by the choice of analgesic technique. The most popular method currently is epidural analgesia, instituted before induction, using either a continuous infusion of opiate, local anaesthetic or a combination of both. Epidural analgesia is said to offer a number of advantages after upper GI surgery, such as a lower incidence of respiratory morbidity compared with systemic opiates, facilitation of early postoperative extubation[68] and it appears to allow the more rapid return of normal GI function with less risk of anastomotic leak, probably by improving gastric tube microcirculation.[69] It has been recommended that epidural analgesia needs to be employed for 5 days after an oesophagectomy for a beneficial effect on postoperative complications to be observed. Any favourable effect secondary to thoracic epidural analgesia on lung volumes, respiratory mechanics and gas exchange are dependent on the extent of the segmental block.

An alternative technique is patient-controlled systemic opiate analgesia (PCA), often in combination with local anaesthetic regional blocks. Although popular opinion holds that effective epidural analgesia is far superior in the immediate postoperative period, a comparative study with systemic opiate PCA failed to identify any difference in morbidity or mortality rates after transthoracic oesophagectomy.[70] A recent editorial has questioned the strength of evidence that epidural analgesia is truly superior to alternative methods of pain relief following major GI surgery.[71]

Epidural analgesia is a potentially hazardous technique and requires a high degree of skill, particularly in the thoracic region. A significant number of epidurals need manipulation in the postoperative period before satisfactory analgesia is achieved and a small number fail to produce adequate analgesia.[71] Patients must be closely observed by competent staff who are totally familiar with possible side-effects, in particular recognising an excessively high block, hypotension, central nervous system and respiratory depression, catheter migration, spinal haematoma and infection. Other complications associated with epidural analgesia include lower limb motor weakness, pruritus, nausea, headache as a consequence of inadvertent dural puncture and hallucinations.

Bilateral sympathetic autonomic blockade and subsequent hypotension is common after extradural bupivacaine, particularly in the thoracic region. Hypotension is exacerbated by hypovolaemia, head-up posture and limited cardiovascular reserve. Epidural opiates are devoid of these cardiovascular effects but can be associated with central respiratory depression of an unpredictable and insidious onset. The risk of respiratory depression by cephalad spread of the epidural opiate appears to be related to the lipid solubility of the drug. Parenteral opiates are contraindicated in the presence of a functioning epidural. For a fuller discussion of epidural analgesia and abdominal surgery the reader should consult Jackson and Loughnane.[72]

Where systemic opiate PCA is used for postoperative analgesia, adequate monitoring of respiratory function and the conscious state is mandatory. Hallucinations, nausea and vomiting, urinary retention, GI ileus and urticaria have all been reported. PCA is only effective if the patient has the ability to cooperate and comprehend.

Both epidural and PCA techniques can be supplemented by non-steroidal analgesia (NSAIDs). Side-effects of NSAIDs are more common with long-term use. Adequate renal function is a prerequisite to their use.

Infiltration of the wound and muscles with local anaesthetic at the end of surgery is more effective for somatic pain than visceral pain, but may help to reduce the patient's opiate requirement. Bupivacaine, 0.25% without epinephrine, to a maximum dose of 2 mg/kg is the most popular.

Postoperative management

Three conditions are implicated in early postoesophagectomy morbidity and mortality that might be directly influenced by anaesthetic management. They are pulmonary and cardiovascular dysfunction,

and anastomotic breakdown secondary to ischaemia. Patients are most at risk of developing serious complications in the first 3–4 postoperative days. Thoracoabdominal and upper abdominal surgery are associated with a high incidence of postoperative hypoxaemia and desaturation during the early postoperative period when oxygen utilisation is high.[39] Appropriate postoperative facilities for the patient's aftercare must be available prior to undertaking upper GI surgery. Typical postoperative medical complications reported following oesophageal surgery are given in Box 4.10. Surgical complications following upper GI surgery are discussed in Chapters 5 and 6.

The need for a patient recovering from upper GI surgery to proficiently clear bronchial secretions and so avoid atelectasis and hypoxia is paramount. Deep-breathing exercises, chest physiotherapy, heated mist inhalation and incentive spirometry have all been shown to be efficacious in reducing the risk of postoperative pulmonary complications.

The aetiology of postoperative hypoxia following upper GI surgery is multifactorial and typically lasts for several days. Postoperative hypoxia correlates with a number of preoperative predictor risk factors including advancing age, ASA grade 2 and above, functional dependence, COPD, smoking, obesity, thoracic surgery and a prolonged operative time. Patients who were marginally hypoxic preoperatively will inevitably become hypoxic postoperatively unless aggressive action is taken.[10] Atelectasis due to an inability to clear retained secretions, the absence of or decreased sighing and the reduction in expiratory reserve volume all compound the situation. Contributory factors include persistent pain, supine posture, a decrease in thoracic compliance, diaphragmatic and intercostal muscle dysfunction and pleural collections.

An obtunded cough reflex will exacerbate respiratory complications following oesophagectomy and increase the risk of pulmonary aspiration. Oxygen consumption rises in the immediate postoperative period.[39] Despite this increase in oxygen utilisation there is no concomitant increase in the oxygen extraction ratio. At arterial oxygen tensions of <8 kPa or 90% oxygen saturation, end-organ hypoxia can ensue if left uncorrected. This can be further exacerbated by haemodynamic instability. Patients whose oxygen delivery was insufficient 6 hours after surgery have an increased incidence of anastomotic leak.[73] It is imperative that the surgical anastomosis is protected from hypoperfusion and ischaemia. All patients must receive humidified oxygen appropriate to their needs postoperatively and have their oxygen saturation monitored as the provision of oxygen by a face mask alone may be insufficient. Several measures to minimise postoperative hypoxia and pulmonary complications following upper GI surgery have been advocated. Adequate analgesia, a semi-erect posture which increases functional residual capacity, particularly in the obese, continuous humidified oxygen for 4 consecutive days and regular physiotherapy are indicated.

Both peripheral and pulmonary inflammatory changes occur after oesophagectomy. The mechanisms of post-thoracotomy lung injury are unknown, similar to those seen in ARDS, and originate during surgery.[18] The incidence of ARDS following oesophagectomy is given as 14–33%[18] and is a major cause of mortality. The perioperative hypoperfusion of the GI tract may be a trigger for the release of systemic inflammatory mediators leading to increased lung permeability to proteins.

> Changes in lung permeability have been reported following oesophagectomy, as has an elevation of pulmonary leucocytes, plasma cytokines, arachidonic acid and thromboxane B_2, all known mediators of ARDS.[60]

The degree of intraoperative hypotension and hypoxaemia during single-lung ventilation does correlate with postoperative lung injury.[18] Other inflammatory triggers include the relative hypoperfusion of the non-ventilated lung leading to ischaemia, and barotrauma to the dependent ventilated lung during the thoracic stage of an oesophagectomy.

Fluid and blood requirements have to be carefully monitored during the immediate postoperative period. Perioperative hypotension and hypoxaemia, as indicated by the need for fluid challenges, blood products, vasopressors and inotropes, is known to be associated with an increased risk of postoperative ARDS.[18] Patients who have undergone a prolonged oesophagectomy often require appreciable volumes of fluid in the immediate postoperative period and a brief period of invasive cardiovascular monitoring is prudent. Central venous pressure and urine output are useful in the evaluation of the patient's fluid requirements.

Between 5% and 10% of patients who have undergone an oesophagectomy will experience cardiovascular complications.[8] Cardiac dysrhythmias are not uncommon within the first 2 postoperative days. All arrhythmias that persist into the postoperative period should be investigated and hypokalaemia and hypomagnesaemia excluded. The most common arrhythmia is atrial fibrillation (AF),[74] the aetiology of which is multifactorial (Box 4.11). Prompt investigation is essential as it may be a systemic manifestation of some serious underlying complication such as mediastinitis secondary to an anastomotic leak. In one study of 427 patients the intraoperative incidence of AF was 17% with a reoccurrence rate of 37% within the first 3 postoperative days.[75] Others have reported an incidence of 20–60% overall.[76]

Postoperative AF associated with sepsis typically starts after day 3, whereas the earlier onset of AF appears to be less sinister. Postoperative AF occurs more frequently in males over 65 years of age with a higher incidence of pulmonary complications. Other contributory factors include a history of pre-existing COPD and cardiac disease, postoperative hypoxia, dilatation of the gastric remnant within the thorax, a cervical anastomosis,[74] poor pulmonary function tests and an elevated central venous pressure.[75]

Neither prophylactic digitalisation or thoracic epidural analgesia appear to have any effect on the incidence of AF following oesophagectomy. Interestingly, in non-cardiac thoracic surgery, statin therapy was associated with a reduced risk of postoperative AF.

Box 4.10 • Typical postoperative medical complications complications following Ivor–Lewis oesophagectomy*

Major

- Bronchopneumonia
- Respiratory failure
- Acute respiratory distress syndrome (ARDS)
- Myocardial infarction
- Unstable angina
- Cardiac failure
- Thromboembolism

Minor

- Arrhythmias
- Psychiatric
- Infective diarrhoea
- Urinary tract infection

*Postoperative surgical complications are discussed in Chapters 5 and 6.

Box 4.11 • Aetiology of postoperative atrial fibrillation following an oesophagectomy

- Anastomotic leak
- Surgical sepsis
- Advancing age
- Pre-existing cardiac and vascular disease
- Intraoperative blood loss
- Extensive high thoracic dissection
- Cervical anastomosis
- Malpositioned chest drains
- Intrathoracic gastric dilatation

- The preoperative physiological state of the patient is one of the most important factors in assessing operative suitability (case selection) and determining outcome following major surgery. Meticulous preoperative evaluation and work-up are a prerequisite to successful surgical outcome.
- All studies agree that coexisting medical conditions, major abdominal or thoracic surgery and increasing age carry a risk of increased perioperative morbidity and mortality.
- The literature fails to identify a specific preoperative risk factor that reliably predicts surgical outcome following upper GI surgery. The aetiology of postoperative complications is multifactorial and may differ between gastric and oesophageal surgery. The data do, however, strongly support the view that patients with a reduced cardiorespiratory reserve tolerate upper abdominal and thoracic surgery poorly.
- Previous myocardial infarction, ischaemia, ventricular hypertrophy, heart failure, conduction and rhythm disturbances appreciably add to the operative risks.
- Upper abdominal and thoracic surgery has a deleterious effect on cardiopulmonary function, which has major implications for postoperative care.
- Significantly impaired preoperative pulmonary function will result in difficulties in maintaining adequate oxygenation during one-lung anaesthesia and in the postoperative period. Abnormal pulmonary function tests alone correlate poorly with the incidence of postoperative complications.
- Diabetes mellitus merits special attention when considering a patient for upper GI surgery. Liver cirrhosis and increasing age are also major risk factors.
- Poor exercise tolerance is associated with an increased risk of perioperative complications independent of age and all other patient characteristics. In selected patients preoperative CPX testing may potentially be of value in stratifying operative risk. Preoperative exercise testing may identify previously unrecognised medical problems, but is probably of limited value in asymptomatic healthy individuals.
- Coexisting remediable risk factors should be identified early and the preoperative period used efficiently to optimise the patient's fitness for anaesthesia, surgery and the postoperative period. Optimisation of cardiac and respiratory function and attention to nutritional status are increasingly important.
- Although there appears to be insufficient evidence to support preoperative spirometry as a tool to stratify pulmonary risk for non-cardiothoracic surgery, it would still be prudent to implement appropriate risk-reduction strategies prior to a thoracotomy when the results of pulmonary function testing suggest suboptimal function, especially when the patient is symptomatic.
- There is continuing interest and research into haemodynamic preoptimisation before major upper GI surgery, although consensus as to how this is best achieved remains debatable. Many published studies are underpowered.
- An appropriately experienced anaesthetist is essential for the safe management of one-lung anaesthesia during the thoracic phase of oesophageal resection.
- Pulmonary and cardiovascular dysfunction and anastomotic breakdown are three conditions that are implicated in early postoesophagectomy morbidity and mortality that might be directly influenced by anaesthetic management.
- The postoperative care of these patients has to be of a high standard if the skills of the anaesthetist and surgeon are to be consolidated. In this regard the first 48–72 hours postoperatively are extremely important.
- Upper GI surgery and one-lung anaesthesia provoke a marked inflammatory response within the GI tract and the lung. There is continuing research into the mechanisms and optimum management of post-thoracotomy lung injury, a significant cause of morbidity and mortality after thoracic surgery.
- Satisfactory postoperative analgesia appears to correlate with an improved outcome. The published evidence to date suggests that adequate postoperative analgesia following oesophagectomy is a prerequisite if a reduction in postoperative cardiopulmonary complications is to be achieved.

- Epidural analgesia is used widely for pain relief in patients undergoing upper abdominal or thoracic incisions. This requires both an experienced anaesthetist and nursing in an appropriate clinical area, ideally with the input of an acute pain team, if complications of this potentially hazardous technique are to be avoided. Epidural analgesia may be superior in the immediate postoperative period, but does not appear to offer any long-term advantages when compared to alternative methods of analgesia following upper GI surgery.
- Successful surgical outcome can only be achieved by a high standard of perioperative care. Timely communication between all the professionals involved is essential.

References

1. Shoemaker WC, Appel PL, Kram HB. Role of oxygen debit in the development of organ failure sepsis, and death in high-risk surgical patients. Chest 1992; 101:208–90.

2. Ferguson MK, Martin TR, Reeder LB et al. Mortality after oesophagectomy: risk factor analysis. World J Surg 1997; 21:599–603.

3. Bartels H, Stein HJ, Siewert JR. Preoperative risk analysis and postoperative mortality of oesophagectomy for resectable oesophageal cancer. Br J Surg 1998; 85:840–4.

4. Nagamatsu Y, Shima I, Yamana H et al. Preoperative evaluation of cardiopulmonary reserve with the use of expired gas analysis during exercise testing in patients with carcinoma of the thoracic oesophagus. J Thorac Cardiovasc Surg 2001; 121:1064–8.

5. Bailey SH, Bull DA, Harpole DH et al. Outcomes after esophagectomy: a ten year prospective cohort. Ann Thorac Surg 2003; 75:210–16.

6. Guidance on Commissioning Cancer Services: improving outcomes in upper GI cancer. The manual. NHS Executive, Department of Health, pp. 26–34.

7. Ferguson MK, Durkin AE. Preoperative prediction of the risk of pulmonary complications after oesophagectomy. J Thorac Cardiovasc Surg 2002; 123:661–8.

8. Griffin SM, Shaw IH, Dresner SM. Early complications after Ivor–Lewis subtotal esophagectomy with two-field lymphadenectomy. Risk factors and management. J Am Coll Surg 2002; 194:285–97.

9. Atkins BZ, Shah AS, Hutcheson KA et al. Reducing hospital morbidity and mortality following esophagectomy. Ann Thorac Surg 2004; 78:1170–6.

10. Tsutsui S, Moriguchi S, Morita M et al. Multivariate analysis of postoperative complications after esophageal resection. Ann Thorac Surg 1992; 53:1052–6.

11. Avendano CE, Flume PA, Silvestri GA et al. Pulmonary complications after esophagectomy. Ann Thorac Surg 2002; 73:922–6.

12. Law S, Wong KH, Kwok KF et al. Predictive factors for postoperative pulmonary complications and mortality after esophagectomy for cancer. Ann Surg 2004; 240:791–800.

13. Abunasra H, Lewis S, Beggs L et al. Predictors of operative death after oesophagectomy for carcinoma. Br J Surg 2005; 92:1029–33.

14. Schroder W, Bollschweiler E, Kossow C et al. Preoperative risk analysis – a reliable predictor of postoperative outcome after transthoracic esophagectomy? Langenbeck's Arch Surg 2006; 391:455–60.

15. Steyerberg EW, Neville BA, Koppert LB et al. Surgical mortality in patients with esophageal cancer: development and validation of a simple risk score. J Clin Oncol 2006; 24:4277–84.

16. Murray P, Whiting P, Hutchinson SP et al. Preoperative shuttle walking testing and outcome after oesophagectomy. Br J Anaesth 2007; 99:809–11.

17. Nagawa H, Kobori O, Muto T. Prediction of pulmonary complications after transthoracic oesophagectomy. Br J Surg 1994; 81:860–2.

18. Tandon S, Batchelor A, Bullock R et al. Perioperative risk factors for acute lung injury after elective oesophagectomy. Br J Anaesth 2001; 86:633–8.

    A study from a specialist unit of lung injury following elective oesophagectomy. The incidence of postoperative adult respiratory distress syndrome was more common in patients who had prolonged one-lung anaesthesia and displayed preoperative instability.

19. Haynes N, Shaw IH, Griffin SM. Comparison of conventional Lewis–Tanner two stage oesophagectomy with synchronous two-team approach. Br J Surg 1995; 82:95–7.

20. Kelley ST, Coppola D, Karl RC. Neoadjuvant chemotherapy is not associated with a higher complication rate vs. surgery alone in patients undergoing esophagectomy. J Gastrointest Surg 2004; 8:277–31.

21. Bollschweiler E, Schroder W, Holscher AH et al. Preoperative risk analysis in patients with adenocarcinoma or squamous cell carcinoma of the oesophagus. Br J Surg 2000; 87:1106–10.

22. Golubovic V, Golubovic S. ASA scores as prognostic criterion for incidence of postoperative complications after transhiatal esophagectomy. Coll Antropol 2002; 26:149–53.

23. Kuwano H, Sumiyoshi K, Sonoda K et al. Relationship between perioperative assessment of organ function and postoperative morbidity in patients with oesophageal cancer. Eur J Surg 1998; 164:581–6.

24. Kinugasa S, Tachibana M, Yoshimura H et al. Esophageal resection in elderly patients: improvement in postoperative complications. Ann Thorac Surg 2001; 71:414–18.

25. Zafirellis KD, Fountoulakis K, Dolan SP et al. Evaluation of POSSUM in patients with oesophageal cancer undergoing resection. Br J Surg 2002; 89:1150–5.

26. Prytherch DR, Whiteley MS, Waever PC et al. POSSUM and Portsmouth POSSUM for predicting mortality. Br J Surg 1998; 85:1217–20.

27. Tekkis PP, McCulloch P, Poloniecki JD et al. Risk adjusted prediction of operative mortality in oesophagogastric surgery with O-POSSUM. Br J Surg 2004; 91:288–95.

28. Lagarde SM, Maris AK, de Castro SM et al. Evaluation of O-POSSUM in predicting in-hospital mortality after resection for oesophageal cancer. Br J Surg 2007; 94:1521–6.

29. Nagabhushan JS, Srinath S, Weir F et al. Comparison of P-POSSUM and O-POSSUM in predicting mortality after oesophagogastric resections. Postgrad Med J 2007; 83:355–8.

30. Lai F, Kwan TL, Yeun WC et al. Evaluation of various POSSUM models for predicting mortality in patients undergoing elective oesophagectomy for carcinoma. Br J Surg 2007; 94:1172–8.

31. Eagle KA, Brundage BH, Chaitman BR et al. Guidelines for perioperative cardiovascular evaluation for non-cardiac surgery. J Am Coll Cardiol 1996; 27:910–48.

32. Eagle KA, Berger PB, Calkins H et al. ACC/AHA guideline update for perioperative cardiovascular evaluation for non-cardiac surgery. Circulation 2002; 105:1257–67.

33. Fleisher LA, Beckman JA, Brown KA et al. ACC/AHA 2007 guidelines on perioperative cardiovascular evaluation and care for non-cardiac surgery: Executive Summary. Circulation 2007; 116:1971–96.

34. Beckman JA, Brown KA, Calkins H et al. ACC/AHA 2006 guideline update on perioperative cardiovascular evaluation for non-cardiac surgery: focused update on perioperative beta-blocker therapy. J Am Coll Cardiol 2006; 47:2345–55.

35. Cohen SL, Goldman L. Preoperative risk evaluation and perioperative management of patients with coronary artery disease. Med Clin North Am 2003; 87:111–36.

36. Lawrence VA, Cornell JE, Smetana GW. Strategies to reduce postoperative pulmonary complications after noncardiac surgery: systematic review for the American College of Physicians. Ann Intern Med 2006; 144:596–608.

37. Fletcher GF, Balady G, Froelicher VF et al. Exercise standards. Circulation 1995; 91:580–615.

38. Girish M, Trayner E, Dammann O et al. Symptom limited stair climbing as a predictor of postoperative cardiorespiratory complications after high risk surgery. Chest 2001; 28:2893–7.

39. Saito H, Minamiya Y, Kawai H et al. Estimation of pulmonary oxygen consumption in the early postoperative period after thoracic surgery. Anaesthesia 2007; 62:648–53.

40. Davies SJ, Wilson RJ. Cardiopulmonary exercise testing for the surgical patient. Care Crit Ill 2007; 23:110–18.

41. Older P, Smith R, Hall F et al. Preoperative cardiopulmonary risk assessment by cardiopulmonary exercise testing. Crit Care Resus 2000; 2:198–208.

42. Dang A, Aguilar J, Riedel B et al. Preoperative chemoradiation impacts physiologic capacity of patients scheduled for esophagectomy. Anesthesiology 2007; 107:A777.

43. Forshaw MJ, Strauss DC, Davies AR et al. Is cardiopulmonary testing a useful test before esophagectomy? Ann Thorac Surg 2007; 85:294–9.

44. Singh SJ, Morgan MDL, Scott S et al. Development of a shuttle walking test of disability in patients with chronic airways disease. Thorax 1992; 47:1019–24.

45. Biccard BM, Sear JW, Foex P. Meta-analysis of the effect of heart rate achieved by perioperative beta-adrenergic blockade on cardiovascular outcomes. Br J Anaesth 2008; 100:23–8.

46. Auerbach AD, Goldman L. Beta-blockers and reduction of cardiac events in non-cardiac surgery. JAMA 2002; 287:1435–45.

47. Hindler K, Shaw AD, Samuels J et al. Improved postoperative outcomes associated with preoperative statin therapy. Anesthesiology 2006; 105:1260–72.

48. Kapoor AS, Kanji H, Buckingham J et al. Strength of evidence for perioperative use of statins to reduce cardiovascular risk: systematic review of controlled studies. Br Med J 2006; 333:1149–52.

49. Wilson J, Wood I, Fawcett J et al. Reducing the risk of major elective surgery: randomised controlled trial of preoperative optimisation of oxygen therapy. Br Med J 1999; 7191:1099–103.

50. Kinsella J. Effect of perioperative fluid therapy on outcome following major surgery. R Coll Anaesth Bull 2001; 8:362–5.

51. Dresner SM, Hayes N, Lamb PJ et al. Prognostic significance of peri-operative blood transfusion following radical resection for oesophageal carcinoma. Eur J Surg Oncol 2000; 26:492–7.

52. Brandstrup B. Fluid therapy in the surgical patient. Best Pract Res Clin Anaesth 2006; 20:265–83.

53. Davies SJ, Wilson RJT. Preoperative optimization of the high-risk surgical patient. Br J Anaesth 2004; 93:121–8.

54. Windsor A, Braga M, Martindale R et al. Fit for surgery. An expert panel review on optimizing patients prior to surgery, with a particular focus on nutrition. Surgeon 2004; 2:315–19.

55. Kondrup J, Rasmussen HH, Hamberg O et al. ESPEN Working Group. Nutritional risk screening: a new method based on an analysis of controlled clinical trials. Clin Nutr 2003; 22:321–36.

56. Murphy PM, Modi P, Bahamim J et al. An investigation into the current perioperative nutritional management of oesophageal carcinoma patients in major centres in England. Ann R Coll Surg Engl 2006; 88:358–62.

57. Sultan J, Di Franco F, Seal CJ et al. The effect of omega-3 fatty acids (O-3FA) on antioxidant status, human leukocyte antigen (HLA)-DR expression on leukocytes and clinical outcome in oesophago-gastric cancer surgery (OGCS). Br J Surg 2008; 95(S3):83.

58. Howard-Ape GM, de Bono J, Hudsmith L et al. Coronary artery stents and non-cardiac surgery. Br J Anaesth 2007; 98:560–74.

59. Vanner R. Arndt endobronchial blocker during oesophagectomy. Anaesthesia 2005; 60:295–6.

60. Cree RT, Warnell I, Staunton M et al. Alveolar and plasma concentrations of interleukin-8 and vascular endothelium growth factor following oesophagectomy. Anaesthesia 2004; 59:867–71.

    A study from a specialist upper gastrointestinal unit demonstrating that oesophageal surgery triggers the release of pulmonary proinflammatory mediators, a potential aetiological factor in subclinical lung injury.

61. Michelet P, D'Journo XB, Roch A et al. Protective ventilation influences systemic inflammation after esophagectomy. Anesthesiology 2006; 105:911–19.

62. Tachibana M, Tabara H, Kotoh T et al. Prognostic significance of perioperative blood transfusion in resectable thoracic esophageal cancer. Am J Gastroenterol 1999; 94:757–65.

63. Langley SM, Alexiou C, Bailey DH et al. The influence of perioperative blood transfusion on survival after esophageal resection for carcinoma. Ann Thorac Surg 2002; 73:1704–9.

64. Craig SR, Adam DJ, Yap PL et al. Effect of blood transfusion on survival after esophagogastrectomy for carcinoma. Ann Thorac Surg 1998; 66:356–61.

65. Herbert PC, Wells G, Blajchman MA et al. A multicenter randomised controlled clinical trial of blood transfusion in the critically ill. N Engl J Med 1999; 340:409–17.

66. Kita T, Mammoto T, Kishi Y. Fluid management and postoperative respiratory disturbances in patients with transthoracic esophagectomy for carcinoma. J Clin Anaesth 2002; 14:252–6.

67. Lanuti M, de Delva PE, Maher A et al. Feasibility and outcomes of early extubation policy after esophagectomy. Ann Thorac Surg 2006; 82:2037–41.

68. Chandrarashekar MV, Irving M, Wayman J et al. Immediate extubation and epidural analgesia allow safe management in a high dependency unit after two-stage oesophagectomy. Br J Anaesth 2003; 90:474–9.

69. Michelet P, Roch A, D'Journo XB et al. Effect of thoracic epidural analgesia on gastric blood flow after oesophagectomy. Acta Anaesthesiol Scand 2007; 51:587–94.

70. Rudin A, Flisberg P, Johansson J et al. Thoracic epidural analgesia or intravenous morphine analgesia after thoracoabdominal esophagectomy: a prospective follow-up of 210 patients. J Cardiothorac Vasc Anesth 2005; 19:350–57.

71. Low J, Johnston N, Morris C. Epidural analgesia: first do no harm. Anaesthesia 2008; 63:1–3.

72. Jackson T, Loughnane F. Regional anesthesia in abdominal surgery. In: Kumar CM, Bellamy M (eds) Gastrointestinal and colorectal anaesthesia. New York: Informa Healthcare, 2007; Chap. 11, pp. 111–25.

73. Kusano C, Baba M, Takao S et al. Oxygen delivery as a factor in the development of fatal postoperative complications after oesophagectomy. Br J Surg 1997; 84:252–7.

74. Ma JY, Wang Y, Zhao YF et al. Atrial fibrillation after surgery for esophageal carcinoma: clinical and prognostic significance. World J Gastroenterol 2006; 12:449–52.

75. Hahm TS, Lee JJ, Yang MK et al. Risk factors for an intraoperative arrhythmia during esophagectomy. Yonsei Med J 2007; 48:474–9.

76. Murthy SC, Law S, Whooley BP et al. Atrial fibrillation after oesophagectomy is a marker for postoperative morbidity and mortality. J Thorac Cardiovasc Surg 2003; 126:1162–7.

5

Surgery for cancer of the oesophagus

S. Michael Griffin

Introduction

Oesophageal cancer is well recognised as being one of the most challenging pathological conditions confronting the surgeon. This is not only due to the versatility required in surgical reconstruction, but also the magnitude of the surgical procedure, dealing with wide areas of the neck, mediastinum and abdomen. Many efforts have been made to increase the cure rate while maintaining the safety of the procedure, but despite this the overall survival for oesophageal cancer remains around 10% in most countries. Whereas management and treatment for cancer of the oesophagus is multidisciplinary, surgery, whenever possible, is still the primary mode of therapy. The surgical approach and extent of resection and dissection required may need to differ in individual cases, depending on the nature of the tumour and the condition of the patient. In the UK 70% of cases are now adenocarcinoma of the lower oesophagus or gastro-oesophageal junction, which represent a different disease from the previously more common squamous carcinoma. This chapter includes the surgical management of adenocarcinoma of the lower oesophagus and the cardia (Siewert types 1 and 2), which are frequently staged and treated as oesophageal cancers, but not subcardial tumours (Siewert type 3), which are described elsewhere (Chapter 7).

Unfortunately the disease often presents late when increasing dysphagia has developed over several months. As a result of poor fitness or unresectable disease only 30–40% of patients are suitable for radical potentially curative treatment, whilst the majority receive non-surgical therapies with the aim of palliation. Outcome is strongly stage dependent; whilst early tumours have excellent results with surgery alone, the majority with transmural or node-positive tumours appear to benefit from multimodality therapy, combining surgery with neoadjuvant chemotherapy or chemoradiotherapy (Chapter 9). The multidisciplinary team must exercise judgement in the choice of the appropriate combination of therapies for each individual patient. This will depend on patient age, fitness, symptoms, prognosis and evidence base, as well as the overall stage and histopathology.

Surgical pathology

The vast majority of oesophageal neoplasms are epithelial in origin. They arise from the squamous lining of the mucosa, but more commonly from metaplastic columnar epithelium, resulting in glandular carcinomas affecting the specialised epithelium in the lower oesophagus. Tumour site and histology are two crucial factors requiring assessment: tumours arising from different sites in the oesophagus vary in their behaviour. Squamous cell carcinoma arising from the cervical and thoracic oesophagus and adenocarcinoma arising in the thoracic oesophagus and cardia differ in their mode of spread and response to therapeutic modalities. It is essential, therefore, that the anatomical regions of the oesophagus are described such that the different therapeutic surgical procedures adopted for tumours at each site can be understood.

Surgical anatomy

The oesophagus is a midline hollow viscus, starting at the cricopharyngeal sphincter at the level of the sixth cervical vertebra, entering the chest at the level of the suprasternal notch, traversing the posterior mediastinum and entering the abdomen through the oesophageal hiatus in the diaphragm to join the stomach at the cardia. It bears a close relationship to the trachea and pericardium in front and the vertebral column posteriorly. The vagus and its branches are in close proximity over its entire length. There is no serosal covering. The thoracic duct enters the posterior mediastinum through the aortic opening in the diaphragm. It lies on the bodies of the thoracic vertebrae posterolateral to the oesophagus and between the aorta and the azygos vein. The left atrium and the inferior pulmonary veins lie in intimate contact with the left wall of the lower third of the oesophagus.

The TNM classification has been proposed and revised in 2002[1] to combine the salient features of the staging process. This classification has divided the oesophagus into discrete anatomical regions (**Fig. 5.1**).

Hypopharynx and cervical oesophagus

The region between the level of the pharyngoepiglottic fold and the inferior border of the cricoid cartilage is known as the hypopharynx, that above as the oropharynx. The cervical oesophagus begins at the lower border of the cricoid cartilage and terminates at the level of the thoracic inlet or jugular notch. Surgical management of carcinomas in these regions differs from that of other parts of the oesophagus, because tumour extension in these two areas commonly overlaps. This is considered separately later in the chapter.

Upper oesophagus

This segment of the oesophagus extends between the level of the jugular notch and the carina.

Middle oesophagus

This section of the oesophagus extends from the tracheal bifurcation to the midpoint between the tracheal bifurcation and the oesophagogastric junction.

Lower oesophagus

This is comprised of both the lower thoracic oesophagus and the hiatal segment of the oesophagus. The latter segment is often termed the 'abdominal oesophagus'. The oesophagogastric junction is a somewhat nebulous term, and the anatomy depends on the differing viewpoints of surgeons, endoscopists, radiologists, pathologists and anatomists. It is further complicated by the presence or absence of a hiatal hernia and the presence or absence of a columnar-lined oesophagus.

Blood supply and lymphatic drainage

The blood supply is derived directly from the aorta in the form of oesophageal vessels together with branches adjacent to or from organs such as the pulmonary hilum, trachea, stomach and thyroid gland. The venous drainage is through tributaries draining into the azygos and hemiazygos system in the chest, via the thyroid veins in the neck and the left gastric vein in the upper abdomen.

The lymphatics of the oesophagus are distributed predominantly in the form of a submucosal

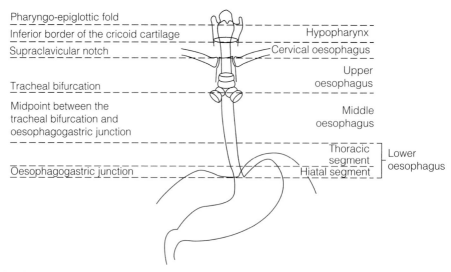

Figure 5.1 • Anatomical regions of the hypopharynx, oesophagus and gastric cardia.

plexus and a paraoesophageal plexus. Both plexuses receive lymph from all parts of the respective layers of the oesophageal wall. The plexuses communicate through penetrating vessels that traverse the longitudinal and circular muscle walls. The paraoesophageal plexus drains into the paraoesophageal lymph nodes, which are situated on the surface of the oesophagus, and also into perioesophageal lymph nodes, situated in close proximity to the oesophagus. Lymphatics also drain from the perioesophageal nodes to the lateral oesophageal nodes or directly from the paraoesophageal to the lateral oesophageal nodes, skipping the perioesophageal group[2] (Box 5.1).

Preoperative surgical preparation

Meticulous preoperative evaluation to accurately stage the tumour and estimate surgical risk is a crucial prerequisite to successful surgical outcome in this disease (see also Chapters 3 and 4).

Nutritional support

Significant malnutrition as well as dehydration are frequently seen in patients with oesophageal narrowing and should be corrected preoperatively. Malnutrition is associated with loss of tissue function, leading to many potential complications during the postoperative period, such as wound breakdown, respiratory failure secondary to poor respiratory muscle function as well as deep vein thrombosis and infective complications.[3] Nutritional deficiency can be corrected either enterally or parenterally. Enteral feeding is simpler and safer, using high-calorie and

high-protein liquid feeds of known volume and composition, given either by mouth via a fine-bore tube placed endoscopically or via a jejunostomy. Perioperative enteral nutrition with the addition of nutrients that can modulate the immune system, termed 'immunonutrition', has been proposed to further reduce postoperative complications and improve outcome.[4]

There is evidence that oesophageal dilatation preoperatively is a high-risk procedure and can affect cure rates if resulting in perforation. For this reason establishment of external nutrition before embarking on multimodal therapy is increasingly standard practice.[5]

The routine use of parenteral feeding (total parenteral nutrition, TPN) is contraindicated on general and immunological grounds and should be avoided in order to minimise nosocomial infections and associated sepsis.

There is evidence that increased nosocomial infections occur when the gastrointestinal (GI) tract is not used for nutrition in the pre- and postoperative periods.[6]

In those patients who have failed to show satisfactory improvement, it may be necessary to construct a feeding jejunostomy, either before or at the time of routine surgery, in order to continue adequate alimentation via the enteral route. Although feeding jejunostomy has a major role to play in alimentation after the perioperative period, routine preoperative and postoperative feeding by jejunostomy in every patient has yet to be proven efficacious on current evidence.[7] A large study from Milan

---

Box 5.1 • Lymph nodes of the oesophagus

Paraoesophageal nodes (on the wall of the oesophagus)*	Left gastric (7)
	Lesser curvature (3)
Cervical (101)	Coeliac (9)
Upper thoracic (105)	Right cardiac (1)
Middle thoracic (108)	Left cardiac (2)
Lower thoracic (110)	
Perioesophageal nodes (in immediate apposition to the oesophagus)	**Lateral oesophageal nodes (located lateral to the oesophagus)**
Deep cervical (102)	Lateral cervical (100)
Supraclavicular (104)	Hilar (109)
Paratracheal (106)	Suprapyloric (5)
Tracheal bifurcation (107)	Subpyloric (6)
Para-aortic or posterior mediastinal (112)	Common hepatic (8)
Diaphragmatic (111)	Greater curvature (4)

* For location see Chapter 3, Fig. 3.3.

suggests that the complications associated with jejunostomy are outweighed by the benefits of early enteral administration.[8]

Respiratory care

Optimisation of respiratory function is vital in preventing the serious pulmonary complications associated with prolonged surgery and thoracotomy. Smoking must be stopped as early as possible, ideally 6 weeks prior to surgery, with the aid of nicotine replacement. Preoperative physiotherapy with coughing exercises and effective use of the diaphragm by restoration of muscle strength through ambulation is encouraged. High-risk patients should also be provided with vigorous physiotherapy with or without bronchodilators prior to surgery. Orodental hygiene is also important in removing a source of chronic sepsis that could disseminate infection to the tracheobronchial tree during intubation.

Prophylactic low-molecular-weight heparin together with antithromboembolism stockings must be provided as soon as the patient comes into hospital to reduce the incidence of thromboembolic complications

Mental preparation/ communication

To minimise fear and apprehension, every effort must be made to familiarise the patient with the hospital environment, including the intensive care unit. Patient cooperation is crucial and can be enhanced by reassurance and meticulous communication. Descriptions of the methods of pain relief, oxygen and intravenous fluid administration, and the awareness of intercostal tube drainage and the likelihood of prolonged periods without oral intake, must be adequately explained. All patients and their relatives should be counselled about the treatment options, paying particular attention to results, limitations and expectations of surgery. The counselling process is greatly enhanced by the involvement of a trained clinical nurse specialist in oesophagogastric cancer.

Detailed perioperative preparation and anaesthetic details are highlighted and explained in depth in Chapter 4.

Surgical objectives

Oesophagectomy for cancer should only be undertaken when a potentially curative R0 resection (complete removal of all macroscopic and microscopic cancer) is expected. Unlike colorectal carcinoma, there is no role for resection in the presence of proven distant metastases (e.g. liver), no matter how localised.

Survival is related to the stage of disease; with stage I disease, 5-year survivals of greater than 80% have been achieved,[9] emphasising the importance of early

detection. Resection alone, therefore, must be the chosen method of therapy in fit patients with T1 tumours of the middle and lower thirds of the oesophagus. In stage III disease, surgery alone produces poor results with prolonged survival for only 10–20% of cases.[10] It appears that both neoadjuvant chemotherapy and radiotherapy provide a benefit for these patients.[11] Further randomised trials must be completed in order to outline the optimal therapeutic strategy.

An attitude of pessimism had prevailed over many years owing to poor surgical results achieved in small series by non-specialised units. The overall results of surgical resection for all stages of tumour have improved over the past 20 years, with falling morbidity and mortality associated with the procedure. The reasons for this are listed in Box 5.2 and have been documented in detail in the COG Guidance Report on Upper GI Cancers.[12] Among these is an increased tendency to concentrate the management of such cases in specialist units, with the numbers treated allowing the development of a multidisciplinary approach that involves surgeons, gastroenterologists, clinical oncologists, anaesthetists, radiologists and intensivists, as well as physiotherapists and clinical and specialist nursing staff. Studies have confirmed that improved results parallel experience in managing this condition,[13] and poor results occur when experience is limited.[14,15] There is now overwhelming evidence to confirm the influence of surgeon case volume on the outcome of site-specific cancer surgery.[14-16] Other reasons for improved outcome include better patient selection, earlier diagnosis by open-access endoscopy, surveillance of Barrett's oesophagus, and improved preoperative, operative and postoperative management.

Principles of oesophagectomy

Resection of primary tumour

Oesophageal cancer spreads longitudinally in the submucosal lymphatics. The incidence of positive resection margins reported in the literature is high. Fortunately, with new advances in endoscopic and radiological techniques such as endoscopic ultrasound, the tumour extent and spread, together with the diagnosis of synchronous lesions, can now be accurately assessed. It is crucial to obtain

---

Box 5.2 • Reasons for improved results for oesophageal resection

- Increase in specialist units
- Multidisciplinary approach
- Earlier diagnosis
- Better patient selection
- Improved perioperative management

accurate information concerning these tumours by careful examination using video endoscopy, endoscopic ultrasound and spiral computed tomography in the preoperative staging process. This will help to determine the exact level of resection. It is still often difficult to ascertain the length required for clear surgical margins, particularly in high lesions, despite exhaustive preoperative investigations.

Rules on resection margins

Most authors would agree that in order to make allowance for intramural submucosal spread of both squamous and adenocarcinomas, a subtotal oesophagectomy should be carried out in patients with tumours of the mid and lower oesophagus. Much discussion has centred around how many centimetres of macroscopically normal oesophagus should routinely be removed either side of the palpable primary lesion. For squamous carcinoma this usually concerns the proximal margins whereas for adenocarcinoma, particularly of the gastrooesophageal junction, the distal margin (gastric) is usually the greater concern. Skinner[17] advocated that a minimum resection margin of 10 cm from the palpable edge of the tumour was essential to minimise the risk of anastomotic recurrence and positive resection margins. This figure, however, does not take into account the nature, pattern and location of the primary cancer. It also fails to discriminate between in vivo margins of resection and resection margins measured by the histopathologist when a considerable degree of shrinkage has occurred after fixation in formalin.[18]

Primary tumours with multicentric lesions require more extensive lengths for safe surgical margins. In squamous cancers, three representative patterns of presentation are encountered (**Fig. 5.2**).[19] Failure to take this into account may explain the finding of positive resection margins in nearly 40% of specimens when the oesophageal resection margin is limited to only 4 cm, and even in 17% when the margin is 10 cm. Therefore, 10 cm is a reasonable resection margin to attain in both directions **if this is possible**. In practice, this rule can rarely be achieved. A 10-cm margin on both sides of a tumour measuring an average of 5.5 cm would require an overall length of specimen exceeding that of the normal human oesophagus.

Many studies have also demonstrated that localised tumours require shorter lengths of clearance for safe surgical margins. Much of the published evidence is conflicting and it has been suggested that a resection margin of as little as 4 cm results in low incidence of anastomotic recurrence. It is the author's opinion that when only a short resection margin can be obtained through the thoracic exposure, a cervical phase with total oesophagectomy is advisable.

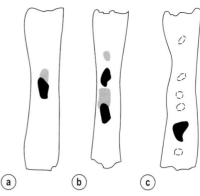

Figure 5.2 • **(a)** A single cancer. **(b)** Multifocal cancer. **(c)** Intramural lymphovascular spread. There is a high risk of positive resection margins in (b) and (c). Shaded areas represent submucosal spread.

Adenocarcinoma of the lower oesophagus commonly infiltrates the gastric cardia, fundus and lesser curve. Extensive sleeve resection of the lesser curve and fundus with the formation of a tubular conduit is necessary to minimise positive distal resection margins. Other studies have demonstrated that patients with microscopically positive margins undergoing palliative resection died of other manifestations before clinical evidence of locoregional recurrence.[20,21] A tumour-free surgical margin is therefore not the only important factor to be considered in radical surgery. Nevertheless, it should remain the main goal of every operation.

Obtaining an adequate tumour-free radial resection margin appears to be equally important, and has been reported to be an independent prognostic factor for oesophageal cancer. Whilst the potential benefits of extended lynphadenectomy are discussed later, these are only relevant if the primary tumour has been adequately excised. An adequate circumferential margin of greater than 1 mm is required to confirm complete resection.[22]

Resection of lymph nodes

As for many other solid-organ tumours, controversy persists as to the value of lymphadenectomy in squamous and adenocarcinoma of the oesophagus. There are two predominant attitudes. First, there is the concept that lymph node metastases are simply markers of systemic disease and the removal of involved nodes will confer no benefit. Consequently, some surgeons advocate removal of the primary lesion alone and claim the same survival as with more extensive resections.[23] Second, there is the belief that cure can be obtained in some patients with positive nodes by a radical surgical approach focusing on wide excision and extended lymphadenectomy using a transthoracic approach.

There is little doubt that some patients with oesophageal cancer who have lymph node involvement could be cured by surgical clearance.[24] The identification of those patients with a low burden of nodal disease who are most likely to benefit is one aspect that provides the preoperative staging process with its greatest challenge.[25] Extensive experience of endoscopic ultrasonography has suggested that this technique is both highly sensitive and specific in detecting lymph node metastases, in both the upper abdominal and paraoesophageal regions. This technique suggests that patients for radical lymph node dissection can be selected more accurately.[26] In addition, recent research surrounding the sentinel node concept in oesophageal adenocarcinoma suggests that this is applicable, in a similar way to breast cancer, in intraoperative evaluation and may be used to tailor the extent of lymphadenectomy to the individual patient and the stage of their disease.[27,28]

Nodal tiers

The description of the tiers of lymph nodes in oesophageal cancer has been designed according to the anatomy of the lymphatic draining system of the oesophagus.[2,29,30]

The extent of lymphadenectomy is demonstrated in **Fig. 5.3**. Many surgeons do not practise a formal lymphadenectomy during either transhiatal or transthoracic approaches to oesophagectomy.

Formal one-field lymph nodal dissection would involve the dissection of the diaphragmatic, right and left paracardiac, lesser curvature, left gastric, coeliac, common hepatic and splenic artery nodes.

Two-field nodal dissection includes the para-aortic (mediastinal nodes) together with the thoracic duct, the right and left pulmonary hilar nodes, the para-oesophageal nodes, tracheal bifurcation and the right paratracheal nodes.

Three-field nodal dissection includes the first and second fields as well as a dissection in the neck to clear the brachiocephalic, deep lateral and external cervical nodes, and including the right and left recurrent nerve lymphatic chains (deep anterior cervical nodes).

The fields of nodal dissection should not be confused with the histopathological staging of nodal involvement (see Chapter 3, Box 3.5). Much of the data available on lymph node dissection in oesophageal cancer suffer from poor definition of the terms 'oesophagectomy' and 'oesophagectomy with lymph node dissection'. It is essential, therefore, that all surgical techniques are standardised such that meaningful data can be derived in the future.

The rationale for lymphadenectomy

The arguments for more extensive surgery are optimal staging, locoregional control and improved cure rates.

Optimal staging

There can be no doubt that lymph node dissection contributes to the accuracy of the final staging of the disease.[31–33]

Locoregional tumour control

More extensive surgery produces prolonged tumour-free survival. In recent years overwhelming evidence has accumulated that R0 resection (no residual tumour left behind) is a very important prognostic variable after surgical excision. To consistently achieve an R0 resection, organ dissection and lymphadenectomy must be radical. Roder et al.[34] showed a statistically significant difference between R0 and R1 (microscopic residual disease) or R2 (macroscopic residual disease) resections for squamous cell carcinoma in a series of 204 resections with 5-year survival rates of 35% and <10% respectively. Lerut et al.[33] demonstrated a 20% 5-year survival for R0 vs. zero 5-year survival for R1 and R2 resections in advanced stage III and stage IV adenocarcinomas and squamous cell carcinomas.

Locoregional disease-free survival is a difficult yet important goal to achieve in oesophageal carcinoma as the majority of patients present with advanced disease. Furthermore, recurrent locoregional mediastinal disease can be very difficult to palliate. Dresner and Griffin[31] described mediastinal and abdominal local recurrence in 21% of patients after two-field nodal dissection in 176 patients. Clark et al.[35] found that nodal recurrence occurred within the area of dissection in only 20% of a small group of 43 patients. In addition, Lerut et al. demonstrated a 4-year survival of 22% in patients with stage IV disease as a result of distant lymph node metastases. This further endorses the apparent beneficial effect of adequate lymphadenectomy in reducing local recurrence.[33] Using a three-field lymphadenectomy, Altorki et al. described a local recurrence rate of 9.7% and a 33% 5-year survival for node-positive oesophageal cancer.[36]

Improved cure rate

The third argument for extended lymphadenectomy is the contribution to an improved survival. This argument suffers from a lack of definite evidence from randomised trials. Many reports describe retrospective series of different extents of lymphadenectomy in squamous and adenocarcinoma of the oesophagus,[17,31,32,37,38] ranging from no formal lymph node dissection to one-field, two-field and three-field lymphadenectomies. Unfortunately, very few prospective randomised trials are available for analysis to determine the extent of lymphadenectomy.[25,39,40]

The long-term outcomes of the Dutch study[25] comparing extended transthoracic with transhiatal oesophagectomy warrant closer examination.

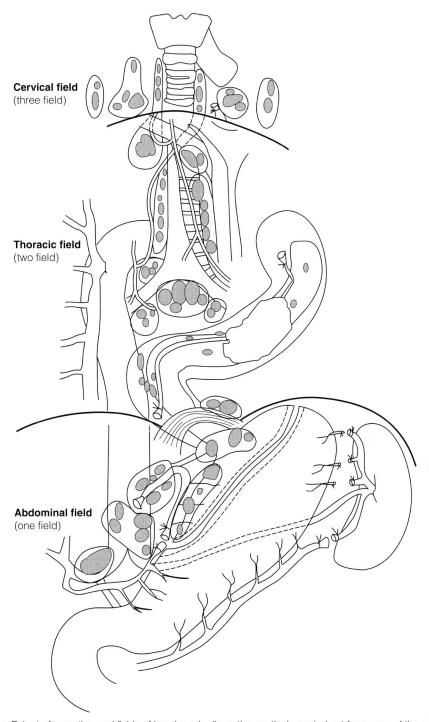

Cervical field
(three field)

Thoracic field
(two field)

Abdominal field
(one field)

Figure 5.3 • Extent of resection and fields of lymph node dissection routinely carried out for cancer of the oesophagus.

Although there was no overall survival benefit for extended transthoracic oesophagectomy over transhiatal oesophagectomy, there was an ongoing trend towards better 5-year survival for type 1 tumours. Moreover, patients with a limited number of posi-

tive nodes (1–8) had a significantly better survival following transthoracic oesophagectomy. This is the group of patients who logically one would expect to be most likely to benefit from extended lymphadenectomy. Node-negative patients did well, and those with a higher nodal burden did poorly, irrespective of the radicality of surgery (see **Fig. 5.4**).

There is some evidence that even patients with early-stage oesophageal carcinoma, in whom a high proportion can have nodal involvement, would also benefit from extensive resection with lymphadenectomy.[41] Nevertheless, some series have described T1 disease as having a zero rate of nodal metastases.[31] The role of radical lymphadenectomy in early-stage disease remains in question, and is clearly dependent on the precise depth of mucosal/submucosal invasion of the primary tumour.[25]

Summary

There is little justification for oesophagectomy to be performed with intent to cure without any attempt to clear the first level of lymph nodes. Patients with either squamous carcinoma or adenocarcinoma of the oesophagus affecting the upper, middle and lower regions have lymph node metastases in the mediastinal nodes in over 70% of cases.[21,31,32,38] Even resections for early tumours have lymph node metastases in up to 20% of cases. Many personal series of oesophageal cancer surgery have confirmed that over three-quarters of patients presenting with lower-third tumours had positive upper abdominal lymph nodes.[27] To perform a potentially curative resection for carcinoma in the middle and lower thirds, a dissection of abdominal and mediastinal lymph nodes is therefore essential. Series from Japan as well as Europe have confirmed that systematic nodal dissection employing meticulous surgical technique can be performed with acceptable operative morbidity and mortality. Despite these advances in lymph node dissection during the last few decades, there is still a mood of scepticism as to whether this really contributes to an improvement in survival.

 It is the author's opinion that a two-field lymph node dissection is justified on the grounds of the histopathological and surgical data presented by both Japanese and European groups.[24,25,31–33,36,38]

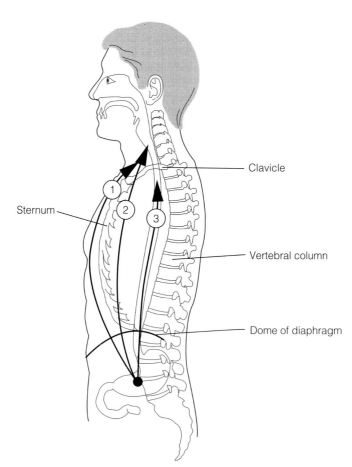

Figure 5.4 • Three routes of oesophageal reconstruction: (1) presternal route; (2) retrosternal route; (3) posterior mediastinal route.

The role of extensive three-field dissection in oesophageal malignancy is less clear. The difference in tumour spread between squamous cell carcinoma and adenocarcinoma needs to be better reported and understood. Many reports combine these quite separate tumours and therefore confuse the results. For cancer of the upper thoracic oesophagus (third field), dissection in the neck does appear to have some justification.[24,32,36] Five-year survival rates showed no significant difference between two-field and three-field dissection for lower-third squamous tumours.[32] In adenocarcinoma of the lower oesophagus, dissection of the cervical nodes cannot be justified, as there is no evidence that three-field nodal dissection provides any survival benefit.

Method of reconstruction of the oesophagus

Route of reconstruction

After resection of the cervical, thoracic or abdominal oesophagus, one of three main paths can be used for reconstruction (Fig. 5.4).

Presternal route

Many years ago the presternal route was the preference of many surgeons. This is approximately 2 cm longer than the retrosternal route, which in turn is approximately 2 cm longer than the posterior mediastinal route. As a result, the popularity of this route of reconstruction has declined over recent years. There seems little indication for using this route unless the thorax is of extremely small capacity such that a bulky oesophageal substitute could compromise effective respiration.

Retrosternal route (anterior mediastinal)

The space between the sternum and the anterior mediastinum is easily created with effective dissection. There is reported to be a lower incidence of cervical anastomotic dehiscence compared with that of the presternal route. Unfortunately its major disadvantage stems from the somewhat unnatural position of the cervical oesophagus in front of the trachea, which results in an unpleasant sensation on swallowing.

A major indication for this extra-anatomical route is for reconstruction following emergency treatment of anastomotic dehiscence or the dehiscence of a gastric substitute that has caused posterior mediastinal sepsis. After incomplete resection (R1 and R2) there is some evidence that a retrosternal conduit would be preferable to the posterior mediastinal route.[42]

The retrosternal route is created by blunt finger dissection through the abdominal and cervical incisions and further developed by insertion of a malleable intestinal retractor. The tip of this instrument is passed up to the neck in direct contact with the back of the sternum. Care is taken not to deviate from the midline. The sternohyoid and sternothyroid muscles are divided in the neck and this allows the passage of the oesophageal substitute easily into the left or right side of the neck.

Posterior mediastinal route

This route provides the shortest distance between the abdomen and the apex of the thorax and also the neck.

 This is the preferred route of reconstruction in the primary surgical excision of oesophageal cancers.[42,43]

Gastric or colonic substitutes are easily passed through the posterior mediastinum after completion of the oesophageal dissection in the thorax. No attempt is made to close the pleura after this route of reconstruction.

Organ of reconstruction

Reconstruction with stomach

The method of reconstruction should be kept as simple as possible, to minimise complications. The oesophageal replacement is determined by the site of the primary lesion. The stomach is the preferred option as this organ is easy to prepare and involves only one anastomosis.

The patient is positioned supine and exposure obtained using an upper midline incision. There are five broad principles and practices that must be observed in the preparation of the stomach as an oesophageal substitute:

1. **The use of isoperistaltic stomach and vascular integrity**. The right gastroepiploic and the right gastric artery and veins are vital in the maintenance of viability of the stomach when used as an oesophageal substitute. The greater omentum is opened and the entire course of the right gastroepiploic artery is carefully identified and preserved. The vascular arcade is interrupted at the junction where the right gastroepiploic artery meets the left. The short gastric vessels are divided and ligated (**Fig. 5.5**).

2. **Excision of the lesser curvature**. Cancers of the lower two-thirds of the oesophagus require complete clearance of the lesser curve lymph nodes as well as the left gastric, common hepatic and proximal splenic artery lymph nodes. The left gastric artery should be ligated at its origin and resection of the proximal half of the lesser curvature of the stomach, including the cardia, is performed. The right gastric artery contributes to the maintenance of the gastric intramural vascular

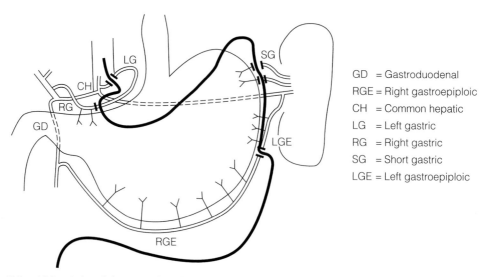

Figure 5.5 • Main arteries of the stomach and points of division of vessels and stomach for oesophageal substitution.

GD = Gastroduodenal
RGE = Right gastroepiploic
CH = Common hepatic
LG = Left gastric
RG = Right gastric
SG = Short gastric
LGE = Left gastroepiploic

network and should be preserved if possible. Although the width of gastric conduit appeared not to impact on outcome in one study,[44] the author recommends using a gastric tube of 5 cm width or greater to minimise the risk of ischaemia as described by A Kryama as early as 1976.

3. **Preservation of the intramural vascular arcade.** Extensive intramural arterial anastomoses between the vascular arcades of the lesser and greater curvatures exist. This has been well demonstrated by el-Eishi et al.[45] and Thomas et al.[46] This vascular network must be preserved dur-

ing resection of the left gastric area of the lesser curvature and the cardia of the stomach. The extent of the resection of the lesser curvature is determined by a line connecting the highest point of the fundus (**Fig. 5.6**) and the lesser curvature at the junction of the right and left gastric arteries. This allows the removal of all potentially involved lymph nodes, yet preserves the arterial network to the fundus. There is no evidence that the trunk and descending branches of the left gastric artery running along the lesser curve need to be preserved and, from an oncological point

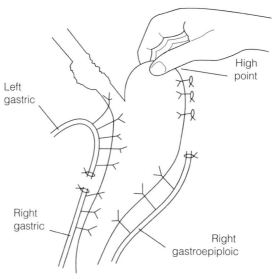

Left gastric

Right gastric

High point

Right gastroepiploic

Figure 5.6 • The high point of the stomach.

of view, it is important that these are excised with the specimen. Care should be taken to ligate the short gastric vessels away from the greater curvature of the stomach to avoid damage to the intramural network and to preserve the extramural vascular network as well. The right gastroepiploic artery provides an adequate blood flow to maintain vascularity in the region of the fundus, which is the area used for anastomosis.

4. **The high point of the stomach.** The stomach is a flexible and capacious organ; its high point is the logical and sensible place at which to fashion an anastomosis with the remaining oesophagus. It is easily identified by applying traction with the surgeon's fingers in an upward direction after all preparations have been completed. The stomach is transected as described previously (Fig. 5.6).

5. **Gastric drainage.** Pyloroplasty or pyloromyotomy after gastric reconstruction is contentious but best evidence suggests it does reduce the incidence of gastric outlet obstruction.[47] As short-term complications of pyloroplasty are minimal, it is the author's view that this should be performed routinely to prevent the life-threatening early complications of gastric stasis and aspiration as well as late vomiting and bloatedness.[48,49]

On occasions the upper anastomosis may need to be as high as the back of the tongue, so the following methods of stomach lengthening must be considered:

1. **Kocher manoeuvre.** This manoeuvre allows the distance between the first part of the duodenum and the hiatus to be reduced.

2. **Excision of lesser curve of stomach.** When the lesser curve of the stomach is unusually short, an increase in length of the gastric substitute can be obtained, by dividing the lesser curve between curved clamps, before its resection. If absolutely necessary, a tense right gastric artery may be sacrificed by division at the level of the pylorus.

3. **Incision of the serosa on the gastric wall.** Multiple incisions placed in the gastric serosa may lengthen the stomach. A longitudinal incision placed along the resection line allows this to occur. The indications for this procedure are extremely rare.

Reconstruction with colon

The principal indication for the use of colonic interposition is for tumours requiring an extensive oesophageal as well as gastric resection. With advances in preoperative staging few of these patients are suitable for resection. A small proportion of patients presenting with oesophageal malignancy will have had a previous gastric resection for peptic ulcer disease, precluding the use of stomach as the oesophageal substitute. The numbers of patients such as this are diminishing. The choice of an oesophageal replacement under these circumstances lies between colon and jejunum. The colon is often recommended because of its advantage in having a greater capacity as a reservoir than the jejunum. Rarely, it may be used in an emergency after failed gastric interposition. The disadvantage of colonic transposition is that the function of the conduit deteriorates over time and is therefore not as durable a substitute as the stomach in the long term.

Indications for colonic reconstruction (Box 5.3). It is preferable to use the colon in an isoperistaltic fashion. Unfortunately the vascular pattern of the colon varies and careful selection of the correct vascular pedicle to ensure viability of the transverse colon is essential. Each case requires evaluation on its own merit because of variations in anatomy. Not infrequently, the marginal artery is found to be of insufficient calibre to maintain viability of the transposed colon. Although the vascular appearance determines the appropriate colonic segment for use in each individual, the two possibilities for effective use of isoperistaltic colon are: (a) transverse colon based on the left colic vessels; (b) right colon based on the middle colic vessels.

The disadvantage of transverse colon is that an abnormally narrow marginal artery may exist at the splenic flexure, thus compromising the blood supply of the proximal colonic segment. Preoperative assessment by angiography of the colonic vascular pathway has been suggested,[50] but careful intraoperative observation of the vascular anatomy with temporary occlusion of vessels before division is a simple manoeuvre that is effective in most cases.

Surgical technique. Preoperative mechanical bowel preparation is necessary, as is oral antibiotic cover to sterilise the bowel for 48 hours prior to surgery. The omentum is freed from the transverse colon and the hepatic and splenic flexures, while the entire colon is mobilised so that it can be placed outside the abdominal cavity for inspection of its vascular blood supply. Mobilising the sigmoid colon provides additional length so that the transverse colon can be tunnelled into the chest, to reach the neck. The proximal colon should be divided

---

Box 5.3 • Indications for colonic reconstruction

- Previous gastric resection
- Tumours with extensive gastric involvement
- Failed gastric transposition

and, after anastomosis to the oesophagus, placed on sufficient stretch to prevent redundancy within the chest or in the substernal area. The colon should then be anchored in the straightened position by sutures to the crural margin of the hiatus, although not circumferentially. Continuity of the large bowel is re-established by end-to-end anastomosis, which is conveniently performed before the colo-jejunostomy or colo-gastrostomy for anatomical reasons. An excellent technical description for the use of various segments of colon has been provided by DeMeester et al.[51]

Reconstruction with jejunum

Replacement of the lower oesophagus is accomplished using either a Roux-en-Y technique or by segmental interposition. Replacement of the upper oesophagus is accomplished by free jejunal transfer with microvascular anastomosis of the jejunal pedicle to neck vessels. It is sometimes possible to create a long loop for replacement of the entire thoracic oesophagus, particularly when the proximal jejunum has adapted after previous gastric surgery. The jejunum should be considered the third choice, after stomach and colon.

No specific measures are required to prepare the small bowel preoperatively other than to ensure that patients are not known to have small-bowel pathology. A loop of jejunum is identified in the upper segments within the first 25 cm after the duodeno-jejunal flexure. The typical jejunal vascular pattern of arterial arcades is encountered in this area, and the veins and arteries are close together but bifurcate at separate levels, making individual division of the veins and arteries essential. Transillumination of the mesentery helps to identify the jejunal vascular tree precisely. It is important to appreciate that during the creation of a jejunal loop, it is the length of the free edge of the mesentery that will determine the length of the loop created rather than the length of the jejunum itself. The jejunum is usually longer than the mesentery and will therefore have a tendency to become redundant.

The technique of microvascular free jejunal transfer for reconstruction of the upper oesophagus is well described elsewhere.[52] The specific indications for such a reconstruction are usually after pharyngo-laryngectomy performed for carcinoma of the hypopharynx, postcricoid region and cervical oesophagus. The operation is usually performed with a radical neck dissection as part of the primary treatment programme or as palliative surgery following recurrence after radiotherapy.

Method of surgical approach

The preceding discussion has described the method and rationale underpinning the surgical objectives in treating oesophageal cancer. The aims of resecting the primary tumour together with the lymph nodes and oesophageal reconstruction must be achieved safely and effectively and with ease of access. The method of surgical approach to obtain these objectives must be considered in each individual case. The choice of the surgical approach is dependent on the tumour location, the extent of spread, the fitness, age and build of the individual patient.

Pharyngolaryngo-oesophagectomy for carcinoma of the hypopharynx and cervical oesophagus

Resection of squamous lesions in this area is achieved by removal of the larynx, the lower pharynx, cervical trachea, one or both lobes of the thyroid gland, and the cervical oesophagus. If the tumour is located in the hypopharynx only (postcricoid region), the thoracic oesophagus may be conserved and a free graft of jejunum transferred by microvascular anastomosis, as previously described. If tumour has extended to the lower part of the cervical oesophagus, a total pharyngolaryngo-oesophagectomy and gastric transposition, with immediate pharyngo-gastric reconstruction, is the treatment of choice.

The patient is placed in the supine position with the neck hyperextended; a U-shaped incision provides excellent access. It allows the construction of a permanent tracheostomy with ease and may be extended into a Y-shaped incision ready for a median sternotomy if required. The resection includes a radical lymph node dissection in the neck. The thyroid and parathyroid glands are also removed en bloc with the internal jugular vein and the deep internal cervical nodes. The common carotid artery, vagus nerve and the sympathetic trunk are carefully protected.

Two-phase subtotal oesophagectomy via a right thoracotomy for carcinomas of the middle and lower thirds of the oesophagus

 Left thoracotomy was the standard approach until the 1960s, and although it provided excellent access to the lower oesophagus, exposure of the upper and middle thoracic oesophagus was restricted by the aortic arch. Two-phase right thoracotomy (initially described by Lewis and Tanner) is now accepted as the open approach of choice to the thoracic oesophagus.[32,48]

The first phase is abdominal mobilisation of the stomach performed through an upper midline laparotomy incision. The second phase is mediastinal dissection and oesophageal resection through a right thoracotomy. The stomach is delivered into the chest and an anastomosis fashioned at the thoracic inlet.

The procedure begins with a laparotomy to assess the primary tumour and exclude the presence of distant metastases. After routine gastric mobilisation, described earlier, the coeliac trunk together with its branches, namely the common hepatic and the roots of the splenic and left gastric arteries, are then skeletonised by complete removal of the surrounding lymph nodes. The left gastric artery is divided and ligated at its origin. The patient is then placed in the left lateral decubitus position and is held firmly in place by a moulding mattress. The right arm is fixed on an armrest while the left is stretched out on an arm-support.

The mediastinal phase is performed via a right posterolateral thoracotomy through the fourth or fifth intercostal space. There is often a tendency to open the chest through too low an incision. It is essential to count the ribs by palpation under the scapula and to go no lower than the fifth intercostal space. In high tumours, such as middle-third squamous lesions, a suprazygous dissection is performed. This is not necessary for lower-third lesions.

So, for tumours of the middle third the superior mediastinal pleura is incised along the course of the right vagus nerve and is extended upwards towards the brachiocephalic and subclavian arteries. The right recurrent laryngeal nerve is preserved and meticulous dissection is then applied to the lymph node chain alongside it. The pleura is incised along the border of the superior vena cava and the right paratracheal lymph nodes located between the trachea and the vein are then dissected free. Care is taken not to dissect circumferentially around the trachea, as this may prejudice its blood supply.

Routine division and/or resection of the arch of the azygos vein is crucial for adequate exposure. The azygos vein marks the line of dissection caudally to the hiatus. The incision through the pleura is deepened to expose the adventitia on the descending aorta. The thoracic duct through which the lymph flows is rarely the site of metastases, except in extensive disease. There are, however, numerous lymph nodes scattered along the length of the duct in the para-aortic region. To remove these an en bloc resection together with the duct is necessary. The duct is easily identified after minimal sharp dissection in the inferior mediastinum on the adventitia of the right aspect of the descending thoracic aorta just above the hiatus. The duct is first ligated at this point and then at the proximal end after resection in the superior mediastinum, along the posterior border of the oesophagus. Chylothorax secondary to inadvertent and undetected damage to the thoracic duct is therefore prevented. Dissection continues on to the right pulmonary hilum, where there is

almost always a small anthracotic lymph node. The right bronchial, carinal and left bronchial nodes are dissected. It is advisable to avoid monopolar diathermy in this region because of the vulnerability of the membranous part of both the trachea and bronchi.

The oesophagus is then transected at the thoracic inlet. The stomach is delivered into the chest and the specimen removed after careful sleeve resection of the lesser curvature, as previously described. Oesophagogastric anastomosis is fashioned in the apex of the thorax. In addition to ensuring adequate resection margins, it is vital that the whole gastric conduit is within the thorax for a good functional outcome. If a lower anastomosis is fashioned differences in abdominal and mediastinal pressure promote reflux and inhibit gastric emptying, resulting in troublesome symptoms and poor quality of life.

Combined synchronous two-team oesophagectomy

Modification of the standard access for oesophagectomy has been described wherein mobilisation of the stomach and abdominal oesophagus proceeds synchronously with mobilisation of the thoracic oesophagus via a right thoracotomy using a second operating team.[53,54] A reduction in operating and anaesthetic time was suggested as a possible reason for decreased operative morbidity and mortality rates in Hong Kong Chinese patients. Patients in the study had a lower incidence of pulmonary and cardiovascular disease than those with oesophageal cancer in the West.

 A comparison of the synchronous two-team approach with conventional two-stage subtotal oesophagectomy was performed in Western patients. Not only was there a higher incidence of complications and a higher mortality rate, but an adequate nodal dissection in larger, more obese patients was technically very difficult because of the limited surgical access.[55]

Three-phase subtotal oesophagectomy for tumours of the upper middle third of the oesophagus

Exposing and dividing the oesophagus in the neck certainly provides excellent access for anastomosis, although it does not allow resection of much more oesophagus than can be removed by the two-phase approach. This is because the cervical oesophagus is relatively short and it is difficult to perform an anastomosis unless a stump of oesophagus is left, hence the term subtotal oesophagectomy. McKeown[56] recommended cervical anastomosis on the grounds that a leak in the neck is less catastrophic than a thoracic leak. This is probably an overstatement and is now of less significance as overall true oesophageal anastomotic leakage is uncommon (approximately 1–2% in experienced hands). The three-phase operation takes longer to complete and is also associated with early postoperative difficulty in swallowing. This is probably because of the extensive proximal mobilisation of the cervical oesophagus. Proponents of the three-phase operation claim that a more complete oesophagectomy is achieved. If the tumour cannot be resected with an adequate proximal longitudinal margin then the three-phase technique ought to be employed.

The first phase of this operation is routine gastric mobilisation with dissection of the nodal groups, as described above. The second phase should mirror the dissection described in the preceding section, but adding the mobilisation of the oesophagus in the apex of the thorax. The right thorax is closed and the patient turned supine once again. Through either a left- or right-sided cervical incision, the whole of the thoracic oesophagus can be removed and the stomach delivered into the neck and an oesophagogastrostomy fashioned. The alternative to reduce operating time is to perform the thoracic phase first and then to turn the patient supine for synchronous abdominal and neck phases.

Left-sided subtotal oesophagectomy for middle- and lower-third oesophageal cancers

A left thoracotomy has been used for many years, particularly by thoracic surgeons, not only for carcinoma of the lower oesophagus and cardia, but also for the mid-thoracic oesophagus. Access to perform a formal abdominal nodal dissection through a diaphragmatic incision is inadequate and advocates of the left thoracotomy approach have failed to quote data about nodal status or the incidence of mucosal resection margins.[57,58] Randomised studies comparing left and right approaches have not been performed. Nevertheless, Molina et al.[59] compared a 10-year experience of both approaches and clearly showed a higher incidence of positive resection margins in patients undergoing left thoracotomy.

The left-sided approach was modified by Matthews and Steel.[60] They described a two-stage procedure with a left thoraco-laparotomy followed by a left-neck approach. Much more extensive access was achieved by dividing the costal margin of the diaphragm peripherally for 15 cm close to its origin on the ribs. Although this should decrease positive resection margins, no data were quoted. This left-sided approach is absolutely contraindicated if the tumour is situated at or above the aortic arch. Although data are few on the incidence of respiratory complications, historical series have suggested an increased incidence of serious chest infections following the left-sided approach. The left thoraco-abdominal approach is still appropriate for selected patients to resect tumours at the cardia.[61] The Japan Clinical Oncology Group trial has shown that for proximal gastric cancer the left thoracoabdominal approach has increased complications and no survival benefit compared to transhiatal gastrectomy.[62]

Transhiatal oesophagectomy for upper- and lower-third tumours of the oesophagus

Controversy still exists about the role of oesophagectomy without thoracotomy in oesophageal cancer surgery. Proponents of the technique argue that outcome is dependent on the stage at presentation rather than the operative technique employed. Opponents claim improvements in survival for some undergoing radical en bloc resection.[33,36] The original technique was a blind procedure, defying the fundamental principle that surgery should always be carried out under direct vision.[63–65] Nevertheless, refinements to the technique have been made and the operation has developed and gained many advocates.[66]

A modified technique of transhiatal oesophagectomy under direct vision has been described[67] using a modification of the transhiatal technique described by Pinotti.[68] Almost the entire procedure is undertaken under direct vision, ensuring adequate local clearance by avoiding direct contact with the tumour, and the anastomosis performed in the neck as a combined synchronous operation. The authors demonstrated no evidence of proximal or distal resection margin involvement with the tumour and an acceptable morbidity and mortality.

Details of the surgical procedure are clearly described elsewhere.[68] At present there are selected indications for transhiatal oesophagectomy:

- **Carcinoma of the hypopharynx and cervical oesophagus.** If the tumour is localised the incidence of mediastinal metastases is low. In this situation oesophagectomy without thoracotomy can therefore be safely performed by blunt dissection. Radical neck dissection with pharyngolaryngo-oesophagectomy is carried out at the same time and reconstruction fashioned using the stomach through the posterior mediastinal route.

- **Intraepithelial squamous carcinoma of the oesophagus.** These tumours rarely disseminate via the lymphatics.[19] With substantial progress in endoscopic techniques using epithelial dye staining and endoscopic ultrasonography, early tumours can be more accurately staged. When tumour penetration is confined to the epithelial layer, resection by transhiatal oesophagectomy is entirely feasible (Chapter 6).

- **Patients with a diagnosis of high-grade dysplasia within a Barrett segment,** who on staging have no evidence of invasion or nodal disease.

The debate will continue over which operative procedure is most appropriate for the treatment of lower-third oesophageal carcinoma. Randomised studies have rarely been performed and no clear survival advantage has emerged for any particular operative technique.

Four randomised controlled trials comparing the transhiatal approach with the transthoracic approach have been published.[25,39,69,70] These have failed to demonstrate significant differences between the two approaches.

The strongest evidence so far comes from the Dutch trial, which included 220 patients with adenocarcinoma of the middle and lower oesophagus. Significantly more nodes were dissected in the thoracic approach, but pulmonary complications were also greater. A trend was noted for increased survival in the radical transthoracic approach, which continued with long-term data. Interestingly, patients with lower oesophageal tumours (Siewert type 1) and those with a low burden (1–8 nodes) of nodal disease appeared to benefit from extended transthoracic oesophagectomy.

Minimally invasive oesophagectomy for cancer

A number of techniques have been described that aim to reduce the severity of the surgical insult and complications produced by formal thoracotomy. These include thoracoscopic dissection within the chest, laparoscopic mobilisation of the stomach for oesophageal replacement, a combined laparoscopic and thoracoscopic approach, a hand-assisted technique and a mediastinoscopic technique. Full details of these developing techniques are provided in Chapter 6. At present the techniques are still in evolution, and complications, immediate outcomes and oncological clearance are still issues to be audited and assessed.

Technique of anastomosis

Meticulous technique is essential in minimising the risk of leakage after oesophageal anastomosis, which is still associated with a significant mortality. The surgical principles relating to oesophageal anastomoses are the same as those in other parts of the alimentary tract. Emphasis is placed on:

- adequate blood supply;
- absence of tension in the anastomosis;

- accurate approximation of epithelial edges;
- precise layer-to-layer suturing with primary healing.

One-, two- and three-layer anastomoses have been described, but no conclusive randomised controlled studies have been reported. A two-layer oesophago-gastric anastomosis is advocated by Akiyama,[19] who emphasises the importance of the absence of a serosal layer, which he believes would reinforce strength at the anastomotic site. He therefore advocates a carefully preserved adventitia, which provides sufficient strength to support sutures.

Stapling devices have been developed for ease of introduction and application, with a low-profile head that permits a larger-diameter anvil to be introduced into the oesophageal stump. A larger-diameter anastomosis is thereby fashioned, reducing the rate of benign anastomotic stricture formation, most commonly seen with a staple ring diameter of 25 mm or less.[9,24,71] The staple head can now also be inserted transorally, allowing a double-staple technique, similar to that in colorectal surgery, to be used.

Anastomotic leakage is more frequent in the neck than in the chest, although the related mortality rates have not been shown to differ between these anastomotic sites.[72] The incidence of leakage does not depend on suture material or technical modalities used to perform the anastomosis. Indeed, there is no evidence that the overall decrease in anastomotic complications is related to the use of a specific conduit approach or route of reconstruction, but is more likely due to progress made in general perioperative management.[73]

No significant difference has been demonstrated between leakage rates using hand-sewn and mechanical anastomoses.[74]

Higher overall leak rates are found in collective reviews rather than in reports from specialist units.

Postoperative management

A detailed account of immediate postoperative care after oesophageal cancer surgery is described in Chapter 4, and a summary is given in Boxes 5.4 and 5.5. Meticulous attention to the maintenance of fluid balance and respiratory care are essential in the immediate postoperative period. Adequate pain control via a thoracic epidural and physiotherapy are crucial. It is the author's routine practice to enterally feed patients undergoing oesophagectomy in the postoperative period, commencing feeding via a jejunostomy on the second postoperative day. Early mobilisation is important in preventing venous thrombosis and pulmonary embolus.

It also enhances ventilation, clearance of sputum and early bowel movement. It is the author's practice to remove the chest drains by the fifth or sixth postoperative days once oral feeding has recommenced, although some surgeons remove them 48 hours after surgery.

The role of routine postoperative radiological imaging of the oesophageal anastomosis has become clearer. There is no evidence that the routine use of contrast radiology is of any value in patients who are asymptomatic in the postoperative phase.[75,76] Patients who are clinically well should be started on oral feeding, while video endoscopy or contrast radiology should be reserved for patients showing signs of sepsis, pleural effusion or haemodynamic instability. Non-ionic contrast media may pick up gross leaks, but if no leak is shown should be followed up by barium investigations or an endoscopy to exclude a small leak.

Routine nasogastric decompression is continued for 5 days until gastrointestinal activity is restored. Patients are allowed 25 mL of water every hour soon after extubation. Subcutaneous low-dose heparin is administered routinely until the patient is discharged. Chest physiotherapy is commenced in intensive care and continued 4-hourly for the first 3 days. Prophylactic antibiotics are commenced on the morning of surgery and continued for two postoperative doses. All patients should be counselled by the surgeon, an oesophageal cancer nurse specialist and a dietician prior to discharge.

Postoperative complications

Postoperative complications may be subdivided into those that are common to any major surgical procedure in an elderly population and those specific to oesophageal resection. The complication rate of oesophageal surgery is relatively high, in the region of 30–40%. Some studies have found increased morbidity rates following neoadjuvant therapy, particularly respiratory problems after chemoradiotherapy. This seems to be further compounded with salvage oesophagectomy after definitive chemoradiotherapy for squamous carcinoma.[77] Early recognition of complications and rapid proactive management is essential to achieve good results for all patients. It has been proposed that postoperative complications are not only associated with poor early outcome, but also, possibly through immunosuppression, with early death from cancer recurrence.[78]

General complications

These complications (see also Chapter 4) may be minimised by improved preoperative patient evaluation. Respiratory complications constitute the largest proportion of this group. Pain is the major contributor to decreased ventilation and atelectasis, which leads to bronchopneumonia and respiratory failure. Extensive lymphadenectomy can cause poor lymphatic drainage of the pulmonary alveoli, leading to parenchymal fluid retention and a consequent acute pulmonary oedema. Significant respiratory complications occur in approximately 24% of cases following subtotal oesophagectomy.[79]

Thromboembolic complications are not uncommon in malignant disease in the elderly. Myocardial ischaemia and cerebral vascular episodes are specific to the age group undergoing surgery and are precipitated by hypoxia, hypotension and underlying vascular occlusive disease.

Major haemorrhage is uncommon and as a result of meticulous technique and the use of new techniques, such as the ultrasonic scalpel during gastric mobilisation, routine blood loss is less than 500 mL, with only a small minority of patients requiring transfusion. Secondary haemorrhage is also rare and is almost always associated with a mediastinal infection from a specific complication such as an anastomotic leakage. The value of minimisation of surgical blood loss should not be underestimated. Perioperative blood transfusion is a significant predictor of decreased overall survival.[80]

Specific complications

The second group of complications following oesophageal surgery for cancer is specific to the procedure.

Anastomotic leakage and leakage from the gastric conduit

Anastomotic leakage is influenced by a variety of factors including cancer hypermetabolism, malnutrition, anastomotic vascular deficit, anastomotic tension and surgical technique. The incidence of anastomotic leakage has decreased significantly over the last 10 years and rates of well under 5% should be expected.[8,73,75]

Early disruption (within 48–72 hours) is the result of a technical error. If early disruption is confirmed and the general condition of the patient is good, then the patient should be re-explored for correction of the technical fault.

 Flexible upper gastrointestinal endoscopy is important in diagnosis and particularly the identification of any conduit necrosis.

Total gastric necrosis can rarely occur with catastrophic consequences. This complication must be diagnosed early by video endoscopy, resuscitation given immediately and the patient returned to theatre for the formation of a cervical oesophagostomy and closing of the viable component of the gastric remnant. The establishment of a feeding jejunostomy is essential if not already in place. At a later date when the patient has stabilised, a colonic interposition is used to restore intestinal continuity. Later disruptions manifest themselves between the fifth and tenth postoperative days and are due to ischaemia of the tissues or tension on the anastomotic line. For leaks from the oesophagogastric anastomosis operative intervention is likely to be hazardous and possibly detrimental. Intensive non-operative treatment with nasogastric suction, radiologically guided chest and mediastinal drainage, therapeutic antibiotic regimens and early enteral nutrition via a jejunostomy are all essential. Late anastomotic leakage should not result in a high mortality if it is aggressively managed.

 The author would strongly urge against the insertion of self-expandable stents in this situation as they prevent adequate drainage of sepsis, are prone to migrate, and may ultimately erode into surrounding structures.

Dehiscence of the gastric resection line is rare but requires re-exploration as the extent of leakage is frequently large.[75]

Chylothorax

The thoracic duct can often be damaged during mobilisation of advanced oesophageal cancers, whether via a right thoracotomy or through the transhiatal route. A comprehensive review reports chylothorax occurring in up to 10% of patients after blunt transhiatal oesophagectomy.[81] An incidence of 2–3% during open resection is commonly reported.[82] Accidental damage to the thoracic duct can be prevented by identification during dissection,

as previously described, and ligating the duct low in the inferior mediastinum on the right lateral aspect of the descending thoracic aorta. Chylothorax usually presents in the first 7 days after surgery, when the patient has commenced oral intake, or jejunostomy feeds, especially of fat-containing nutrients. A massive increase in chest drainage occurs that if left untreated results in malnutrition and significant immune suppression, with a markedly reduced CD4 count, from the subsequent white-cell loss. It is difficult to predict whether a chylous leak will spontaneously heal despite attempts to quantify the size of the leak.[83] Immediate re-exploration is therefore recommended for major leaks, as the damaged thoracic duct is usually easily identified, following a bolus of cream, at the time of re-exploration.[82] Leaks of less than 500 mL/day may resolve with enteral feeding using medium-chain triglycerides. Prolonged total parenteral nutrition has been used but patients who rapidly become malnourished are prone to nosocomial infections and frequently require a long hospital stay. Prophylactic antibiotic cover with co-trimoxazole for *Pneumocystis* is essential for the lymphopenic patient.[84] On rare occasions, chylothorax can be resistant to treatment, whether re-exploration or conservative therapy. This is often due to abnormal lymph anatomy around the hiatus. The author has documented up to three large ducts in the posterior mediastinum in such patients. Pleuroperitoneal shunting has resulted in successful outcomes in resistant chylous leaks. This allows reabsorption of chyle and prevents the sequelae of immune suppression.

Recurrent laryngeal palsy

The incidence of recurrent laryngeal palsy has increased over recent years due to the increase of cervical oesophagogastric anastomoses. It is extremely rare when the anastomosis is constructed in the apex of the chest via the thoracotomy route for subtotal oesophagectomy. If the palsy is transient but unilateral, the opposite cord may well compensate. If the palsy is permanent, Teflon injection of the cord or a formal thyroplasty can restore adequate voice volume and a satisfactory cough.[85]

Gastric outlet obstruction

Gastric outlet obstruction is prevented by the routine use of a pyloroplasty or a pyloromyotomy. Emptying problems are kept at a minimum when the anastomosis is in the apex of the thorax. Procedures that leave part of the stomach as an abdominal organ and part of the stomach as a thoracic organ predispose to duodeno-gastro-oesophageal reflux. Prokinetic agents such as low-dose erythromycin can improve gastric emptying and minimise these complications. Dumping syndrome after oesophagogastric reconstruction is relatively common but usually resolves in the 12 months following surgery. It is adequately treated by the avoidance of high carbohydrate loads.

Duodeno-gastro-oesophageal reflux

Acid or alkaline reflux is common[86,87] and, although it may be controlled by motility agents and acid suppressants, can be troublesome. There is some evidence that performing a modified fundoplication as an antireflux manoeuvre at the time of oesophagectomy is effective in controlling postoesophagectomy reflux in the majority of patients.[88]

Benign anastomotic stricture

These strictures are not uncommon but usually respond to a single dilatation performed with the flexible video endoscope under image intensification and sedation.[9]

Overall results of single-modality resectional therapy

Overall results of surgical therapy in oesophageal cancer can be analysed in terms of hospital mortality and patient survival. Assessment of quality of life (patient-related outcomes) as an outcome measure is essential as there is increasing evidence relating it to overall survival.[89] The fact that it takes 9 months for quality of life to recover following surgery illustrates the scale of trauma that oesophagectomy produces. Very little new data have become available on single-modality surgery for oesophageal cancer. Increasingly, published results include patients subjected to multimodality treatments.

Hospital mortality

Although individual units have achieved considerably better results, three comprehensive reviews during the last two decades shed some light on trends in both hospital mortality and overall survival.[8,90,91]

The review of Jamieson et al.[91] confirmed that the average hospital mortality rate following oesophagectomy had continued to decrease, from 28% (1953–1978), to 13% (1980–1988), to 8.8% (1990–2000).

This may be attributed to improvements in anaesthesia, surgical technique, perioperative care, and the specialisation and centralisation of oesophageal cancer services. No evidence has been provided to relate tumour biology to mortality rate following oesophageal resection and there is no difference in mortality rates between resections for squamous cell carcinoma and adenocarcinoma. Overall mortality rates in many series can be confusing because of variations in definitions. 'In-hospital' and not 30-day mortality rates should be quoted in all papers, but unfortunately this continues not to be the case. Series from specialist centres in the last few years cite operative hospital mortality rates of less than 5%.[24,31,75] This includes a huge series of over 20 000 oesophagectomies from China.[92] There is no longer any place for the occasional oesophagectomist in the management of this disease. There is clearly still further room for improvement as data from a large multicentre UK audit recently reported mortality rates of over 10%.[93]

Comparisons of hospital mortality rates for different resection techniques reveal only minor differences. In the review by Muller et al.,[8] the lowest mortality rate was for transhiatal oesophagectomy, with a median figure of 8%. These data, however, are not strictly comparable because transhiatal resection was the most recent surgical development and therefore benefited from the experience of recent advances in perioperative care.

Nevertheless, preoperative risk analysis using a composite scoring system to predict operative risk managed to show a decrease in mortality in a large series from 9.4% to 1.6%.[16] No overall difference was noted in the randomised controlled trial of transthoracic vs. transhiatal approaches in the Dutch study.

Rigorous preoperative assessment will continue to reduce hospital mortality from this major thoraco-abdominal operation (see Chapter 4).

Survival figures

In a review of the 1980s, Muller et al. found that 56% of all resected patients survived the first postoperative year, 34% the second, 25% the third, 21% the fourth and 20% the fifth year after resection. It was depressing to note that these figures were very similar to those collected by Earlam and Cunha Melo, revealing that despite improved hospital mortality, the overall long-term prognosis had remained unchanged. No differences in the 5-year survival rates were noted between different techniques of resection but en bloc resections showed a significantly better long-term prognosis.[30,63] More recent data from the Dutch trial[25] revealed 5-year survival was 36% and 34% after transhiatal and transthoracic resection respectively. There is some evidence to suggest that adenocarcinomas tend to fare worse than squamous lesions, although this may simply reflect the more advanced stage at which these lesions tend to present.[60] With increasing numbers of early tumours being diagnosed on surveillance programmes for Barrett's oesophagus, this hypothesis will be tested. The primary determinants of overall outcome appear to be the stage of the tumour and the cell type.

Overall survival is, of course, strongly stage dependent. There are many case series describing stage-specific survival but there has been no systematic review of these reports. The author's published results confirm a greater than 90% 5-year survival for stage 0 and stage 1 disease. For stage 2a, 2b and stage 3 disease, 5-year survival is 60%, 16% and 13% respectively.[31] Other specialist units have achieved similar results with resection and two-field lymphadenectomy as unimodality therapy.[17,24,25,31,36,39,41] The poor outcome for patients with node-positive disease has led to multimodality therapy becoming the standard of care for these patients. A recent meta-analysis demonstrated a greater 2-year survival benefit for both neoadjuvant chemoradiotherapy and chemotherapy, although the standardisation of the staging investigations and surgical resection has been questioned in many of these trials[77] (see Chapter 9).

Summary and future research

The main areas of progress and interest in surgery for oesophageal cancer have been the introduction of a multidisciplinary approach, improved disease staging, the development of new surgical and endoscopic techniques for the management of early tumours including minimally invasive oesophagectomy, and the introduction of multimodality therapy for locally advanced disease. The future of oesophageal cancer surgery will be based on procedures tailored to the individual patient. Certain patients with early adenocarcinoma may initially undergo endoscopic resection to identify those requiring a formal oesophagectomy. These patients may undergo sentinel node mapping[27] such that patients potentially can be spared radical node dissection. Patients with locally advanced adenocarcinoma, particularly those with a low burden of nodal disease, will be targeted with increasingly effective multimodality regimens including, based on the Dutch trial, a radical en bloc oesophagectomy with two-field lymph node dissection. Neoadjuvant regimes should be tailored, possibly by genetic profiling, to determine the best therapeutic strategy for each patient. Despite all this, significant improvements in long-term outcome for oesophageal cancer will only be achieved if focus is placed on earlier detection of what continues to be a very aggressive disease.

Key points

- The overall results of surgical resection for all stages of tumour have improved over the past 20 years.
- Meticulous preoperative evaluation and estimation of surgical risk is a prerequisite to successful surgical outcome in this disease.
- There is now overwhelming evidence to confirm the influence of surgeon case volume on the outcome of site-specific cancer surgery.
- Enteral feeding is preferred over parenteral feeding (TPN) for nutritional support.
- Subtotal oesophagectomy should be carried out in patients with tumours of the middle and lower oesophagus to make allowance for intramural submucosal spread of squamous and adenocarcinomas.
- The stomach is the preferred conduit for oesophageal reconstruction.
- Two-phase oesophagectomy with two-field lymphadenectomy is recommended for lower oesophageal adenocarcinoma, particularly those with a low nodal burden.
- Multimodality therapy including high-quality surgery should be considered for patients with >T2 N0 tumours.
- Outcome is strongly stage dependent – the focus must be on early detection.

References

1. Sobin LH, Wittenkind CH (eds) UICC classification of malignant tumours, 6th edn. New York: John Wiley, 2002.

2. Japanese Society for Oesophageal Diseases. Guidelines for the clinical and pathological studies on carcinoma of the oesophagus. Part 1: clinical classification. Jpn J Surg 1976; 6:64–78.

3. Tetteroo GW, Wagenvoort JH, Castelein A et al. Selective decontamination to reduce gram-negative colonisation and infections after oesophageal resection. Lancet 1990; 335(8691):704–7.

4. Gianotti L, Braga M, Nespoli L et al. A randomized controlled trial of preoperative oral supplementation with a specialized diet in patients with gastrointestinal cancer [see comment]. Gastroenterology 2002; 122(7):1763–70.

5. Heslin MJ, Latkany L, Leung D et al. A prospective, randomized trial of early enteral feeding after resection of upper gastrointestinal malignancy. Ann Surg 1997; 226(4):567–77; discussion 577–80.

   This small trial questions routine feeding jejunostomy in all operative patients.

6. Moore FA, Feliciano DV, Andrassy RJ et al. Early enteral feeding, compared with parenteral, reduces postoperative septic complications. The results of a meta-analysis. Ann Surg 1992; 216(2): 172–83.

   This meta-analysis emphasises the benefits of enteral feeding in the perioperative period.

7. Braga M, Gianotti L, Gentilini O et al. Feeding the gut early after digestive surgery: results of a nine-year experience. Clin Nutr 2002; 21(1):59–65.

8. Muller JM, Erasmi H, Stelzner M et al. Surgical therapy of oesophageal carcinoma. Br J Surg 1990; 77(8):845–57.

   This large trial reviewed oesophageal surgical publications published in the 1980s, and demonstrated improvements in operative mortality from the previous decade, but no better overall survival.

9. Griffin SM, Woods SD, Chan A et al. Early and late surgical complications of subtotal oesophagectomy for squamous carcinoma of the oesophagus. J R Coll Surg Edinb 1991; 36(3):170–3.

10. Lerut T. Oesophageal carcinoma – past and present studies. Eur J Surg Oncol 1996; 22(4):317–23.

11. Gebski V, Burmeister B, Smithers BM et al. Survival benefits from neoadjuvant chemoradiotherapy or chemotherapy in oesophageal carcinoma: a meta-analysis. Lancet Oncol 2007; 8(3):226–34.

12. Department of Health. Guidance on commissioning cancer services. Improving outcomes in uppergastrointestinal cancers. The manual. London: NHS Executive, 2001.

13. Sutton DN, Wayman J, Griffin SM. Learning curve for oesophageal cancer surgery. Br J Surg 1998; 85(10):1399–402.

14. Finlayson EV, Goodney PP, Birkmeyer JD et al. Hospital volume and operative mortality in cancer surgery: a national study. Arch Surg 2003; 138(7):721–5; discussion 726.

15. Kuo EY, Chang Y, Wright CD et al. Impact of hospital volume on clinical and economic outcomes for esophagectomy. Ann Thorac Surg 2001; 72(4):1118–24.

16. Begg CB, Cramer LD, Hoskins WJ et al. Impact of hospital volume on operative mortality for major cancer surgery [see comment]. JAMA 1998; 280(20):1747–51.

17. Skinner DB. En bloc resection for neoplasms of the esophagus and cardia. J Thorac Cardiovasc Surg 1983; 85(1):59–71.

18. Siu KF, Cheung HC, Wong J et al. Shrinkage of the esophagus after resection for carcinoma. Ann Surg 1986; 203(2):173–6.

19. Akiyama H. Surgery for cancer of the oesophagus. Baltimore: Williams & Wilkins, 1990.

20. Mandard AM, Chasle J, Marnay J et al. Autopsy findings in 111 cases of esophageal cancer. Cancer 1981; 48(2):329–35.

21. Sons HU, Borchard F. Cancer of the distal esophagus and cardia. Incidence, tumorous infiltration, and metastatic spread. Ann Surg 1986; 203(2):188–95.

22. Dexter SP, Sue-Ling H, McMahon MJ et al. Circumferential resection margin involvement: an independent predictor of survival following surgery for oesophageal cancer. Gut 2001; 48(5):667–70.

23. Orringer MB, Marshall B, Iannettoni MD. Transhiatal esophagectomy for benign and malignant esophageal disease. World J Surg 2001; 25(2):196–203.

24. Lerut T, Coosemans W, De Leyn P et al. Is there a role for radical esophagectomy. Eur J Cardiothorac Surg 1999; 16(Suppl 1):S44–7.

25. Hulscher JB, van Sandick JW, de Boer AG et al. Extended transthoracic resection compared with limited transhiatal resection for adenocarcinoma of the esophagus. N Engl J Med 2002; 347(21):1662–9.

   These trials suggest that both techniques are safe but that there is lower morbidity in the transhiatal group and a trend to longer survival in the extended transthoracic groups.

26. Preston SR, Clark GW, Martin IG et al. Effect of endoscopic ultrasonography on the management of 100 consecutive patients with oesophageal and junctional carcinoma. Br J Surg 2003; 90(10):1220–4.

27. Lamb PJ, Griffin SM, Burt AD et al. Sentinel node biopsy to evaluate the metastatic dissemination of oesophageal adenocarcinoma. Br J Surg 2005; 92(1):60–7.

28. Kitagawa Y, Fujii H, Mukai M et al. Intraoperative lymphatic mapping and sentinel lymph node sampling in esophageal and gastric cancer. Surg Oncol Clin North Am 2002; 11(2):293–304.

29. Sato T, Sacamoto K. Illustrations and photographs of surgical oesophageal anatomy, specially prepared for lymph node dissection. In: Sato T, Sacamoto K (eds) Colour atlas of surgical anatomy for oesophageal cancer. Toyko: Springer, 1992; pp. 25–90.

30. Tanabe G, Baba M, Kuroshima K et al. Clinical evaluation of the esophageal lymph flow system based on RI uptake of dissected regional lymph nodes following lymphoscintigraphy [in Japanese]. Nippon Geka Gakkai Zasshi 1986; 87(3):315–23.

31. Dresner SM, Griffin SM. Pattern of recurrence following radical oesophagectomy with two-field lymphadenectomy. Br J Surg 2000; 87(10):1426–33.

32. Akiyama H, Tsurumaru M, Udagawa H et al. Radical lymph node dissection for cancer of the thoracic esophagus. Ann Surg 1994; 220(3): 64–72; discussion 372–3.

33. Lerut T, De Leyn P, Coosemans W et al. Surgical strategies in esophageal carcinoma with emphasis on radical lymphadenectomy. Ann Surg 1992; 216(5):583–90.

34. Roder JD, Busch R, Stein HJ et al. Ratio of invaded to removed lymph nodes as a predictor of survival in squamous cell carcinoma of the oesophagus. Br J Surg 1994; 81(3):410–13.

35. Clark GW, Peters JH, Ireland AP et al. Nodal metastasis and sites of recurrence after en bloc esophagectomy for adenocarcinoma. Ann Thorac Surg 1994; 58(3):646–53; discussion 653–4.

36. Altorki N, Kent M, Ferrara C et al. Three-field lymph node dissection for squamous cell and adenocarcinoma of the esophagus. Ann Surg 2002; 236(2):177–83.

37. Orringer MB. Transthoracic versus transhiatal esophagectomy: what difference does it make? Ann Thorac Surg 1987; 44(2):116–18.

38. Siewert JR, Roder JD. Lymphadenectomy in oesophageal cancer surgery. Dis Esophagus 1992; 2:91–7.

39. Goldminc M, Maddern G, Le Prise E et al. Oesophagectomy by a transhiatal approach or thoracotomy: a prospective randomized trial. Br J Surg 1993; 80(3):367–70.

40. Kato H, Watanabe H, Tachimori Y et al. Evaluation of neck lymph node dissection for thoracic esophageal carcinoma. Ann Thorac Surg 1991; 51(6):931–5.

41. Kato H, Tachimori Y, Mizobuchi S et al. Cervical, mediastinal, and abdominal lymph node dissection (three-field dissection) for superficial carcinoma of the thoracic esophagus. Cancer 1993; 72(10):2879–82.

42. Gawad KA, Hosch SB, Bumann D et al. How important is the route of reconstruction after esophagectomy: a prospective randomized study. Am J Gastroenterol 1999; 94(6):1490–6.

43. Bartels H, Thorban S, Siewert JR. Anterior versus posterior reconstruction after transhiatal oesophagectomy: a randomized controlled trial. Br J Surg 1993; 80(9):1141–4.

These trials confirm that the mediastinal route is the preferred route for reconstruction after curative resection.

44. Tabira Y, Sakaguchi T, Kuhara H et al. The width of a gastric tube has no impact on outcome after esophagectomy. Am J Surg 2004; 187(3):417–21.

45. el-Eishi HI, Ayoub SF, el-Khalek MA. The arterial supply of the human stomach. Acta Anat (Basel) 1973; 86(3):565–80.

46. Thomas DM, Langford RM, Russell RC et al. The anatomical basis for gastric mobilization in total oesophagectomy. Br J Surg 1979; 66(4):230–3.

47. Khan OA, Manners J, Rengarajan A et al. Does pyloroplasty following esophagectomy improve early clinical outcomes? Interact Cardiovasc Thorac Surg 2007; 6(2):247–50.

48. Cheung HC, Siu KF, Wong J. Is pyloroplasty necessary in esophageal replacement by stomach? A prospective, randomized controlled trial. Surgery 1987; 102(1):19–24.

This randomised trial failed to show significant differences in morbidity and mortality between pyloroplasty and no drainage after gastric transposition.

49. Law S, Cheung MC, Fok M et al. Pyloroplasty and pyloromyotomy in gastric replacement of the esophagus after esophagectomy: a randomized controlled trial. J Am Coll Surg 1997; 184(6):630–6.

50. Ventemiglia R, Khalil KG, Frazier OH et al. The role of preoperative mesenteric arteriography in colon interposition. J Thorac Cardiovasc Surg 1977; 74(1):98–104.

51. DeMeester TR, Johansson KE, Franze I et al. Indications, surgical technique, and long-term functional results of colon interposition or bypass. Ann Surg 1988; 208(4):460–74.

52. Sasaki TM, Baker HW, McConnell DB et al. Free jejunal graft reconstruction after extensive head and neck surgery. Am J Surg 1980; 139(5):650–3.

53. Nanson EM. Synchronous combined abdomino-thoraco-cervical (oesophagectomy). Aust NZ J Surg 1975; 45(4):340–8.

54. Chung SC, Griffin SM, Wood SD et al. Two team synchronous esophagectomy. Surg Gynecol Obstet 1990; 170(1):68–9.

55. Hayes N, Shaw IH, Raimes SA et al. Comparison of conventional Lewis–Tanner two-stage oesophagectomy with the synchronous two-team approach. Br J Surg 1995; 82(3):426.

This small randomised trial demonstrated higher complication and mortality rates in Western patients operated on by the synchronous technique.

56. McKeown KC. The surgical treatment of carcinoma of the oesophagus. A review of the results in 478 cases. J R Coll Surg Edinb 1985; 30(1):1–14.

57. Lu YK, Li YM, Gu YZ. Cancer of esophagus and esophagogastric junction: analysis of results of 1,025 resections after 5 to 20 years. Ann Thorac Surg 1987; 43(2):176–81.

58. Pradhan GN, Eng JB, Sabanathan S. Left thoracotomy approach for resection of carcinoma of the esophagus. Surg Gynecol Obstet 1989; 168(1):49–53.

59. Molina JE, Lawton BR, Myers WO et al. Esophagogastrectomy for adenocarcinoma of the cardia. Ten years' experience and current approach. Ann Surg 1982; 195(2):146–51.

60. Matthews HR, Steel A. Left-sided subtotal oesophagectomy for carcinoma. Br J Surg 1987; 74(12):1115–17.

61. Forshaw MJ, Gossage JA, Ockrim J et al. Left thoracoabdominal esophagogastrectomy: still a valid operation for carcinoma of the distal esophagus and esophagogastric junction. Dis Esophagus 2006; 19(5):340–5.

62. Sasako M, Sano T, Yamamoto S et al. Left thoracoabdominal approach versus abdominal–transhiatal approach for gastric cancer of the cardia or subcardia: a randomised controlled trial. Lancet Oncol 2006; 7(8):644–51.

63. Le Quesne LP, Ranger D. Pharyngolaryngectomy, with immediate pharyngogastric anastomosis. Br J Surg 1966; 53(2):105–9.

64. Turner GG. Excision of thoracic oesophagus for carcinoma with construction of an extra thoracic gullet. Lancet 1933; 1:1315–16.

65. Ong GB. Carcinoma of the hypo-pharynx and cervical oesophagus. In: Smith RE (ed.) Progress in clinical surgery. London: J & A Churchill, 1969; pp. 155–78.

66. Orringer MB, Sloan H. Esophagectomy without thoracotomy. J Thorac Cardiovasc Surg 1978; 76(5):643–54.

67. Alderson D, Courtney SP, Kennedy RH. Radical transhiatal oesophagectomy under direct vision. Br J Surg 1994; 81(3):404–7.

68. Pinotti HW. A new approach to the thoracic esophagus by the abdominal transdiaphragmatic route. Langenbecks Arch Chir 1983; 359(4):229–35.

69. Chu KM, Law SY, Fok M et al. A prospective randomized comparison of transhiatal and transthoracic resection for lower-third esophageal carcinoma. Am J Surg 1997; 174(3):320–4.

70. Jacobi CA, Zieren HU, Muller JM et al. Surgical therapy of esophageal carcinoma: the influence of surgical approach and esophageal resection on cardiopulmonary function. Eur J Cardiothorac Surg 1997; 11(1):32–7.

These two small randomised studies failed to demonstrate differences in cardiopulmonary complications between the transhiatal and transthoracic approaches.

71. Dresner SM, Lamb PJ, Wayman J et al. Benign anastomotic stricture following transthoracic subtotal oesophagectomy and stapled oesophago-gastrostomy: risk factors and management. Br J Surg 2000; 87(3):362–73.

72. Egberts JH, Schniewind B, Bestmann B et al. Impact of the site of anastomosis after oncologic esophagectomy on quality of life – a prospective, longitudinal outcome study. Ann Surg Oncol 2008; 15(2):566–75.

73. Lerut T, Coosemans W, Decker G et al. Anastomotic complications after esophagectomy. Dig Surg 2002; 19(2):92–8.

74. Law S, Fok M, Chu KM et al. Comparison of hand-sewn and stapled esophagogastric anastomosis after esophageal resection for cancer: a prospective randomized controlled trial. Ann Surg 1997; 226(2):169–73.

This small study showed no difference in anastomotic integrity between stapled and hand-sewn anastomosis but confirmed a higher rate of strictures using the stapler for anastomosis.

75. Griffin SM, Lamb PJ, Dresner SM et al. Diagnosis and management of a mediastinal leak following radical oesophagectomy. Br J Surg 2001; 88(10):1346–51.

76. Lamb PJ, Griffin SM, Chandrashekar MV et al. Prospective study of routine contrast radiology after total gastrectomy. Br J Surg 2004; 91(8):1015–19.

77. Smithers BM, Cullinan M, Thomas JM et al. Outcomes from salvage esophagectomy post definitive chemoradiotherapy compared with resection following preoperative neoadjuvant chemoradiotherapy. Dis Esophagus 2007; 20(6):471–7.

78. Lagarde SM, de Boer JD, ten Kate FJ et al. Postoperative complications after esophagectomy for adenocarcinoma of the esophagus are related to timing of death due to recurrence. Ann Surg 2008; 247(1):71–6.

79. Tandon S, Batchelor A, Bullock R et al. Peri-operative risk factors for acute lung injury after elective oesophagectomy. Br J Anaesth 2001; 86(5):633–8.

80. Dresner SM, Lamb PJ, Shenfine J et al. Prognostic significance of peri-operative blood transfusion following radical resection for oesophageal carcinoma. Eur J Surg Oncol 2000; 26(5):492–7.

81. Wemyss-Holden SA, Launois B, Maddern GJ. Management of thoracic duct injuries after oesophagectomy. Br J Surg 2001; 88(11):1442–8.

82. Merigliano S, Molena D, Ruol A et al. Chylothorax complicating esophagectomy for cancer: a plea for early thoracic duct ligation. J Thorac Cardiovasc Surg 2000; 119(3):453–7.

83. Dugue L, Sauvanet A, Farges O et al. Output of chyle as an indicator of treatment for chylothorax complicating oesophagectomy. Br J Surg 1998; 85(8):1147–9.

84. Thaker H, Snow MH, Spickett G et al. *Pneumocystis carinii* pneumonia after thoracic duct ligation and leakage. Clin Infect Dis 2001; 33(11):E129–31.

85. Griffin SM, Chung SC, van Hasselt CA et al. Late swallowing and aspiration problems after esophagectomy for cancer: malignant infiltration of the recurrent laryngeal nerves and its management. Surgery 1992; 112(3):533–5.

86. Dresner SM, Griffin SM, Wayman J et al. Human model of duodenogastro-oesophageal reflux in the development of Barrett's metaplasia. Br J Surg 2003; 90(9):1120–8.

87. Aly A, Jamieson GG. Reflux after oesophagectomy. Br J Surg 2004; 91(2):137–41.

88. Aly A, Jamieson GG, Pyragius M et al. Antireflux anastomosis following oesophagectomy. Aust NZ J Surg 2004; 74(6):434–8.

89. Blazeby JM, Brookes ST, Alderson D. The prognostic value of quality of life scores during treatment for oesophageal cancer. Gut 2001; 49(2): 227–30.

90. Earlam R, Cunha-Melo JR. Oesophageal squamous cell carcinoma: I. A critical review of surgery. Br J Surg 1980; 67(6):381–90.

91. Jamieson GG, Mathew G, Ludemann R et al. Postoperative mortality following oesophagectomy and problems in reporting its rate. Br J Surg 2004; 91(8):943–7.

92. Liu JF, Wang QZ, Ping YM et al. Complications after esophagectomy for cancer: 53-year experience with 20,796 patients. World J Surg 2008; 32(3):395–400.

93. McCulloch P, Ward J, Tekkis PP. Mortality and morbidity in gastro-oesophageal cancer surgery: initial results of ASCOT multicentre prospective cohort study. Br Med J 2003; 327(7425):1192–7.

6

Treatment of early oesophageal cancer

Burkhard H.A. von Rahden
Hubert J. Stein

Introduction

'Early oesophageal cancers' appear in clinical practice with increasing frequency.[1,2] This may be attributable to epidemiological changes,[3,4] as well as to improved diagnostic tools[5,6] and surveillance strategies.[7]

The definition of 'early oesophageal cancer' covers pT1 lesions as well as high-grade intraepithelial neoplasia (HG-IN), and is irrespective of lymph node metastases, which may be present in a substantial number of cases, particularly in tumours infiltrating the submucosal layer. Especially with respect to 'early cancers', distinction of the two main oesophageal tumour entities – adenocarcinoma (AC) and squamous cell carcinoma (SCC) – is of utmost importance.[2,8] Differences in aetiology, pathophysiology, tumour biology, pattern of lymphatic spread, presence of multifocal lesions, prevalence of synchronous/metachronous cancers at other locations and type of affected patients have major impact on management strategies.

Substantial differences between early oesophageal AC and SCC can be noted between West and East,[9] with oesophageal AC now prevailing in America and Europe and oesophageal SCC still the almost exclusive oesophageal cancer entity in Asia/Japan.

 In sharp contrast to advanced oesophageal malignancies, which can only rarely be cured,[10] the chances for cure in patients with early oesophageal cancers are excellent. Survival equals that of the general population, provided that an appropriate therapeutic approach is pursued.[2]

In many institutions the standard of care for early oesophageal neoplasms is still radical oesophagectomy and lymphadenectomy. In the past years, a number of limited surgical procedures have been suggested as alternatives to radical resection and are currently under clinical investigation. More recently some interventional endoscopists have completely questioned the need for surgical resection of early oesophageal cancer and propose the use of endoscopic resection/ablation techniques as 'curative treatment'.[11]

Histological tumour entities of early oesophageal cancer

Oesophageal adenocarcinoma and Barrett's oesophagus

In the Western world, we are now dealing predominantly with oesophageal adenocarcinomas, an entity that has seen a dramatic and largely unexplained rise in incidence among white males.[3,4] Chronic gastro-oesophageal reflux disease (GORD) and Barrett's oesophagus have been recognised as the underlying precancerous condition and precursor lesion of these tumours.[12] The characterisation of the malignant progression from Barrett's metaplasia through intraepithelial neoplasia to invasive carcinoma sequence opened the door for screening and surveillance strategies, which are currently recommended by guidelines.[7]

Chapter 6

Oesophageal squamous cell carcinoma

Early oesophageal squamous cell carcinomas (SCCs) are uncommon in the Western world,[9] due to the low and probably decreasing overall incidence of this tumour entity. In contrast to Japan and China, where screening strategies for early SCC are effective, detection of these tumours in the West is a chance phenomenon. The major risk factors for oesophageal SCC are smoking and alcohol abuse. About 10% of patients with head and neck cancers suffer from a secondary oesophageal SCC.

Defining early oesophageal cancer

'Early oesophageal cancer' is defined as locally limited tumour growth, with depth of invasion no further than the submucosal layer (pT1 or pTis according to the TNM staging system of the UICC/AJCC[13]) and irrespective of nodal involvement.

'Intraepithelial neoplasia' (IN) is the currently recommended nomenclature by the 'WHO Classification of Tumours of the Digestive Tract'[14] for what was formerly, and is still frequently, addressed as 'dysplasia'. The new term was chosen to distinguish these lesions from inflammatory changes and clearly stress their (pre-)malignant potential.

Mucosal tumours (pT1a or pT1m, category 5.1 of the 'Vienna classification'), submucosal tumours (pT1b or pT1sm; category 5.2 of the 'Vienna classification') as well as high-grade intraepithelial neoplasia (HG-IN, category 4 of the 'Vienna classification') are all included under the term 'early oesophageal cancer'.

This 'Vienna classification' of gastrointestinal epithelial neoplasia[15] (see Table 6.1) has been designed to standardise distinction of these subgroups by different pathologists and correct for the well-known inter-observer bias.

 However, there is plenty of evidence to suggest that, despite the use of such standardised classification systems, grading of intraepithelial neoplasia (low grade, LG-IN, category 3 vs. high grade, HG-IN, category 4) and invasive carcinomas is still severely biased. Blinded analyses of representative histopathological specimens have shown substantial variation, even with respect to distinction between invasive and non-invasive growth.[15,16]

Establishing the diagnosis

The diagnosis of early oesophageal cancer is based on histopathological evaluation of endoscopically retrieved biopsies, with the issues of histopathological

Table 6.1 • The Vienna classification of gastrointestinal epithelial neoplasia

Category 1	Negative for neoplasia/dysplasia
Category 2	Indefinite for neoplasia/dysplasia
Category 3	Non-invasive neoplasia low grade (low-grade adenoma/dysplasia)
Category 4	Non-invasive neoplasia high grade:
4.1	High-grade adenoma/dysplasia
4.2	Non-invasive carcinoma (carcinoma in situ)
4.3	Suspicious for invasive carcinoma
Category 5	Invasive neoplasia:
5.1	Intramucosal carcinoma
5.2	Submucosal carcinoma

Reproduced from Schlemper RJ, Riddell RH, Kato Y et al. The Vienna classification of gastrointestinal epithelial neoplasia. Gut 2000; 47:251–5. With permission from BMJ Publishing Group Ltd.

grading as discussed above. Because the diagnosis is based on biopsy retrieval, this raises the next problem with respect to where and when to retrieve these biopsies. Since early oesophageal malignancies are usually asymptomatic, the diagnosis is often made by chance (during endoscopy for another indication) or more commonly during surveillance endoscopies performed in patients with known Barrett's oesophagus. A standardised biopsy protocol for Barrett's is recommended to control for the 'sampling error'. Biopsies should be taken every 1–2 cm in every quadrant along the whole length of the Barrett's mucosa. Macroscopically suspect lesions should be biopsied in addition.[7]

The diagnostic yield for detection of oesophageal SCC may be improved by the use of **Lugol stain**, as oesophageal SCCs do not take up 0.8% Lugol iodine. Although oesophageal SCC can be found in any part of the oesophagus, the majority of early SCC is localised in the mid-thoracic oesophagus.

Depth of invasion is usually determined with **endoscopic ultrasound**. However, even with the use of new technologies (high-resolution probes, etc.), this method has poor accuracy defining submucosal invasion.[17-19] The only means of accurately defining depth of invasion is currently to perform a **diagnostic endoscopic mucosal resection**. We and others have already adopted this strategy into treatment algorithms.[20,21]

Lymph node metastases

Early oesophageal **adenocarcinomas** and **squamous cell cancers** differ greatly with respect to their pattern and prevalence of lymphatic spread.[2] This may be attributed to the different biological behaviour of these tumours but may, at least in part, also be

116

an effect of the different tumour location, with AC arising almost exclusively in the distal third and SCC originating predominantly in the middle third.

 While lymph node metastases are always absent in patients with HG-IN (irrespective of the histological tumour type), about 2% of patients with pT1a AC and up to 10% of patients with pT1a SCC may already have lymphatic spread. The likelihood of lymphatic spread rises to about 25% for submucosal (pT1b) AC and may exceed 40% in patients with submucosal SCC.[2,22–27]

Attempts at further subdivision of the mucosal and submucosal layers have revealed that the likelihood for lymphatic spread rises substantially (to about 60%) when the tumour invades the deep submucosal layers.[27,28] Of note, these data are based on evaluation of the surgical specimen and are irrespective of the difficulties in establishing the diagnosis preoperatively. Because of the inaccuracy of current staging modalities to predict depth of tumour infiltration preoperatively, the potential of lymphatic spread must thus always be kept in mind when making therapeutic decisions.

Screening and surveillance

Endoscopic screening for Barrett's oesophagus is performed among patients with GORD. **Endoscopic surveillance** is performed for patients harbouring Barrett's oesophagus. Although the effectiveness of both strategies to improve patients' life expectancy is disputed,[29,30] it seems clear that they are currently the only available tools for detection of early oesophageal adenocarcinomas.[7,31,32]

It is recommended that **endoscopic screening** is performed at least once in all patients with symptomatic GORD.[7] If Barrett's oesophagus is suspected, the diagnosis requires histological confirmation by means of intensive endoscopic mapping (four-quadrant biopsies along the entire length of columnar mucosa and additional biopsy of macroscopically suspicious areas). After initial diagnosis of Barrett's oesophagus, the endoscopic work-up should be repeated within the first year.[7,33] When the epithelium is non-dysplastic, an **endoscopic surveillance** interval of every 5 years seems appropriate. When the diagnosis is LG-IN, a more thorough work-up is recommended. The diagnosis of HG-IN is an indication for intervention.

Low-grade and high-grade dysplasia (intraepithelial neoplasia)

Histopathological detection and grading of intraepithelial neoplasia (dysplasia) as 'low-grade' (LG-IN) and 'high-grade dysplasia' (HG-IN) according to WHO criteria[14] is still the most reliable currently available marker for stratification of the risk for malignant progression of Barrett's oesophagus. The vast majority of intraepithelial neoplasias (92.4%) and even many invasive adenocarcinomas (32.7%) cannot be detected by means of endoscopy and are only seen on biopsy.[34]

The malignant potency of LG-IN and HG-IN is, however, not easy to evaluate, because of numerous forms of bias:

- the endoscopists' sampling error;
- the pathologists' intra- and inter-observer bias;
- the clinicians' mal-adherence to guidelines;
- patients' mal-compliance.

However, it seems clear that LG-IN is associated with a substantially higher rate of malignant progression to invasive adenocarcinoma as compared to non-dysplastic Barrett's oesophagus.[33] Consequently, surveillance should be intensified once LG-IN is diagnosed.

Histological differentiation of HG-IN from invasive carcinoma (and to a lesser degree from LG-IN) carries even more intra- and inter-observer bias, even when standardised criteria (e.g. the Vienna classification) are used. This makes 'HG-IN' a rather unsafe diagnosis. HG-IN is, however, regarded as a clear (pre-)malignant lesion that may originate uni- or multifocally within entirely non-neoplastic Barrett's epithelium[35] and is frequently already associated with synchronous invasive Barrett's carcinoma.[36–38]

Although 'watchful waiting' is still recommended by some investigators in patients with HG-IN in Barrett's oesophagus,[39] most agree that these patients should be treated as patients with histologically proven mucosal or submucosal cancer.[40] Because of these far-reaching therapeutic consequences, and the difficulties in establishing the diagnosis, the diagnosis should be established and confirmed by two specialised gastrointestinal pathologists ('second opinion').

Treatment of early oesophageal cancer

Radical surgical resection, by means of oesophagectomy and systematic lymphadenectomy, is still the standard treatment for early oesophageal cancer.[11,40] However, this standard is currently challenged because the associated morbidity and mortality are deemed to be high, especially for early oesophageal adenocarcinomas. On the one hand, limited surgical procedures have been suggested. These include limited resection of the oesophagogastric junction,[41] vagal-sparing oesophagectomy[42,43] and minimally invasive oesophagectomy.[44] On the other hand, interventional endoscopists have questioned the necessity of surgical resection at all. A variety of techniques for mucosal ablation (photodynamic therapy, argon plasma coagulation) and endoscopic resection (endoscopic mucosal resection and endoscopic submucosal dissection) have been proposed.[11,45]

Standard treatment: radical surgical resection and lymphadenectomy

The long-term survival with radical oesophagectomy and systematic mediastinal and upper abdominal lymphadenectomy in patients with early oesophageal cancer exceeds 80–90% in most series.[2,11,25] However, even in experienced hands, perioperative mortality is up to 5%, postoperative complications occur in 30% or more, and less than 20% of patients are completely free of symptoms 2 years after undergoing radical oesophageal resection for early oesophageal carcinoma. The main persistent symptoms are weight loss, reflux and dysphagia.[46]

Limited surgical approaches to early oesophageal cancer

Because of the morbidity and long-term side-effects of radical oesophagectomy, limited surgical approaches to early oesophageal cancer have recently been proposed, particularly in patients with early adenocarcinoma arising in Barrett's oesophagus, i.e. close to the oesophagogastric junction. These include:

- limited resection of the distal oesophagus and oesophagogastric junction and reconstruction with a pedicled isoperistaltic jejunal loop (the so-called modified Merendino procedure);[2,41,47]
- vagal-sparing oesophagectomy (VSO);[42,43]
- minimally invasive oesophagectomy (MIO).[44,48]

Limited resection of the oesophagogastric junction and jejunal interposition

This operation employs a pure transabdominal approach, with splitting of the oesophageal hiatus. The distal oesophagus can thus be dissected transhiatally up to the level of the tracheal bifurcation without thoracotomy. The procedure can incorporate a systematic lower mediastinal and upper abdominal lymphadenectomy with or without preservation of the vagal innervation of the distal stomach. After resection of the distal oesophagus, cardia and proximal stomach the gastrointestinal continuity is restored by means of interposition of an isoperistaltic pedicled jejunal loop to prevent postoperative reflux. This operation is considered oncologically

adequate for early adenocarcinomas arising within short segments of Barrett's mucosa, because:

- complete tumour removal (R0 resection) is possible in all cases;
- a systematic regional lymphadenectomy is performed;
- Barrett's mucosa up to 5 cm in length can be included in the specimen.

The outcome of more than 100 such procedures now performed for early Barrett's cancer shows that this procedure compares very favourably to radical oesophagectomy in terms of long-term survival and is associated with substantially lower peri- and postoperative morbidity, and a very good postoperative quality of life. The procedure offers preservation of healthy oesophagus and gastric function but is technically challenging and requires attention to detail to achieve good long-term functional results.

Vagal-sparing oesophagectomy (VSO)

Another attempt to reduce the negative side-effects of an oesophagectomy is the use of a VSO, which had first been described by Akiyama et al.[49] and was further developed and used for pT1a adenocarcinoma and HG-IN lesions by the DeMeester group in Los Angeles.[42,43] The rationale to develop this procedure was an attempt to reduce the negative physiological impacts of oesophagectomy, elimination of the need for a pyloroplasty and minimising the risk of dumping and postvagotomy diarrhoea in patients who do not require lymphadenectomy (i.e. pT1a/HG-IN adenocarcinoma).

The VSO is performed through an upper abdominal incision and a left neck approach. Both vagal trunks are identified and protected with vessel loops. A highly selective vagotomy is performed along the lesser curvature of the stomach from the crow's foot on the incisura up to the gastro-oesophageal junction. No formal abdominal lymphadenectomy is performed and the left gastric artery is preserved. Through a left neck incision, the cervical oesophagus is isolated and divided. A standard vein stripper is passed retrograde through a gastrotomy just below the gastro-oesophageal junction. The distal cervical oesophagus is secured around the stripper and then slowly pulled back into the abdomen, inverting the oesophagus in on itself and out of the gastrotomy. This manoeuvre strips the branches of the oesophageal plexus off the longitudinal muscle and preserves the integrity of the vagal nerves. Reconstruction is performed with a gastric tube or an isoperistaltic left colon graft that is interposed between the cervical oesophagus and the intact innervated stomach. No pyloroplasty procedure is performed because the antral innervation is preserved. The DeMeester group[43] report a 2% mortality with VSO and a significantly decreased morbidity in comparison with more radical oesophagectomy procedures. Major complications were reported in 35% of patients. Postvagotomy symptoms like diarrhoea and dumping were substantially reduced.

> The major disadvantage of VSO is that lymphadenectomy is completely omitted. This makes it suitable only for pT1a and HG-IN lesions in Barrett's oesophagus, where lymphatic spread is virtually absent. An exact preoperative discrimination of pT1b lesions, which are often associated with lymphatic spread, is thus mandatory.

This is currently only possible with the routine use of a preoperative diagnostic endoscopic mucosal resection and in unifocal lesions.

Minimally invasive oesophagectomy (MIO)

MIOe is a now increasingly employed approach to reduce morbidity of oesophagectomy, irrespective of tumour stage. Its broadest application, however, is in patients with early disease. Most minimally invasive oesophagectomies are hybrid operations (thoracotomy/laparoscopy or thoracoscopy/laparotomy or require some 'hand-assist' access ports).

The greatest experience with a totally minimally invasive technique avoiding the need for 'access' laparotomy and thoracotomy has been reported from Pittsburgh.[44,48] This is a three-stage operation with the oesophageal specimen removed through a left neck incision. Following the insertion of a double-lumen tube for single-lung ventilation, the operation commences with a right thoracoscopic approach for complete thoracic mobilisation of the oesophagus, including resection of the mediastinal pleura, and paraoesophageal and subcarinal lymph node groups. This is followed by a laparoscopic approach for gastric mobilisation and upper abdominal lymphadenectomy. The final stage is a cervical anastomosis of the gastric tube to the oesophagus in the left side of the neck. Luketich and co-workers from Pittsburgh have reported the largest series of MIO for oesophageal cancer with favourable results in terms of perioperative morbidity, mortality and time to recovery. Since this approach only aims at reducing access trauma and immediate perioperative morbidity, and since the extent of the procedure matches that of a conventional oesophagectomy, the negative long-term sequelae should also be identical.

Endoscopic approaches to early oesophageal cancer

Several endoscopic techniques have been reported for elimination of early neoplastic lesions in the oesophagus. These can in principle be categorised into **ablative techniques** and **resective techniques**.[11,45,50] The key feature of this strategy is 'organ preservation' with minimal mortality and procedure-related morbidity.

> The technical feasibility of these methods has been clearly demonstrated. However, their efficacy and oncological adequacy for early oesophageal cancer therapy remain to be determined.

While endoscopic resection techniques in combination with ablation of Barrett's oesophagus are already propagated by some as a 'curative treatment' option for early oesophageal cancer,[45,51] several concerns remain.

Endoscopic ablation

Ablation techniques using argon plasma coagulation, laser therapy, photodynamic therapy or radiofrequency result in destruction of the mucosa.[11,45,50] The problem with all these techniques is that a specimen for histopathological examination is not obtained. This makes evaluation of the completeness of the intervention impossible. This is also problematic because the diagnosis 'HG-IN' and distinction from mucosal and submucosal tumours can only be based on histopathological evaluation of a surgical specimen.

Even when an endoscopic ablation appears 'complete' with restitution of a normal squamous epithelium, it is not guaranteed that the tumour growth will not continue underneath this epithelium in remnants of Barrett's/intraepithelial neoplasia/invasive carcinoma.[52] Furthermore, ablation of Barrett's mucosa may be associated with substantial morbidity, as it may cause severe oesophageal strictures and stenoses. Ablative strategies can thus only be recommended in patients who are not amenable to surgical or endoscopic resection.

Endoscopic resection

Because of the shortcomings of endoscopic ablation, several techniques for 'endoscopic resection' of oesophageal mucosa have been developed. In principle one needs to distinguish between so-called endoscopic mucosal resection (EMR)[45] and endoscopic submucosal dissection (ESD).[53,54]

EMR is performed in various techniques with or without submucosal injections to lift up the tumour and with or without the use of a suction device ('suck and cut technique' vs. 'simple snare resection' using a diathermy snare, also called 'strip biopsy').

ESD is a newer technique that has been introduced for endoscopic removal of gastric lesions, and has recently also been applied in patients with oesophageal neoplasms.[53,54] The technique utilises an insulated-tip knife to dissect the submucosal layer underneath the carcinoma in order to obtain a large resection specimen with the neoplasm resected en bloc. ESD is technically demanding, particularly in the region close to the oesophagogastric junction. There is a substantial learning curve with long procedure times. Complications are frequent and include perforations requiring surgery, bleeding and severe stenosis, particularly when circumferential or long-segment resections are performed.

Endoscopic intervention versus surgical resection for early oesophageal cancer

With the advent of interventional endoscopic techniques the time-proven principles and standards of surgical therapy for early neoplasms in the oesophagus have been challenged. Because of the potential of 'organ preservation', endoscopic intervention is now vehemently propagated by some as the treatment of choice for early oesophageal adenocarcinoma in Barrett's oesophagus and squamous cell carcinoma.[45,51] This view is based on the assumption that the neoplastic lesions can be entirely removed with a local approach and that lymphatic spread is absent.

However, in the majority of patients undergoing endoscopic resection removal of the tumour-infiltrated mucosa is only possible in a piecemeal fashion, which neglects the principle of surgical oncology to never cut through a tumour in situ. The consequence is a high rate of incomplete 'R1' resections at the lateral margins. The protagonists of endoscopic resection suggest that these 'lateral R1 situations' do not matter and hypothesise that only the basal margin is relevant. However, especially with respect to the basal margin, the appropriateness of the use of the R classification in its current sense must be critically discussed, because it is questionable if the small (at maximum microscopic) submucosal basal margin is wide enough to classify the 'resection' as R0.[50]

Since endoscopic intervention does not allow for a lymphadenectomy, only patients with a zero or very low risk of lymphatic spread are potential candidates, i.e. it is theoretically only applicable in patients with unifocal HG-IN or mucosal cancer in Barrett's oesophagus. However, at present depth of invasion cannot be predicted with sufficient accuracy, even with the use of new and sophisticated staging tools.

Furthermore, even after complete endoscopic removal of early neoplastic lesions, segments with precancerous Barrett's mucosa are usually left behind. Additional treatment modalities like photodynamic therapy have so far not been proven useful. EMR for oesophageal neoplasms within Barrett's oesophagus has therefore been described as 'similar to pulling weeds out of a garden and expecting them never to grow again'.[20]

In fact, even in experienced hands tumour recurrence rates after endoscopic resection may exceed 30%, particularly in patients with piecemeal resection, long-segment Barrett's oesophagus, no ablative therapy of residual Barrett's oesophagus and those with multifocal neoplasia.[55] Endoscopic intervention thus currently appears more than questionable if not a priori inadequate. Patients with early oesophageal neoplasms should not be denied a high chance of being cured by means of an appropriate surgical resection. Endoscopic interventions should be considered only in patients who may not tolerate a surgical intervention or have, for other reasons, limited chances for cure by means of adequate oncological resection.

Key points

- Early oesophageal adenocarcinomas and squamous cell cancers are different entities with different therapeutic implications.
- Barrett's oesophagus is regarded as the precancerous lesion of early oesophageal adenocarcinomas. Endoscopic surveillance with a standardised schedule and biopsy protocol is recommended.
- Endoscopic surveillance for Barrett's oesophagus should be tailored to the presence of low-grade intraepithelial neoplasia.
- High-grade intraepithelial neoplasia – similar to invasive carcinoma – is an indication for surgical resection.
- The resection specimen in early oesophageal adenocarcinomas must include the entire segment of underlying Barrett's mucosa.
- Radical resection with systematic lymphadenectomy is the standard treatment for early oesophageal carcinoma, particularly when submucosal tumour infiltration is present.
- In experienced hands and selected patients, limitations of the surgical approach (e.g. limited resection of the oesophagogastric junction, vagal-sparing oesophagectomy, minimally invasive oesophagectomy) are justified.
- Endoscopic treatment modalities are still experimental and should not be considered as curative treatment because recurrence rates are unacceptably high.

References

1. Stein HJ, von Rahden BHA, Siewert JR. Survival after surgery of cancer of the esophagus. Langenbeck's Arch Surg 2004; 390:280–5.

2. Stein HJ, Feith M, Bruecher BL et al. Early esophageal cancer: pattern of lymphatic spread and prognostic factors for long-term survival after surgical resection. Ann Surg 2005; 242:566–73.

3. Pohl H, Welch HG. The role of overdiagnosis and reclassification in the marked increase of esophageal adenocarcinoma incidence. J Natl Cancer Inst 2005; 97:142–6.

4. Devesa SS, Blot WJ, Fraumeni JF Jr. Changing patterns in the incidence of esophageal and gastric carcinoma in the United States. Cancer 1998; 83:2049–53.

5. Dubuc J, Legoux JL, Winnock M et al. Société Française d'Endoscopie Digestive. Endoscopic screening for esophageal squamous-cell carcinoma in high-risk patients: a prospective study conducted in 62 French endoscopy centers. Endoscopy 2006; 38:690–5.

6. Connor MJ, Sharma P. Chromoendoscopy and magnification endoscopy for diagnosing esophageal cancer and dysplasia. Thorac Surg Clin 2004; 14:87–94.

7. Sampliner RE. The Practice Parameters Committee of the American College of Gastroenterology. Updated guidelines for the diagnosis, surveillance, and therapy of Barrett's esophagus. Am J Gastroenterol 2002; 97:1888–95.

8. Siewert JR, Stein HJ, Feith M et al. Histologic tumor type is an independent prognostic parameter in esophageal cancer: lessons from more than 1,000 consecutive resections at a single center in the Western world. Ann Surg 2001; 234:360–7.

9. Siewert JR, von Rahden BHA, Stein HJ. Current status of esophageal cancer – West versus East: the European point of view. Esophagus 2004; 1:147–59.

10. von Rahden BHA, Stein HJ. Staging and treatment of advanced esophageal cancer. Curr Opin Gastroenterol 2005; 21:472–7.

11. Conio M, Cameron AJ, Chak A et al. Endoscopic treatment of high-grade dysplasia and early cancer in Barrett's oesophagus. Lancet Oncol 2005; 6:311–21.

12. von Rahden BHA, Stein HJ. Barrett's esophagus and Barrett's carcinoma. Curr GERD Rep 2007; 1:125–32.

13. Sobin LH, Wittekind Ch (eds). UICC TNM classification of malignant tumors, 6th edn. New York: Wiley-Liss, 2002.

14. Werner M, Flejou JF, Hainaut P et al. Adenocarcinoma of the oesophagus. In: Hamilton SR, Aaltonen L (eds) World Health Organization classification of tumours: pathology and genetics – tumours of the digestive system. Lyon: IARC Press, 2000; pp. 20–5.

15. Schlemper RJ, Riddell RH, Kato Y et al. The Vienna classification of gastrointestinal epithelial neoplasia. Gut 2000; 47:251–5.

16. Ormsby AH, Petras RE, Henricks WH et al. Observer variation in the diagnosis of superficial oesophageal adenocarcinoma. Gut 2002; 51:671–6.

17. Chemaly M, Scalone O, Durivage G et al. Miniprobe EUS in the pretherapeutic assessment of early esophageal neoplasia. Endoscopy 2008; 40:2–6.

18. May A, Günter E, Roth F et al. Accuracy of staging in early oesophageal cancer using high resolution endoscopy and high resolution endosonography: a comparative, prospective, and blinded trial. Gut 2004; 53:634–40.

19. Pech O, May A, Günter E et al. The impact of endoscopic ultrasound and computed tomography on the TNM staging of early cancer in Barrett's esophagus. Am J Gastroenterol 2006; 101:2223–9.

20. DeMeester SR. New options for the therapy of Barrett's high-grade dysplasia and intramucosal adenocarcinoma: endoscopic mucosal resection and ablation versus vagal-sparing esophagectomy. Ann Thorac Surg 2008; 85:S747–50.

21. Stein HJ, Feith M. Surgical strategies for early esophageal adenocarcinoma. Best Pract Res Clin Gastroenterol 2005; 19:927–40.

22. Nishimaki T, Suzuki T, Kanda T et al. Extended radical esophagectomy for superficially invasive carcinoma of the esophagus. Surgery 1999; 125:142–7.

23. Kodama M, Kakegawa T. Treatment of superficial cancer of the esophagus: a summary of responses to a questionnaire on superficial cancer of the esophagus in Japan. Surgery 1998; 123:432–9.

24. Natsugoe S, Baba M, Yoshinaka H et al. Mucosal squamous cell carcinoma of the esophagus: a clinicopathologic study of 30 cases. Oncology 1998; 55:235–41.

25. Nigro JJ, Hagen JA, DeMeester TR et al. Occult esophageal adenocarcinoma: extent of disease and implications for effective therapy. Ann Surg 1999; 230:433–8.

26. Buskens CJ, Westerterp M, Lagarde SM et al. Prediction of appropriateness of local endoscopic treatment for high-grade dysplasia and early adenocarcinoma by EUS and histopathologic features. Gastrointest Endosc 2004; 60:703–10.

27. Liu L, Hofstetter WL, Rashid A et al. Significance of the depth of tumor invasion and lymph node metastasis in superficially invasive (T1) esophageal adenocarcinoma. Am J Surg Pathol 2005; 29:1079–85.

28. Westerterp M, Koppert LB, Buskens CJ et al. Outcome of surgical treatment for early adenocarcinoma of the esophagus or gastro-esophageal junction. Virchow's Arch 2005; 446:497–504.

29. van Blankenstein M. Barrett's esophagus: so what! Dis Esoph 2002; 15:1–4.

30. Dellon ES, Shaheen NJ. Does screening for Barrett's esophagus and adenocarcinoma of the

esophagus prolong survival? J Clin Oncol 2005; 23:4478–82.

31. van Sandick JW, van Lanschot JJ, Kuiken BW et al. Impact of endoscopic biopsy surveillance of Barrett's oesophagus on pathological stage and clinical outcome of Barrett's carcinoma. Gut 1998; 43:216–22.

32. Peters JH, Clark GW, Ireland AP et al. Outcome of adenocarcinoma arising in Barrett's esophagus in endoscopically surveyed and nonsurveyed patients. J Thorac Cardiovasc Surg 1994; 108:813–21.

33. von Rahden BHA, Stein HJ, Weber A et al. Critical reappraisal of current surveillance strategies for Barrett's esophagus: analysis of a large German Barrett's database. Dis Esoph 2008; 21:685–9.

34. Vieth M, Stolte M. Barrett's mucosa, Barrett's dysplasia and Barrett's carcinoma: diagnostic endoscopy without biopsy-taking does not suffice. Dis Esoph 2000; 13:23–7.

35. Buttar NS, Wang KK, Sebo TJ et al. Extent of high-grade dysplasia in Barrett's esophagus correlates with risk of adenocarcinoma. Gastroenterology 2000; 120:1630–9.

36. Sujendran V, Sica G, Warren B et al. Oesophagectomy remains the gold standard for treatment of high-grade dysplasia in Barrett's oesophagus. Eur J Cardiothorac Surg 2005; 28:763–6.

37. Tharavej C, Hagen JA, Peters JH et al. Predictive factors of coexisting cancer in Barrett's high-grade dysplasia. Surg Endosc 2006; 20:439–43.

38. Heitmiller RF, Redmond M, Hamilton SR. Barrett's esophagus with high-grade dysplasia. An indication for prophylactic esophagectomy. Ann Surg 1996; 224:66–71.

39. Schnell TG, Sontag SJ, Chejfec G et al. Long-term nonsurgical management of Barrett's esophagus with high-grade dysplasia. Gastroenterology 2001; 120:1607–19.

40. Spechler SJ. Barrett's esophagus. N Engl J Med 2002; 346:836–42.

41. Stein HJ, Feith M, Mueller J et al. Limited resection for early adenocarcinoma in Barrett's esophagus. Ann Surg 2000; 232:733–42.

42. Banki F, Mason RJ, DeMeester SR et al. Vagal-sparing esophagectomy: a more physiologic alternative. Ann Surg 2002; 236:324–35.

43. Peyre CG, DeMeester SR, Rizzetto C et al. Vagal-sparing esophagectomy: the ideal operation for intramucosal adenocarcinoma and Barrett with high-grade dysplasia. Ann Surg 2007; 246:665–71.

44. Luketich JD, Alvelo-Rivera M, Buenaventura PO et al. Minimally invasive esophagectomy: outcomes in 222 patients. Ann Surg 2003; 238:486–94.

45. Pech O, May A, Rabenstein T et al. Endoscopic resection of early oesophageal cancer. Gut 2007; 56:1625–34.

46. Headrick JR, Nichols FC 3rd, Miller DL et al. High-grade esophageal dysplasia: long-term survival and quality of life after esophagectomy. Ann Thorac Surg 2002; 73:1697–702.

47. Stein HJ, Hutter J, Feith M et al. Limited surgical resection and jejunal interposition for early adenocarcinoma of the distal esophagus. Semin Thorac Cardiovasc Surg 2007; 19:72–8.

48. Ashrafi AS, Keeley SB, Shende M et al. Minimally invasive esophagectomy. Eur Surg 2007; 39:141–50.

49. Akiyama H, Tsurumaru M, Ono Y et al. Esophagectomy without thoracotomy with vagal preservation. Am Coll Surg 1994; 178:83–5.

50. von Rahden BHA, Stein HJ. Barrett's esophagus with high-grade intraepithelial neoplasia: observation, ablation or resection? Eur Surg 2007; 39:249–54.

51. Ell C, May A, Pech O et al. Curative endoscopic resection of early esophageal adenocarcinomas (Barrett's cancer). Gastrointest Endosc 2007; 65:3–10.

52. Satodate H, Inoue H, Fukami N et al. Squamous reepithelialization after circumferential endoscopic mucosal resection of superficial carcinoma arising in Barrett's esophagus. Endoscopy 2004; 36:909–12.

53. Fujishiro M, Yahagi N, Kakushima N et al. Endoscopic submucosal dissection of esophageal squamous cell neoplasms. Clin Gastroenterol Hepatol 2006; 4:688–94.

54. Saito Y, Takisawa H, Suzuki H et al. Endoscopic submucosal dissection of recurrent or residual superficial esophageal cancer after chemoradiotherapy. Gastrointest Endosc 2008; 67:355–9.

55. Pech O, Behrens, A, May A et al. Long-term results and risk factor analysis for recurrence after curative endoscopic therapy in 349 patients with high-grade intraepithelial neoplasia and mucosal adenocarcinoma in Barrett's oesophagus. Gut 2008; 57:1200–6.

Surgery for cancer of the stomach

Simon A. Raimes

Introduction

This chapter describes the development of modern gastric cancer surgery for patients with advanced (T2–T4) gastric cancer. Radical gastric cancer surgery is based on the principles first defined by the Japanese and then adapted to take into account the different factors that affect Western patients, including the higher frequency of diffuse-type and proximal cancers and also their age, build and increased comorbidity. The drive has been towards procedures with a lower mortality but retaining the principles of a radical resection in a rational way – balancing radicality with risk. This has led to the concept of 'tailored' operations and it is important to understand how the decision-making process has developed in recent years.

Patients with advanced gastric cancer now frequently receive neoadjuvant or adjuvant therapies, but the most important factor in producing potential cure is the quality of the surgery. There is now a move towards laparoscopic or laparoscopic-assisted surgery, but the principles of resection should remain the same whichever approach is used. The aim of this chapter is to describe the theory and practice of modern gastric cancer surgery.

Modes of spread and areas of potential failure after gastric cancer surgery

A rational approach to surgery for gastric cancer requires an understanding of the modes of spread of this cancer and how it recurs after surgery. This knowledge is essential to be able to define the aims and limitations of radical surgery.

Metastatic pathways

Direct extension

Where direct extension occurs to affect adjacent organs or structures, these may be excised en bloc with the stomach as part of a potentially curative resection.

Lymphatic spread

Lateral spread occurs in the submucosal and subserosal lymphatic plexuses, depending on the depth of penetration of the cancer. Drainage is then to the perigastric nodes and subsequently along the lymphatics that accompany the arteries to the stomach back to the coeliac trunk. This is discussed in more detail below in the section on lymphadenectomy. Lymphatic spread can occur at any stage, but becomes more likely the deeper the invasion through the stomach wall. Lymphatic spread is the most common mode of dissemination in both intestinal and diffuse types of gastric cancer. This emphasises the potential importance of adequate nodal excision as there is good-quality evidence to show that patients with nodal spread can still be cured by radical surgery. Unlike some other cancers, spread to lymph nodes may not necessarily be a marker of disseminated disease, although this concept remains hotly debated.

Peritoneal spread

This should only occur once the cancer has breached the serosal surface, when cells can then be shed into the peritoneal cavity. Up to 70% of cancers in the West are serosa-positive and thus a large number of patients have the potential for intraperitoneal recurrence by cell implantation in the gastric bed or elsewhere in the peritoneal cavity. The risk of peritoneal spread increases with the area of the serosa that is involved. Peritoneal seeding is much more common in diffuse-type cancers (45–75% vs. 10–30% for the intestinal type).[1] In general, surgery has no curative role in treating this mode of spread. Surgery that includes removal of the intact lesser sac peritoneum may possibly be of value for a localised cancer with only posterior wall serosal invasion, though this has never been proven. It is very important to appreciate this limitation in treating the majority of patients with gastric cancer in the West.

Haematogenous spread

Despite the rich vascular supply of the stomach, liver metastases at the time of diagnosis are relatively uncommon, even in advanced cancers. It has been postulated that gastric cancer is inefficient in metastasising via the haematogenous route and this may apply to the diffuse type in particular. The alternative explanation is that diffuse-type cancers spread rapidly by other routes and that, while haematogenous spread may occur, the patient dies of other metastatic disease before liver and distant metastases become clinically apparent.

Concept of gastric cancer as a locoregional disease

It has been observed that even when gastric cancer is locally advanced at the time of diagnosis the disease is still confined to the area of the stomach and the retroperitoneum. Liver and distant metastases are often not detected. Cancers that have breached the serosal surface frequently metastasise within the peritoneal cavity. Recurrence in patients who have had serosa-positive (T3 and T4) cancers is rarely in the liver and distant sites alone. While about a third of patients will have evidence of haematogenous spread, the majority of these patients will have multiple sites of recurrence within the peritoneal cavity, including the gastric bed, anastomoses and distant seedlings.

The pattern of recurrence is different in serosa-negative (T1 and T2) cancers and, especially, early gastric cancers. Unlike serosa-positive cancers, which tend to recur early (within 2 years), if recurrence does occur it does so later and more frequently as haematogenous metastases without local recurrence.

The high incidence of serosa-positive cancers in the West explains why the overall outlook after gastric resection is still poor. Recurrence occurs early and within the abdomen – most of these patients probably do not live long enough to show evidence of blood-borne metastases. It is possible that improved locoregional control of serosa-positive cancers will not prevent patients dying later of distant metas-

tases. However, control of locoregional recurrence would improve the prognosis in a large number of patients even if cure were not achieved. The value of the symptom-free interval in those patients who cannot be cured by surgery should not be underestimated.

It has been postulated that there is a biphasic pattern of recurrence in gastric cancer. There is an initial early phase of local failure in the gastric bed, anastomosis and peritoneal surfaces that is most commonly seen in serosa-positive cancers, in particular the diffuse-type cancers. The second, later phase of failure is due to haematogenous metastases to the liver or distant organs. This is more commonly seen in earlier cancers and intestinal-type cancers that have not recurred locally in the first phase. It is important to appreciate that the two Lauren histological types of gastric cancer have different patterns of metastasis and that this should influence the approach to surgical treatment.[2]

The role of surgery is limited to complete removal of curable lesions that have not disseminated at the time of diagnosis and to minimising the early phase of locoregional recurrence.

Strategies to minimise locoregional failure

Local or gastric bed recurrence

There are three factors to consider:

1. Complete resection of the primary lesion to ensure that all resection margins are free of malignant cells. This includes extending the resection line in continuity to adjacent structures and organs if feasible and safe.
2. En bloc resection of all potentially involved lymph nodes within the normal lymphatic pathways from the stomach.
3. Prevention of implantation of free cancer cells in the gastric bed.

It is apparent that appropriate radical surgery has a definite role in the control of the first two factors. However, it will have only a minimal effect in preventing cell implantation on the gastric bed, especially in serosa-positive and more advanced cancers with lymphatic spread into the second tier of nodes or beyond.

Peritoneal dissemination

Cunliffe and Sugarbaker have proposed a 'tumour cell entrapment hypothesis', which suggests that cells shed before or during surgery can implant on and remain viable in the deperitonealised resection site. These cells may already be present in the peritoneal cavity at the time of surgery in serosa-positive cancers or may be shed during resection from the tumour surface and cut lymphatics and blood vessels.[3] Meticulous surgical technique with en bloc resection of the stomach, affected adjacent organs and intact gastric lymphatic chains is important to prevent 'iatrogenic' cell spillage into the peritoneal cavity.

Measures to destroy free cells in the perioperative period will be required in addition to surgery in patients who have serosal involvement and/or metastases in the second tier of lymph nodes. There is increased interest in intraperitoneal chemotherapy in the West. This is already commonly utilised in Japan as part of the multimodality treatment of advanced cancers.[4,5] This treatment is of most value if started during or immediately after surgery. Delayed postoperative treatment does not improve survival. This is thought to be because cells have already implanted in the gastric bed and are protected by a fibrinous coagulum.[6]

Summary

It is important for the surgeon to define the point of diminishing returns in gastric cancer surgery. Radical surgery has a place in controlling local disease, and for patients with localised disease this will lead to cure, particularly for serosa-negative cancer. In others, radical surgery can prolong symptom-free survival time.[7] However, it is important to realise that surgery is increasingly only one part of the multimodality treatment of advanced gastric cancer.[8] The potential roles of chemotherapy and radiotherapy are discussed in more detail in Chapter 9.

The concept of radical gastric cancer surgery

Having established the potential role of surgery in the treatment of gastric cancer, it is now important to understand the development of the concept of radical surgery. Although radical surgery has been attempted in many centres worldwide, it is the Japanese surgeons who have been at the forefront of the practice of radical gastric resection and lymphadenectomy.

Gastric cancer surgery in Japan

Stomach cancer is the most common cause of cancer death in Japan. Fifty years ago the survival rates were little different to those reported in the West. However, three important changes subsequently occurred that have led to improved rates of survival.

National screening programme for gastric cancer

This national programme was established in 1960. Initial population screening is with high-quality

barium studies and then gastroscopy of those with abnormalities. Over 60% of screen-detected cancers are early (T1) lesions (see Chapters 2 and 8).

Japanese Research Society for Gastric Cancer (JRSGC)

This was established in 1961 to promote the research and management of gastric cancer. The initial objective was to collect standardised data on clinical (macroscopic) staging at the time of surgery and subsequent pathological (microscopic) staging to allow accurate comparison of results. Recommended surgical techniques and rules for documentation of surgery were published and are regularly updated.[9] Pathological assessment is rigidly standardised and similarly updated.

Radical gastric cancer surgery

Radical excision of the stomach and the related lymphatic drainage had previously been practised in specialist centres in both Japan and the West. Publication by the JRSGC of precise definitions of radicality and standardisation of operations in the 'General Rules' reinforced this concept and led to the widespread adoption of radical gastric surgery, which includes a 'systematic' or D2 lymphadenectomy in Japan. It has been proposed that this surgical attitude has been a major factor in the improvement in results. Remarkably, this has never been tested in a randomised trial and Japanese surgeons feel that to try and do so now would be unethical.

The real question is to what extent each of the above factors has contributed to the overall improvement in survival. These measures were introduced concurrently and the Japanese have not been able to separate the respective contributions of earlier diagnosis, improved pathological staging and radical surgery. This analysis is very important in understanding how practice is evolving in the West.

Development of gastric cancer surgery in the West

This has varied between different countries and even varies between centres within the same country. Many specialist centres in Western countries have now developed and undertake radical surgery along the lines proposed by the Japanese.[10]

Screening for gastric cancer

A UICC Workshop held in the UK in 1990 concluded that asymptomatic screening of the population for gastric cancer was only cost-effective in countries with a high incidence of the disease. It could not be recommended as a public health policy in the West.

Screening of symptomatic 'dyspeptic' patients does increase the proportion of early gastric cancers that are diagnosed.[11] However, it must be emphasised that there is a significant difference in outcome between symptomatic cancers diagnosed at an earlier stage and that of screen-detected asymptomatic cancers and this has been proven in Japanese series.[12] This has been labelled the 'shift to the left phenomenon'. The presentation of gastric cancer can be considered to produce a spectrum of disease, with the worst stages to the right. Asymptomatic screening, and to a lesser extent symptomatic screening, not only increases the proportion of early cancers at the far left of the spectrum, but may also shift the whole spectrum to the left. Staging simply divides the spectrum of the disease into four sections. The shift to the left phenomenon may mean that all stages contain a higher proportion of patients in the more favourable left side of the stage. This may partly explain why the survival of all stages of gastric cancer is better in screened populations. It is also postulated that increased population awareness of the risk of gastric cancer, such as has occurred in Japan, also contributes to a shift to the left phenomenon even in the non-screened population, as more patients recognise the potential significance of their symptoms and report them earlier. Increased awareness of Western populations to significant gastrointestinal symptoms linked to the increased availability of diagnostic services should shift the spectrum of disease to the left, although it will never have the same impact as asymptomatic screening.

It may be more meaningful to compare Western results with those of symptomatic Japanese patients only – this would allow a more accurate prediction of the likely effects of the widespread adoption of radical surgery in the West.

Effects of radical surgery and improved pathology on staging

The staging systems previously used in the West were not as clearly defined or standardised as those in Japan. Accurate comparison of results was not possible until 1985, when the UICC and AJCC agreed a unified staging system (see Chapter 3).

It should be recognised that there are also other, more subtle effects on the process of staging that affect comparison of Western and Japanese practice, and the concept of 'stage migration factor' is discussed later.

Different disease in the West?

There is little evidence to support the hypothesis that gastric cancer in the West may be a different disease to that in Japan. Comparison of the results of gastric cancer treatment in racially similar Tokyo and Honolulu Japanese shows poorer results for those treated by Western methods.[13] The natural course of the disease, the modes of spread and sites of recurrence are similar. However, a more recent study has

shown that Asians living in the USA present with less advanced disease and may actually have a less aggressive tumour biology.[14]

Three factors that may be of major significance are discussed below.

Lauren histological type

Many studies show a higher proportion of intestinal-type cancer in Japan. This type has a better prognosis than the diffuse type that is more commonly seen in the West, particularly when diagnosed at an advanced stage.

Proximal cancers

Cancers of the proximal third of the stomach have a worse prognosis than those in the distal two-thirds.[15] Results of surgery are significantly worse in cancers of the proximal third in Japan.[16] Recent Western series report a >50% incidence of proximal cancers compared with 20–30% in Japan. The incidence of proximal cancers continues to increase in the West and it is possible that this will negate the beneficial effects of other factors that are being improved.

Perioperative mortality of radical surgery in the West

While the Japanese specialist centres report mortality rates of 1–3% for radical gastric surgery, this is considerably higher in the West and particularly for total gastrectomy.[17] Until fairly recently centres of excellence in the West were reporting a mortality rate of 5–10% for curative surgery.[18] The results are improving and there are now a number of series with mortality rates well below 5%.[19,20] However, recent larger audits in the UK still show a mortality around 10%.[21,22] While there are other factors apart from throughput, there is some evidence that units with a higher caseload achieve lower mortality and morbidity figures.[23]

It is unlikely that mortality will ever be equal to the Japanese figures because Western patients are on average 10 years older and have a higher incidence of cardiovascular disease than those with gastric cancer in Asia.[24,25] Japanese patients are thinner and also have a very low incidence of postoperative thromboembolic complications. There is increasing evidence that obesity increases the morbidity of gastric cancer surgery, even in Japanese patients.[26,27] A recent study from Korea also reported a direct relationship between obesity and postoperative complications.[28] It is thus likely that results in the West will be significantly affected by the increasing incidence of obesity. A comparison of the outcome after anastomotic leak has shown that the mortality at the National Cancer Centre Hospital (NCCH) in Tokyo is only a third of that reported in the Dutch Gastric Cancer Study.[29] This probably reflects both the greater experience of the Japanese in managing postoperative complications and also the higher risk of the Western population. The higher incidence of proximal cancers in the West means that the proportion undergoing a total gastrectomy is considerably higher, and it should be remembered that this operation is associated with a mortality of about twice that of a subtotal resection.

 It is apparent that the results obtained in gastric cancer treatment in Japan are superior to those in the West for multiple reasons. It has to be accepted that comparison of overall survival rates is of little value.

Role of radical surgery in Western practice

Past experience with radical gastric resection in the West produced variable and usually disappointing results, with any therapeutic gain being negated by the higher mortality of more extensive surgery. Until recently gastric cancer surgery has remained within the remit of the 'general surgeon' in much of the West. Many non-specialist surgeons restricted their surgical effort to limited resections that could be achieved with an acceptable operative mortality. Only a few specialist centres pursued the concept of radical excision as practised by the Japanese. The Leeds group were the first to report stage-specific survival rates nearer to those of best Japanese practice, at least for the earlier stages of the disease. They showed an acceptable mortality, so demonstrating that Japanese practice could be adopted in the West (Table 7.1).[30,31] Other centres in the USA and Europe subsequently reported similarly impressive results for a radical surgical approach.[32–35]

It seems reasonable to assume that radical gastric cancer surgery does produce some survival benefit, but that this may be variable depending on the stage of the disease. However, if that advantage is only small for Western patients then it could be offset by the increased mortality of more radical surgery. In addition, more extensive resections are associated

with increased postoperative morbidity, long-term sequelae and nutritional consequences.

Modern radical gastric cancer surgery is still evolving and only when the benefits of this approach outweigh the increased risks of more extensive resection will this become standard practice. It has become clear that the concept of a 'one size fits all' approach to gastric cancer surgery is unsuitable in Western patients. There is an increasing move towards 'tailoring' operations so that they are not just appropriately radical for the stage of disease but take the patient-related factors into account.[36] This forms the basis for understanding the modern principles of gastric cancer surgery.

Principles of radical gastric cancer surgery

There are certain basic principles on which to base the radical surgical treatment of gastric cancer. There is now considerable evidence for the standardised procedures. However, each case is different and there are multiple factors that affect the operative tactics. The stage of the cancer, evidence of spread, mode of spread and the patient's health, age and build all have to be taken into account in 'designing' the appropriate procedure for each patient. We can now talk in terms of a 'rational gastric resection' based on the standardised procedures, but taking these other factors into account. The components of a gastric cancer resection are considered under the following headings:

- Extent of the gastric resection
- Lymphadenectomy
- Splenectomy
- Distal pancreatectomy
- Extended resections
- Lesser resections.

Extent of gastric resection

The primary objective of gastric cancer surgery is to adequately excise the primary lesion with clear longitudinal and circumferential margins. The type of

Table 7.1 • Five-year survival after potentially curative gastric cancer surgery: comparison of results from Leeds[30] and Tokyo[31]

	Cumulative 5–year survival (%)	
	Tokyo	Leeds
All potentially curative resections	75	54
Early gastric cancer	91	91
Stage I	91	87
Stage II	72	65
Stage III	44	18

gastrectomy required to achieve this depends on the position of the cancer and the margin necessary to be certain not to leave malignant cells at the anastomotic line.

Lateral spread in the gastric wall occurs by direct invasion and by spread within the submucosal and subserosal lymphatics. Once the submucosa has been penetrated there may be extensive lateral spread within the abundant lymphatic plexus. Diffuse-type cancers are particularly prone to spread in this way and in the most aggressive forms most or all of the submucosa may be infiltrated, so producing a linitis plastica. It is important to realise that both the oesophagus and duodenum can be infiltrated by spread in the mural lymphatics – in the former via the submucosal channels and in the latter via the subserosal channels. This must be taken into account when planning the extent of resection if there is palpable tumour at either end of the stomach.

It is often stated that diffuse-type cancers require a wider resection margin than the intestinal type. This concept is debatable, as examination of resection margins has shown that a 5-cm margin from the palpable edge of the tumour is sufficient for both intestinal and diffuse types.[37] Cancers that have penetrated the serosa may require a wider margin, and 6 cm from the palpable edge of the tumour or infiltrated wall has been recommended.[38] Serosa-negative cancers, particularly of the intestinal type, may be resected with a smaller margin in elderly or high-risk patients. The place of limited resections is discussed later.

Type of gastrectomy (Fig. 7.1)

This depends on the location of the cancer: **Fig. 7.1**

Distal-third cancer (A and AM)

A subtotal (80%) gastrectomy with resection of the first part of the duodenum is recommended. A total gastrectomy is only indicated for large tumours or when there is submucosal infiltration to within 7–8 cm of the oesophagogastric junction.

Middle-third cancer (M and MA)

In many cases a total gastrectomy will be necessary, but this depends on the amount of stomach remaining below the oesophagogastric junction after excising an adequate margin of stomach proximal to the palpable edge of the tumour. A minimum of 2 cm

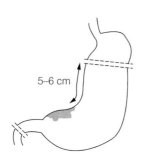

Antral carcinoma
Subtotal gastrectomy and resection of first part of duodenum

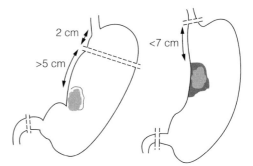

Carcinoma of middle third
Subtotal or total gastrectomy depending on proximal margin of resection

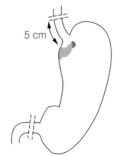

Carcinoma of cardia
Total gastrectomy and resection of lower oesophagus

Figure 7.1 • Extent of gastric resection.

is needed, and so for a serosa-negative cancer there must be a 7-cm margin from the oesophagogastric junction. A smaller margin might be accepted in the elderly and particularly for intestinal-type cancers.

Proximal-third cancer (C, CM and MC)

The standard operation is a total gastrectomy, and this is certainly indicated if the cancer margin crosses the line between the upper and middle thirds of the stomach. However, a total gastrectomy does lead to significant long-term nutritional problems and affects the performance status and quality of life of the patient. There has been a move in recent years to look at the possibility of a limited proximal partial gastrectomy. Many surgeons are reluctant to use this procedure as anastomosis of the distal stomach to the oesophagus tends to produce a poor functional result; alkaline reflux in particular can be very troublesome and difficult to control. However, some specialist centres routinely use a proximal partial resection without apparently compromising survival rates or producing unacceptable side-effects.[39]

There is increasing use of a limited proximal resection for early gastric cancer in Japan. Studies arising from this new practice confirm that the functional results, including ability to eat a normal meal and maintenance of nutritional state, are better than a total gastrectomy.[40] The reconstruction after proximal gastrectomy can be by using a jejunal interposition, jejunal pouch or creating a tube from the remaining stomach (**Fig. 7.2**). A small non-randomised study suggests that the gastric tube technique has advantages over a jejunal interposition and leads to fewer troublesome side-effects.[41] The use of a jejunal interposition also produces a good functional result and significantly improves the maintenance of body weight compared with a total gastrectomy.[42]

Apart from concerns over bile reflux after proximal gastrectomy, the other major factor to consider is whether the lesser resection compromises the chance of cure. Cancer of the proximal third of the stomach tends to be more advanced for both T and N stages when compared with distal cancers.[43] Analysis of one large series has shown that, even allowing for stage of presentation, proximal gastric cancer behaves in a more aggressive way compared with distal cancer.[44] It is important that a sufficient margin of stomach is resected and that the lymph nodes most likely to be affected are resected en bloc. There is evidence that resection of the distal stomach is not required on an oncological basis as those patients with advanced cancers with positive nodes around the distal stomach do not actually show any benefit from the extended resection.[45] This is discussed further in the section on lymphadenectomy (see below).

Cancer of the cardia poses a particular problem in terms of surgical approach, extent of resection and lymph node excision.[46] If an adequate proximal margin can be obtained then the preferred approach is a total gastrectomy with excision of the crural muscles around the hiatus and transhiatal excision of the lower mediastinal nodes.[47] In patients with diffuse-type, poorly differentiated or large-diameter (>5 cm) cardia cancers then extended resection of the lower oesophagus is recommended, and this requires a thoracic or thoracoabdominal approach. The alternative approaches to cancer around the oesophago-gastric junction are also discussed in Chapter 6.

 In the absence of a good prospective randomised study, total gastrectomy is presently recommended for proximal-third gastric cancer in Western patients as it is in theory a better cancer operation. This supposition may well be flawed on the basis of recent Japanese data and the experience of some specialist centres in the West. The functional side-effects and long-term nutritional problems associated with a total gastric resection may outweigh the risk of reflux after a limited proximal resection. A prospective randomised study for patients with locally advanced proximal cancer (type 2 and limited type 3 junctional cancer) is required.

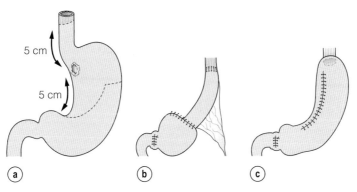

Figure 7.2 • Proximal partial gastrectomy and techniques of reconstruction.

Extensive cancers (CMA)

Total gastrectomy is indicated provided there is a chance of worthwhile palliation in this type of advanced cancer, which is usually of the linitis plastica type, provided there are no peritoneal seedlings and the cytology of peritoneal washings is negative (see Chapter 3). In cases where there is no detectable distant spread, surgical resection is probably indicated even if invaded adjacent organs have to be removed en bloc. Importantly, wide resection margins have to be incorporated as there are malignant cells in the submucosal lymphatic plexuses well away from the palpable edge of the cancer. It has been argued that surgery is not worthwhile for this type of gastric cancer and certainly the poor results suggest that resection is only providing limited palliation. In the absence of any other effective treatment then resection, possibly combined with intraoperative or postoperative adjuvant treatment (see Chapter 8), is indicated in younger patients with disease confined to the stomach and perigastric tissues. There is a real need to explore novel ways of treating this increasingly frequent form of diffuse-type gastric cancer.

Total gastrectomy 'de principe' for distal cancers

The absolute indications for removal of the whole stomach have been listed above – in these circumstances this is termed a 'total gastrectomy de nécessité'. There are surgeons in some European centres who argue that all cancers of the stomach, even those in the distal third, should be treated in the same way – 'total gastrectomy de principe'. It is important to understand the arguments for and against such a policy:

Less risk of positive proximal resection margin

Provided the rules on safe margins of resection are adhered to, a positive proximal resection margin is rare. If the margins are still positive despite an adequate margin then this usually indicates an aggressive malignancy and anastomotic recurrence as the only site of recurrence is unusual.

Multicentric cancer and gastric mucosal 'field change'

The incidence of stump cancer is low, even in long-term survivors. However, an important part of the preoperative work-up before a subtotal gastrectomy is careful endoscopic examination and biopsy of the proximal stomach. If this shows evidence of a premalignant field change, the presence of multiple gastric polyps, or if the patient has pernicious anaemia then total gastrectomy is advised.[48]

Adequacy of lymphadenectomy

It has been argued that total gastrectomy allows a more certain D2 lymphadenectomy. The only difficult nodes to remove en bloc in a subtotal gastrectomy

are the left paracardial group. While it is still possible to resect these nodes, there is not really a significant therapeutic advantage in doing so as they are positive in less than 5% of distal cancers. In addition, survival of the patients with positive left paracardial nodes is very poor and there is no demonstrable therapeutic advantage in resection of them.

There are no studies that prove a significant survival benefit for total gastrectomy de principe – one well-conducted randomised study has shown no survival benefit.[49] Against this is a higher mortality for total gastrectomy. Even in the best hands the mortality of total gastrectomy is up to 5%. There is an increased risk of long-term nutritional problems after total gastrectomy, particularly in older patients and even when a jejunal pouch is constructed.[50] Quality-of-life assessments also show a significant benefit for subtotal gastrectomy in the long term.[51]

 On the basis of good-quality data there is no support for the concept of total gastrectomy de principe for cancers in the lower half of the stomach. The standard operation for distal gastric cancer is a subtotal gastrectomy.

Lymphadenectomy

Lymph node metastasis is the most common mode of spread in gastric cancer. It is now recognised that lymphatic spread can occur in the absence of haematogenous spread and that gastric cancer may remain a localised disease even when nodes are involved.

The pattern of lymphatic spread should in theory divide into four zones based on the arterial blood supply of the stomach. Detailed pathological studies show that lymphatic involvement is not this predictable, mainly due to the abundant blood and lymphatic plexuses in the submucosal layer of the stomach.

The Japanese have extensively investigated the distribution of lymph node involvement. As described in Chapter 3, the nodes have been grouped into 16 stations (see Fig. 3.2 in Chapter 3) and these are listed in Box 7.1. Studies of large numbers of patients treated at the NCCH in Tokyo have shown the likelihood of involvement of each node station for cancers in different parts of the stomach[52] (see Table 7.2). In planning the extent of lymphadenectomy three factors have to be considered:

1. The likelihood of metastasis at each node station.
2. The possible survival benefit of removing all nodes at that station.
3. The additional risk of mortality and serious morbidity in removing the nodes.

Box 7.1 • Lymph node stations: names and locations of the regional lymph nodes of the stomach

1. Right cardiac nodes
2. Left cardiac nodes
3. Nodes along the lesser curvature
4. Nodes along the greater curvature:
   4sa – nodes along the short gastric arteries
   4sb – nodes along the left gastroepiploic artery
   4d – nodes along the right gastroepiploic artery
5. Suprapyloric nodes
6. Infrapyloric nodes
7. Nodes along left gastric artery
8. Nodes along the common hepatic artery
9. Coeliac artery nodes
10. Splenic hilum nodes
11. Nodes along the splenic artery
12. Nodes in the hepatoduodenal ligament
13. Nodes on the posterior of the pancreas
14. Nodes at the root of the mesentery
15. Nodes on the middle colic artery
16. Para-aortic nodes
110. Lower thoracic paraoesophageal nodes
111. Diaphragmatic nodes

The JRSGC database has shown that only resection of stations 1–12 produces any worthwhile benefit in terms of 5-year survival. The improvement in survival after removal of stations 13–16 is so small

that any possible benefit is almost certainly negated by the increased mortality and morbidity associated with the extended radical resection. The station-12 hepatoduodenal ligament nodes are in the third tier for all thirds of the stomach. These nodes are involved in 9% of lower-third and 4% of middle-third cancers. Five-year survival rates of up to 25% have been reported in Japan for patients who have had positive station-12 nodes resected. This manoeuvre is probably worthwhile in distal cancers where N2 nodes appear involved. Some surgeons resect these nodes routinely as part of a D2 resection.

Definition of extent of lymphadenectomy

The Japanese introduced the concept of tiers of lymph nodes with lymphatic spread occurring progressively through the tiers. The tiers are allocated an N number:

- N1 – perigastric nodes closest to the primary lesion.
- N2 – distant perigastric nodes and the nodes along the main arteries supplying the stomach.
- N3 – nodes outside the normal lymphatic pathways from the stomach, involved in advanced stages or by retrograde lymphatic flow due to blockage of normal pathways.

The tiers are different for each third of the stomach (see Table 7.3).

Table 7.2 • Incidence of metastasis at each node station for cancers in the proximal, middle and distal thirds of the stomach

Node station	Percentage risk of nodal metastases for advanced gastric cancers		
	Distal (A)	Middle (M)	Proximal (C)
1	7	16	31
2	0	1	13
3	38	40	39
4	35	31	11
5	12	3	2
6	49	15	3
7	23	22	19
8	25	11	7
9	13	8	13
10	0	2	10
11	4	4	12
12	8	2	1
13–16	(0–5% for all)		

Data from the National Cancer Centre Hospital in Tokyo.[52]

Table 7.3 • Lymph node tiers according to the rules of the Japanese Research Society for Gastric Cancer (JRSGC)

Location	AMC, MAC, MCA, CMA	A, AM	MA, M, MC	C, CM
First tier (N1)	1	3	3	1
	2	4	4	2
	3	5	5	3
	4	6	6	4s
	5		1	
	6			
Second tier (N2)	7	7	2	4d
	8	8	7	7
	9	9	8	8
	10	1	9	9
	11		10	10
		11	11	
			5	
			6	
Third tier (N3)	12	2	12	12
	13	10	13	13
	14	11	14	14
	110	12		110
	111	13		111
		14		

Stations 2 and 10 should be excised in a D2 resection for an MC cancer but are optional for M and MA.
Station 5 and 6 resection is optional for C and CM and if not resected the operation is still classified as a D2 resection.

It is important to understand the nomenclature as all too often the extent of nodal dissection is wrongly described in the literature.

- **D1 – Limited lymphadenectomy:** all N1 nodes removed en bloc with the stomach.
- **D2 – Systematic lymphadenectomy:** all N1 and N2 nodes removed en bloc with the stomach. If most, but not all, of the second-tier stations are resected then this is technically a D1 resection, although it is sometimes represented as a D1/D2 resection.
- **D3 – Extended lymphadenectomy:** a more radical en bloc resection including the third-tier nodes. This more commonly includes only some stations, such as the station-12 nodes.

In the Japanese Rules for Gastric Cancer Surgery the minimum requirement for an effective resection of gastric cancer is a systematic D2 lymphadenectomy.

Lymphadenectomy and cure of gastric cancer

This concept is strictly defined in the Japanese Rules:

- **Absolute curative resection** – the surgical D number is greater than the pathological N number, e.g. D2 lymphadenectomy for N0 or N1 disease.
- **Relative curative resection** – the D number equals the N number.

Effect of the international unified TNM staging system on the definition of lymphadenectomy

As explained in Chapter 3, the introduction of the 1997 UICC TNM unified staging system has been important in allowing the direct comparison of treatment results. Unfortunately this has also introduced considerable scope for confusion, especially when describing the extent of lymphadenectomy. The unified staging system should be used for **pathological staging** of the cancer. It is recommended that the JRSGC Rules are still used for **planning the extent of the lymphadenectomy** and, in particular, the node groups that should be removed. The new agreed definition of a D2 lymphadenectomy (removal of more than 15 nodes irrespective of node stations) adds a further confounding factor. This new definition for a D2 lymphadenectomy does allow comparison of results of surgery from different countries and does appear to correlate well with the JRSGC Rules (see Chapter 3).

However, with the widespread acceptance of the new definition there is now recognition that a D2 lymphadenectomy is the minimum requirement in radical curative gastric cancer surgery.

D2 lymphadenectomy

No aspect of gastric cancer surgery has proved more controversial in recent years than the merits or otherwise of D2 systematic lymphadenectomy. While the Japanese continue to advocate this as a basic requirement of surgery, surgeons in other countries have been reluctant to adopt this radical approach. However, many specialist units in other countries, including the UK, Europe and to a lesser extent the USA, now perform a more extensive lymphadenectomy as part of a radical curative gastric resection.

The evidence base

This can be divided into Japanese data and that from other countries – the latter have increased significantly over the last 15 years. The Japanese database is huge and contains an accumulation of data from many large specialised surgical units. The Japanese have never performed randomised studies comparing D2 with a lesser extent of lymphadectomy, but have accumulated many thousands of patients in observational studies and have compared the results of D2 lymphadenectomy with historical controls. In interpreting the evidence base it is necessary to balance the results of more powerful non-Japanese randomised controlled trials (RCTs) with these observational data. In addition, there is now a considerable number of observational studies from non-Japanese countries that appear to confirm the Japanese experience. In assessing the evidence base it is important to appreciate two factors that have an effect on stage-related survival after surgery. These are the accuracy and quality of pathological assessment and the stage migration factor.

The Japanese Rules for Pathology require very detailed sampling of each defined node group and multiple sections of each node. The detection of nodal metastases by this type of detailed sampling is more likely than in historical Japanese and standard Western pathological assessment. If the same principles were applied in the West a proportion of cancers would be allocated to a worse stage on the basis of the true N factor (see Chapter 3). Present pathological analysis in many Western centres produces over-optimistic staging of cancers and this may be one reason why long-term survival is not as good as the comparable Japanese figures for the same stage. Many specialist centres have already addressed this shortcoming and nodal staging is now much more accurate.

Stage migration factor (SMF) explains how the improved stage-specific survival of patients who have undergone a more extensive lymphadenectomy is actually in part due to correct staging rather than the surgery. If only the first tier of nodes is excised in a gastric cancer resection then the N factor could not be more than N1. In most Japanese centres all second-tier and possibly some third-tier nodes are also excised en bloc and so if there are metastases in these nodes the cancer will be correctly staged N2 or N3. Examination of 5-year survival rate (5YSR) in Japan reveals the importance of correctly determining the N factor by a more radical lymphadenectomy, as shown, for example, by the following:[53]

T2N1M0	71% 5YSR
T2N2M0	52% 5YSR
T3N1M0	46% 5YSR
T3N2M0	23% 5YSR

The correct staging of a node-positive cancer may thus decrease the 5-year survival expectancy by about 20%. It is still not clear what proportion of the 'benefit' of radical lymphadenectomy is due to removal of nodal tissue as opposed to that attributable to the correct pathological staging of the cancer. This not only affects comparison of radical lymphadenectomy with historical control groups, but is also an important factor that should be allowed for in randomised studies comparing stage-specific survival of D1 and D2 lymphadenectomy. With the new TNM staging there is no longer reliance on deciding which tier an involved node lies within but on number of involved nodes and so the effects of SMF are to some extent reduced. This may be further improved by using the ratio of involved to non-involved nodes.[54] However, surgical effort to remove nodes in the second tier and beyond will still improve stage-specific survival and the real test in randomised trials is whether it produces an overall survival benefit.[55]

Japanese evidence

The extent of lymphadenectomy correlates well with survival in Japanese studies. Multivariate analysis has shown that this is an independent positive variable for survival.[53] There are many other Japanese reports of improved survival after D2 compared with lesser resections.[31] In Table 7.4 the stage-specific 5YSR of patients treated by D2 lymphadenectomy at the NCCH in Tokyo is shown.[56] The widespread adoption of systematic lymphadenectomy in Japan was based on comparison of the results of this type of resection with historical control data. However, as already discussed, this simple type of analysis does not take into account the more accurate pathological staging that is inevitable with more extensive nodal resections. As such this is a statistically weak method with which to draw conclusions about more extensive lymph node resection.

Although the Japanese data are of only limited statistical value they can be used to help demonstrate the likely value of more extensive lymphadenectomy by examining the outcome of patients with different levels of nodal spread:

N2 disease

It is apparent from Table 7.4 that for each T stage some patients with N2 survive at least 5 years after surgery. It is reasonable to assume that they would not have survived as long after a lesser resection that left malignant nodes in the gastric bed. While only a very small proportion of T1 cancers have spread to N2 nodes, up to 31% of T2 cancers and more than 40% of T3 cancers have second-tier nodal spread.[31] It can be calculated that a 5YSR of 52% for T2N2 should equate to an improvement of up to 15% for all T2 disease if a D2 lymphadenectomy rather than

Table 7.4 • Five-year survival (5YSR) related to stage of gastric cancer: per cent survivors corresponding to new unified TNM categories

Stage	TNM	5YSR (%)
Ia	pT1 pN0 M0	99
Ib	pT1 pN1 M0	90
	pT2 pN0 M0	88
II	pT1 pN2 M0	79
	pT2 pN1 M0	71
	pT3 pN0 M0	69
IIIa	pT2 pN2 M0	52
	pT3 pN1 M0	46
	pT4 pN0 M0	52
IIIb	pT3 pN2 M0	23
	pT4 pN1 M0	26
	pT4 pN2 M0	16
IV	M1	10

a lesser resection is performed for all T2 cancers. The improvement for T3 cancers is less as the 5YSR is only 23% for T3N2, but this would still equate to about a 10% improvement for all T3 disease if all underwent a D2 lymphadenectomy. The improvement in Japanese patients is mainly seen in those with small areas of serosal involvement, and there was no benefit for Borrmann type IV cancers.[57] There are now non-Japanese series showing a similar trend for the survival of N2 patients,[32] although radical lymphadenectomy has not proved as beneficial for those with serosal invasion.[58]

N1 disease

One of the ways to examine the benefit of systematic lymphadenectomy from the Japanese data is to compare the survival difference for patients with N1 node involvement only. An incomplete D1 (D0) resection produces a 4% 5YSR, rising to 46% for a D1 resection and with a further 10% benefit for a D2 resection.[59] Most importantly, this emphasises the value of complete resection of the first tier of nodes. The smaller benefit with D2 lymphadenectomy is also partly explained by the SMF.

N0 disease

There is evidence of an improvement in survival of node-negative (N0) patients after D2 compared with D1 lymphadenectomy.[60] This seems to be explained by the failure of standard histological stains to identify micrometastases in nodes.[61] It is likely that a proportion of node-negative cases should be classified as having node-positive disease with malignant cells identified in first-tier nodes. There are now similar reports from specialist Western units.[62] It is likely that on the same hypothesis a proportion of N1 cancers do actually have N2 disease and so this may partly explain the possible benefit of a D2 against a lesser lymphadenectomy.

Non-Japanese evidence

Many Western surgeons have been unable to reproduce the beneficial effects of radical lymphadenectomy. In attempting to incorporate Japanese practice they have encountered higher mortality and morbidity rates than for less radical operations. There are now a number of prospective controlled studies comparing the different operative strategies. These provide valuable evidence for the role of radical node dissection in gastric cancer surgery.

German Gastric Cancer Study [35]

This was a prospective non-randomised study of the practice of D1 ($n = 558$) and D2 ($n = 1096$) lymphadenectomy in specialist German surgical units between 1986 and 1989. The definition of a level of lymphadenectomy was based on the number of nodes retrieved from the specimen rather than the surgeon's description or analysis of node stations. This definition makes it difficult to compare this directly with Japanese practice at that time. The mortality and complication rates were very similar for the two groups. Multivariate analysis revealed that D2 lymphadenectomy was an independent positive factor for survival. More detailed analysis showed that this only applied for those patients who were N0 or N1 and not N2 – this also explains why a significant survival benefit was only detected for stages II and IIIA. Interestingly, the Japanese have produced very similar results from the same type of analysis.[52] Ten-year results have shown a statistically significant independent effect of D2 resection for both the subgroups of stage II disease only. This effect appears to be independent of the SMF.[63]

Dutch Gastric Cancer Trial[64]

This was a multicentre prospective randomised trial comparing D1 and D2 lymphadenectomy. It involved 33 surgical departments coordinated by Leiden University Hospital and recruited 380 patients in the D1 group and 331 in the D2 limb. Because most Dutch surgeons were not familiar with the D2 operation a Japanese surgeon from the NCCH in Tokyo taught and supervised eight coordinating surgeons who then continued the supervision of the other participating surgeons. The main findings are shown in Table 7.5.

Pathological assessment of resected lymph nodes demonstrated the difficulty in adhering rigidly to the JRSGC Rules. Disappointingly, 81% of patients who had undergone a D2 resection had absence of node groups that should have been resected ('non-compliance'), and in 48% of the D1 patients there were nodes present that should not have been resected ('contamination').[65] It is possible that these technical protocol violations have affected the survival results. Importantly, many of the participating surgeons contributed only relatively small numbers of patients at a time when they were still in their 'learning curve' for the D2 operation. This factor may have affected the completeness of the nodal resection and is also likely to have contributed to the increased mortality and morbidity of the more radical operation.

What is accepted is that the improvements in survival with D2 resection detected in the subgroup stages II and IIIa are largely attributable to stage migration. It is also recognised that the increased mortality and morbidity of the D2 resections were largely due to the threefold increase in splenectomy and 10-fold increase in distal pancreatectomy in this group compared with the D1 group. Analysis of risk factors showed that splenectomy was an important risk factor for overall complications, while pancreatectomy and type of gastrectomy were the only factors significantly influencing the occurrence of major surgical complications.[66]

MRC Gastric Cancer Surgical Trial (STO1)[67]

This was a prospective randomised multicentre study comparing D1 and D2 lymphadenectomy, with 200 patients in each limb. Uniformity of surgical technique was ensured by the use of standardised descriptions and videos and by monitoring the surgeons' reports. This quality control was not nearly as rigorous as that employed in the Dutch trial.

The mortality and incidence of adverse events are remarkably similar to the Dutch trial and also largely related to resection of the spleen and pancreas (Table 7.6). It was also accepted that many of the surgeons were in their 'learning curve' for the D2 operation. Patients who had both pancreas and spleen resected had a significantly poorer survival than those who had neither organ resected. The hazard ratio for those having only their spleen removed fell just below the significance level.[68] In a subgroup

Table 7.5 • Comparison of results of D1 and D2 lymphadenectomy in the Dutch Gastric Cancer Trial[64]

	D1	D2	Significance
Perioperative mortality (%)	4	10	$P = 0.004$
Significant complications (%)	25	43	$P < 0.001$
Median hospital stay (days)	18	25	$P < 0.001$
5-year survival (%)	45	47	NS

Table 7.6 • Comparison of results of D1 and D2 lymphadenectomy in the MRC Gastric Cancer Surgical Trial[67]

	D1	D2	Significance
Perioperative mortality (%)	6.5	13	$P = 0.04$
Overall morbidity (%)	28	46	$P < 0.001$
Median (range) hospital stay (days)	14 (6–101)	14 (10–147)	NS
5-year survival (%)	35	33	NS

analysis, patients undergoing a D2 lymphadenectomy without resection of their spleen or distal pancreas had the best long-term survival, although these were mainly patients with distal cancers.

Publications since the Dutch and MRC studies

Although regarded by many as the definitive research in establishing the role of radical gastric cancer surgery in the West, it should be remembered that these studies were published in the mid-1990s and as such are already out of date. A smaller Italian multicentre prospective randomised trial comparing D1 and D2 resection reported preliminary results showing a mortality of 3.1% for the D2 procedure and a much lower rate of serious morbidity than the MRC and Dutch studies. There was only a trend to improved survival in the D2 group in patients who did not have a pancreatectomy.[69] There are now reports of European and UK series with a mortality rate of less than 5%, including a number with a rate of 2% or less.[19,20,32,70] The emphasis in recent publications has been on the expertise of the participating surgeons and the avoidance of pancreatic and splenic resection unless specifically indicated. While the role of surgical skill and expertise is recognised as a risk factor for mortality, Sasako has also emphasised that this expertise has to extend to the management of complications; this is a very important factor for maintaining a low mortality rate in radical surgery.[71]

There are reports from non-Japanese centres of improved survival for patients undergoing a D2 lymphadenectomy compared with a lesser resection in historical control groups. While these papers have the same failings as the Japanese reports, it is of interest to examine the fate of patients with positive second-tier nodes (N2). In the Dutch trial 20% of the D2 group with N2 nodes were still alive at 11 years.[72] Others have reported up to 30% of N2 patients alive at 5 years.[20,73] Although this is relatively soft evidence, it cannot be ignored as about a quarter of Western patients with resectable gastric cancer have positive second-tier nodes.

Summary

There is a very large body of evidence on which to base a decision about D2 lymphadenectomy.[74] The following summarises the present position:

1. At present there is no evidence from randomised trials that routine use of a D2 resection confers a survival benefit over a D1 resection. None of these trials is from Japan and a major criticism is the lack of experience of the participating surgeons in the D2 technique and subsequently the high rates of serious complications, mortality and trial protocol violations. Most participating surgeons only performed small

numbers of cases and it is now accepted that there is a significant learning curve for radical gastric cancer surgery.[75] There has been much criticism of the Dutch and MRC trials, but both have failed to show a benefit for the routine use of D2 resections. Both have shown the detrimental effects on postoperative complications and long-term survival of resecting the distal pancreas and spleen as part of a D2 operation in Western patients. This has also been recognised in Japan, where there has also been a change in practice away from pancreatic and splenic resection in recent years (see below).

2. Results of large non-randomised studies from Japan and other countries, including Germany, support a significant survival benefit for D2 resection. Analysis of results suggests that the benefit is largely confined to those with N0 and N1 disease. A small subgroup with N2 disease should also theoretically benefit. The increase in 5-year survival is most obvious for stages II and IIIa.

3. Comparison of results for the TNM stages does not allow for the 'stage migration phenomenon' produced by improved pathological data from more extensive nodal resections. The relative contributions of the surgical effort and correct pathological staging have been tested in hypothetical models and suggest that perhaps half the apparent improvement is related to correct staging/stage migration.

4. It is proposed that resection of second-tier nodes should decrease the incidence of local recurrence in the gastric bed in node-positive patients. This benefit is more likely to be apparent when the cancer has not penetrated the serosal layer. Series from both Japan and the West show that a significant proportion of patients with N2 disease survive for more than 5 years after a D2 resection – it is unlikely that they would survive as long after a lesser lymphadenectomy.

5. The mortality and morbidity of D2 resection is higher than D1 resection. In the West there are the additional factors of the age and general health of gastric cancer patients. Non-Japanese centres with experience of the technique of radical lymphadenectomy and the subsequent management of postoperative complications are now reporting mortality rates well under

5% and not significantly different to lesser resections.

6. Until we have the quality of evidence to make a definite decision about D2 lymphadenectomy, the operation should only be performed when the surgeon can be confident that the mortality of the operation they perform will not be increased by attempts to remove second-tier (or beyond) nodes.

Conclusions

Gastrectomy with D2 lymphadenectomy should not be used *routinely* in the surgical treatment of gastric cancer in Western patients.

Gastrectomy with D2 lymphadenectomy should only be performed by surgeons with proven experience of this type of radical surgery.

The added risks of D2 lymphadenectomy over a lesser nodal dissection are minimal for cancers in the distal half of the stomach. In the absence of any evidence of distant spread (including evidence of third-tier nodal involvement) this is the operation of choice. This is supported by a large number of non-randomised studies from Japanese and Western specialist centres and from subgroup analysis of the randomised MRC trial and the Dutch trial.

The situation for cancers in the proximal half of the stomach is more complicated. There is some evidence to support the use of a D2 or modified D2 lymphadenectomy in stages II and IIIa, but probably only in those with no or minimal serosal involvement. Those who are serosa positive or have N2 nodal involvement will require adjuvant or possibly neoadjuvant treatment and nodal resections that are modified to minimise morbidity and mortality.[1]

The future

The future trend will be towards radical node resections that are tailored to the preoperative and operative staging of each case and to the age and fitness of the patient.[19,36] Improvements in staging techniques should allow a more rational approach to specific node station resections based on the likelihood of involvement and the potential benefit of en bloc removal of each station.[76] Many centres now follow this approach. The place of splenic and pancreatic removal as part of a radical lymphadenectomy is now doubtful and is discussed at length in the next two sections.

Splenectomy

The addition of a splenectomy increases the rate of septic and thromboembolic complications after a gastrectomy.[77] It also affects the immunological response to certain bacteria and possibly to gastric cancer.[78] However, this is controversial and a recent study has found that splenectomy is not an independent variable for postoperative septic problems.[79] The evidence for a lasting adverse immunological effect in cancer patients is theoretical rather than proven. There are both univariate and multivariate analyses that suggest lack of survival benefit or even a negative prognostic effect in all stages of gastric cancer except possibly stage IV.[80] However, there are also studies that have not confirmed an independent effect on survival. The evidence that removal of station-10 nodes improves survival is conflicting.[81,82] In view of these concerns there is an increasing trend to avoid splenectomy unless specifically indicated.

Indications for splenectomy

Direct invasion of spleen or tail of pancreas

If all macroscopic disease can be resected and the operation is potentially curative then en bloc splenectomy or pancreato-splenectomy is worthwhile. If the operation is obviously palliative then the likely benefit of splenectomy has to be weighed against the increased risk of morbidity and mortality.

Removal of splenic hilum (station-10) lymph nodes

There are two factors to consider:

1. **The likelihood of station-10 nodal metastases.**
   There are a number of Japanese papers documenting the incidence of splenic nodal metastases in advanced gastric cancer. The summarised mean incidences for the different parts of the stomach are:

Distal third (A): <1%
Middle third (M): 10%
Upper third (C): 15–20%
Whole stomach: 25%.

This analysis can be further refined for proximal cancers by taking into account whether the cancer involves the greater curve, in which case positive nodes are more likely.[52,83] Smaller tumours (<4 cm diameter) are less likely to involve nodes in the splenic hilum.[81] The incidence of nodal involvement is also related to the depth of invasion and is significantly lower in T1 and T2 cancers. The incidence of positive nodes in proximal-third cancers may be higher in Western patients due to the greater proportion of more advanced cancers – in the MRC trial 25% of cases with C or CM cancers had positive station-10 nodes.[67]

2. **The likely survival benefit of removing all station-10 nodes.** Even if the splenic nodes are removed the survival of patients with distal cancers and positive station-10 nodes is minimal. In proximal cancers with positive nodes the 5-year survival is up to 25% at the NCCH in Tokyo.[52] A high proportion of those with positive nodes also have positive para-aortic nodes and so a D3 or D4 nodal dissection is recommended by some if the spleen is to be removed as part of a radical gastric cancer operation.[84]

It is simple to calculate that if the spleen was removed in all Western patients with proximal-third cancer then the survival benefit, without subgroup analysis, is just 6% and then only if Japanese results can be reproduced.

The indications for splenectomy to allow complete removal of station-10 lymph nodes have been tightened in recent years. This should only be considered for cancers in the upper stomach and possibly even then restricted to larger cancers involving the greater curve and fundus of the stomach. There is a need to test this recommendation in a randomised trial.[67] In view of the suspected adverse immunological effects of splenectomy in the earlier stages of gastric cancer there is now a good case for not removing the spleen in T1 or T2 cancers. Further evidence is required.

 The spleen should not be removed for cancers confined to the distal half of the stomach.

 The role of splenectomy as part of a D2 lymphadenectomy for proximal cancer requires further research.

Clearance of station-10 nodes with splenic preservation

This was previously thought not to be feasible. The Japanese have reported a technique of dissecting out the splenic hilar nodes and have confirmed the removal of all lymphatic tissue.[85] This procedure is still controversial in Japan and there are doubts that the technique can be consistently performed in Western patients.

 At present splenic hilar dissection is not recommended in Western patients.

Distal pancreatectomy

En bloc pancreatic resection is associated with a significant increase in morbidity and mortality when compared with gastrectomy with or without splenectomy. This has been consistently demonstrated in studies of radical gastric surgery in both the West and Japan.[86] Complications include pancreatic leakage, abscess formation, fistula and acute pancreatitis. A few patients will become diabetic after distal pancreatectomy. The complications of the associated splenectomy have to be added to those of the pancreatic resection.

Indications for distal pancreatectomy

In view of the high complication rate, the indications for resection of the left side of the pancreas have to be carefully analysed:

Direct invasion of tail of pancreas

As previously discussed, distal pancreatectomy should only be contemplated if all macroscopic disease can be removed. There is some evidence that this can improve the prognosis in selected patients.[87,88]

Removal of splenic artery (station-11) lymph nodes

There are two factors to consider:

1. **The likelihood of station-11 nodal metastases.** About 10% of patients with proximal cancers have positive splenic artery nodes. As with station-10 nodes the highest incidence is seen with greater curve and advanced cancers. In some patients only the nodes closest to the coeliac trunk are involved, this being due to retrograde lymphatic spread from nodes around the origins of the left gastric and common hepatic arteries rather than antegrade spread along the normal lymphatic pathway. This type of involvement is seen in advanced cancers affecting any part of the stomach. In such cases resection of the nodes around the origin of the artery may reduce local gastric bed recurrence and increase the disease-free interval, but there is no evidence that it improves the chance of cure.

2. **The likely survival benefit of removing all station-11 nodes.** The 5-year survival of patients undergoing resection of positive splenic artery nodes is reported to be 15–20% in Japan.[52]

The decision to resect station-10 and -11 nodes, necessitating distal pancreatectomy and splenectomy, has to be made with the realisation that in Western gastric cancer practice the benefit is at best only marginal. The benefit for proximal-third cancers can be calculated to be only about 2% if all patients had a distal pancreatectomy – less than the increased mortality. The Japanese have now confirmed that there is no survival benefit even for localised proximal-third cancers.[89] This procedure is not indicated for cancers in the distal half of the stomach, although nodes along the proximal part of the splenic artery (11p nodes) are excised as part of a radical D2 excision of the coeliac trunk nodes.[89] En bloc pancreatic excision should now only be considered in the younger and fitter patient with an advanced proximal cancer where a lesser procedure is anticipated to leave residual cancer.

There is no place for *routine* resection of the distal pancreas in gastric cancer surgery.

Pancreas-preserving gastrectomy

This has been described in Japan for excision of station-11 nodes in patients with proximal cancers.[90] It requires splenectomy as the splenic artery and accompanying nodes are dissected off the pancreas and the artery ligated just distal to the branching of the dorsal pancreatic artery. Lymphangiographic studies show that the splenic artery lymphatics lie within the subserosal space on the upper and posterior aspect of the pancreas and never within the parenchyma. The arterial supply to the distal pancreas is adequate after ligation of the distal splenic artery. Preservation of the pancreas significantly reduces the incidence of postoperative complications. There is increasing experience with this technique in Japan. It is contraindicated if there is direct invasion of the pancreas. A prospective randomised study from Japan has shown that the pancreas-preserving operation is associated with less intraoperative blood loss and fewer pancreatic leaks, without any adverse effect on survival compared with pancreatico-splenectomy.[91] A study from Italy has confirmed that this procedure can be safely performed in Western patients, as part of a total gastrectomy with D2 lymphadenectomy, with a mortality of only 3.9%.[92] The place of this operation is not yet confirmed, but it is probably the procedure of choice when station-11 nodes are thought to be positive, providing the surgeon has the necessary experience.

Extended resections

The concept of gastric cancer remaining a locoregional disease with relatively late distant spread has already been discussed. It is possible that in some patients with locally advanced disease it is still possible to produce prolonged survival and perhaps cure by radical surgery, though such cases have to

be carefully selected.[93] Extended resection is defined as any dissection beyond a D2 subtotal or total gastrectomy. It is advocated by the Japanese for resectable advanced cancers with no evidence of distant spread.

There are two categories of extended resection to consider, namely the resection of involved adjacent organs and extended lymphadenectomy.

En bloc resection of involved adjacent organs

Spread into adjacent organs can occur in two different ways:

1. **Intramural spread** – either by direct growth or via lymphatics into the oesophagus or duodenum. Extending the resection margin either proximally or distally is certainly worthwhile as cure is still possible.

2. **Transmural spread** – into adjacent organs, e.g. pancreas, spleen, left lobe of liver and transverse mesocolon. Pathological assessment in cases of apparent invasion shows that in about one-third the adherence to another organ is inflammatory rather than neoplastic. In one recent study only 14% had pathologically confirmed invasion of the adjacent organ.[94] However, trial dissection and intraoperative biopsy carries a risk of disseminating malignant cells. Resection of the adjacent organ is thus recommended provided the patient is fit enough to undergo the extended procedure. If the patient is unfit or too elderly for a radical excision then gastrectomy may still be worthwhile as a high proportion may still have a clear lateral resection margin.

The results of surgical series of extended resections must be interpreted with care. Transmural spread has a much worse prognosis than intramural spread, and series may include different proportions of each.[95] It is also important to determine whether the paper includes only patients with pathological confirmation of transmural invasion or all patients with adherence to adjacent organs. It is not entirely surprising that analysis of the late results of extended resection has produced conflicting results. Overall it appears that there is a small survival advantage, but this is only realised if operative mortality is minimised in what are usually very major operations. In two papers from the USA the 5YSR of patients with invasion of a single adjacent organ was about 25%, although with a significant perioperative mortality.[94,96] The 5YSR for resections where two adjacent organs are invaded is only 4% and thus lower than the increased mortality risk. Extended resection should only be considered when there will be no evidence of macroscopic residual disease after the resection. The risks in older patients and those with concomitant diseases must be carefully weighed up against the potential survival benefit. It must be remembered that these more advanced gastric cancers are usually node positive and the minimum level of node dissection in an extended resection should be a D2 lymphadenectomy.[35]

Extended lymphadenectomy

Removal of node stations 13–16 has only been reported to be of benefit in Japan.[31] Resection of third- and fourth-tier para-aortic nodes does potentially decrease the risk of gastric bed recurrence and prolong the symptom-free interval. It is uncertain whether this potential benefit is worthwhile in Western patients because of the increased risks of radical resection. Two multicentre randomised trials in Japan comparing D2 and D4 lymphadenectomy for advanced cancer have recently reported their results.[97,98] Both trials concluded that a D4 resection did not improve survival but did increase operation-related risks.

Extended D4 lymphadenectomy does not provide any survival benefit over D2 lymphadenectomy for advanced gastric cancer.

A recent Polish RCT looked at extending nodal dissection beyond the second tier and found no survival benefit but increased risk.[99] A study from Taiwan comparing D1 with D3 lymphadenectomy did demonstrate a survival benefit for the extended resection.[100]

There are limited indications for extended surgery in Western patients. The differentiation between curative and palliative surgery for locally advanced cancers is often blurred. It is likely that extended resections do improve symptom-free survival in some patients even if cure is not achieved.[101] However, this surgery has to be performed with low mortality and morbidity to produce benefit.

An extended resection for advanced gastric cancer should be preceded by neoadjuvant chemotherapy in those fit enough to receive multimodality therapy and probably avoided in those who are not fit enough (see Chapter 9).

Resection of liver metastases

The success of hepatic resection in treating metastatic colorectal cancer has led to interest in a similar approach for gastric cancer. There is now an increasing evidence base of observational studies. It is apparent that patients with synchronous liver metastases do badly, though there are reports of long-term survivors with a single metastasis at presentation.[102] It is of note that some of the larger series show a 5YSR of >30% for patients with a solitary metachronous secondary lesion.[103,104] Lesions under 5 cm in diameter that can be resected with a clear 10-mm margin have the best prognosis.[105] Patients with multiple metastases do poorly after resection and should be treated non-surgically. Recurrence after resection of liver metastases is usually within the liver.

Limited gastric resections in advanced gastric cancer

In the elderly or unfit patient it is reasonable to consider a less radical gastric resection, accepting that while the chance of cure may be reduced there is a lower risk of mortality and serious morbidity. There are both Japanese and non-Japanese papers that show the mortality of radical gastric surgery is not increased in well-selected elderly patients.[106–108]

There is no doubt that quality of life is better after limited gastric resections and particularly in terms of postprandial symptoms and nutritional sequelae. It is important to remember the cost–benefit ratio for elderly patients is very different to that of a younger patient – at NCCH in Tokyo the 5YSR rate in those over 80 with early gastric cancer was only 53.8%, with most dying of diseases other than recurrent cancer.[109] A recent survey showed that the majority of cancer centres in Japan now use some form of limited resection for older and less fit patients. Use of these procedures in the West may be limited by the lower incidence of early gastric cancer and the higher incidence of nodal spread in such cases. The increasing use of endoscopic ultrasound may open up this treatment option for older Western patients with both early and advanced cancers.

Technique of gastric resection with D2 lymphadenectomy

The aim of this section is not to provide a detailed operative manual, but to summarise the basic steps of the main procedures. A more detailed description that can be recommended is that of McCulloch.[110] This description was strongly influenced by the work of Keiichi Maruyama from the NCCH in Tokyo.

Incision

Gastric cancers below the cardia can be resected via an upper midline incision. In obese or heavily built patients it is usually necessary to extend the incision below the umbilicus to gain adequate exposure and room to operate. Some surgeons use a left thoraco-abdominal approach (LTA) for radical excision of the upper stomach, but there is an increased morbidity and mortality associated with disrupting the left costal margin and diaphragm and entering the left chest. This type of approach should be reserved for cancers in the cardia where it is necessary to resect more than 5 cm of the lower oesophagus to obtain adequate proximal clearance. Increasingly those with specialist experience are using the abdominal transhiatal approach.[47] This involves excision of the crura and oesophagophrenic ligament en bloc with the cardia. In addition, the diaphragm is divided anterior to the hiatal opening, thus allowing a wide exposure of the lower mediastinum. With appropriate retraction it is possible to resect 6–8 cm of lower oesphagus together with associated lymphatic tissue. A recent Japanese RCT comparing abdominal transhiatal with LTA was closed after interim analysis when no survival improvement was detected but LTA caused increased morbidity.[111] The bilateral subcostal or 'rooftop' incision also provides excellent exposure of the upper stomach and hiatus.

Intraoperative staging

This has been discussed in detail in Chapter 3. Meticulous staging is essential in deciding the appropriate type of resection and lymphadenectomy. Evidence of serosal invasion, invasion of an adjacent organ, peritoneal seedlings, apparent nodal involvement beyond the second tier and liver metastases must be sought. If any of these is found then radical surgery alone may not cure the patient and a decision has to be made about whether to proceed with the planned dissection, modify the operation with a view to adjuvant therapy or to opt for a lesser palliative procedure.

Operative strategy after staging

Three types of resection are considered:

1. subtotal D2 gastrectomy;
2. total D1/D2 gastrectomy without splenectomy and distal pancreatectomy;
3. total D2 gastrectomy with splenectomy and distal pancreatectomy.

Variations on these procedures and extended or limited versions may all be indicated in certain circumstances. These three operations fulfil the requirements for radical treatment of gastric cancer in the majority of patients and are the basic armaments of the specialist gastric cancer surgeon. The initial part of the dissection is common to all three procedures.

Initial dissection

1. Mobilise hepatic flexure of colon and fully Kocherise the duodenum and head of pancreas.

This allows examination of retropancreatic and para-aortic nodes.

2. Mobilise splenic flexure of colon and carefully divide any adhesions between omentum and spleen so that the capsule is not torn during the dissection.

3. Separate the greater omentum from the transverse colon along a bloodless line about 1 cm from the bowel. This plane of dissection is continued onto the anterior leaf of the transverse mesocolon. This leaf can be completely separated from the posterior leaf so that the lesser sac remains intact. This is not always an easy dissection in Western patients and requires some patience. It is especially important for cancers that breach the serosa of the posterior wall of the stomach. The line of dissection continues between the peritoneum over the pancreas and the gland itself and care must be taken not to damage the parenchyma.

4. At the right side this line of dissection leads onto the right gastroepiploic vessels and subpyloric nodes. These nodes are swept up on the vessels, which are bared and ligated at their origins.

5. The lesser omentum is divided along the line of the reflection on the liver capsule. There is usually an accessory left hepatic artery in the omentum and this should be ligated close to the liver. The line of dissection is continued upwards proximally over the oesophagogastric junction to include the oesophagophrenic ligament and, in cancers of the cardia, part of the diaphragm. Distally the line of dissection passes down the peritoneum over the hepatoduodenal ligament to the upper border of the duodenum.

6. At this stage the surgeon should perform the optional dissection of the lymphatic tissue in the hepatoduodenal ligament (station-12) nodes. This is only done for cancers in the lower half of the stomach and particularly if there is evidence of involvement of the suprapyloric or common hepatic nodes. The dissection starts at the reflection of the peritoneum in the porta hepatis and includes the peritoneum and all lymphatic tissue from both front and back of the bile ducts, common and right and left hepatic arteries and the portal vein down to the neck of the pancreas. The gallbladder may be removed as part of this dissection.

7. Whether or not the hepatoduodenal ligament has been dissected out, the line of dissection brings the surgeon down onto the common hepatic artery and the origin of the often insubstantial right gastric artery. This is ligated at its origin taking care not to damage or occlude the hepatic artery.

8. The first part of the duodenum is now freed from the head of the pancreas. There are several small vessels running between the gastroduodenal and superior pancreaticoduodenal arteries and the duodenal wall. It is important to ligate these individually and not use diathermy in this area as both the pancreas and duodenum can suffer damage leading to leakage. The duodenum should be divided at least 2 cm distal to the pylorus – a wider margin is needed for cancers in the distal stomach.

9. Lifting the distal stomach up and to the left, the dissection of the lymphatics and peritoneum on the posterior wall of the lesser sac is continued to the left. This includes the tissue on the upper border of the body of the pancreas, along the common hepatic artery and to the left of the portal vein. Troublesome bleeding is often encountered near the pancreas, and the left gastric vein sometimes passes down behind the upper border of the pancreas to the splenic vein. Great care is needed in this area, and again vessels should be ligated or transfixed rather than diathermised close to pancreatic parenchyma. The retroperitoneal nodes to the left of the inferior vena cava tend to bleed quite profusely and dissection of these nodes should only be contemplated for upper-third cancers – in other cases the peritoneal dissection is continued up onto the posterior aspect of the proximal lesser curve, thus exposing the right crus of the diaphragm. Inferiorly the dissection reaches the junction of common hepatic and splenic arteries on the upper border of the pancreas.

10. The lymphatic tissue around the origin of the splenic artery is divided and swept up towards the left gastric artery if the operation is for a distal cancer or if the spleen and pancreas are not to be removed. The nodal tissue around the coeliac trunk is carefully dissected off the artery, trying to avoid entering the tough neural and fibrous tissue around the origin of the trunk on the anterior aorta. All this tissue is swept upwards with the lymphatic tissue on the left gastric artery. The left gastric artery is then ligated at its origin, leaving the distal coeliac trunk and the origins of the common hepatic and splenic arteries bared completely. The left gastric vein is variable and there may be more than one – it is ligated as found.

At this point the operation strategy depends on the extent of the planned resection.

Subtotal gastrectomy

All the tissue on the proximal lesser curve from the oesophagogastric junction downwards should be removed with the left gastric pedicle. This starts with ligation of the ascending branch of the artery and vein at the hiatus. Small vessels passing to the stomach wall are individually ligated. If involved nodes are detected in this tissue it is preferable to do a total gastrectomy.

The final part of the dissection involves separating the left side of the greater omentum from the splenic flexure of the colon and following the line of resection up to the lower pole of the spleen. The dissection of the anterior leaf of the mesocolon is completed between the middle colic vessels and the splenic flexure. This continues over the distal pancreas up towards the hilum of the spleen. At this point the left gastroepiploic vessels are identified, with the artery being the first branch of the splenic artery visible at the hilum. The inferior two or three short gastric arteries are also ligated nearer to the stomach to allow full mobilisation of the greater curve. The blood supply of the stomach remnant is entirely from the proximal short gastric arteries (**Fig. 7.3**).

Total gastrectomy without splenectomy and distal pancreatectomy

The resection is the same thus far. The ligation of the short gastric arteries should be as close to the hilum as is safe. In order to achieve this it is best to divide the peritoneum (lienorenal ligament) lateral to the spleen and mobilise the spleen and tail of pancreas. If there appear to be involved nodes in the hilum, the splenic artery and vein should be dissected off the tail of the pancreas, transfixed and divided, so removing the spleen with the stomach.

The nodal dissection is continued up the front of the aorta from the coeliac trunk up into the hiatus, the assistant lifting the stomach up to allow a good view of this area. Two significant vessels are encountered in removing this tissue en bloc with the stomach. The first is the posterior gastric or short gastric artery, which passes to the posterior proximal stomach from the splenic artery. The

D2 subtotal gastrectomy

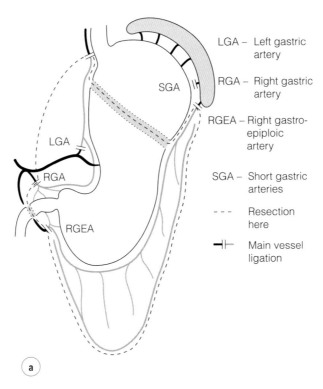

LGA – Left gastric artery

RGA – Right gastric artery

RGEA – Right gastro-epiploic artery

SGA – Short gastric arteries

- - - Resection here

⊣⊢ Main vessel ligation

D2 total gastrectomy with preservation of spleen and pancreas

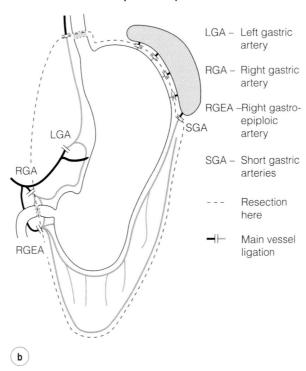

LGA – Left gastric artery

RGA – Right gastric artery

RGEA –Right gastro-epiploic artery

SGA – Short gastric arteries

- - - Resection here

⊣⊢ Main vessel ligation

Figure 7.3 • (a) D2 subtotal gastrectomy. **(b)** D2 total gastrectomy with preservation of spleen and pancreas.

other is the left phrenic artery, which should be divided near the upper border of the left adrenal gland to allow the left cardial nodal tissue to be dissected completely off the left crus. The left subphrenic branch of this vessel is divided as it reaches the diaphragm, so freeing the lymphatic tissue on the left aspect of the oesophagogastric junction. It is often not appreciated that the cardia is retroperitoneal in this area and the resection must include all the tissue in the triangle between the upper border of the tail of the pancreas, the left crus and the upper pole of the spleen. Both vagi and the other small vessels around the lower oesophagus are divided so that only the oesophagus attaches the stomach. The length of oesophagus mobilised depends on the resection margin required. The transhiatal approach for cardia cancers has already been described (Fig. 7.3).

Total gastrectomy with splenectomy and distal pancreatectomy

Resection of the spleen and pancreas via an abdominal incision is not technically easy because of limited space. One commonly used manoeuvre is to divide the peritoneum laterally and mobilise the spleen and distal pancreas to the right. The alternative is to mobilise the pancreas where the splenic artery joins it and to divide the pancreas, artery and vein at this point. The dissection is then continued to the left posterior to the pancreas until the lienorenal ligament is divided, so freeing the spleen. The dissection is then continued up in the retroperitoneum above the tail of the pancreas as described. When the decision has been made to do a complete D2 resection for a proximal cancer the author finds this latter manoeuvre easier and less bloody than mobilisation of the spleen and pancreas to the right with the limited exposure provided by an abdominal approach. An essential step in the distal pancreatectomy is ligation of the pancreatic duct.

Laparoscopic gastric resection

This is fully described in Chapter 8. There has been increasing interest in the potential for laparoscopic resection of gastric cancer recently, with the procedures being either totally laparoscopic or more usually laparoscopic-assisted. There are now studies that show the safety of the laparoscopic procedures and that confirm that a D2 lymphadenectomy can be performed to the same standard.[112,113] It should be noted that most of the published studies are from Asia and largely comprise of patients with T1 or T2 cancers and so we do not yet have definitive information about this approach for the more advanced cancers. A meta-analysis of open versus laparoscopic-assisted gastrectomy (LADG) yielded only a small

number of suitable RCTs and showed no differences between the groups except for a longer operating time and a reduced nodal yield in LADG.[114] There was a trend to faster postoperative recovery and discharge after LADG. The authors did note when searching the literature the small sample sizes and the sparsity of RCTs together with limited duration of follow-up.

 It is likely that the laparoscopic procedures will continue to be developed and the most important message is that the lessons learnt during the development of safe open gastric cancer surgery should not be forgotten as the new techniques are adopted. Further RCTs in Western patients with advanced cancers and with a sufficient follow-up period are still needed.

Reconstruction after gastric resection

The two main dangers for a patient undergoing a major gastric resection for cancer are recurrence of the cancer and significant malnutrition. There is a tendency to concentrate mainly on the former and to forget that weight loss and inadequate absorption of essential nutrients can severely affect quality of life after a gastrectomy. In recognising that many patients will not be cured by radical surgery it is most important to maximise quality of life while the patient is free of symptomatic recurrence. This is achieved by appropriate reconstruction of the upper gastrointestinal tract and then close follow-up of nutritional status.

Aims of reconstruction

The aims of reconstruction are as follows:

1. The construction of the least complex anastomosis to allow adequate nutritional intake.
2. The procedure should be safe and not add to the mortality and morbidity of the gastric resection.
3. The alteration in upper gastrointestinal physiology should be minimised.
4. The procedure should not be prone to long-term complications such as bacterial overgrowth.
5. It should prevent the reflux of bile and alkaline duodenal juices into the oesophagus.
6. It should not obstruct at an early stage if there is gastric bed recurrence.

Reconstructions can be broadly divided into two groups – duodenal bypass and duodenal continuity.

Duodenal bypass

The duodenal stump is closed and the proximal jejunum used to provide continuity. This results in a less physiological mixing of food with bile and pancreatic enzymes and a significant alteration in neurohumoral feedback from the duodenum. This latter abnormality is not so important after excision of the antrum and pylorus and in any case is probably more important in theory than in reality. The best clinical results are obtained using the Roux-en-Y technique with a 40–60 cm limb of proximal jejunum. There are many variations on this technique, but the important thing is that all prevent the reflux of duodenal contents into the gastric remnant and oesophagus. The disadvantage of a Roux reconstruction is that this segment of proximal jejunum is important for optimum digestion and absorption, but food passing through it has not mixed with bile and pancreatic enzymes. Use of a long jejunal loop instead of a Roux limb 'wastes' even more proximal jejunum and unless a very long loop is used it is associated with a high incidence of bile reflux problems.

Duodenal continuity

Duodenal continuity is maintained either by joining the gastric remnant to the duodenal stump (Billroth 1) or interposing a segment of proximal jejunum between the oesophagus or gastric remnant and the duodenal stump. It allows a more physiological mixing of food with bile and enzymes, though this is by no means normal because of rapid passage of unprepared food through the duodenum. The main disadvantages are an increased risk of symptomatic bile and alkaline reflux and a higher rate of postoperative complications, particularly with the more complex interposition procedures. This type of procedure is not advisable for locally advanced cancers that tend to recur in the gastric bed and may lead to early obstruction of the anastomoses or interposed jejunum.

There is no evidence that preservation of duodenal continuity improves nutritional parameters, weight or quality of life.[115] Recent studies from Japan have shown that a Roux reconstruction has both symptomatic and functional advantages over a Billroth 1 reconstruction.[116,117]

Examples of the various reconstruction procedures for subtotal and total gastrectomy are shown in **Fig. 7.4**.

Jejunal pouch reconstruction

The most common symptom after total gastrectomy is early satiety. This restricts food intake and makes it difficult for patients to maintain an adequate cal-orie intake. Various operations have been devised to increase the reservoir capacity of the proximal jejunum. Initially such operations were used as remedial procedures in patients with severe restriction of intake or with disabling postprandial symptoms. They are now used routinely by some gastric cancer surgeons, either as modifications of the Roux limb or as formal jejunal pouches, supported by the results of randomised trials.[118,119] However, while there are many trials these all involve small numbers of patients. A recent review of the best-quality studies identified only 19 randomised trials comparing a simple Roux-en-Y with a pouch reconstruction; together these only included 866 patients (only two trials had more than 30 patients in each arm).[120] This review shows that construction of a pouch entails a small increase in operative time, but does not increase morbidity or mortality. Early postoperative meal capacity is better with a pouch and weight is better maintained. In the longer term the only significant finding was an improved quality of life in those with a pouch. It is likely that rigorous dietetic surveillance is of more value than the actual type of reconstruction in ensuring optimal nutrition after a gastrectomy.[50,121]

While the evidence is not strong, it is apparent that construction of a jejunal pouch is as safe as a simple reconstruction in the hands of experienced surgeons. There is evidence that early postoperative eating capacity and weight are better maintained with a pouch. In the longer term a pouch reconstruction is associated with an improved quality of life.

Early postoperative complications

As with any abdominal surgical procedure the complications can be divided into general complications and those specifically associated with gastric resection and reconstruction. The general complications of major gastric surgery are covered in Chapter 4. The complication rate is higher after total gastrectomy and particularly if the spleen and distal pancreas have been resected. There is very little in the literature about the management of complications, though a review by the surgeons of the NCCH in Tokyo is recommended.[29]

A basic principle in radical gastric surgery is to recognise complications early and deal with them in a proactive way. This is especially important for intra-abdominal complications within the first few days of surgery. One of the important lessons learnt is to 'look and see' rather than 'wait and see'.

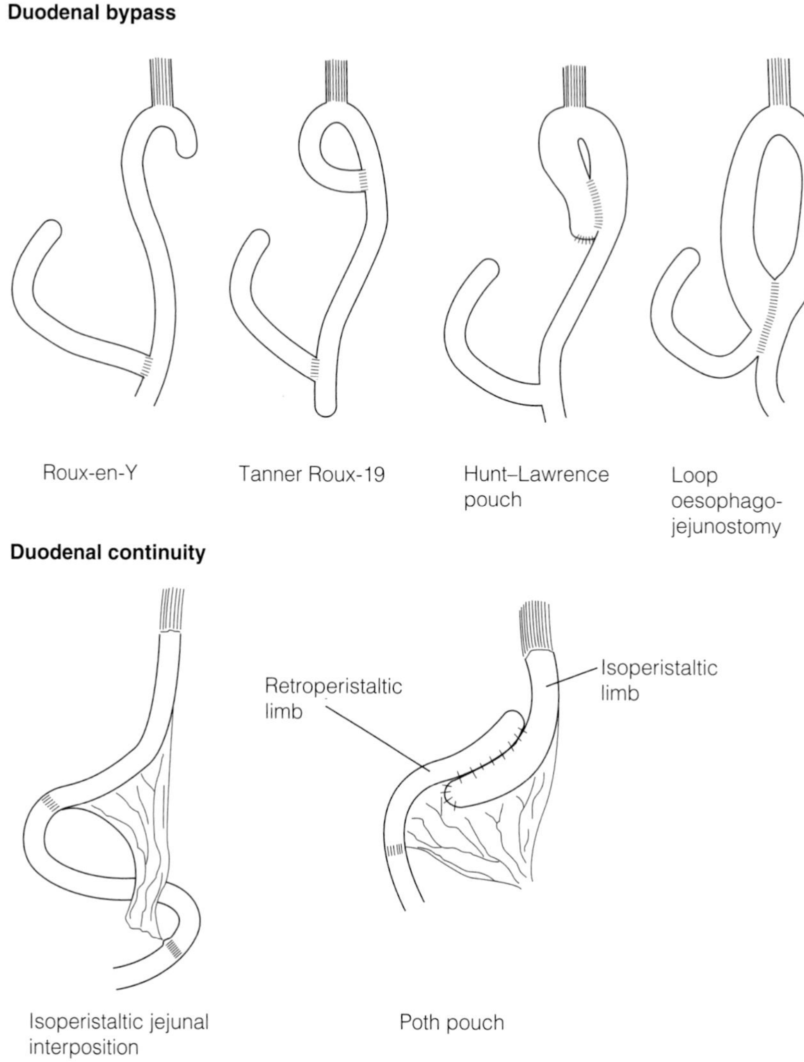
Duodenal bypass
Roux-en-Y
Tanner Roux-19
Hunt–Lawrence pouch
Loop oesophago-jejunostomy
Duodenal continuity
Retroperistaltic limb
Isoperistaltic limb
Isoperistaltic jejunal interposition
Poth pouch

Figure 7.4 • Reconstruction after gastrectomy.

A second-look laparotomy when the patient is still stable is considerably safer than waiting until the condition of the patient has deteriorated and sepsis has developed. An early operation may allow correction of the problem while a delay may make this impossible. Increasingly there is a move towards the use of interventional radiology for the treatment of septic complications. After the first two or three postoperative days re-operation becomes much more dangerous and so radiological treatment should be the first-line approach.

The following are the more common intra-abdominal complications specific to gastrectomy for cancer.

Haemorrhage

This may be either reactive, within the first few hours of surgery, or secondary, caused by partially or inadequately treated intra-abdominal sepsis. Early re-laparotomy is advocated for definite or even suspected reactive haemorrhage. It must be remembered that drains can occlude with blood clot and the clinical suspicion of bleeding in a haemodynamically unstable patient is sufficient indication to operate.

Secondary haemorrhage is truly life-threatening and every effort should be made to prevent this occurring. Any intra-abdominal sepsis must be treated aggressively, in particular collections around the coeliac trunk, as erosion of the main arteries in this area is extremely dangerous. If the radiological facilities are adequate then embolisation may be attempted. The author's experience is that in full-blown secondary haemorrhage there is little time to take definitive action and immediate laparotomy is a safer option. This is not to say that surgical control of secondary haemorrhage is easy, but temporary control may save the patient's life while preparation is made for definitive control. Haemorrhage from the coeliac trunk vessels may require cross-clamping of the aorta. Since the hiatus is filled by the reconstruction it is often safer to clamp the aorta above the diaphragm using a left thoracic or thoraco-abdominal approach and so avoid damage, or further damage, to the anastomoses. This complication most commonly occurs about two or more weeks after the gastrectomy when postoperative adhesions are dense and maturing – in the heat of the moment significant damage can occur. Suture of the eroded vessels is often difficult in the presence of infection, and a non-absorbable monofilament material is recommended. It is most important that the infected area is adequately debrided and drained prior to closure. The organisms causing the infection must be rapidly identified and appropriate antibiotics administered.

Duodenal stump leak

This may be due to technical error, afferent limb obstruction or ischaemia of the duodenal margin. The role of drains in abdominal surgery is always debatable, but a silastic tube drain to the duodenal stump is strongly recommended. In early leaks the appearance of bile-stained fluid in the drain is an indication for re-exploration, and it is frequently possible to correct the problem completely. Conservative management of early leaks produces a less predictable outcome and so intervention is far safer.

Delayed leaks can often be treated conservatively if the duodenal contents come out through the drain and the patient is not obviously septic. In this situation it may be safer to apply gentle suction to the drain for the first few days to ensure the leak remains localised and a fistulous tract is established. Parenteral nutrition is not necessary if the leak is controlled as it is preferable to give an enteral elemental-type diet and to suppress pancreatic secretion with a subcutaneous somatostatin analogue infusion. Drainage should be continued for at least 14 days and the drain then gradually pulled back from the duodenum. Provided the tract has matured, the resistance in the tract will be greater than that in the duodenum and the fistula

should close. If the fistula output is greater than 200 mL/24 hours without suction, then drainage should be continued for longer and contrast studies obtained to determine whether there is a technical problem with the reconstruction leading to a degree of obstruction in the short limb. In delayed leakage that does not appear in the drain the patient usually presents with a subhepatic abscess. In this situation percutaneous radiological drainage may be sufficient provided the patient's clinical condition responds to drainage. Drainage is continued until the fistula dries up, and although this may take weeks, it is worthwhile persevering. The patient can continue on enteral nutrition, with or without a subcutaneous somatostatin analogue, and need not stay in hospital if otherwise well. Any patient who remains septic and unwell despite drainage requires surgical exploration, debridement of the cavity and placement of a drain close to the point of leakage. If there is a major defect then a Foley-type catheter can be placed in the duodenum with a plan to form a controlled fistula. It is unwise to try to suture the duodenum if the presentation is delayed because of the poor tissue condition due to associated sepsis.

Anastomotic leak

This may occur because of technical error, ischaemia of the tissues or tension on the anastomotic line. In fact all these causes are 'technical errors'. Leakage is associated with a high mortality. It is of interest that the mortality of patients with an anastomotic leak in the Dutch D1 vs. D2 study was 43.1%, and that this is about three times greater than the mortality of this complication at the NCCH in Tokyo. Achieving a low mortality in Western patients requires reduction of the mortality of anastomotic leaks to the same level as the Japanese.[19] While part of this difference may be due to patient factors, it is likely that the more important factor is the experience and approach of the Japanese surgeons.[29] The Japanese emphasise the importance of using appropriately placed prophylactic drains for high-risk anastomoses. If a leak is identified within the first 72 hours then re-operation is advised. At worst this will allow placement of a drain right up against the point of leakage and also the construction of a more distal feeding jejunostomy. At best the anastomosis can be repaired or patched before sepsis is established in the surrounding tissues. Early leakage in more complex reconstructions may be from any of several suture lines and, more importantly, may be due to jejunal ischaemia. This must be dealt with before complete disruption occurs, when the chance of survival diminishes rapidly.

The management of a delayed-presentation anastomotic leak is more controversial. If the leak is contained and only identified on a contrast study prior to beginning enteral feeding then it is wise to keep the patient on a liquid diet and repeat the contrast study every 7 days to confirm resolution of the cavity. However, if the patient is septic then a drain must be placed in the cavity. The dilemma is whether to do this radiologically and risk incomplete drainage or to explore the cavity surgically and risk a very difficult operation. Surgical exploration has the advantage that a feeding jejunostomy can be constructed and the septic area debrided, but the whole upper abdomen is often 'glued up' with new adhesions at this time – it is not an operation for the inexperienced surgeon.

There is no doubt that with appropriate surgical action, modern antibiotics, expert radiological assistance and enteral feeding techniques, anastomotic leakage is no longer a surgical disaster. However, it is still the most common surgical cause of death and can be avoided by adhering to basic surgical principles.

Intra-abdominal sepsis

This may present at any time in the first 2 weeks after a gastrectomy. It may be due to anastomotic or duodenal leakage, pancreatic necrosis due to pancreatic parenchymal damage during the resection, or leakage from the pancreatic stump. Sepsis is statistically more common after splenectomy, although whether this is an immunological effect or simply reflects damage to or resection of the pancreas as part of the operation is unclear.

Computed tomography with both intravenous and intraluminal contrast is important in defining the site and cause of the sepsis. The choice between radiological and surgical drainage has already been discussed. The dangers of incompletely drained sepsis leading to deterioration of the patient's condition and the risk of secondary haemorrhage makes adequate drainage essential.

It is not unreasonable to start with radiological drainage unless there is significant tissue necrosis identified on the scans. Percutaneous drainage may be only a temporising measure while the patient's condition is improved, and the surgeon must always be prepared to abandon this method of drainage and opt for surgical debridement.

Pancreatic fistula

Whenever the tail of the pancreas is resected it is advisable to place a drain close to the stump. Minor pancreatic leaks are relatively common and can be controlled by the drain. Uncontrolled leakage usually presents as a left upper quadrant abscess. It may occur after damage to the tail of the pancreas during splenectomy or following distal pancreatectomy.

There is often associated necrosis of the pancreatic and peripancreatic tissue. The principle of treatment is as outlined above – surgical drainage with debridement of necrotic tissue and placement of a silastic tube drain to the point of leakage is recommended. Since the proximal pancreatic duct is not obstructed this type of leak will close spontaneously. Subcutaneous infusion of a somatostatin analogue is helpful in reducing the volume of the leaked juice in a higher output fistula.

Postsplenectomy infections

Left subphrenic abscess after splenectomy has already been discussed. There is increasing evidence that splenectomy predisposes the patient to an increased risk of bacterial infections in both the early postoperative period and probably for the remainder of their life. Immediate prophylaxis with twice daily oral penicillin is now recommended for patients of all ages. The patient should also be immunised with vaccines against pneumococci, meningococcus and *Haemophilus influenzae*. If the splenectomy has been planned as part of a radical procedure these vaccines are most effective if administered preoperatively. The patient should have an annual influenza vaccine and an updated pneumococcal vaccine about every 3 years.

Late sequelae and complications

The place of follow-up clinics after cancer surgery is a subject that generates considerable discussion and debate. In this section it should become apparent that methodical follow-up of patients who have had a gastrectomy for cancer is mandatory if they are to realise their maximum quality of life, even if survival is likely to be limited. Regular follow-up by trained personnel is the best way of identifying and solving problems that affect the patient's physical and psychological well-being after major cancer surgery.

The main long-term problems and complications can be divided into three groups:

- side-effects and postprandial sequelae;
- nutritional problems;
- recurrence of cancer.

Side-effects and postprandial sequelae

Early fullness

Loss of the reservoir function of the stomach results in a feeling of early satiety and, in some patients, upper abdominal pain. Although the proximal jejunum dilates after a gastrectomy it can never completely replace the gastric reservoir, and all patients have to limit their meal size to some extent. Good dietary advice is important to ensure an adequate calorie intake taken in more frequent smaller meals. The role of gastric pouches has already been discussed and they do apparently decrease the incidence of early satiety. Early dumping is a common cause of postprandial fullness and requires appropriate dietary manipulation. A less common cause of fullness in some patients who have had a Roux-en-Y reconstruction is a defect of normal peristalsis in the long limb. This produces hold-up in the propulsion of the meal and results in an unpleasant pain during eating and involuntary, or often voluntary, regurgitation of the meal.

Early dumping syndrome

The rapid filling of the proximal small intestine with hypertonic food leads to rapid movement of fluid into the gut from the extracellular fluid compartment. It also triggers a complex neurohumoral response that in some patients produces a variety of unpleasant gastrointestinal and cardiovascular symptoms. The main importance of the dumping syndrome is that it leads to food avoidance, whether because of fullness or other unpleasant symptoms. In severe cases the patient is incapacitated after eating or suffers profuse diarrhoea that prevents normal activities after meals. Quality of life may be very severely restricted and malnutrition can occur rapidly in these patients.

It is perhaps fortunate that patients who have had a total or subtotal gastrectomy have a small reservoir and are usually unable to eat a large hypertonic load. The syndrome is much more common and troublesome in those who have an intact stomach, with the pylorus destroyed or bypassed, or after a partial gastrectomy. Many gastrectomy patients have some dumping symptoms in the first few weeks after surgery, but in most these are relatively mild and improve considerably with simple dietary adjustments that the patients often discover for themselves. During early follow-up it is important to identify significant dumping symptoms. A careful history should be taken and in less clear cases the patient asked to keep a diary recording foods eaten and symptoms experienced. Most patients can be treated quite simply by appropriate dietary adaptation. It is important to involve an experienced dietician in the management of patients with dumping.

Reactive hypoglycaemic attacks

This is often incorrectly termed 'late dumping'. In many patients this occurs without early dumping symptoms. Symptoms of hypoglycaemia, which include, in the most profound cases, blackouts and grand mal fits, occur about 2 hours after the last meal. The patient often experiences a craving for sweet food early in the attack.

Dietary assessment is the first step and the patient is then advised to decrease the carbohydrate load in their main meals and to take small amounts of carbohydrate between main meals. Careful explanation of the problem is usually sufficient to reassure the patient they do not have a serious disorder. Those with frequent attacks should carry dextrose tablets to eat at the first sign of symptoms.

Diarrhoea

There are several possible causes for diarrhoea after a gastrectomy for cancer.

Truncal vagotomy

This is discussed in Chapter 18.

Early dumping

Diarrhoea not infrequently occurs towards the end of or even after a dumping attack and is part of the symptom complex. Unlike postvagotomy diarrhoea the attack follows a large hypertonic load and has other associated symptoms.

Bacterial overgrowth

While a theoretical problem after gastrectomy when there are complex reconstructions or pouches producing a blind limb, it is not often clinically significant. Overgrowth in the proximal small intestine may also occur after a Roux-en-Y reconstruction. It is the combination of the loss of gastric acid, which destroys pathogenic ingested bacteria, and the formation of 'blind loops' that allows overgrowth of both aerobic and anaerobic organisms. These faecal-type bacteria produce toxins that damage the brush border enzymes vital for digestion. They may also utilise important nutrients such as the B vitamins. Pathogenic anaerobes deconjugate and dehydroxylate bile acids, which are essential for normal fat absorption in the proximal small intestine. Faecal fat levels can become markedly elevated and in the worst cases the patient has steatorrhoea and loses weight rapidly.

Steatorrhoea

This may be due to bacterial overgrowth or relative pancreatic insufficiency caused by poor mixing of duodenal contents with food in reconstructions where the duodenum is excluded. Patients with fat malabsorption complain of unpleasant flatus and large-bowel colic and pass bulky greasy stools that float and are difficult to flush away. A carefully taken history will identify the problem. If bacterial overgrowth has been excluded then persistent fat malabsorption may respond to pancreatic enzyme supplements taken before or preferably mixed with food.

Bile reflux

Reflux of bile and alkaline juices into the stomach remnant and oesophagus may cause epigastric discomfort, heartburn and vomiting or regurgitation of bile. In the worst cases patients may avoid eating for fear of exacerbating their symptoms. Persistent oesophageal reflux may produce stricturing.

The diagnosis is usually made on clinical grounds. Gastroscopy is important to confirm whether there is mucosal damage and to exclude any other cause for the symptoms. Objective evidence can be obtained with a technetium-99m-HIDA scan.

Treatment is often unsatisfactory and prevention of the problem by a bile-diverting reconstruction in the first place is important. Unremitting symptoms are an indication for further surgery to divert the duodenal contents by changing the reconstruction or lengthening the Roux limb.

Nutritional problems

These can be divided into general malnutrition, reflected by weight loss, and deficits of specific nutrients.

General malnutrition and weight loss

It is important to recognise that malabsorption is a rare cause of malnutrition after a subtotal or total gastrectomy, unless there is bacterial overgrowth. With few exceptions patients who lose weight, or fail to regain their preoperative weight, do so because they fail to ingest sufficient calories. Early satiety and the dumping syndrome are the most common causes, and correction of these symptoms is usually sufficient to correct malnutrition.

Patients undergoing a subtotal gastrectomy rarely experience serious problems with weight loss. It is a fallacy that patients who have undergone a total gastrectomy invariably lose weight after the initial few months, although most fail to completely regain their pre-illness weight.[122] Women, and particularly those over 70, do frequently have difficulty maintaining their weight after total gastrectomy. While patients will take sufficient calories under close supervision in hospital, their intake usually decreases on first going home.[123] Nutrition then improves over the first 6 months after surgery, by which time more than half of the patients are taking their recommended calorie intake.[124] It is advised that all patients are kept under close dietary surveillance for at least 12 months after surgery.

Carbohydrate absorption is nearly complete even after total gastrectomy, but the pattern of absorption is abnormal. Protein absorption is decreased, as reflected by an increase in faecal nitrogen, but this is rarely clinically important. Fat malabsorption is the main cause of inadequate calorie absorption. On average postgastrectomy patients absorb about 80% of ingested fat – easily enough to provide adequate calories provided intake is sufficient.

Specific deficiencies

Vitamin B$_{12}$

Gastric acid is necessary to release B$_{12}$ from foodstuffs and, more importantly, gastric parietal cell intrinsic factor is essential for absorption of this vitamin in the terminal ileum. After total gastrectomy patients absorb virtually no vitamin B$_{12}$ and body stores are gradually depleted, although this may take up to 24 months to become clinically apparent. All patients should receive 1 mg of hydroxycobalamin intramuscularly every 3 months for life.

Other B vitamins

Deficiency only becomes clinically important if there is intestinal bacterial overgrowth. Treatment of the underlying cause of overgrowth is the priority, but oral B complex supplements should be given during treatment and for several weeks afterwards.

Fat-soluble vitamins

Malabsorption is similar to that of fat. Vitamin A deficiency is detectable but remains a subclinical problem even many years after surgery. There is evidence that vitamin E deficiency can occur after total gastrectomy and may rarely lead to neurological symptoms, and so this should be kept in mind in long-term survivors.[125]

Vitamin D malabsorption is of much more importance and particularly in postmenopausal women and long-term survivors. There is evidence of an increasing incidence of metabolic bone disorders from 2 years after surgery.[126] Vitamin D and calcium metabolism disorders are common after total gastrectomy and supplementation of both may prevent age-related loss of bone mass.[127] Postmenopausal women and all patients over 70 should take an oral calcium and vitamin D supplement twice a day for life after a total gastrectomy. At 5 years a full assessment for signs of developing subclinical metabolic bone disease should be undertaken in all patients.

Iron

Absorption is surprisingly normal after total gastrectomy and even if the duodenum has been bypassed. It appears that the jejunum can adapt to absorb iron provided that there are sufficient naturally occurring chelating agents in the food. Iron absorption shows a gradual improvement after gastrectomy and, provided intake is adequate, is near normal 12 months after surgery. If indicated an oral iron supplement in combination with vitamin C may be given once or twice a day for the first year, but only continued thereafter in those with a poor intake of iron-containing foodstuffs.

Recurrence of cancer

The detection and treatment of recurrent gastric cancer remains a complex issue affected by multiple factors. The mode of recurrence can often be predicted by the stage of the original disease.[128] Cancers that have not penetrated the serosa recur later and usually as liver or distant metastases, whereas those that have invaded through the serosa often recur earlier and within the gastric bed on the peritoneal surfaces.

There have been no randomised trials of different follow-up protocols. It remains a stark fact that most patients with 'late' gastric cancer have persisting microscopic disease after 'curative' surgery and at some time this will manifest as recurrent disease. Until it is known whether the detection of asymptomatic recurrence confers any benefit in terms of survival or, more importantly, overall quality of life measured over the remainder of the patient's life, the place of follow-up will remain contentious. Recent research has demonstrated that early detection does not affect overall survival even if actively treated.[129,130] Further research is needed to establish the best method for detecting early recurrence and also to be able to measure the effects of early treatment before the recurrence causes significant symptoms.[131]

It is now recognised that follow-up of patients is important for other complex reasons and often for psychological support for the patient and their family. The role of the clinical nurse specialist is especially important in this phase of the patient's ongoing treatment.[132]

While radiotherapy or chemotherapy may occasionally be indicated, the majority of patients with clinical recurrence will simply be treated symptomatically. Further surgery for obstructive symptoms is worthwhile, not least because some patients will be found to have another cause for obstruction that is treatable. Malignant obstruction may be relieved by a bypass procedure, but there are often multiple areas of intestinal involvement and the prognosis is generally very poor. The terminal care of patients with recurrent cancer is a subject in itself and does not fall within the scope of this chapter.

Key points

- The pattern of recurrence is different in serosa-negative (T1 and T2) and serosa-positive (T3 and T4) gastric cancers. Serosa-positive cancers tend to recur early (within 2 years) and within the peritoneal cavity, especially in the gastric bed. Serosa-negative cancers recur later and more frequently as haematogenous metastases without local recurrence, provided all local disease is resected.
- The high incidence of serosa-positive cancers in the West explains why the overall outlook after gastric resection is still poor.
- The role of surgery is limited to complete removal of curable lesions that have not disseminated at the time of diagnosis and to minimising the early phase of locoregional recurrence.
- Measures to destroy free cells in the perioperative period will be required in addition to surgery in patients who have significant serosal involvement. Further work is needed on the role of intraperitoneal chemotherapy in the West.
- The balance of evidence is that radical gastric cancer surgery does produce some survival benefit, but that this is variable depending on the stage of the disease. However, if that advantage is only small for Western patients then it could be offset by the increased mortality of more radical surgery.
- On the basis of good-quality data there is no support for the concept of 'total gastrectomy de principe' for cancers in the lower half of the stomach. The standard operation for distal gastric cancer is a subtotal gastrectomy.
- In the absence of good evidence, total gastrectomy is presently recommended for proximal gastric cancer in Western patients. Randomised studies for patients with locally advanced proximal cancer (type 2 and limited type 3 junctional cancer) are required to determine whether a proximal partial gastrectomy has advantages over a total gastrectomy.
- There is good evidence to show that D2 lymphadenectomy should not be used routinely in the surgical treatment of gastric cancer in Western patients. Only selected patients are likely to benefit from this type of resection. The risks of D2 compared with D1 lymphadenectomy for distal gastric

cancer are smaller and so this is currently recommended for patients with localised disease without significant serosal involvement.

- Gastrectomy with D2 lymphadenectomy should presently only be performed by surgeons with proven experience of this type of radical surgery.
- The spleen should not be removed for cancers confined to the distal half of the stomach. The role of splenectomy as part of a D2 lymphadenectomy for proximal cancer requires further research.
- There is no place for routine resection of the distal pancreas in gastric cancer surgery. Resection is only indicated when a posterior wall gastric cancer invades the pancreas and there is no other evidence of dissemination.
- Randomised trials show that extended lymphadenectomy does not provide any survival benefit over D2 lymphadenectomy for advanced gastric cancer.
- There is no evidence that preservation of duodenal continuity improves nutritional parameters, weight or quality of life. Recent studies from Japan have shown that a Roux reconstruction has both symptomatic and functional advantages over a Billroth 1 reconstruction.
- While the evidence is not strong, it is apparent that construction of a jejunal pouch is as safe as a simple reconstruction in the hands of experienced surgeons. There is evidence that early postoperative eating capacity and weight are better maintained with a pouch. In the longer term a pouch reconstruction is associated with an improved quality of life.

References

1. Averbach AM, Jacquet P. Strategies to decrease the incidence of intra-abdominal recurrence in resectable gastric cancer. Br J Surg 1996; 83:726–33.

2. Marrelli D, Roviello F, de Manzoni G et al. Different patterns of recurrence in gastric cancer depending on Lauren's histological type: longitudinal study. World J Surg 2002; 26:1160–5.

3. Cunliffe WJ, Sugarbaker PH. Gastrointestinal malignancy: rationale for adjuvant therapy using early postoperative intraperitoneal chemotherapy. Br J Surg 1989; 76:1082–90.

4. Yu W, Whang I, Suh I et al. Prospective randomized trial of early postoperative intraperitoneal chemotherapy as an adjuvant to resectable gastric cancer. Ann Surg 1998; 228:347–54.

5. Yonemura Y, Ninomiya I, Kaji M et al. Prophylaxis with intraoperative chemohyperthermia against peritoneal recurrence of serosal invasion-positive gastric cancer. World J Surg 1995; 19:450–4.

6. Sautner T, Hofbauer F, Depisch D et al. Adjuvant intraperitoneal cisplatin chemotherapy does not improve long-term survival after surgery for advanced gastric cancer. J Clin Oncol 1994; 12:970–4.

7. Hanazaki K, Sodeyama H, Mochizuki Y et al. Efficacy of extended lymphadenectomy in the non-curative gastrectomy for advanced gastric cancer. Hepatogastroenterology 1999; 46:2677–82.

8. Dickens BJ, Bigam DL, Cass C et al. Gastric adenocarcinoma: review and considerations for future directions. Ann Surg 2005; 241:27–39.

9. Nakajima T. Gastric cancer treatment guidelines in Japan. Gastric Cancer 2002; 5:1–5.

10. Schwarz RE, Karpeh MS, Brennan MF. Surgical management of gastric cancer: the Western experience. In: Daly JM, Hennessey TPJ, Reynolds JV (eds) Management of upper gastrointestinal cancer. London: WB Saunders, 1999; pp. 83–106.

11. Hallissey MT, Allum WH, Jewkes AJ et al. Early detection of gastric cancer. Br Med J 1990; 301:513–15.

12. Hisamichi S. Screening for gastric cancer. World J Surg 1989; 13:31–7.

13. Hundahl SA, Stemmermann GN, Oishi A. Racial factors cannot explain superior Japanese outcomes in stomach cancer. Arch Surg 1996; 131:170–5.

14. Theuer CP, Kurosaki T, Ziogas A et al. Asian patients with gastric carcinoma in the United States exhibit unique clinical features and superior overall and cancer specific survival rates. Cancer 2000; 89:1883–92.

15. Roder JD, Bonenkamp JJ, Craven J et al. Lymphadenectomy for gastric cancer in clinical trials: update. World J Surg 1995; 19:546–53.

16. Kunisaki K, Shimada H, Ono H et al. Comparison of results of surgery in the upper third and more distal stomach. J Gastrointest Surg 1996; 10: 718–26.

17. Allum WH, Powell DJ, McConkey CC et al. Gastric cancer: a 25-year review. Br J Surg 1989; 76:535–40.

18. Macintyre IM, Akoh JA. Improving survival in gastric cancer: review of operative mortality in English language publications from 1970. Br J Surg 1991; 78:771–6.

19. Lamb P, Sivashanmugam T, White M et al. Gastric cancer surgery – a balance of risk and radicality. Ann R Coll Surg Engl 2008; 90:235–42.

20. Roviello F, Marrelli D, Morgagni P et al. Survival benefit of extended D2 lymphadenectomy in gastric cancer with involvement of second level lymph nodes: a longitudinal multicenter study. Ann Surg Oncol 2002; 9:894–900.

21. McCulloch P, Ward J, Tekkis PP. Mortality and morbidity in gastro-oesophageal cancer surgery: initial results of ASCOT multicentre prospective cohort study. Br Med J 2003; 327:1192–7.

22. Pye JK, Crumplin MK, Charles J et al. One-year survey of carcinoma of the oesophagus and stomach in Wales. Br J Surg 2001; 88:278–85.

23. Bachmann MO, Alderson D, Edwards D et al. Cohort study in South and West England of the influence of specialization on the management and outcome of patients with oesophageal and gastric cancers. Br J Surg 2002; 89:914–22.

24. Kodera Y, Sasako M, Yanamoto S et al. Identification of risk factors for the development of complications following extended and superextended lymphadenectomies for gastric cancer. Br J Surg 2005; 92:1103–9.

25. Park DJ, Lee HJ, Kim HH et al. Predictors of operative morbidity and mortality in gastric cancer surgery. Br J Surg 2005; 92:1099–102.

26. Tsukada K, Miyazaki T, Kato H et al. Body fat accumulation and postoperative complications after abdominal surgery. Am Surg 2004; 70:347–51.

27. Tsujinaka T, Sasako M, Yamamoto S et al. Influence of overweight on surgical complications for gastric cancer: results from a randomized control trial comparing D2 and extended para-aortic lymphadenectomy. Ann Surg Oncol 2007; 14:355–61.

28. Lee JH, Paik YH, Lee LS et al. Abdominal shape of gastric cancer patients influences short-term surgical outcomes. Ann Surg Oncol 2007; 14:288–94.

29. Sasako M, Katai H, Sano T et al. Management of complications after gastrectomy with extended lymphadenectomy. Surg Oncol 2000; 9:31–4.

    An important paper regarded as the 'gold standard' for management of gastrectomy complications.

30. Sue-Ling HM, Johnston D, Martin IG et al. Gastric cancer: a curable disease in Britain. Br Med J 1993; 307:591–6.

    The first UK paper to show results of gastric cancer surgery nearer to Japanese results.

31. Maruyama K, Okabayashi K, Kinoshita T. Progress in gastric cancer surgery in Japan and its limits of radicality. World J Surg 1987; 11:418–25.

32. Roukos DH, Lorenz M, Encke A. Evidence of survival benefit of extended (D2) lymphadenectomy in western patients with gastric cancer based on a new concept: a prospective long-term follow-up study. Surgery 1998; 123:573–8.

33. Marubini E, Bozzetti F, Miceli R et al. Lymphadenectomy in gastric cancer: prognostic role and therapeutic implications. Eur J Surg Oncol 2002; 28:406–12.

34. Volpe CM, Koo J, Miloro SM et al. The effect of extended lymphadenectomy on survival in patients with gastric adenocarcinoma. J Am Coll Surg 1995; 181:56–64.

35. Siewert JR, Bottcher K, Roder JD et al. Prognostic relevance of systematic lymph node dissection in gastric carcinoma. German Gastric Carcinoma Study Group. Br J Surg 1993; 80:1015–18.

    An important study of German gastric cancer surgery – not randomised.

36. Sano T. Tailoring treatments for curable gastric cancer. Br J Surg 2007; 94:263–4.

37. Hornig D, Hermanek P, Gall FP. The significance of the extent of proximal margins on clearance in gastric cancer surgery. Scand J Gastroenterol 1977; 22(Suppl 133):69–71.

38. Bozzetti F, Bonfanti G, Bufalino R et al. Adequacy of margins of resection in gastrectomy for cancer. Ann Surg 1982; 196:685–90.

39. Harrison LE, Karpeh MS, Brennan MF. Total gastrectomy is not necessary for proximal gastric cancer. Surgery 1998; 123:127–30.

40. Hinoshita E, Takahashi I, Onohara T et al. The nutritional advantages of proximal gastrectomy for early gastric cancer. Hepatogastroenterology 2001; 48:1513–16.

41. Shiraishi N, Adachi Y, Kitano S et al. Clinical outcome of proximal versus total gastrectomy for proximal gastric cancer. World J Surg 2002; 26:1150–4.

42. Katai H, Sano T, Fukagawa T et al. Prospective study of proximal gastrectomy for early gastric cancer in the upper third of the stomach. Br J Surg 2003; 90:850–3.

43. Siewert JR, Bottcher K, Stein HJ et al. Problem of proximal third gastric carcinoma. World J Surg 1995; 19:523–31.

44. Harrison LE, Karpeh MS, Brennan MF. Proximal gastric cancers resected via a transabdominal-only approach. Results and comparisons to distal adenocarcinoma of the stomach. Ann Surg 1997; 225:678–83.

45. Kobayashi T, Sugimura H, Kimura T. Total gastrectomy is not always necessary for advanced gastric cancer of the cardia. Dig Surg 2002; 19:15–21.

46. Siewert JR, Stein HJ, Sendler A et al. Surgical resection for cancer of the cardia. Semin Surg Oncol 1999; 17:125–31.

47. Wayman J, Dresner SM, Raimes SA et al. Transhiatal approach to total gastrectomy for adenocarcinoma of the gastric cardia. Br J Surg 1999; 86:536–40.

48. Bozzetti F. Total versus subtotal gastrectomy in cancer of the distal stomach: facts and fantasy. Eur J Surg Oncol 1992; 18:572–9.

49. Bozzetti F, Marubini E, Bonfanti G et al. Subtotal versus total gastrectomy for gastric cancer: five-year survival rates in a multicenter randomized Italian trial. Italian Gastrointestinal Tumor Study Group. Ann Surg 1999; 230:170–8.

   A prospective randomised trial regarded as the definitive study on the type of gastrectomy necessary for distal gastric cancer.

50. Svedlund J, Sullivan M, Liedman B et al. Quality of life after gastrectomy for gastric carcinoma: Controlled study of reconstructive procedures. World J Surg 1997; 21:422–33.

51. Davies J, Johnston D, Sue-Ling H et al. Total or subtotal gastrectomy for gastric carcinoma? A study of quality of life. World J Surg 1998; 22:1048–55.

52. Maruyama K, Gunven P, Okabayashi K et al. Lymph node metastases of gastric cancer. General pattern in 1931 patients. Ann Surg 1989; 210:596–602.

   This is the largest and most detailed study of lymph node involvement in gastric cancer and is regarded as a seminal work.

53. Maruyama K, Sasako M, Kinoshita T et al. Effectiveness of systematic lymph node dissection in gastric cancer surgery. In: Nishi M, Ichikawa H, Nakajima T et al (eds) Gastric cancer. Tokyo: Springer Verlag, 1993; pp. 293–305.

54. Marchet A, Mocellin S, Ambrosi A et al. The ratio between metastatic and examined lymph nodes (N ratio) is an independent prognostic factor in gastric cancer regardless of the type of lymphadenectomy: results from an Italian multicentric study. Ann Surg 2007; 245:543–52.

55. Yoshikawa T, Sasako M, Sano T et al. Stage migration caused by D2 dissection with para-aortic lymphadenectomy for gastric cancer from the results of a prospective randomized controlled trial. Br J Surg 2006; 93:1526–9.

56. Maruyama K. Results of surgery correlated with staging. In: Preece PE, Cuschieri A, Wellwood JM (eds) Cancer of the stomach. London: Grune & Stratton, 1986; pp. 145–63.

57. Seto Y, Nagawa H, Muto T. Results of extended lymph node dissection for gastric cancer cases with N2 lymph node metastasis. Int Surg 1997; 82:257–61.

58. Hayes N, Ng EK, Raimes SA et al. Total gastrectomy with extended lymphadenectomy for 'curable' stomach cancer: experience in a non-Japanese Asian center. J Am Coll Surg 1999; 188:27–32.

59. Nakajima T, Nishi M. Surgery and adjuvant chemotherapy for gastric cancer. Hepatogastroenterology 1989; 36:79–85.

60. Maehara Y, Tomoda M, Tomisaki S et al. Surgical treatment and outcome for node-negative gastric cancer. Surgery 1997; 121:633–9.

61. Siewert JR, Kestlmeier R, Busch R et al. Benefits of D2 lymph node dissection for patients with gastric cancer and pN0 and pN1 lymph node metastases. Br J Surg 1996; 83:1144–7.

62. Harrison LE, Karpeh MS, Brennan MF. Extended lymphadenectomy is associated with a survival benefit for node-negative gastric cancer. J Gastrointest Surg 1998; 2:126–31.

63. Siewert JR, Bottcher K, Stein HJ et al. Relevant prognostic factors in gastric cancer: ten-year results of the German Gastric Cancer Study. Ann Surg 1998; 228:449–61.

64. Bonenkamp JJ, Hermans J, Sasako M et al. Extended lymph-node dissection for gastric cancer. Dutch Gastric Cancer Group. N Engl J Med 1999; 340:908–14.

   A multicentre RCT of D1 vs. D2 lymphadenectomy in Dutch patients.

65. Bunt AM, Hermans J, Boon MC et al. Evaluation of the extent of lymphadenectomy in a randomized trial of Western–Japanese-type surgery in gastric cancer. J Clin Oncol 1994; 12:417–22.

66. Sasako M. Risk factors for surgical treatment in the Dutch Gastric Cancer Trial. Br J Surg 1997; 84:1567–71.

67. Cuschieri A, Fayers P, Fielding J et al. Postoperative morbidity and mortality after D1 and D2 resections for gastric cancer: preliminary results of the MRC randomised controlled surgical trial. The Surgical Cooperative Group. Lancet 1996; 347:995–9.

   A multicentre RCT of D1 vs. D2 lymphadenectomy in Western patients.

68. Cuschieri A, Weeden S, Fielding J et al. Patient survival after D1 and D2 resections for gastric cancer: long-term results of the MRC randomized surgical trial. Surgical Co-operative Group. Br J Cancer 1999; 79:1522–30.

69. Degiuli M, Sasako M, Ponti A et al. Survival results of a multicentre phase II study to evaluate D2 gastrectomy for gastric cancer. Br J Cancer 2004; 90:1727–32.

   A multicentre RCT of D1 vs. D2 lymphadenectomy in Italian patients.

70. Yildirim E, Celen O, Berberoglu U. The Turkish experience with curative gastrectomies for gastric carcinoma: is D2 dissection worthwhile. J Am Coll Surg 2001; 192:25–37.

71. Sasako M. Principles of surgical treatment for curable gastric cancer. J Clin Oncol 2003; 21:274s–5s.

72. Peeters KC, van de Velde CJ. Improving treatment outcome for gastric cancer: the role of surgery and adjuvant therapy. J Clin Oncol 2003; 21: 272s–3s.

73. Wu CW, Hsieh MC, Lo SS et al. Results of curative gastrectomy for carcinoma of the distal third of the stomach. J Am Coll Surg 1996; 183:201–7.

74. McCulloch P, Nita ME, Kazi H et al. Gastrectomy with extended lymphadenectomy for primary treatment of gastric cancer. Br J Surg 2005; 92:5–13.

A comprehensive meta-analysis of available data on the merits of D2 lymphadenectomy.

75. Parikh D, Johnson M, Chagla L et al. D2 gastrectomy: lessons from a prospective audit of the learning curve. Br J Surg 1996; 83:1595–9.

76. Kampschoer GH, Maruyama K, van de Velde CJ et al. Computer analysis in making preoperative decisions: a rational approach to lymph node dissection in gastric cancer patients. Br J Surg 1989; 76:905–8.

77. Otsuji E, Yamaguchi T, Sawai K et al. Total gastrectomy with simultaneous pancreaticosplenectomy or splenectomy in patients with advanced gastric carcinoma. Br J Cancer 1999; 79:1789–93.

78. Griffith JP, Sue-Ling HM, Martin I et al. Preservation of the spleen improves survival after radical surgery for gastric cancer. Gut 1995; 36:684–90.

79. Fujita T, Matai K, Kohno S et al. Impact of splenectomy on circulating immunoglobulin levels and the development of postoperative infection following total gastrectomy for gastric cancer. Br J Surg 1996; 83:1776–8.

80. Wanebo HJ, Kennedy BJ, Winchester DP et al. Role of splenectomy in gastric cancer surgery: adverse effect of elective splenectomy on long-term survival. J Am Coll Surg 1997; 185:177–84.

81. Kikuchi S, Nemoto Y, Natsuya K et al. Which patients with advanced, proximal gastric cancer benefit from complete clearance of spleno-pancreatic lymph nodes. Anticancer Res 2002; 22:3513–17.

82. Schmid A, Thybusch A, Kremer B et al. Differential effects of radical D2-lymphadenectomy and splenectomy in surgically treated gastric cancer patients. Hepatogastroenterology 2000; 47:579–85.

83. Monig SP, Collet PH, Baldus SE et al. Splenectomy in proximal gastric cancer: frequency of lymph node metastasis to the splenic hilus. J Surg Oncol 2001; 76:89–92.

84. Chikara K, Hiroshi S, Masato N et al. Indications for pancreaticosplenectomy in advanced gastric cancer. Hepatogastroenterology 2001; 48:908–12.

85. Sugimachi K, Kodama Y, Kumashiro R et al. Critical evaluation of prophylactic splenectomy in total gastrectomy for the stomach cancer. Gann 1980; 71:704–9.

86. Kitamura K, Nishida S, Ichikawa D et al. No survival benefit from combined pancreaticosplenectomy and total gastrectomy for gastric cancer. Br J Surg 1999; 86:119–22.

87. Piso P, Bellin T, Aselmann H et al. Results of combined gastrectomy and pancreatic resection in patients with advanced primary gastric carcinoma. Dig Surg 2002; 19:281–5.

88. Maehara Y, Oiwa H, Tomisaki S et al. Prognosis and surgical treatment of gastric cancer invading the pancreas. Oncology 2000; 59:1–6.

89. Kodera Y, Yamamura Y, Sasako M et al. Lack of benefit of combined pancreaticosplenectomy in D2 resection for proximal-third gastric carcinoma. World J Surg 1997; 21:622–7.

90. Maruyama K, Sasako M, Kinoshita T et al. Pancreas-preserving total gastrectomy for proximal gastric cancer. World J Surg 1995; 19:532–6.

91. Furukawa H, Hiratsuka M, Ishikawa O et al. Total gastrectomy with dissection of lymph nodes along the splenic artery: a pancreas-preserving method. Ann Surg Oncol 2000; 7:669–73.

92. Doglietto GB, Pacelli F, Caprino P et al. Pancreas-preserving total gastrectomy for gastric cancer. Arch Surg 2000; 135:89–94.

93. Kodama I, Takamiya H, Mizutani K et al. Gastrectomy with combined resection of other organs for carcinoma of the stomach with invasion to adjacent organs: clinical efficacy in a retrospective study. J Am Coll Surg 1997; 184:16–22.

94. Martin RC, Jaques DP, Brennan MF et al. Extended local resection for advanced gastric cancer: increased survival versus increased morbidity. Ann Surg 2002; 236:159–65.

95. Kockerling F, Reck T, Gall FP. Extended gastrectomy: who benefits. World J Surg 1995; 19:541–5.

96. Shchepotin IB, Chorny VA, Nauta RJ et al. Extended surgical resection in T4 gastric cancer. Am J Surg 1998; 175:123–6.

97. Sasako M, Sano T, Yamamoto S et al. D2 lymphadenectomy alone or with para-aortic nodal dissection for gastric cancer. N Engl J Med 2008; 139:453–62.

A multicentre RCT of D2 vs. D4 lymphadenectomy.

98. Yonemura Y, Wu CC, Fukushima N et al. Randomized clinical trial of D2 and extended paraaortic lymphadenectomy in patients with gastric cancer. Int J Clin Oncol 2008; 13:132–7.

A multicentre RCT of D2 vs. D4 lymphadenectomy.

99. Kulig J, Popiela T, Kolodziejczyk P et al. Standard D2 versus extended D2 (D2+) lymphadenectomy for gastric cancer: an interim safety analysis of a multicenter, randomized, clinical trial. Am J Surg 2007; 193:10–15.

A multicentre RCT of D2 vs. D3 lymphadenectomy in Polish patients.

100. Wu CW, Hsiung CA, Lo SS et al. Nodal dissection for patients with gastric cancer: a randomized controlled trial. Lancet Oncol 2006; 7:309–15.

101. Doglietto GB, Pacelli F, Caprino P et al. Palliative surgery for far-advanced gastric cancer: a retrospective study on 305 consecutive patients. Am Surg 1999; 65:352–5.

102. Koga R, Yanamoto J, Ohyama S et al. Liver resection for metastatic gastric cancer: experience with 42 patients including eight long-term survivors. Jpn J Clin Oncol 2007; 37:836–42.

103. Okano K, Maeba T, Ishimura K et al. Hepatic resection for metastatic tumors from gastric cancer. Ann Surg 2002; 235:86–91.

104. Sakamoto Y, Ohyama S, Yamamoto J et al. Surgical resection of liver metastases of gastric cancer: an analysis of a 17–year experience with 22 patients. Surgery 2003; 133:507–11.

105. Ambiru S, Miyazaki N, Ito H et al. Benefits and limits of hepatic resection for gastric metastases. Am J Surg 2001; 181:279–83.

106. Kunisaki C, Akiyama H, Nomura M et al. Comparison of surgical outcomes of gastric cancer in elderly and middle-aged patients. Am J Surg 2006; 191:216–24.

107. Tsujitani S, Katano K, Oka A et al. Limited operation for gastric cancer in the elderly. Br J Surg 1996; 83:836–9.

108. Bittner R, Butters M, Ulrich M et al. Total gastrectomy. Updated operative mortality and long-term survival with particular reference to patients older than 70 years of age. Ann Surg 1996; 224: 37–42.

109. Sasako M, Kinoshita T, Maruyama K. Prognosis of early gastric cancer. Stomach Intestine 1993; 28:139–46.

110. McCulloch P. Description of the Japanese method of radical gastrectomy. Ann R Coll Surg Engl 1994; 76:110–14.

111. Sasako M, Sano T, Yamamoto Y et al. Left thoraco-abdominal versus abdominal-transhiatal approach for gastric cancer of the cardia or subcardia: a randomized trial. Lancet Oncol 2006; 8: 644–51.

A multicentre Japanese RCT that ceased at interim analysis.

112. Tanimura S, Higashino M, Fukunaga Y et al. Laparoscopic gastrectomy with regional lymph node dissection for upper gastric cancer. Br J Surg 2007; 94:204–7.

113. Huscher CG, Mingoli A, Sgarzini G et al. Laparoscopic versus open subtotal gastrectomy for distal gastric cancer: five-year results of a randomized prospective trial. Ann Surg 2005; 241:232–7.

An RCT with adequate follow-up but numbers too small to reach a statistically sound conclusion.

114. Memon MA, Khan S, Yunus RM et al. Meta-analysis of laparoscopic and open distal gastrectomy for gastric carcinoma. Surg Endosc 2008; 22:1781–9.

115. Yu W, Seo BY, Chung HY. Postoperative body-weight loss and survival after curative resection for gastric cancer. Br J Surg 2002; 89:467–70.

116. Nunobe S, Okaro A, Sasako M et al. Billroth 1 versus Roux-en-Y reconstruction: a quality-of-life survey at 5 years. Int J Clin Oncol 2007; 12:433–9.

117. Kojima K, Yamada H, Inokuchi M et al. A comparison of Roux-en-Y and Billroth-1 reconstruction after laparoscopic-assisted distal gastrectomy. Ann Surg 2008; 247:962–7.

118. Buhl K, Lehnert T, Schlag P et al. Reconstruction after gastrectomy and quality of life. World J Surg 1995; 19:558–64.

119. Nakane Y, Okumura S, Akehira K et al. Jejunal pouch reconstruction after total gastrectomy for cancer. A randomized controlled trial. Ann Surg 1995; 222:27–35.

120. Lehnert T, Buhl K. Techniques of reconstruction after total gastrectomy for cancer. Br J Surg 2004; 91:528–39.

A comprehensive review of all the studies of pouch reconstruction.

121. Liedman B et al. Food intake after gastrectomy for gastric carcinoma: the role of a gastric reservoir. Br J Surg 1996; 83:1138–43.

122. Liedman B, Andersson H, Bosaeus I et al. Changes in body composition after gastrectomy: results of a controlled, prospective clinical trial. World J Surg 1997; 21:416–20.

123. Bradley ELIII, Isaacs J, Hersh T et al. Nutritional consequences of total gastrectomy. Ann Surg 1975; 182:415–29.

124. Braga M, Zuliani W, Foppa L et al. Food intake and nutritional status after total gastrectomy: results of a nutritional follow-up. Br J Surg 1988; 75:477–80.

125. Rino Y, Susuki Y, Kuroiwa Y et al. Vitamin E malabsorption and neurological consequences after gastrectomy for gastric cancer. Hepatogastroenterology 2007; 54:1858–61.

126. Rino Y, Takanashi Y, Yamamoto Y et al. Bone disorder and vitamin D after gastric cancer surgery. Hepatogastroenterology 2007; 54:1596–600.

127. Glatzle J, Piert M, Meile T et al. Prevalence of vertebral alterations and the effects of calcium and vitamin D supplementation on calcium metabolism and bone mineral density after gastrectomy. Br J Surg 2005; 92:579–85.

128. Maehara Y, Emi Y, Baba H et al. Recurrences and related characteristics of gastric cancer. Br J Cancer 1996; 74:975–9.

129. Kodera Y, Ito S, Yamamura Y et al. Follow-up surveillance for recurrence after curative gastric cancer surgery lacks survival benefit. Ann Surg Oncol 2003; 10:898–902.

130. Bohner H, Zimmer T, Hopfenmuller W et al. Detection and prognosis of recurrent gastric cancer – is routine follow-up after gastrectomy worthwhile? Hepatogastroenterology 2000; 47:1489–94.

131. Whiting J, Sano T, Saka M et al. Follow-up of gastric cancer: a review. Gastric Cancer 2006; 9:74–81.

132. Allum WH, Griffin SM, Watson A et al. Guidelines for the management of oesophageal and gastric cancer. Gut 2002; 50(Suppl 5):v1–23.

8

Endoscopic and surgical treatment of early gastric cancer

Geoffrey W.B. Clark

Early gastric cancer

Definition

Early gastric cancer (EGC) is defined as a tumour that is limited to the mucosa or submucosa of the gastric wall independent of the presence of lymph node metastases.[1] EGC is a curable condition with more than 90% of patients surviving 5 years after treatment. Fifty years ago less than 20% of patients with stomach cancer who presented to the National Cancer Centre in Tokyo, Japan had early-stage disease. However, as a consequence of the widespread use of screening programmes currently over 60% of all gastric cancers in Japan are diagnosed as EGC.[2] The high frequency of EGC is one of the main reasons why the overall 5-year survival rates for stomach cancer approach 70% in Japanese patients. In Europe and the USA the incidence of EGC is much lower at around 10% (range 5–20%) and overall 5-year survival rates are less than half those observed in Asia. EGC occurs at a mean age of 58 in Japanese patients and 60 years in Western patients. There is a male predominance of 2:1.[3]

Symptoms of early gastric cancer

In Japan over 50% of patients with EGC are asymptomatic, the lesion being identified during surveillance. In the remaining Japanese patients the commonest presentation is with vague epigastric discomfort while classical ulcer-type epigastric pain affects <20%. Weight loss is present in <5% of patients. In contrast epigastric pain and dyspepsia affect 60–90% of European patients who are diagnosed with EGC and weight loss affects up to 40%.

Risk factors

The risk factors for EGC are similar to those for the more advanced stage of the disease. *Helicobacter pylori* is considered to be the predominant risk factor worldwide and has been listed as a class 1 carcinogen by the World Health Organisation.[4] More than 50% of the world's population have the infection but the lifetime risk of developing gastric cancer is less than 2%. *Helicobacter pylori* induces two patterns of gastritis. Antral predominant non-atrophic gastritis is associated with normal or high gastric acid secretion and duodenal ulcer disease but rarely gastric cancer. Atrophic pan gastritis is associated with reduced levels of gastric acid secretion and is associated with the development of gastric cancer.[5] It is possible to detect atrophic pan gastritis serologically as these patients have low concentrations of pepsinogen I and low pepsinogen I:II ratios. Watabe et al. followed up 6983 patients enrolled in a gastric screening programme in Japan.[6] Patients had serological testing for *H. pylori* and pepsinogen on enrolment with the programme. Patients who did not have atrophic gastritis had a very low risk of developing gastric cancer, 0.04% per annum if *H. pylori* negative and 0.06% if *H. pylori* positive. Patients with atrophic gastritis were at significantly increased risk of developing gastric cancer, 0.35% annual incidence if positive for *H. pylori* and 0.6% annual risk if negative for *H. pylori*.

Patients with autoimmune atrophic gastritis associated with pernicious anaemia are at increased risk of intestinal pattern EGC. Patients who have undergone previous gastric resection are at risk of developing gastric stump carcinoma that affects

2.4% of patients after 5 years and 6.1% after 10 years.[7] Western authors have indicated that endoscopic surveillance was not effective in reducing cancer-related deaths in this patient population.[8] Ohashi et al. reviewed 108 Japanese patients who had cancer of the gastric stump at a mean of 7.5 years after undergoing a distal gastrectomy for cancer.[9] They stressed the importance of endoscopic surveillance because 67/108 (62%) were diagnosed with EGC, in whom the 5-year survival rate was 76%. Further, patients who were diagnosed with advanced gastric stump cancer had a very poor outcome (10% 5-year survival) even when resection was undertaken.

Recent interest has focused on identifying patients who are genetically predisposed to develop gastric cancer. Germ-line mutations of the E-cadherin (CDH1) gene are associated with the development of diffuse-type gastric cancer that is transmitted in an autosomal dominant manner. Huntsmand et al. first reported the outcome of prophylactic total gastrectomy in patients with hereditary diffuse-type gastric cancer carrying the CDH1 gene mutation.[10] Multiple foci of poorly differentiated EGC were found in the gastrectomy specimens of four out of five young asymptomatic family members who underwent pre-emptive surgery. Similar results were reported by other groups, with all 11 patients treated with prophylactic total gastrectomy having foci of intramucosal adenocarcinoma in their gastrectomy specimens.[11,12] Newman and Mullholland[13] did not identify any cancer in two patients who underwent prophylactic total gastrectomy for CDH1 mutations, but Lewis et al.[14] reported that they had needed to perform between 150 and 250 tissue blocks from their prophylactic gastrectomy patient specimens before identifying foci of invasive intramucosal cancer.

Macroscopic appearance

Fifty percent of EGCs are located in the gastric antrum, 40% arise in the gastric body and 10% arise in the proximal stomach. Between 5% and 10% are multifocal in origin. The term EGC does not bear any relationship to the size of the lesion. Most EGCs are 1–3 cm in size but giant EGCs of 10 cm or more in diameter have been described. Endoscopic detection of EGC requires careful scrutiny of the whole gastric mucosa using sufficient distension with air to flatten the gastric rugal folds. Gastric peristalsis can be interrupted by intravenous administration of buscopan or glucagon. Subtle features of EGC include either increased or decreased colour differences compared to the normal gastric mucosa, a propensity for lesions to haemorrhage, friability and reduced vascularity. The detection

of EGC can be facilitated by vital dye spraying of suspicious lesions using 10 mL of indigo carmine dye mixed with 20 mL of normal saline and 10 mL of air. Application of the dye provides contrast that allows easier identification of the endoscopic abnormality and an improved ability to accurately locate the margins of the lesion.

EGCs are classified by their endoscopic appearance according to Murakami (**Fig. 8.1**).[1] Type I cancers are elevated from the surrounding mucosa. Type II cancers are of the flat variety and are subgrouped as: IIa, slightly elevated; IIb, absolutely flat; IIc, slightly depressed. Type III cancers are ulcerated or excavated. Type III cancers make up 65–75% of all EGCs, 20% are type I and 5–10% are type II. Morphologically, many lesions are a combination of the above and are described with the predominant appearance first, for example IIa and III.

Microscopic appearance

EGC is classified as being of the intestinal type or diffuse type according to Lauren.[15] EGCs are all stage T1 but the lesions are subdivided into mucosal cancers and submucosal cancers dependent upon whether the tumour has invaded beyond the muscularis mucosa. This histological distinction is important, as the prevalence of lymphatic spread is five- to sixfold higher in submucosal lesions.

There is considerable controversy between Japanese and Western pathologists regarding the diagnosis of mucosal-type EGC.[16,17] The high incidence of EGC reported in Japan has been criticised by some in the West as being attributable to over-

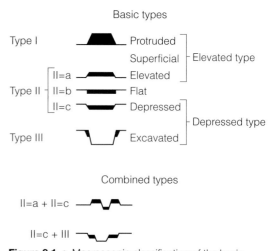

Figure 8.1 • Macroscopic classification of the basic types of EGC according to Murakami. Representative examples of common combined types are shown.

diagnosis of dysplastic lesions as invasive cancer. Western pathologists require definite invasion of solitary malignant cells into the lamina propria before they consider that the basement membrane has been breached and invasive cancer can be diagnosed. In the absence of this evidence, the lesion is termed severe dysplasia. In Japan, nuclear factors (enlargement, pleomorphism, prominent nucleoli and loss of polarity) and glandular architectural abnormalities (complex budding, branching and back-to-back glands) are sufficient for establishing the diagnosis of cancer. Two factors suggest that the Western approach may be too restrictive. Firstly it is recognised that invasive tumours may produce their own basement membrane and secondly there is a high incidence of invasive carcinoma when patients who are diagnosed as having severe dysplasia by Western criteria undergo resection of the affected organ. In order to resolve these difficulties two classification systems of gastrointestinal epithelial neoplasia have emerged from consensus conferences, the Padova classification[18] and the Vienna classification.[19] It is the latter system that has been more universally adopted (Box 8.1). This new classification system facilitates improved agreement between Western and Japanese pathologists.

Growth patterns of early gastric cancer

EGC grows in two directions, horizontally within the mucosa and vertically into the deeper layers.

The superficially spreading tumours are termed SUPER, whereas the vertically spreading tumours are termed PEN (penetrating). Kodama et al.[20] have classified EGCs according to the growth pattern by combining both macroscopic appearance and histological features. This classification groups EGCs into three categories:

1. SUPER type >4 cm. This includes mucosal tumours and those that invade just beyond the muscularis mucosa.
2. Small mucosal cancers <4 cm or small submucosal tumours <4 cm that have invaded just beyond the muscularis mucosa.
3. PEN type <4 cm that penetrate deeply into the submucosa. The PEN A subtype completely destroys the submucosa whereas the PEN B subtype infiltrates the submucosa by fenestration of the muscularis mucosa. The classification is helpful in predicting the natural history, with the PEN A subtype carrying the poorest prognosis.

Lymphatic spread

Nodal metastases occur in 3% (range 0.7–21%) of mucosal tumours and in 20% (range 10.6–64%) of submucosal tumours.[21-27] The depth of submucosal invasion can be divided into SM1, SM2 and SM3 for tumours involving the upper, middle and lower thirds of the submucosal layer. Lymph node metastasis occurs in 10% of SM1 tumours, 19% of SM2 and 33% of SM3 lesions.[28] SM1 tumours are subdivided into SM1a, <200 μm from the muscularis mucosa, which have a 5% risk of nodal metastasis and SM1b, >200 μm from the muscularis mucosa, with a 15% risk of nodal metastasis.

There are a number of macroscopic and microscopic characteristics of EGCs that may predict the presence of lymph node metastasis, as shown in Table 8.1.[21-26,29,30] The size of the tumour is predictive of the presence of nodal metastasis. Tumours <2 cm in size have a low incidence of metastasis of 1–3%. Depressed and ulcerated tumours (type IIc and III lesions) have a two- to threefold higher rate of nodal metastasis compared to elevated or flat tumours (types I, IIa and IIb). Histologically, the presence of ulceration or permeation of the mucosal or submucosal lymphatics are significant risk factors for nodal metastasis. By combining the known risk factors it has been demonstrated that mucosal tumours <3 cm in size, with no ulceration and no histological lymphatic permeation, have only a 0.36% chance of nodal metastasis.[29]

Table 8.1 • Characteristics of early gastric cancers that are associated with statistically increased risk of lymph node metastases by multivariate analysis

Macroscopic			Microscopic
Size	<2 cm	2.5% positive nodes	Submucosal invasion[21–26]
	2–4.9 cm	9.7% positive nodes	
	>5 cm	21.7% positive nodes	
			Lymphatic permeation[29]
Multifocal disease[22]			Undifferentiated/signet cell type[22] *
Murakami types: IIc and III[22–25]			Abnormal staining for E-cadherin
Kodama type: PEN A[24]			and β-catenin[30]

* This is controversial as some papers report a higher incidence of node metastasis in the well-differentiated type.

Most nodal metastases from EGC are perigastric, located within the first tier of nodes. Metastasis to the second tier of lymph nodes from mucosal EGC is rare, accounting for <1% of all patients. Yamao et al. reported 1196 Japanese patients with EGC limited to the mucosa who underwent D2 gastrectomy.[29] Only 7/1196 (0.6%) had nodal metastasis in the level 2 nodes. In EGC with submucosal involvement 2.3–8.9% of metastases reach the second tier of nodes, which are removed during a D2 resection. Further, skip metastases have been demonstrated that would have been missed if a D1 resection were undertaken. Arai et al.[31] showed that 138 (10%) of 1381 patients who underwent D2 gastrectomy for EGC had nodal metastases. Fifty-four patients (4%) had one solitary node involved but in nine patients (0.65%) the solitary nodal metastasis was in the level 2 nodes.

Natural history of early gastric cancer

It has been proposed that EGC is a pseudo-tumour with little potential for malignant invasion. Tsukuma et al. showed that the 5-year survival rate for patients with untreated EGC was 63%.[32] The majority (36/56, 70%) of EGC progressed to advanced gastric cancer after a median of 44 months. Progression to the advanced form was inevitably fatal. In patients with EGC who underwent delayed surgical resection there was a better 5-year survival rate of 78% compared to the untreated patients. Thus EGC has a long natural history but in general it progresses to the advanced stage with time and results in death from gastric cancer if left untreated. Bando et al. have reported that age and sex are important indicators of outcome in EGC.[33] Ten-year survival in EGC patients over 80 years of age was only 30%, with most patients dying from causes unrelated to their cancer. The trend was strongest for Japanese men whose life expectancy was almost 5 years less than for Japanese women.

Staging of patients with suspected early gastric cancer

Contrast-enhanced abdominal computed tomography (CT) imaging excludes liver metastases but does not provide useful imaging of the primary tumour. Endoscopic ultrasound (EUS) using the standard radial scanning probe at 7.5 MHz frequency has a 90% accuracy in T staging gastric cancer but higher scanning frequencies (12 or 20 MHz) are required to differentiate between mucosal and submucosal lesions.

 EUS has an accuracy of 70% in differentiating T1 lesions. It tends to overstage mucosal as submucosal lesions, possibly due to submucosal fibrosis and ulceration.[34]

It is not possible to rely on EUS to predict N0 tumours because >50% of nodal metastases from EGC are <5 mm in size.[31] Conversely when EUS identifies round, hypoechoic nodes >1 cm in size the positive predictive value is >85%, which would preclude local therapy. Laparoscopy is unnecessary when the abdominal CT is normal and EUS demonstrates a T1 lesion.

Treatment of early gastric cancer

In Japan the gold standard treatment for EGC has been surgical resection in the form of a D2 gastrectomy. This strategy was associated with high cure rates of >90% but with significant morbidity and a small risk of mortality. However, with the huge experience that has come out of Japanese centres, it is now recognised that the majority of EGCs do not have nodal metastasis. Consequently, the treatment of EGC has now shifted from a policy of uniform radical surgery to a more sophisticated stage-oriented or tailored therapy applied to individual cases.

The treatment options include endoscopic mucosal resection (EMR), endoscopic submucosal dissection (ESD), the destructive therapies of phototherapy or argon-beam ablation, or surgery, which can be performed open but is now increasingly performed with laparoscopic assistance. Endoscopic treatment of EGC is attractive since it is non-invasive, associated with a short period of hospitalisation and less expensive than surgical resection.

Local therapies are only suitable for mucosal tumours. This raises the question as to how accurately the depth of invasion can be diagnosed prior to instituting treatment. Standard endoscopy can measure the size of the tumour using the open biopsy technique and the morphology of these lesions can be accurately described (Murakami clas-sification). Elevated tumours, <2 cm in diameter and free of ulceration, are usually mucosal whereas ulcerated tumours usually invade the submucosa; however, there is a significant degree of overlap in the distinction that makes clinical decision-making unreliable.[35] Overall the accuracy of diagnosing sub-mucosal invasion in non-ulcerated cancers is 55% by endoscopy, 58% by barium meal and 85% by EUS.[36] Therefore, histological examination of the entire tumour is the only reliable way of differenti-ating mucosal from submucosal invasion in EGC.

Endoscopic mucosal resection

The strip technique of EMR was described by Tada et al.[37] and is shown in **Fig. 8.2**. EMR is performed

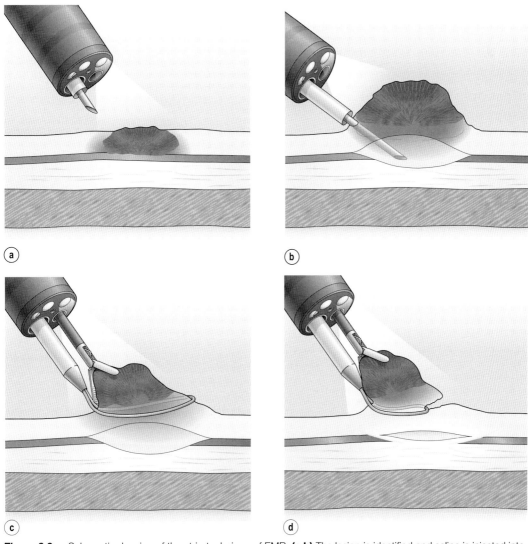

(a)

(b)

(c)

(d)

Figure 8.2 • Schematic drawing of the strip technique of EMR. **(a,b)** The lesion is identified and saline is injected into the submucosal plane to elevate the tumour. **(c)** The snare is placed around the lesion, which is elevated by use of the grasping forceps. **(d)** The snare is tightened around the base producing a polyp that is removed with diathermy.

under i.v. sedation and may be facilitated by injection of 20 mg of buscopan. Using a dual-channel endoscope the margins of the tumour are defined with 0.1% indigo carmine dye and the resection margin is marked with a diathermy needle knife. An endoscopic needle is used to inject 3–5 mL of physiological saline into the submucosal layer, allowing the lesion to be elevated, providing a clear plane for the resection. Difficulty lifting the lesion may indicate submucosal invasion. Ulcerated tumours do not lift up easily as a result of submucosal fibrosis and are therefore unsuitable for EMR. Grasping forceps are passed through the loop of the endoscopic snare. The grasping forceps are used to retract the elevated lesion and the diathermy snare is placed around the base of the specimen, allowing it to be removed following application of the coagulating current. The specimen is retrieved via the endoscope and pinned out on a cork board for histological analysis. EMR can be technically difficult for proximal and high posterior tumours, particularly if it is necessary to retroflex the scope to gain exposure.

Endoscopic submucosal dissection

Many Japanese centres routinely resect EGCs with an insulated tipped electrosurgical knife. At the tip is a Teflon-coated ball that helps limit the depth of cut to the plane underneath the submucosa, leaving the underlying muscle layer intact. Initially the edges of the resection are marked with a diathermy knife. Submucosal injection of 1:10 000 adrenaline solution is used to elevate the lesion. Initial cuts are made with the diathermy knife but then the continued dissection of the lesion is carried out with elevation via grasping forceps and careful dissection with the tipped knife under direct vision to remain in the correct plane. The technique is preferred for lesions >15 mm in diameter as this facilitates the removal of the specimen in one piece 'en bloc', allowing for more accurate pathological assessment and determination of the depth of invasion of the tumour. Box 8.2 shows the essential

Box 8.2 • Pathological reporting requirements in assessment of lesions resected by EMR/ESD

Depth of invasion
Degree of differentiation
Lymphatic permeation
Vascular invasion
Clear margin of resection

Box 8.3 • Microscopic and histological characteristics of tumours that are suitable for treatment by EMR or ESD

Elevated or flat lesions <2 cm size
Depressed lesions <1 cm without ulceration
Mucosal invasion
Well differentiated
No lymphatic permeation

pathological reporting requirements for lesions removed by EMR or ESD.

The absolute indications for EMR and ESD are shown in Box 8.3. Larger tumours can be resected in patients who are unfit for surgical therapy; this is classed as a relative indication.[38] Ono et al. have extended the absolute indications to include tumours up to 3 cm in size.[39] As the indications for EMR/ESD are broadened and larger lesions are resected, the chances of obtaining tumour-free margins are reduced and the risk of complications increase.[40] Fifteen percent of tumours resected by EMR/ESD are found to have submucosal invasion following histological analysis.[39] These tumours carry a significant risk of lymph node metastasis that requires subsequent surgical therapy. EMR can achieve clear lateral resection margins in 84% of mucosal tumours <2 cm in size and 69% of those <3 cm in size.[39,41] Provided there is no histological lymphatic permeation treatment can be regarded as curative and only regular endoscopic follow-up is required. Local recurrence rates are 2%. Thirty percent of mucosal tumours resected by EMR have a positive lateral margin. The favoured option for treatment in the presence of a positive lateral margin is by re-endoscopy with ablative therapy by either laser or argon beam. Under these circumstances ablative therapy is associated with good long-term results but the local recurrence rates are higher at around 10%. Surgical therapy or a further EMR are also appropriate options to treat mucosal EGC with lateral margin involvement according to physician or patient preference. Ono et al.,[39] from the National Cancer Centre in Tokyo, have demonstrated that EMR is an appropriate therapeutic strategy for mucosal EGC. They treated 445 patients over an 11-year period with a median follow-up of 38 months and there were no cancer-related deaths.

Complications following EMR/ESD are uncommon. Bleeding occurs in 5% and can usually be controlled by endoscopic haemostatic techniques. Perforation is a serious risk and occurs in 5%. When the expertise is available this can be treated endoscopically by the application of endoscopic clips, otherwise urgent surgical therapy is required.

Ablative techniques for the treatment of mucosal-type early cancer

 Because histological assessment is the only reliable method to accurately measure the depth of invasion of EGC, the use of ablative therapies that destroy the primary tumour must be viewed with caution.

These techniques have been employed in a few centres with good results but they are unlikely to gain widespread acceptance because of the risk of missing a curable submucosal tumour with local nodal involvement. Their place is in the treatment of tumours that are not easily accessible to EMR in patients unfit for surgical resection. Ablative techniques are useful to treat the residual margins of mucosal tumours that have a positive lateral margin after EMR.

Sagawa et al. reported 27 patients with 'intramucosal' EGC who were treated with argon plasma coagulation.[42] Ninety-six percent of the patients were rendered tumour free during a median follow-up of 30 months and no complications were reported. No long-term follow-up is available. Treatment with Nd:YAG laser[43] and photodynamic therapy[44] is unlikely to confer any additional advantage over argon-beam therapy, in view of the significant costs and the risks of photosensitivity for the latter technique.

Traditional open surgical therapy

EGC located in the gastric antrum is treated by subtotal gastrectomy. A subtotal gastrectomy is suitable treatment for intestinal-type EGC located in the mid-gastric body provided a 2-cm clear proximal margin is obtained. For diffuse-type EGC located in the mid-gastric body and proximal EGC a total gastrectomy is undertaken.

The extent of lymph node dissection is considered D1 when the first tier (group I) nodes are removed and D2 when the second tier (group II) nodes are removed. In Japanese centres D2 gastrectomy has been standard practice to treat EGC since the 1960s, although there are no randomised trials to support this strategy. The results of radical surgery have been excellent, with 5-year survival figures regularly reported as high as 90–95%.[45,46] There is controversy over the benefits of D2 lymphadenectomy for EGC and in most Japanese centres there has been a move away from radical surgery to a more tailored approach. This is important because of three factors: (i) the low prevalence of nodal metastasis in

EGC; (ii) the good long-term survival rates following EMR; and (iii) the risks of reduced quality of life after radical surgery in patients with the potential for long-term survival.

The results of the large randomised MRC and Dutch trials comparing D1 and D2 gastrectomy both showed no survival benefit for D2 resection of EGC compared to the D1 resection.[47,48] The 5-year survival rates for T1 gastric cancer were 77% for D2 in the Dutch study. In the Dutch study the survival rate for node-negative EGC was 81% for patients undergoing D1 resection and 81% in those undergoing D2 resection. These data indicate that the role of D2 gastrectomy in the treatment of EGC is unproven and that in node-negative tumours the operation is unlikely to confer any surgical advantage.

 These two studies were large, randomised, prospective trials of D1 vs. D2 gastrectomy. Both studies demonstrated similar results, with neither showing a survival advantage for the D2 resection. The morbidity and mortality was significantly higher following the D2 resection, which was largely attributable to performing a splenectomy and distal pancreatectomy. These extended resections are not indicated when operating for EGC.[47,48]

Baba et al. reported that D2 gastrectomy conferred a survival advantage at 5 and 10 years over the D1 resection for the treatment of EGC.[49] The 5-year survival figures were D2 95.4% and D1 81.1%, with a higher recurrence rate in the D1-treated group. The survival advantage was evident for both mucosal and submucosal tumours. In contrast, Tsujitani et al. reported no survival advantage when D2 resection was used to treat patients with mucosal disease.[50] They showed that for patients with submucosal cancer the 10-year survival rate was 78.3% following D2 resection and 56.8% following the D1 procedure. The improved survival was not related to tumour recurrence but rather to the fact that patients who received the D1 resection were older and died from other causes. Otsuji et al. reported that D2 gastrectomy was associated with a significant survival advantage in the treatment of EGC located in the antrum.[51] The outcomes following D1 and D2 dissections were comparable for proximal or middle-third EGCs.

 Given the conflicting reports a practical approach has to be adopted. EGCs that are estimated to be mucosal by endoscopy and EUS should be resected by EMR provided they are well differentiated, <2 cm in size and not ulcerated. Gastrectomy is indicated for the treatment of

patients with EGC that do not meet the criteria for EMR and for tumours that are removed by EMR and are subsequently found to have submucosal invasion (**Fig. 8.3**). For healthy patients a D2 resection is preferred. Since there is no indication for splenectomy, distal pancreatectomy or an omental bursectomy, the risk of mortality and morbidity should be very low. Because the risk of metastasis to the second tier of nodes is relatively low a D1 resection is a reasonable option for patients with significant cardiovascular or respiratory disease.

A number of less radical surgical techniques have been described to treat EGC. These include the open limited gastric resections (proximal gastrectomy, segmental gastrectomy and pylorus-preserving distal gastrectomy) and laparoscopic procedures (local resections, laparoscopic distal gastrectomy and laparoscopic lymphadenectomy). A number of Japanese centres have used sentinel node technology to guide the extent of surgical therapy in the treatment of EGC with varying degrees of success.

Proximal gastrectomy with jejunal interposition

Standard treatment of proximal gastric cancer is by total gastrectomy with D2 lymphadenectomy. In patients with EGC in the proximal stomach that is not suitable for EMR this procedure is usually curative but it is associated with significant long-term morbidity with significant weight loss, often >20% of initial body weight, reflux oesophagitis, dumping

and nutritional failure. It is recognised that nodal metastasis in the distal gastric nodes (groups 5 and 6) from EGC in the proximal stomach is extremely rare, which supports retaining the distal stomach in these patients. However, proximal gastrectomy with primary oesophagogastric anastomosis has been abandoned because of the resulting intractable symptoms of reflux oesophagitis and bilious vomiting. Katai et al. have reported excellent results with proximal gastrectomy with a short isoperistaltic jejunal limb reconstruction.[52] The procedure involves removal of the upper half of the stomach, along with nodes in groups 1, 2, 3, 4s, 7, 8a, 9 and 11p. The spleen is preserved and with experience the hepatic and pyloric branches of the vagus nerves can be preserved. Reconstruction is with a 10–20 cm segment of proximal jejunum, stapled to the oesophagus with a circular stapler and with a hand-sewn jejunogastric anastomosis.[52,53] Katai et al. undertook this procedure in 45 patients with no mortality and minimal morbidity. Long-term survival was not compromised and postgastrectomy symptoms were minimised.[52]

Segmental gastrectomy

For EGC involving the mid portion of the stomach, or even those in the upper stomach >2 cm distal to the gastro-oesophageal junction, segmental resection with lymphadenectomy followed by a two-layered, hand-sewn, end-to-end gastro-gastric anastomosis has been reported.[54,55] The technique involves removal of the tumour and mid portion of the stomach as far proximally as 2 cm below the gastro-oesophageal junction. Lymphadenectomy

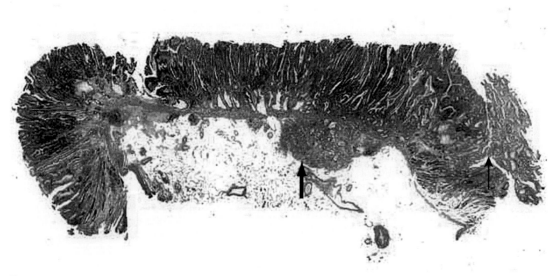

Figure 8.3 • Histological section of endoscopic mucosa resection of an EGC. The lateral margins are clear of tumour (small arrow) but there is submucosal invasion (large arrow).

includes the group 1, 2, 3 and 4s nodes, along with group 7, 8a, 9 and 11p nodes above the pancreas. The hepatic and pyloric branches of the vagus are preserved along with the coeliac branches of the posterior vagus, by dividing the left gastric artery >1 cm above its origin. The technique is easy to perform and is associated with a shorter operating time than for proximal gastrectomy with jejunal interposition. Lymph node harvest is reported to be high, well above 30 nodes, and the frequency of post-gastrectomy symptoms is low.[55]

Pylorus-preserving gastrectomy

The operation of pylorus-preserving gastrectomy (PPG) is similar to standard distal gastrectomy except that the distal transection is made 1.5 cm proximal to the pylorus rather than 1 cm distal to the pylorus as in the standard procedure. The hepatic and pyloric branches of the vagus are preserved, as are the suprapyloric nodes (group 5). The operation is indicated for EGC located in the mid-body or antrum with a distal tumour margin that is >4 cm proximal to the pylorus. By retaining the pyloric sphincter there is a reduced incidence of postoperative dumping and gastric protection against bile reflux. Nishikawa et al. showed that following PPG pyloric function was maintained, allowing control over the gastric emptying of solids with better long-term functional results compared to standard D2 distal gastrectomy.[56]

Laparoscopic local resections

This approach is recommended for the treatment of mucosal-type EGC as an alternative to EMR. As no lymph node dissection is performed the selection criteria are theoretically the same as for EMR. Two techniques are described:

1. The transperitoneal approach is used to resect tumours located on the anterior aspect of the stomach or on the lesser or greater curvatures. The lesion is located endoscopically and marked by the injection of carbon dye, making it visible from the outside of the stomach. The stomach is distended with air. Three laparoscopic ports are used. The anterior wall of the stomach is raised to the abdominal wall and a needle is passed into the stomach adjacent to the tumour. Small metal bars are passed down the needle sheath and used to lift up the tumour. The anterior gastric wall is then excised with several firings of the endoscopic stapler cutter. The specimen is removed laparoscopically.
2. A transgastric approach is adopted for tumours of the posterior wall of the stomach. Following insertion of a laparoscope via a subumbilical

port, three balloon trocars are placed in the upper abdomen. The stomach is distended with air via an endoscope and each of the balloon trocars is passed through the anterior gastric wall. Once inside the gastric lumen the balloons are inflated on each of the trocars maintaining gastric distension and the pneumoperitoneum is released. The laparoscope is passed through one of the three intragastric ports and the tumour is resected through the other two ports with electrocautery after injection of 3–5 mL of saline to elevate the tumour in a similar fashion to that performed by EMR. The specimen is removed via the gastroscope. The balloons are deflated and the trocars are removed. The trocar holes on the anterior gastric wall are each closed with intracorporal suturing.

The advantage of these two approaches compared to EMR is that a large cuff of clear margin can be resected by both techniques. Ohgami et al. reported that they achieved clear resection margins in all patients with mucosal EGC who were resected using these techniques.[57] The transgastric approach can be used for tumours of the cardia and those high on the posterior gastric wall, sites which are difficult for EMR.

Laparoscopic-assisted distal gastrectomy (Billroth I)

Laparoscopic-assisted distal gastrectomy (LADG) with Billroth I reconstruction has become the preferred treatment for Japanese patients with EGC of the distal stomach that cannot be cured by EMR. Kitano et al. have reported the results of 1185 patients who underwent LADG for EGC in one of 16 leading Japanese centres between 1994 and 2003, concluding that short- and long-term outcomes were excellent and preferable to open surgery.[58]

Briefly, the technique requires the placement of four to five laparoscopic ports. The gastrocolic omentum is divided caudal to the gastroepiploic arcade using an ultrasonic scalpel. The limits of the dissection are the origin of the left gastroepiploic artery that is clipped and divided, down to the right gastroepiploic vessels that are clipped and divided on the surface of the pancreas. The gastrohepatic omentum is divided and the right gastric artery clipped and divided. The duodenum is Kocherised with the assistance of a 45° angled laparoscope. The stomach is elevated and the left gastric vein clipped and divided. The left gastric artery is divided with an endovascular GIA or transfixed with sutures prior to division. This completes the gastric mobilisation. A 4–8 cm transverse incision is made in the epigastrium and the stomach is delivered into the wound. An automatic purse string device is placed across the duodenum prior to division. The anvil of a CEEA size 31 gun is placed in the duodenum and the purse string tightened. The site of transaction of the stomach is selected and a GIA 80 linear stapler fired across 50% of the way from the lesser to the greater curvature. The stomach is turned back on itself. The CEEA gun is passed through the distal opening (pylorus) and a gunned gastroduodenal anastomosis is fashioned through the back wall of the stomach. The GIA 80 linear stapler cutter is fired again across the remaining 50% of the greater curvature to complete division of the distal stomach and remove the specimen.

LADG removes group 3, 4, 5, 6 and 7 nodes (D1 + α) with many surgeons also removing the group 8 and 9 nodes (D1 + β). Those performing a full laparoscopic D2 dissection will endeavour to remove the 11p, 12a and 14v nodes.[59–62] Most early reports showed that a mean of 15 nodes were removed, less than the nodal harvests obtained after open D2 distal gastrectomy.[59,60,63,64] However, with increasing experience many authors are now routinely reporting harvests of more than 30 nodes after LADG.[61,62,65]

The laparoscopic operation is associated with less postoperative pain, improved postoperative respiratory function, earlier return of gastrointestinal function and a shorter hospital stay.[60,64] The laparoscopic operation takes longer but has less blood loss. Weight gain after the laparoscopic approach is improved compared to the open operation.

These two small randomised controlled trials both showed significant benefits following laparoscopic Billroth I gastrectomy compared with open surgery. The advantages were in a faster postoperative recovery with less postoperative pain.[60,64]

Long-term survival after LADG is comparable to that following open D2 distal gastrectomy, with Kitano et al. reporting 5-year disease-free survival figures of 99.8% for stage IA disease and 98.7% for stage IB disease.[58] Mochiki et al. reported an overall 5-year survival rate of 98% for EGC treated with LADG.[66]

Laparoscopic lymphadenectomy

Many patients who require surgery for EGC have already undergone some form of endoscopic therapy for the primary tumour such as EMR or ESD. It is often the case that the primary lesion has been completely excised but that submucosal invasion deems that additional surgery is required because of the significant risk of nodal metastasis. Consequently, Abe et al. have postulated that such patients do not require further gastric resection but simply need a lymphadenectomy.[67] They have reported five patients who had previously undergone ESD for submucosal EGC who underwent a laparoscopic lymphadenectomy alone, removing an average of 15 lymph nodes from the appropriate sites according to primary tumour location. The lymphatics and relevant accompanying gastric arteries were removed en bloc. The procedures took on average 240 minutes to perform and were associated with minimal blood loss and no ischaemic complications. Following surgery the patients who were node negative required no further intervention and clearly retained their stomach. The authors suggest that if the patient is node positive then further radical surgery would be recommended. Whether such a strategy is feasible in Western patients with a relatively higher body mass index is controversial.

Sentinel node-directed surgery for EGC

The sentinel node hypothesis is that the first site of draining nodes will be the first site for lymph node metastases from a tumour and that if the sentinel node is negative for metastases then the more distant nodes will also not contain metastatic disease. Ichikura et al. injected the tumour margins of EGC with ^{99m}Tc-labelled tin colloid solution the day before open surgery.[68] Using a hand-held gamma camera probe they assessed each of the nodal stations for evidence of increased activity. In this study indocyanine green solution was also injected close to the tumour to assist in visually identifying sentinel nodes. The authors identified an average of five sentinel nodes per patient, which were sent for frozen section. In the presence of nodal metastases a standard D2 gastrectomy was performed. However, in 61 of 73 patients the sentinel nodes were free of tumour. In these patients the authors carried out limited gastric resections (segmental or pylorus-preserving gastrectomy) with vagal nerve preservation without formal lymphadenectomy. Of these patients, 58 were node negative on final histology but three were node positive. Otani et al. have reported the use of sentinel node biopsy combined with laparoscopic-assisted, vagal-sparing segmental gastrectomy for patients with EGC.[69] They examined the nodes from the resected specimen with the gamma camera probe and sent positive nodes for frozen section. When the nodes were negative no further intervention was required. At present further studies with long-term follow-up will be required to confirm the value of sentinel node navigated surgery in the treatment of EGC.

Conclusions

EGC is a common diagnosis in Japan as a consequence of successful endoscopic surveillance for gastric cancer. Because of the vast experience of EGC patients a tailored approach to the therapy of this lesion has evolved over the past two decades. Radical resection of EGC has largely been replaced by endoscopic therapy by means of EMR and ESD for mucosal cancers with excellent long-term survival while retaining full gastric function. For submucosal EGC the risk of lymphatic spread requires additional therapy to EMR/ESD. The standard of care has become laparoscopic-assisted distal gastrectomy with limited open surgery being performed for more proximal tumours. Advances in laparoscopic expertise will facilitate even less invasive procedures in the future, including sentinel node navigated surgery and laparoscopic lymphadenectomy without gastrectomy for suitable patients. Because of the low incidence of EGC in the West and because of the increasingly obese population it is inevitable that most of the developments in this disease will come from the major Japanese centres and that Western surgeons will need to apply this new knowledge on a selective basis to their patients with EGC.

Key points

- As a consequence of endoscopic surveillance more than 60% of Japanese patients present with early gastric cancer (EGC).
- EGC has a long natural history, but in general it progresses to the advanced stage with time and results in death if left untreated.
- In EGC nodal metastases occur in 3% (range 0.7–21%) of mucosal tumours and in 20% (10.6–64%) of submucosal tumours.
- Most nodal metastases from EGC are perigastric, located in the first tier of nodes. Less than 1% of mucosal cancers have spread to the second tier of nodes, but 2–9% of submucosal cancers have spread beyond the first tier.
- Endoscopic mucosal resection is the preferred treatment for mucosal EGC <15 mm in size. For larger, non-ulcerated lesions endoscopic submucosal dissection allows removal of lesions en bloc.
- Histological assessment is the only reliable way of differentiating mucosal from submucosal cancer.
- Treatment of EGC by open D2 subtotal or total gastrectomy is associated with 90–95% 5-year survival, but because of the associated risks of morbidity these techniques have been largely replaced by tailored, more limited, surgical techniques.
- Open surgery for EGC includes proximal gastrectomy with jejunal interposition for upper-third EGC, central segmental gastrectomy for middle-third EGC and pylorus-preserving gastrectomy for lower-third EGC that is >4 cm away from the pylorus.
- Laparoscopic-assisted distal gastrectomy has become the standard of care for the treatment of distal EGC in Japan, with the outcome of nearly 1200 procedures showing a 98% 5-year survival rate for stage IA disease.
- With experience laparoscopic-assisted distal gastrectomy provides adequate lymph node harvests (>30 nodes) equivalent to those obtained by open D2 subtotal gastrectomy.
- Laparoscopic lymphadenectomy alone may become a suitable treatment option for patients who have undergone complete excision of their EGC by prior ESD.
- Sentinel node guided surgery may hold promise for the future but the long-term outcomes of this technique in the management of EGC remain to be established.

References

1. Murakami T. Pathomorphological diagnosis, definition, and gross classification of early gastric cancer. Gann Monogr Cancer Res 1971; 11:53–5.

2. Hisamichi S. Screening for gastric cancer. World J Surg 1989; 13:31–7.

3. Everett SM, Axon ATR. Early gastric cancer in Europe. Gut 1997; 41:142–50.

4. Asaka M, Takeda H, Sugiyama T et al. What role does *Helicobacter pylori* play in gastric cancer? Gastroenterology 1997; 113:S56–60.

5. Uemura N, Okamoto S, Yamamoto S et al. *Helicobacter pylori* infection and the development of gastric cancer. N Engl J Med 2001; 345:784–9.

6. Watabe H, Mitsushima T, Yamaji Y et al. Predicting the development of gastric cancer from combining *Helicobacter pylori* antibodies and serum pepsinogen status: a prospective endoscopic cohort study. Gut 2005; 54:764–8.

7. Hosokawa O, Kaizaki Y, Watanabe K et al. Endoscopic surveillance for gastric remnant cancer after early gastric cancer surgery. Endoscopy 2002; 34:469–73.

8. Stael von Holstein C, Ericksson S, Huldt B et al. Endoscopic screening during 17 years for gastric stump carcinoma. A prospective clinical trial. Scand J Gastroenterol 1991; 26(10):1020–6.

9. Ohashi M, Katai H, Fukagawa T et al. Cancer of the gastric stump following distal gastrectomy for cancer. Br J Surg 2007; 94:92–5.

10. Huntsmand DG, Carneiro F, Lewis FR et al. EGC in young asymptomatic carriers of the germ-line mutation E-cadherin mutations. N Engl J Med 2001; 344:1904–9.

11. Chun YS, Lindar NM, Smyrk TC et al. Germline E-cadherin gene mutations: is prophylactic total gastrectomy indicated? Cancer 2001; 92: 181–187.

12. Norton JA, Ham CM, Van Dam J et al. CDH1 truncating mutations in the E-cadherin gene; an indication for total gastrectomy to treat hereditary diffuse gastric cancer. Ann Surg 2007; 245:873–9.

13. Newman EA, Mulholland MW. Prophylactic gastrectomy for hereditary diffuse gastric cancer syndrome. J Am Coll Surg 2006; 202:612–17.

14. Lewis FR, Mellinger JD, Hayashi A et al. Prophylactic total gastrectomy for familial gastric cancer. Surgery 2001; 130:612–17.

15. Lauren P. The two histological main types of gastric carcinoma: diffuse and so called intestinal-type carcinoma. Acta Pathol Microbiol Scand 1965; 64:31–49.

16. Schlemper RJ, Itabashi M, Kato J et al. Differences in diagnostic criteria for gastric carcinoma between Japanese and Western pathologists. Lancet 1997; 349:1725–9.

17. Lauwers GY, Riddell RH, Kato Y et al. Evaluation of gastric biopsies for neoplasia: differences between Japanese and Western pathologists. Am J Surg Pathol 1999; 23:511–18.

18. Rugge MC, Dixon P, Hattori MF et al. Gastric dysplasia; the Padova International Classification. Am J Surg Pathol 1999; 24:167–76.

19. Schlemper RJ, Riddell RH, Kato Y et al. The Vienna classification of gastrointestinal epithelial neoplasia. Gut 2000; 47:251–5.

20. Kodama Y, Inokuchi K, Soejima K et al. Growth patterns and prognosis in early gastric carcinoma. Superficially spreading and pentrating growth types. Cancer 1983; 51:320–6.

21. Sano T, Kobori O, Muto T. Lymph node metastasis from early gastric cancer: endoscopic resection of tumour. Br J Surg 1992; 79:241–4.

22. Popiela T, Kulig J, Kolodziejczyk P et al. Long-term results of surgery for early gastric cancer. Br J Surg 2002; 89:1035–42.

23. Hioki K, Nakane Y, Yamamoto M. Surgical strategy for early gastric cancer. Br J Surg 1990; 77: 1330–4.

24. Folli S, Dente M, Dell'Amore D et al. Early gastric cancer: prognostic factors in 233 patients. Br J Surg 1995; 82:952–6.

25. Ichikura T, Uefuji K, Tomimatsu S et al. Surgical strategy for patients with gastric carcinoma with submucosa invasion. Cancer 1995; 76:935–40.

26. Hayes N, Karat D, Scott DJ et al. Radical lymphadenectomy in the management of early gastric cancer. Br J Surg 1996; 83:1421–1423.

27. An Y, Baik YH, Choi MG et al. Predictive factors for lymph node metastasis in early gastric cancer with submucosal invasion: analysis of a single institutional experience. Ann Surg 2007; 246:749–53.

28. Shimada S, Yagi Y, Shiomori K et al. Characterization of early gastric cancer and proposal of the optimal therapeutic strategy. Surgery 2001; 129:714–19.

29. Yamao T, Shirao K, Ono H et al. Risk factors for lymph node metastases from intramucosa gastric carcinoma. Cancer 1996; 77:602–6.

30. Tanaka M, Kitajima Y, Edakuni G et al. Abnormal expression of E-cadherin and β-catenin may be a molecular marker of submucosal lymph node metastasis in early gastric cancer. Br J Surg 2002; 89:236–44.

31. Arai K, Iwasaki Y, Takahashi T. Clinopathological analysis of early gastric cancer with solitary lymph node metastases. Br J Surg 2002; 89:1435–7.

32. Tsukuma H, Oshima A, Narahara H et al. Natural history of early gastric cancer: a non-concurrent, long term, follow up study. Gut 2000; 41:618–21.

33. Bando E, Kojima N, Kawamura T et al. Prognostic value of age and sex in early gastric cancer. Br J Surg 2004; 91:1197–201.

34. Yanai H, Noguchi T, Mizumachi S et al. A blind comparison of the effectiveness of endoscopic ultrasonography and endoscopy in the staging of early gastric cancer. Gut 1999; 44:361–5.

35. Sano T, Okuyama Y, Kobori O et al. Early gastric cancer. Endoscopic diagnosis of depth of invasion. Dig Dis Sci 1990; 35:1340–44.

36. Nakamura T, Suzuki T, Matsura A et al. Assessment of the depth of invasion of gastric carcinoma by endoscopic ultrasonography (EUS) focussed upon peptic ulceration within the cancerous area. Stom Intest 1999; 24:1105–17.

37. Tada M, Murakami A, Yania H et al. Endoscopic resection of early gastric cancer. Endoscopy 1993; 25:445–450.

38. Hiki Y, Shimao H, Mieno H et al. Modified treatment of early gastric cancer: evaluation of endoscopic treatment of early gastric cancers with respect to treatment indication groups. World J Surg 1995; 19:517–522.

39. Ono H, Gotoda T, Shirao K et al. Endoscopic mucosal resection for treatment of early gastric cancer. Gut 2001; 48:225–9.

40. Miyata M, Yokoyama Y, Okoyama N et al. What are the appropriate indications for endoscopic mucosal resection of early gastric cancer? Endoscopy 2000; 32:773–8.

41. Takekoshi T, Baba Y, Ohta H et al. Endoscopic resection of early gastric carcinoma: results of a retrospective analysis of 308 cases. Endoscopy 1994; 26:352–358.

42. Sagawa T, Takayama T, Oku T et al. Argon plasma coagulation for successful treatment of early gastric cancer with intramucosa invasion. Gut 2003; 52:334–9.

43. Sibille A, Descamps C, Jonard P et al. Endoscopic Nd:YAG treatment of superficial gastric carcinoma: experience of 18 Western inoperable patients. Gastrointest Endosc 1995; 42:340–345.

44. Ell C, Gossner L, May A et al. Photodynamic ablation of early cancers of the stomach by means of mTHPC and laser irradiation: preliminary clinical experience. Gut 1998; 43:345–9.

45. Nishi M, Ishihara S, Nakajima T et al. Chronological changes of characteristics of early gastric cancer and therapy: experience in the Cancer Institute Hospital of Tokyo 1950–1994. J Cancer Res Clin Oncol 1995; 121:535–41.

46. Endo M, Habu H. Clinical studies of early gastric cancer. Hepatogastroenterology 1990; 37:408–10.

47. Cuschieri A, Wedden S, Fielding J et al. Patient survival after D1 and D2 resections for gastric cancer: long-term results of the MRC randomised surgical trial. Br J Cancer 1999; 79:1522–30.

48. Bonenkamp JJ, Hermans J, Sasako M et al. Extended lymph-node dissection for gastric cancer. N Engl J Med 1999; 340:908–14.

49. Baba H, Maehara Y, Takeuchi H et al. Effect of lymph node dissection on the prognosis in patients with node-negative early gastric cancer. Surgery 1994; 117:165–9.

50. Tsujitani S, Oka S, Saito H et al. Less invasive surgery for early gastric cancer based on the low probability of lymph node metastasis. Surgery 1999; 125:148–54.

51. Otsuji E, Toma A, Kobayashi S et al. Long-term benefit of extended lymphadenectomy with gastrectomy in distally located early gastric carcinoma. Am J Surg 2000; 180:127–32.

52. Katai H, Sano T, Fukagawa T et al. Prospective study of proximal gastrectomy for early gastric cancer in the upper third of the stomach. Br J Surg 2003; 90:850–3.

53. Takeshita K, Saito N, Saeki I et al. Proximal gastrectomy and jejunal pouch interposition for the treatment of early cancer in the upper third of the stomach: surgical techniques and evaluation of post operative function. Surgery 1997; 121:278–86.

54. Ohwada S, Nakamura S, Ogawa T et al. Segmental gastrectomy for early gastric cancer in the mid-stomach. Hepatogastroenterology 1999; 46:1229–33.

55. Shinohara T, Ohyama S, Muto T et al. Clinical outcome of high segmental gastrectomy for early gastric cancer in the upper third of the stomach. Br J Surg 2006; 93:975–80.

56. Nishikawa K, Kawahara H, Yumiba T et al. Functional characteristics of the pylorus in patients undergoing pylorus-preserving gastrectomy for early gastric cancer. Surgery 2002; 131:613–624.

57. Ohgami M, Otani Y, Kumai K et al. Curative laparoscopic surgery for early gastric cancer. Five years experience. World J Surg 1999; 23:187–193.

58. Kitano S, Shiraishi N, Uyama I et al. and the Japanese Laparoscopic Surgery Study Group. A multicenter study on oncological outcome of laparoscopic gastrectomy for early gastric cancer. Ann Surg 2007; 245:68–72.

59. Nagai Y, Tanimura H, Takifuji K et al. Laparoscopic-assisted Billroth I gastrectomy. Surg Laparosc Endosc 1995; 5:281–7.

60. Kitano S, Shiraishi N, Fujii K et al. A randomised controlled trial comparing open vs laparoscopy-assisted distal gastrectomy for the treatment of early gastric cancer: an interim report. Surgery 2002; 131:S306–11.

61. Lee SI, Choi YS, Park DJ et al. Comparative study of laparoscopic-assisted distal gastrectomy and open distal gastrectomy. J Am Coll Surg 2006; 202:874–80.

62. Huscher CGS, Mingoli A, Sgarzini G et al. Totally laparoscopic total and subtotal gastrectomy with extended lymph node dissection for early and advanced gastric cancer: early and long-term results of a 100-patient series. Am J Surg 2007; 194:839–44.

63. Shimizu S, Uchiyama A, Mizumoto T et al. Laparoscopically assisted distal gastrectomy for early gastric cancer. Surg Endosc 2000; 14:27–31.

64. Mochiki E, Nakabayashi T, Kamimur H et al. Gastrointestinal recovery and outcome after laparoscopy-assisted versus conventional open distal gastrectomy for early gastric cancer. World J Surg 2002; 26:1145–9.

65. Shimizu S, Noshiro H, Nagai E et al. Laparoscopic gastric surgery in a Japanese institution: analysis of the initial 100 procedures. J Am Coll Surg 2003; 197:372–8.

66. Mochiki E, Kamiyama Y, Aihara R et al. Laparoscopic assisted distal gastrectomy for early gastric cancer: five years' experience. Surgery 2005; 137:317–22.

67. Abe N, Mori T, Takeuchi H et al. Laparoscopic lymph node dissection after endoscopic submucosal dissection: a novel and minimally invasive approach to treating early-stage gastric cancer. Am J Surg 2005; 190:496–503.

68. Ichikura T, Chochi K, Sugasawa H et al. Individualized surgery for early gastric cancer guided by sentinel node biopsy. Surgery 2006; 139:501–7.

69. Otani Y, Furukawa T, Kitagawa Y. New method of laparoscopic-assisted function preserving surgery for early gastric cancer: vagus-sparing segmental gastrectomy under sentinel node navigation. J Am Coll Surg 2004; 198:1026–31.

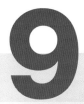

Radiotherapy and chemotherapy in treatment of oesophageal and gastric cancer

Adrian Crellin

Introduction

The treatment of oesophagogastric cancer has become more complex, with evidence of the benefits of multimodality therapy. The limitations of single-modality approaches in producing acceptable long-term survival rates have driven the changing patterns of management of both oesophageal and gastric cancer. Early-stage disease can be treated with excellent outcomes. However, improvements in staging, imaging and pathology have demonstrated that the majority of patients present with either locally advanced or metastatic disease. High local recurrence rates and early failure with metastatic disease are easier to understand in past series of patients who would have been accepted as operable and treated as potentially curable.

The changing pattern of disease with rapidly increasing rates of adenocarcinoma of the distal oesophagus and oesophagogastric junction but reducing numbers of cancers of the body and antrum of the stomach may require a different approach to treatment.

Improvements in staging with spiral computed tomography (CT), magnetic resonance imaging, endoscopic ultrasound (EUS) and positron emission tomography (PET) now allow patients to be selected for specific approaches to treatment. The early identification of metastases can allow a palliative approach to be followed, avoiding the potential mortality and morbidity associated with resection as well as the significant effect on quality of life. Equally, the demonstration of early-stage disease can allow the selected use of single-modality therapy. There are undoubtedly limitations to the use of imaging, particularly in predicting the response to primary non-surgical treatment, chemotherapy or

chemoradiotherapy (CRT), but the addition of new techniques such as PET, in addition to better use of and understanding of molecular markers, offers promise for the future.

An increasingly elderly population tends to have more comorbid conditions and so present particular challenges. It is possible to reduce postoperative mortality by the appropriate selection of patients.[1] Some of these, although not fit for a transthoracic approach to resection, may be appropriate for primary non-surgical treatment such as CRT and so may still be offered a reasonable chance of long-term disease control.

In oesophageal cancer the changing pattern of squamous cell carcinoma and adenocarcinoma has meant some mixed series of cases and variable results. The variable inclusion of lower oesophageal cancer with cancer of the oesophagogastric junction and with gastric adenocarcinoma has also brought about some difficulty in interpreting the true role of chemotherapy and radiotherapy from the literature.

The identification of improved activity when chemotherapy and radiotherapy are given synchronously has already led to CRT becoming the primary approach in anal cancer, with surgery now used for salvage.[2,3] There is now good evidence that primary CRT has a role in oesophageal cancer treatment.

With mounting evidence of the benefit of a multidisciplinary approach to care and assessment, and of selected multimodality treatment, it is important for surgeons and oncologists to understand more of the strengths and weaknesses of their own and each other's treatments. Only then can treatment be truly integrated and improved outcomes achieved with minimal morbidity.

Both oesophageal and gastric cancers have high response rates to chemotherapy. There is a clearly established role for chemotherapy in palliative treatment of advanced and metastatic disease. However, it has taken longer to define a role for its use in the neoadjuvant or adjuvant setting.

The definition of adjuvant treatment and potentially curative therapy is worth stressing. Adjuvant therapy usually means additional treatment given after potentially curative therapy, in an attempt to improve the long-term outcome. Neoadjuvant therapy is the use of either chemotherapy and/or radiotherapy prior to surgery. The role of chemotherapy and radiotherapy should be seen in the context of how they combine with surgery to alter patterns of relapse and improve survival or provide a viable alternative to surgery. In this context, surgery can really only be described as potentially curative if the tumour is resected with no residual macroscopic disease and clear histological margins (R0), in the absence of metastatic disease.

The following sections are intended to allow the role of chemotherapy and radiotherapy to be put into context, and the strength of evidence assessed. The sections on potentially curative approaches are more detailed. This is the area in which most treatment will be integrated with surgery in current or future approaches.

Oesophageal cancer

Potentially curative treatment

Preoperative radiotherapy

Theoretical advantages of preoperative radiotherapy treatment include:

- a more easily defined target volume;
- improved tumour oxygenation at the time of treatment;
- the potential to improve resectability and reduce the impact of tumour cell spillage at surgery;
- minimisation of the impact of microscopic residual disease and reduction of local recurrence.

This approach has been shown to be of value in rectal cancer.[4]

There have been six randomised trials of preoperative radiotherapy. Three trials were restricted to squamous carcinoma. One of these, by Gignoux et al., reported an improvement in local/regional recurrence (46% vs. 67%).[5] Nygaard et al. report improved survival,[6] but this series is complicated by the inclusion of some patients also receiving chemotherapy. One trial included both squamous and adenocarcinoma,[7] and two do not specify the histology. Overall it is difficult to draw firm conclusions from these trials.

A meta-analysis of updated individual patient data from 1147 patients in randomised trials reported a hazard ratio of 0.89 (95% CI 0.78–1.01) with an absolute survival benefit of 4% at 5 years.[8] This result did not reach conventional statistical significance. The benefit seems likely therefore to be small, if present, and with little evidence of improved resectability.

Postoperative radiotherapy

The main attraction of postoperative radiotherapy is that it can be restricted to selected patients who may have a higher risk of recurrence, particularly of local/regional failure. There are four randomised trials in the literature. The numbers are small (totalling 843 adjuvant patients), and three out of the four include only squamous carcinoma. Teniere et al.[9] showed no survival advantage in 221 patients. There was a small improvement in the failure rate but at the cost of significant side-effects. The benefit appears to be limited to node-negative patients. Fok et al.[10] included both adenocarcinoma and squamous carcinoma. Whilst both curative and palliative resections were included, the patients were separately analysed and received different radiotherapy doses. The results show a significant morbidity (37%) and mortality related to bleeding from the transposed intrathoracic stomach. It should be noted that the dose per fraction of the radiotherapy was high (3.5 Gy), which may be significant. There was a lower intrathoracic recurrence rate, particularly relating to tracheo-bronchial disease.

A larger randomised study from China[11] included 495 well-staged patients with squamous carcinoma randomised to receive either surgery alone (S) or surgery and postoperative radiotherapy (S + R). Whilst there are significant concerns about the ethics (the patients were not aware they were in a trial and so did not give appropriate consent), the study was still published because of its significant results. The surgery appears to be of a high standard and included a lymph node dissection. The radiotherapy was wide field and included the bilateral supraclavicular fossae (SCF), mediastinum and anastomosis to an initial dose of 40 Gy. A further 10 Gy was given to the SCF and 20 Gy to the mediastinum by a different technique, allowing a maximum dose to the transposed stomach of 50 Gy. There was a relatively high proportion of earlier stage IIA disease in the study compared with a UK population. The analysis showed a highly significant difference in 1-, 3- and 5-year survival in stage III disease between the S and S + R arms (67.5%, 23.3%, 13.1% vs. 75.5%, 43.2%, 35.1% respectively). The pattern of relapse was different between the two arms, with significantly fewer recurrences in the neck, SCF and mediastinum. Unlike other studies, toxicity to the transposed stomach was minimal.

There is thus reasonable evidence that postoperative radiotherapy may be offered to pathological stage III squamous carcinoma of the oesophagus. To translate the results into UK practice, where many patients will have had preoperative chemotherapy, would require a step away from a pure evidence base, but is perhaps justifiable given the effect on relapse patterns. For adenocarcinoma the justification is less clear outside the context of a clinical trial. The known poor prognosis for a positive circumferential radial margin but with a low nodal burden might identify a suitable subset of patients to study.

Preoperative chemotherapy

The rationale behind preoperative chemotherapy is to improve operability by tumour shrinkage and downstaging and to treat occult metastatic disease as early as possible, thereby trying to reduce late metastatic disease as a cause of failure. A useful additional benefit may be that some patients will improve their swallowing and so gain weight and a better nutritional status in the preoperative phase. Non-responders to chemotherapy, however, will have surgery delayed and the possibility of chemotherapy side-effects. Preoperative chemotherapy in both squamous and adenocarcinoma appears to achieve consistently good clinical response rates, ranging from 47%[12] to 61%.[13]

Early studies, predominantly in squamous carcinoma, used combinations of cisplatin, vindesine and bleomycin. More recently cisplatin and 5-fluorouracil (5-FU) combinations have been used in important randomised trials. New 5-hydroxytryptamine-3 ($5-HT_3$) antagonist antiemetic drugs have allowed cisplatin to be used with dramatically reduced toxicity. Protracted venous infusion (PVI) 5-FU in combination with cisplatin and epirubicin (the ECF regimen) has produced increased response rates in non-randomised studies. These more modern cisplatin–5-FU combinations seem to be active in both squamous[14] and adenocarcinoma.[13]

Randomised trials of preoperative chemotherapy

There are three older randomised trials in the literature. Roth et al.[15] reported the results of 39 patients treated with cisplatin, vindesine and bleomycin. There was no survival advantage between the two arms but responders did seem to have a longer median survival (>20 months vs. overall 9 months

vs. non-responders 6.2 months). Schlag[12] randomised 75 patients to receiving cisplatin and 5-FU. The trial was stopped early due to increased postoperative morbidity and mortality in the chemotherapy-treated patients. Nygaard et al.[6] showed no survival advantage at 3 years. These trials were all small and so were only powered to reliably demonstrate large differences in outcome. A meta-analysis published in 1996[16] did not show a survival benefit to preoperative chemotherapy.

However, since then the results from three larger trials have become available, which are influential in suggesting that preoperative chemotherapy does have a role. In a randomised study undertaken by the Rotterdam Esophageal Tumor Study Group,[17] 160 patients with squamous carcinoma were randomised to receive two courses of cisplatin and etoposide or surgery (transhiatal resection) alone. Those patients who demonstrated a good clinical response (69/74) then went on to receive two further courses. Data on 148 patients were analysed with a median follow-up of 15 months. There was a significant difference ($P = 0.002$) in the median survival between the chemotherapy + surgery and the surgery alone arm (18.5 months vs. 11 months). The conclusion was that neoadjuvant chemotherapy improves survival.

The American Intergroup Trial (INT 0113)[18] produced data on 440 randomised patients with a median follow-up of 46.5 months. Adenocarcinoma (54%) was the predominant histology. The chemotherapy given was three preoperative courses (cisplatin and 5 days of infusional 5-FU) and in stable or responding patients two postoperative courses. Overall, 83% of patients received the intended two preoperative cycles of chemotherapy. However, only 32% of patients received both postoperative chemotherapy cycles. There was no difference in treatment-related mortality between the two arms (6% surgery (S) vs. 7% chemotherapy (C) + surgery (S); $P = 0.33$). On an intent-to-treat basis there was no difference in median survival (16.1 months C + S vs. 14.9 months S), and 1-, 2- and 3-year (23% C + S vs. 26% S) survivals. Disappointingly, there was no difference in the pattern of metastatic disease between the two arms. However, there was a significantly higher rate of R1 resections in the surgery alone arm.

The Medical Research Council (MRC) OEO2 study is the largest and arguably the most influential trial in this area.[19] A total of 802 patients were randomised to receive two courses of cisplatin and a 4-day infusion of 5-FU followed by surgery (CS) after 3–5 weeks or immediate surgery alone (S) and showed a significant survival advantage for patients receiving preoperative chemotherapy.

The majority of patients (66%) had adenocarcinoma histology. The two arms appear balanced and criticisms of the staging, which was relatively poor by modern standards and could have been as little as a chest radiograph and an abdominal ultrasound, are largely mitigated by the size of the study. The majority of patients in the CS arm received both of the cycles of chemotherapy (90%), with another 6% having just one cycle. The overall operation rate was similar in both arms (94%) but there was a significant difference in the microscopic complete resection rate (60% CS vs. 53% S; $P < 0.0001$). There was good evidence for a downstaging effect in terms of size of primary and extent of nodal involvement. The postoperative mortality was equivalent in both arms at 10%.

The overall survival rate was significantly improved with preoperative chemotherapy ($P = 0.004$; hazard ratio 0.79, CI 0.67–0.93), with an estimated reduction in risk of death of 21% and 2-year survival figures of 43% CS vs. 34% S. There was no evidence that the effect of chemotherapy varied with histology. Long-term follow-up with a median follow-up of 6 years has confirmed these results, with 5-year survivals of 23% CS vs. 17% S.[20]

The differing results between the two US and European trials is difficult to explain. Concerns about a low operation rate of 80% in the chemotherapy arm of the Intergroup Trial may reflect the more ambitious and prolonged chemotherapy regime, leading to more toxicity. In the MRC trial there was no real difference in the rate of death from cancer and one could hypothesise that the important determinant of survival is the achievement of a potentially curative R0 resection, enhanced by the local downstaging effect of chemotherapy. Any factor that precludes such a resection, resulting from chemotherapy, such as excess toxicity or delay in surgery in non-responding patients, might counter any gains in the responding patients.

An updated Cochrane review of 11 randomised trials involving 2051 patients concludes that there was a 21% increase in survival at 3 years with preoperative chemotherapy, but that statistical significance was not reached until 5 years.[21] Increased toxicity and mortality due to chemotherapy were evident and the pathological complete response (pCR) rate was a disappointing 3%. Preoperative chemotherapy has been adopted as a standard of care in the UK, although chemoradiation is more widely used in the USA.

The current MRC/NCRI trial in the UK (OEO5) compares OEO2 chemotherapy with four cycles of ECX (epirubicin–cisplatin–capecitabine) in adenocarcinoma alone. The high completion rate and positive results of preoperative chemotherapy in the MRC MAGIC (ST02)[22] study for gastric and gastro-esophageal cancer pointed to the strategy of using a modified ECF regimen, which is accepted in the UK as the best standard of care for advanced gastroesophageal cancer, and using it in a neoadjuvant setting to try and improve on the results of OEO2. The results of the REAL2 study,[23] a phase III trial of palliative chemotherapy, showed that the oral fluoropyrimidine (capecitabine) could be substituted for infusional 5-FU with safety and at least equivalent efficacy. The advantage of easier chemotherapy delivery without the use of Hickman lines and their associated morbidity is a step forward. This study is also important in that it places an emphasis on high-quality assurance of staging, surgery, chemotherapy and pathology. There is little doubt that at least one of the reasons for differing results in trials in the whole area of gastro-oesophageal cancer has been a wide variation in the quality of staging modalities and surgery. The trial sets high standards which should translate into improved patient selection and outcomes, even within the control arm. Recruitment is good and the intial trial target is for 1300 randomised patients.

Postoperative chemotherapy

There are few useful trials that address the question of adjuvant postoperative chemotherapy. The trials reported by Roth et al.[15] and Kelsen et al.[18] both have an adjuvant component, coupled with preoperative treatment. The fact that only 32% completed the postoperative phase in the Intergroup study[18] underlines a problem with this approach. Patients undergoing major resections for oesophageal carcinoma often have a prolonged postoperative phase. The start of chemotherapy may be delayed due to performance status. Patients may also choose not to continue. A strategy that relies solely on postoperative treatment may have significant problems. Improved patient selection and postoperative supportive care may allow this approach to be practical. The MAGIC gastric cancer trial latterly included tumours of the gastro-oesophageal junction and lower oesophagus and intended three postoperative courses of ECF as well as three given preoperatively in the protocol. Again, only 40% completed the postoperative chemotherapy. The trial has shown an improvement in overall survival, as described in the section on gastric cancer,[22] which lends further support for the concept of neoadjuvant chemotherapy for cancers of the oesophagus or gastro-oesophageal junction. Our centre's policy on postoperative chemotherapy has been to reserve it for situations in which a primary resection has been undertaken for tumours staged as T2N0 or less, and so not receiving preoperative chemotherapy, but where unexpected higher stage pathology arises. Then, two cycles of postoperative OEO2 chemotherapy are given on an empirical basis.

Preoperative chemoradiotherapy

The rationale in using chemotherapy and radiotherapy together is that enhanced tumour cell kill might lead to improved outcomes. Chemotherapy can lead to a decreased ability of tumour cells to repair radiation-induced DNA damage. Many of the commonly used chemotherapy drugs with significant activity in oesophageal and gastric cancer appear to be radiation sensitisers (5-FU, cisplatin, mitomycin C, taxanes). There is good evidence that pCR rates are significantly higher with CRT than with radiotherapy or chemotherapy given alone. There is the significant attraction of achieving enhanced local therapy coupled with a systemic benefit as sought with preoperative chemotherapy alone. When added to surgery, it is not clear that pCR is necessarily the only useful end-point. Preoperative CRT has the added advantage in providing direct evidence to guide the process of developing and optimising combination chemotherapy and radiotherapy schedules for use as definitive treatments.

Both radiotherapy and chemotherapy rely on achieving an acceptable balance between increased response rates in the tumour on one hand and normal tissue morbidity coupled with patient tolerance on the other. Whilst many of the side-effects of chemotherapy are relatively early in presentation, for example hair loss, emesis and myelosuppression, radiotherapy side-effects can present late, from 6 months to years out from treatment. If radical surgery is added in combined modality therapy the potential for high levels of morbidity become significant.

Non-randomised studies of CRT have appeared in the literature since the late 1980s. The review article by Geh et al.[24] summarises 46 trials containing 20 patients or more. Overall, pooled data from these studies show that out of 2704 patients (squamous 68% and adenocarcinoma 32%), 79% were operated on with a pCR rate of 24% of those treated and 32% of those resected. As experience with this modality of treatment has grown, lessons have been learned. Attempts to escalate the dose of radiotherapy can lead to unacceptable rates of morbidity, especially if higher doses per fraction are used.[25,26] Reported CRT-related deaths in the non-randomised series ranged from 0% to 15% (mean 3%). Postoperative deaths ranged from 0% to 29% (mean 9%). Adult respiratory distress syndrome, anastomotic leak and breakdown, pneumonia and sepsis were the commonest causes of death following oesophageal resection. Treatment-related deaths ranged from 3% to 25% (mean 9%) of all patients treated. It seems clear that the risk of chemotherapy-related toxicity, particularly myelosuppression, rises with the number of drugs used and the intensity of the CRT regimen.[27,28] An increased risk of tracheobronchial fistula has been reported.[29] However, most of the reported series did not have the latest sophisticated radiotherapy techniques that allow greater precision and sparing of organs and tissues to within normal tissue tolerance.

Consistent reporting of pathology is important, and a grading of CRT response has been described by Mandard et al.[30] Five grades of response ranging from no identifiable tumour to complete absence of regression allow a more objective approach to be adopted. In this paper the significant predictor of disease-free survival after multivariate analysis was the tumour regression grade. There is evidence that pCR confers a survival advantage over those patients not achieving pCR.[31–36] In **Fig. 9.1**, different comparative outcomes such as median survival in months, overall or disease-free survival in years, are plotted together in the series, quoting outcomes separately. The importance is in the consistent nature of the difference in outcomes in

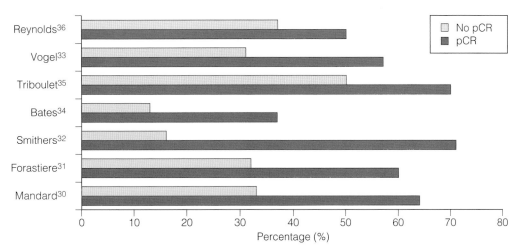

Figure 9.1 • Relative survival outcomes – pathological complete response (pCR) to CRT.

each series. It becomes clear that prediction of this response prior to treatment either through molecular markers or PET activity after induction chemotherapy alone might allow very different algorithms of treatment modalities.

Table 9.1 summarises eight reported randomised trials of preoperative CRT compared with surgery alone. In three of these the chemotherapy was given sequentially to the radiotherapy and in four synchronously. Two trials using sequential treatment in squamous carcinoma[6,37] received relatively low doses of radiotherapy and showed no convincing evidence of improved survival with the combined treatment. In a larger European Organisation for Research and Treatment of Cancer (EORTC) trial[26] involving 282 patients, the cisplatin chemotherapy was given in close sequence with the radiotherapy. The radiotherapy was given in a split course and at a relatively high dose per fraction (two courses of 18.5 Gy in five daily fractions split 2 weeks apart). The CRT patients were more likely to have a curative resection. The disease-free survival was significantly longer (3-year CRT + S 40% vs. S 28%). There was no difference in the overall survival, largely due to a significantly higher postoperative mortality in the CRT arm (12% vs. 4%). Apinop et al.[38] reported a synchronous CRT series of 69 squamous histology patients with no improvement in survival.

There are three larger trials of preoperative synchronous CRT.

The Walsh study[39] has been influential in changing practice, particularly in the USA. In 113 patients with adenocarcinoma, cisplatin and 5-FU were given with 40 Gy in 3 weeks of radiotherapy. There was an overall survival benefit in favour of the CRT arm (median 16 months vs. 11 months; 3-year survival 32% vs. 6%). Morbidity in this series was not inconsiderable. The radiotherapy technique and fractionation may explain this. Most open to question, however, is the noticeably poor survival in the surgery alone control arm. The basic standards of staging could potentially have led to an imbalance of true staging in the treatment arms.

The University of Michigan trial[40] randomised 100 patients with both squamous and adenocarcinoma. The surgery was a transhiatal resection. Patients in the CRT arm received 45 Gy in 30 fractions with cisplatin, 5-FU and vinblastine. At first analysis there was no significant difference between the arms but at 3 years a statistically significant benefit to the combined treatment emerged, with overall survival of 32% vs. 15%. A final analysis has shown no survival advantage and demonstrates the danger of early publication of a trial that was essentially underpowered.

The results of the Australasian Gastro-Intestinal Trials Group (AGITG)[41] have been criticised for having a low radiotherapy dose and only one cycle of cisplatin and 5-FU chemotherapy. Although the trial was negative overall there are some clues for the direction of future approaches. There was a significant survival difference in patients with squamous histology (36% of the total) with the addition of CRT and a much higher pathological complete response rate.

Not only do trials need to be larger, but attention to the quality assurance of all components of treatment and staging is required to ensure that the rather variable results of the past are not replicated. One such trial unfortunately closed in the USA, NCCTG-C9781 (CALGB 9781). The results of the Intergroup Study INT-0116 (SWOG 9008)[42] were presented at the American Society of Clinical Oncologists (ASCO) 2000 Meeting. Whilst this was predominantly a trial of postoperative CRT in gastric cancer, it included tumours of the gastro-oesophageal junction. It was felt that the positive results of the SWOG 9008 trial would preclude further randomisation to a trial with a surgery-only control arm. In addition, recruitment was already poor due to preoperative CRT becoming adopted as a standard of care in the USA. However, mature results from CALGB 9781[43] are available and despite small numbers show a significant improvement in overall survival in preoperative CRT compared to surgery alone (5-year survival of 39% vs. 16%). Resection rates were high in the preoperative CRT arm (87%) and there was no increase in operative mortality. The trial included higher quality staging and surgery.

A systematic overview of preoperative CRT[44] has looked at factors influencing pCR rates. There is evidence that increasing radiotherapy dose, cisplatin and 5-FU doses are linked to higher pCR rates. However, having optimised some standard chemotherapy drug combinations, the use of induction chemotherapy prior to CRT, radiotherapy dose and technology delivery, it may be that a plateau will be reached in pCR rates and the next step is the addition of biological agents.

Neoadjuvant chemoradiotherapy or chemotherapy?

There are still major questions to be answered, but a surgery-alone arm is not likely to be considered acceptable in the UK or in the USA for stage III disease. The good outcomes from surgery alone in stage I and II disease make neoadjuvant therapy difficult to justify.

Early experience with neoadjuvant CRT in the UK was very variable in terms of its impact on operative risk and toxicity. The results of OEO2 have meant that the UK has continued with a chemotherapy approach in the current OEO5 study.

Table 9.1 • Randomised trials of preoperative chemoradiation

Reference	Sequential or concurrent	Squamous or adenocarci-noma	Patients	Chemo*	RT dose (Gy)	Resection rate	Mortality in CRT arm	Result†
Nygaard et al.[6]	Seq	Sq	88	Cis–Bleo	35	66%	24%	Negative
Le Prise et al.[37]	Seq	Sq	86	Cis–5-FU	20	85%	8%	Negative
Bosset et al.[26]	Seq	Sq	282	Cis	37	78%	12%	Improved DFS only
Apinop et al.[38]	Con	Sq	69	Cis–5-FU	40	74%	12%	Negative
Walsh et al.[39]	Con	Adeno	113	Cis–5-FU	40	90%	10%	Improved OS
Urba et al.[40]	Con	Adeno/Sq	100	Cis–5-FU–Vbl	45	Not reported	Not reported	Negative
Burmeister et al.[41]	Con	Adeno/Sq	256	Cis–5-FU	35	85%	4.6%	Negative
Tepper et al.[43]	Con	Adeno/Sq	56	Cis–5-FU	50.4	87%	0%	Improved OS

*Bleo, bleomycin; Cis, cisplatin; 5-FU, 5-fluorouracil; Vbl, vinblastine.
†DFS, disease-free survival; OS, overall survival.

A recent meta-analysis[45] of both chemotherapy and CRT raises some interesting questions. It included 10 randomised neoadjuvant CRT vs. surgery-alone trials and eight neoadjuvant chemotherapy vs. surgery alone trials. It concluded that the hazard ratio for CRT was 0.81 (corresponding to a 13% absolute difference in survival at 2 years), with similar results for adencarcinoma and squamous carcinoma. The hazard ratio for chemotherapy was 0.90 (corresponding to a 7% absolute difference in survival at 2 years), with a marked difference between a benefit demonstrated for adenocarcinoma and no benefit for squamous carcinoma.

There is rightly a clear separation in future trials for adenocarcinoma and squamous carcinoma. As the trend moves towards squamous cancers being treated with primary CRT, the role of preoperative CRT may be revisited as a means of improving the outcome for patients with adenocarcinoma who can be predicted to still have adverse prognostic features such as a predicted positive circumferential margin, similar to the rectal cancer management philosophy. The undoubted extra toxicity may be justified for this selected group and is infinitely preferable to postoperative treatment. New radiotherapy technology allows more accurate treatment delivery and lower morbidity, and when coupled with higher quality sugery and perioperative care should allow the sort of overall results from CALGB 9781 to be reproduced. Whatever improvements in locoregional treatments are proposed, the highest risk to be faced and addressed with new trials for stage III adenocarcinoma is ultimate systemic relapse. Trials with new biological agents added to standard chemotherapy or selective CRT are likely to be the next step with advance knowledge from their use in the advanced and metastatic disease setting.

At present preoperative CRT should only be considered within the context of a clinical trial.

Definitive radiotherapy and chemoradiotherapy

Surgery as a local treatment modality with neoadjuvant chemotherapy or CRT for stage III disease still remains a gold standard against which new approaches to potentially curative treatment must be compared. However, it is clear that there are long-term survivors in series of definitive non-surgical treatment. With an ageing population it must be remembered that 'inoperable' due to the nature of local disease or comorbidity and performance status does not mean treatment is therefore palliative.

Definitive radiotherapy

With an increasingly elderly population it is not uncommon to be faced with patients who have localised disease on staging, particularly squamous cancers, but who clearly are not candidates for an operation and who because of comorbidity may not tolerate the chemotherapy component of a CRT treatment. There still is a role for radical radiotherapy alone.

Classical quoted figures of survival from radical radiotherapy come from the paper from Earlam and Cunha-Melo.[46] Here mean survival figures of 8489 patients at 1, 2 and 5 years were 18%, 8% and 6% respectively. Approximately 50% of patients were treated with curative intent. Older series tend to be of squamous carcinoma treated with radiotherapy alone. Modern radiotherapy in more selected patients can produce impressive survival results. In a series of 101 patients treated at the Christie Hospital in Manchester[47] between 1985 and 1994, 3- and 5-year survival figures of 27% and 21% respectively were recorded. There was a slightly better survival for adenocarcinoma, but not reaching statistical significance. The majority of tumours (96/101) were of 5 cm or less in length. Importantly, the only significant prognostic factor was the use of diagnostic CT, introduced during the latter part of the study. This was used to plan the radiotherapy and led to an increase in field sizes. The conclusion of the paper was that radiotherapy provided an effective alternative to surgery and that modern radiotherapy planning techniques may improve results.

There is no reason to compromise on staging or treatment planning standards and with modern technology high doses can be given with low morbidity. A selected series[48] of 51 patients 80 years and over with squamous carcinoma treated with 66 Gy of radiotherapy in Japan produced median survival of 30 months and a 3-year survival rate of 39%.

Definitive chemoradiotherapy

The adoption of CRT stems from high response rates and in particular high pCR rates seen in patients going on to resection. There are four randomised trials comparing radiotherapy alone with CRT. Three of these use low doses or low intensity of chemotherapy. A small series of 59 patients from Brazil[49] did not demonstrate a significant survival advantage. The response rates and 5-year survival rates (6% vs. 16%) were better in the CRT arm but at a cost of increased acute toxicity. An important non-randomised series is reported by Coia et al.[50] Treatment was with infusional 5-FU and mitomycin C with 60 Gy of radiotherapy. Patients with early-stage disease are reported separately. The respective 5-year survival and local failure rate, in clinical stages I and II combined, were 30% and 25%. There was no treatment-related mortality, although there was increased acute toxicity (22% grade III and 6% grade IV).

The biggest series with a major impact on treatment patterns has been the RTOG 85-01, Herskovic study.[51] A total of 123 patients were randomised to receive either radiotherapy alone to a dose of 64 Gy or two courses of cisplatin and infusional 5-FU concurrent with 50 Gy of radiotherapy. Two more courses of chemotherapy were scheduled after the completion of the radiotherapy. A summary of the results of the randomised patients is shown in Table 9.2.

In a confirmatory study, 69 non-randomised patients were treated with the CRT protocol and achieved similar results in terms of median survival and a 3-year survival of 26%. The acute toxicity in the combined treatment arm was significantly higher, with notably haematological and renal pathology and mucositis as the major problems. There was no significant difference in the late complication rates. In all, 80% of patients in the combined modality arm received the protocol treatment. The poor overall survival in the radiotherapy-alone control arm remains a question mark against the study.

The high local failure rate of 45% in the Herskovic trial led to the Intergroup study 0122.[52] The dose of radiotherapy was increased to 64.8 Gy and the intensity of the chemotherapy increased in this 45-patient toxicity and survival phase II study. The results showed increased toxicity, with 11% treatment-related deaths as compared with 2% in the Herskovic study. The protocol was not adopted into a phase III study. Another approach to improve local control was to use brachytherapy to intensify the radiotherapy dose to the tumour. Study RTOG 92-07[53] used the 50-Gy external beam and chemotherapy protocol from the Herskovic protocol and added an intraluminal brachytherapy boost with one of two methods of delivery, high dose rate or low dose rate. Six of the 35 patients developed an oesophageal fistula. This toxicity was deemed unacceptable.

Following successful CRT or radiotherapy alone there is a significant rate of benign stricture formation. This ranges from 12%[54] to 25%[50] in more modern studies. However, good swallowing function can be maintained in the majority of patients. Even in those with a benign stricture a full or soft diet in 71% of cases[55] can be maintained by dilations. The treatment of post-CRT benign stricture with stents has not been successful in the author's experience and gives rise to mediastinal pain.

The higher pCR rates seen with CRT, the improved local control rates and altered patterns of failure in the literature have all contributed to CRT being largely adopted as a standard of care. The management of patients with CRT is complex and requires good support from specialist nurses and dieticians and high standards of technical radiotherapy. The risk of morbidity is real but can be overcome. It should be seen as a single integrated modality of therapy rather than two different treatments that happen to be delivered at the same time.

Future directions in definitive chemoradiation

The ability to predict which patients will respond to chemotherapy or CRT would allow greater certainty in a primary non-surgical approach. Molecular markers predicting response to chemotherapy hold some promise.[56–58] Conventional reassessment following treatment, with a negative endoscopic biopsy[35] and CT,[59] appear unreliable. However, the use of a positive surveillance endoscopic biopsy to direct salvage surgery in squamous carcinoma treated with definitive CRT has been reported.[60] Reports of the value of endoscopic ultrasound are more variable, with some showing a good correlation with final pathological stage[61] and others suggesting it is not reliable.[62] There are reports advocating that this failure to reliably predict pCR necessitates resection.[34]

There is increasing evidence to show that PET scanning may be extremely useful in predicting which patients are responding to chemotherapy and CRT.[63] Changes in metabolic activity on PET, 14 days after the start of treatment, appear to be significantly correlated with tumour response and patient survival. The ability to predict response in this way might be an attractive tool to determine if definitive CRT should be continued or a change made to a policy of resection. This would avoid surgical delay and increase morbidity in patients who are unlikely to benefit from chemotherapy or CRT. Such a policy would clearly need validation in a trial setting.

Table 9.2 • Summary of results of the RTOG 85-01 study of Al-Sarraf et al. (1997)[51]

	RT	RT + CT	P value
Median survival (months)	9.3	14.1	
Overall survival (%):			
1-year	34	52	
2-year	10	36	
5-year	0	30	0.0001
Rate distant metastases (%)	37	21	0.0017
2-year local recurrence rate (%)	59	45	0.0125
Overall disease free (%)	11	36	<0.001

CT, chemotherapy; RT, radiotherapy.

Improvements in CRT outcomes are likely to come from refinements in chemotherapy and radiotherapy technique. Results from preoperative phase II studies suggest a steady improvement in pCR rates with more acceptable toxicity. The rates of pCR range from 24%[31] in 1993 to reports of 56%[64] in 1998. Care must be taken in interpreting the literature as pCR rates can vary depending upon whether rates are quoted as intent to treat or of completed resections. Careful staging can ensure that patients with established metastatic disease are appropriately managed. There has been a trend to accept lower standards of staging in non-surgical series. It is important that all patients who are deemed to have a potentially curative therapy have access to comparable staging, including EUS. In the preoperative setting new protocols can be assessed for toxicity and response rates[65] before use in a phase III randomised setting.

Central to improving treatment strategies is an understanding of patterns of treatment failure. An important series of a detailed analysis of CRT has been published from Australia using combined data from Trans-Tasman Radiation Oncology Group studies.[66] This looks at results from 274 patients treated with definitive CRT and 92 patients treated with preoperative CRT. A summary of survival and recurrence patterns is given in Table 9.3. The overall local control rate for definitive CRT is almost 55%, rising to 70% in upper squamous cancers. The striking difference in outcome for these upper cancers includes an apparently lower distant failure rate and improved overall survival. It may be that these tumours are inherently different and respond more like squamous carcinomas of the head and neck. The persisting high distant failure rate in adenocarcinoma treated with CRT and surgery underlines a need for either earlier diagnosis and treatment or improved systemic therapy. There is no doubt that the success of CRT as definitive treatment is determined by similar factors to the outcomes of surgery, namely stage, performance status and the length of the tumour.

There are huge changes in the technology available for radiotherapy treatment. The development of 3-D and conformal radiotherapy treatment planning systems directly linked to spiral CT data allows the shape of radiotherapy fields to be individually tailored to an irregular-shaped target volume. In order for this to be successful, however, reliable imaging techniques are essential, including using EUS[67] and PET[68] to help delineate the gross tumour volume. A reduction in normal tissue damage and so potentially the toxicity of combining therapy will be possible. The ability to define varying dose intensity within a radiotherapy field (intensity-modulated radiotherapy treatment, IMRT) may be helpful in being able to grade the dose between a primary tumour and its associated nodal areas. There is no doubt that even better distributions of dose can be achieved with proton therapy but availability and cost may preclude this being feasible for some years. Improvements in CRT will also come from a better understanding of the effects on normal tissue near the clinical target volume such as heart and lung.

The use of new radiosensitising chemotherapy drugs in combination with radiotherapy may allow some small incremental gains in response rates (oxaliplatin/taxanes/capecitabine) and hence local control. Lastly more attention to the treatment of elective nodal irradiation, perhaps wider fields to a lower dose, may reduce locoregional failure.

The current NCRI study of definitive CRT (SCOPE 1) aims to compare cisplatin and capecitabine with 50 Gy of radiotherapy in the control arm and add the epidermal growth factor receptor (EGFR) monoclonal antibody cetuximab to the investigational arm. There is evidence that one mechanism of radiotherapy resistance is through activation of the EGFR

Table 9.3 • Five-year survival and cumulative incidence of relapse in the study of Denham et al. (2003)[66]

Treatment regimen*	Site	Histology	Number	Survival (%)	Local failure (%)	Distant failure (%)
Def CRT	All	All	274	28.8	42.4	33.5
Def CRT	Upper	Squamous	54	49.2	29.9	26.0
Def CRT	Middle	Squamous	81	24.7	41.8	37.3
Def CRT	Lower	Squamous	68	22.0	44.4	29.2
Def CRT	Lower	Adenocarcinoma	54	18.2	50.7	31.9
CRT + surgery	All	All	92	22.5	28.4	43.2
CRT + surgery	Middle	Squamous	31	26.7	30.3	36.4
CRT + surgery	Lower	Squamous	18	23.7	16.7	44.4
CRT + surgery	Lower	Adenocarcinoma	26	3.8	38.5	57.7

* Def CRT, definitive chemoradiation; CRT + surgery, preoperative chemoradiation + surgery.

pathways and clinical evidence from a randomised trial in squamous cancer of the head and neck of improved local control and overall survival.[69] This study is important in also defining very high radiotherapy technical standards for the UK, ensuring the accuracy of target volume definition and minimising normal tissue morbidity. It is open to both adenocarcinoma and squamous carcinoma selected by multidisciplinary teams as being suitable.

Definitive CRT vs. surgery

Definitive CRT treatments now report good survival figures[51,59] rivalling those of surgery, stage for stage.[70,71]

In squamous carcinoma there seems to be increasing evidence that a policy of primary CRT with surgery as salvage may be the direction for the future.[72]

Many squamous cancers are in the mid and upper oesophagus and their pattern of lymph node spread is less predictable. These areas can be safely treated with CRT with increasing sophistication. For adenocarcinoma, there is a fundamental difficulty in such a policy of primary non-surgical therapy. The stomach and small bowel have more distinct dose-limiting toxicity, and extending radiotherapy fields to cover wider areas below the diaphragm and potential lymph node spread seem likely to produce higher levels of morbidity but may be safely covered by the extent of a surgical resection. Tumours primarily of the lower oesophagus or limited to the gastro-oesophageal junction might be candidates for CRT but target volumes are more difficult and perhaps CRT should be reserved where a surgical approach is ruled out by age, performance status or comorbidity. Tumours with significant extension to the cardia or primarily of the stomach will require surgery.

There have been few trials that allow a direct comparison between a primary CRT policy and surgery and indeed CRT studies may have had a selection bias against them. The results of CRT alone tend to have 5-year survival figures generally comparable to those seen in Tables 9.2 and 9.3, of the order of 30% overall, which are close to surgical figures. Squamous cancers in particular of the mid and upper thirds have better outcomes. It does allow CRT to be considered as a viable option to chemotherapy and surgery for adenocarcinoma and as primary treatment for squamous carcinoma.

There are two trials that address the additional value of surgery after CRT and would give some support to a selective approach to its use, particularly in squamous carcinoma.

In a French study patients were assessed after induction CRT using 5-FU and cisplatin.[73] If they had achieved an objective response they were randomised (295 of 455 patients) to carry on with CRT or go to surgery. There was no significant difference between the 2-year survival rates for patients who had surgery (33.6%) and those who had CRT alone (39.8%). There were more early deaths in the surgery arm but CRT required more dilatations and stents.

In a German trial[74] 177 patients with T3 or T4 squamous carcinoma were randomised to receive CRT + surgery or CRT alone. The rate of response to initial CRT was the same for both arms. There was a strong trend towards improved local tumour control in the arm with surgery. In responding patients the 3-year survival (45% and 44% respectively) was equivalent in both arms, whereas in non-responding patients the rates were 18% and 11%. The 3-year survival rate improved to 35% in non-responding patients undergoing complete tumour resection, implying that a subgroup of non-responding patients may benefit from surgery as an elective salvage procedure. Longer-term results confirm no clear survival difference between a surgical versus CRT approach. It did show a clinical response to induction chemotherapy may be a valuable surrogate for predicting prognosis.

There is evidence collected from the literature[75] that selected salvage surgery is possible after CRT failure with acceptable operative mortality of 11.4% and 5-year survival rates of 25–35%. Clearly such a high-risk policy should be after CT-PET restaging.

It may be then that for squamous carcinoma only selected groups of patients may benefit from surgery.

Small-cell oesophageal cancer

Small-cell oesophageal cancer (SCOC) is a rare (up to 2.5% of primary oesophageal cancer) entity with a poor prognosis due to a high rate of metastatic disease. It thus requires a distinct approach to management with similarities to primary small-cell lung cancer (SCLC), which has similar histological features.

The literature is made up of small retrospective series from major institutions. It tends to have male preponderance and occur in the mid and lower oesophagus. Series vary but most, even with staging that would be considered less than optimum today, have a majority of patients with metastases at presentation. The median survival of untreated metastatic patients is less than 3 months.

The treatment of SCOC is dependent on a separation between limited disease and extensive disease. Table 9.4 shows the outcomes in two of the larger and most recent series[76,77] in the literature. Both have good references and discussion.

Table 9.4 • Outcomes of small-cell oesophageal cancer series

Date	Series	Patient numbers	Median survival LD	Median survival ED	Overall median survival
2007	Hudson et al.[76]	16	24.4	9.1	13.2
2008	Ku et al.[77]	25	22.5	8.5	19.8

ED, extensive disease; LD, limited disease.

The treatment of patients with extensive disease is palliative chemotherapy based on etoposide- and platinum-containing regimens if the performance status allows. Response rates to treatment are high and there is definite improvement in overall survival, but outcomes are universally poor with median survivals of 8–11 months.

Due to the very high rate of systemic relapse, limited stage disease requires primary treatment with chemotherapy, again based on etoposide- and platinum-containing regimes. There is a role for consolidation treatment to enhance local control and to prevent local symptomatic progression. There are surgical series with good local control rates, but the majority of series concentrate on radiotherapy (doses up to 50 Gy) or chemoradiotherapy as would be considered for SCLC, thus avoiding the mortality risk and morbidity of surgery.

Local control rates with surgery are high but overall prognosis poor, with survival dictated by metastatic disease and median survivals in the range of 15–24 months. There is no literature on prophylactic cranial irradiation, which has been shown to be an advantage in SCLC after successful systemic and local therapy.

Gastric cancer

Potentially curative treatment

Perioperative adjuvant chemotherapy

The goal of systemic therapy for gastric cancer is to reduce the late patterns of failure following successful surgical resection. The pattern of spread includes nodal and liver metastases. A significant proportion of patients will fail with intra-abdominal, peritoneal or omental disease. Extended lymphadenectomy has been advocated to improve the local/regional control rates. Chemotherapy, either systemic or intraperitoneal, has been used to try to reduce the incidence of widespread recurrence. Despite encouraging results of chemotherapy in advanced disease, proof of a benefit for adjuvant postoperative chemotherapy has been elusive. Standard approaches have been with postoperative chemotherapy but

more recent studies have looked at a combination of preoperative and postoperative treatment.

There have been a wide range of randomised adjuvant chemotherapy trials. Regimens with significant activity in the advanced disease setting have been tested since the 1980s. There are variations in the surgery used, the timing of the start of chemotherapy and the toxicity, which all make interpretation and comparisons difficult.

An early trial using 5-FU and the nitrosourea compound methyl-CCNU showed promise. In the Gastrointestinal Tumour Study Group trial,[78] a significant benefit became apparent 2 years post-surgery in 142 randomised patients. The 5-year survival was 50% vs. 31% in favour of the chemotherapy arm. These results were not, however, confirmed in two subsequent studies[79,80] using the same regimen, which together included 314 patients. A regimen using a combination of 5-FU, doxorubicin and mitomycin C (FAM) was seen to be active in advanced disease[81] with a good response rate (35%), including 5% complete responses. When used as adjuvant treatment, however, no survival benefit was seen.[82,83]

A large randomised trial of 2873 patients, reported by Hattori et al. in 1986, compared 5-FU with mitomycin C against mitomycin C alone.[84] Again, no difference was seen in overall survival. New orally active prodrugs of 5-FU are now available and have been seen to be active in gastrointestinal cancer. This form of chemotherapy has obvious attractions as an adjuvant therapy in terms of patient acceptability and the scope for longer duration of therapy. The drug tegafur is absorbed orally and is converted to 5-FU in the liver. A combination with uracil, acting to potentiate the 5-FU, is called UFT. Recent trials have attempted to make use of these drugs. In a trial reported by Nakajima et al.,[85] 579 patients who had undergone a curative resection with serosa-negative gastric cancer were randomised to have no further treatment or intravenous mitomycin and 5-FU immediately after surgery for 3 weeks. Then oral UFT was given for 18 months. There was no difference in survival. The survival of the T1 patients was 92–95% in the two arms. One of the conclusions was that these patients can be excluded from future trials as their outlook was already so good. In an attempt to use the same approach in Western patients of AJCCC stage III, Circera et al.[86] used a large single dose of mitomycin and 3 months of tegafur. The reported improvement in overall 5-year survival of 46% in the control group and 56% in the treated group (*P* = 0.04), however, is open to question because a non-stratified sealed envelope randomisation was used and there was an imbalance in node-negative patients in the groups.

Three meta-analyses exist. The first,[87] in 1993, excluded trials before 1980 and only included those with a surgery-only control arm. The conclusion was that there was a small benefit, with a common odds ratio of 0.77 (95% CI 0.65–0.88) in favour of adjuvant chemotherapy. The second, published in 1999,[88] found 13 trials meeting the eligibility criteria. The odds ratio for death in the treated group was 0.80 (95% CI 0.66–0.97). There was thus a small survival benefit of borderline significance which was more marked in trials with greater than two-thirds of patients having node-positive disease. The third,[89] pooling data from 3658 patients, again concludes that there is a small survival advantage but, given the limitations of a literature-based meta-analysis, reasons that adjuvant chemotherapy should still be considered investigational. Thus there is probably a small benefit from adjuvant chemotherapy for some patients.

However, many of the regimes in the older studies have low response rates (10–30%) in advanced disease, compared with the higher expected response of more modern regimes such as ECF.

The MRC STO2 (MAGIC) trial[22] was opened in 1994 and aimed to recruit 500 patients testing the role of three courses of ECF before and after resection in operable gastric cancer. The results suggest a significant downstaging effect of the chemotherapy.

As the MRC OEO2 neoadjuvant oesophageal trial was completed, the eligibility criteria were widened in 1999 to include adenocarcinoma of the lower oesophagus. The type of resection was left to the discretion of the participating surgeon and the staging was relatively permissive by modern standards. The arms of the study were well balanced and included 74% stomach, 14% oesophageal and 12% junctional cancers. Toxicity of the chemotherapy was acceptable but only 40% of patients received both cycles of postoperative treatment. In fact the majority of resections were at least D1, with 40%

having a D2. The proportion deemed to have had a potentially curative resection was 10% higher with chemotherapy (79% vs. 69%). There was a significant effect on tumour size, T stage and nodal status. Recent results with a median follow-up of >3 years have demonstrated an improvement in overall survival (hazard ratio of 0.75, *P* = 0.009), with 5-year survival rates of 36% for chemotherapy and surgery vs. 23% for surgery alone. Progression-free survival was also significantly prolonged.

It is thus reasonable to adopt a standard approach using chemotherapy for tumours other than early-stage gastric cancer.

The current NCRI study ST03 or 'MAGIC 2' compares three cycles of pre- and postoperative ECX with the addition of bevacizumab and three cycles of maintainence bevacizumab, a humanised monoclonal antibody against vascular endothelial growth factor (VEGF). High levels of VEGF expression in gastric adenocarcinoma have been shown to correlate with poor 5-year survival rates, lymph node metastasis and vascular invasion.

Intraperitoneal chemotherapy

The pattern of peritoneal and hepatic recurrence in gastric cancer makes the early use of intraperitoneal chemotherapy attractive. The most positive trial is from Japan[90] using mitomycin C adsorbed onto activated charcoal, acting as a delayed-release preparation. Fifty patients with serosal involvement were randomised to immediate treatment or observation. A highly significant difference in survival at 2 years was seen (68.6% vs. 26.9%), with the treatment group maintaining its advantage at 3 years. The treatment was reported to be well tolerated. However, when an attempt was made to repeat these results, in an Austrian multicentre study,[91] serious toxicity caused the trial to be suspended. A significantly higher postoperative complication rate (35% vs. 16%) and 60-day mortality rate (11% vs. 2%) were seen in the treatment arm of the study. No benefits were found in overall or recurrence-free survival.

Postoperative chemoradiotherapy

Radiotherapy has not been routinely used in the management of stomach cancer. However, local recurrence can be a significant problem. The stomach and nodal areas are close to many crucial normal tissues with dose-limiting susceptibility to toxicity, such as kidney, spinal cord and small bowel.

In the British Stomach Cancer Group trial[83] postoperative radiotherapy was one of the arms of the study. The other arms were FAM chemotherapy and a control surgery-only group. There was no difference in survival but the local recurrence rate was significantly better (54% surgery vs. 32% with radiotherapy; $P < 0.01$).

The American Intergroup INT 0116 (SWOG 9008) study (commonly referred to as the Macdonald study) has produced important results. Postoperative CRT has been reported to show a significant benefit to survival following gastric resection.[42]

The regimen consisted of 5-FU–leucovorin (folinic acid) given in the first and last weeks of radiotherapy (45 Gy) and two 5-day courses of 5-FU–leucovorin given monthly. With a median follow-up of 3.3 years both the disease-free survival (49% vs. 32%) and overall survival (52% vs. 41%) were improved in the CRT arm. There was some significant haematological and gastrointestinal morbidity. However, the treatment-related mortality was only 1%. The need for great care in the technical quality and placement of the radiotherapy was apparent. However, a significant proportion of the patients (54%) had only a D0 resection and the survival in the surgery-alone arm was relatively poor (41% 3-year survival). It is possible that the CRT is making up for less than adequate surgery, and may not translate into routine practice where more extensive surgery is undertaken. It is the most obvious source of criticism of the trial. However, multivariate analysis did not find the 'D level' to be a significant prognostic factor. However, in a subsequent paper,[92] using a different surgical quality assurance measure for the likelihood of undissected disease (the Maruyama Index), the group concluded that surgical undertreatment clearly undermines survival. Major concerns about the toxicity and chemotherapy used and the poor radiotherapy technique are being addressed, which should significantly reduce the potential for long-term morbidity and make the most of sophisticated IMRT and radiotherapy planning techniques. Despite criticisms postoperative CRT has been patchily adopted throughout the world.

Thus there are now two major trials demonstrating improved survival with the addition of perioperative therapy in gastric cancer. One study (MAGIC)[22] involves pre- and postpperative chemotherapy, and the other (INT 0116)[42] the use of postoperative CRT. Whilst one can argue the relative merits of each approach, one certain conclusion is that for all but early-stage tumours surgery alone is no longer a standard of care.

Palliative chemotherapy

Squamous carcinoma of the oesophagus

Cisplatin-containing combination chemotherapy is the standard for the treatment of advanced and recurrent squamous carcinoma. The indications for use are limited by the relative infrequency of the disease, and in particular the age and performance status of patients requiring palliation. Very often the indication to improve symptoms and quality of life are local, and local therapy with a stent or radiotherapy will be adequate. However, good response rates of the order of 35% can be achieved with cisplatin and 4- or 5-day 5-FU infusion.[93] Response duration is variable and can range from 3 to 6 months. Consideration should be given to consolidation palliative radiotherapy after successful chemotherapy to improve local control where recurrent growth may produce symptoms for patients with a better performance status and expectation of life. There is some evidence that the improved response rates seen with PVI 5-FU in adenocarcinoma can be achieved in squamous carcinoma.[14] New agents such as paclitaxel are clearly active as single agents but have yet to demonstrate their clear superiority in combination regimens. Some results are promising, with response rates nearer 50%.[94]

Adenocarcinoma of the oesophagus and stomach

Whilst earlier literature tends to report activity in pure gastric cancer, the changing pattern of disease has meant that more recent reports deal with oesophagogastric cancer. The single agents most commonly used in the treatment of advanced oesophagogastric cancer include 5-FU, methotrexate, mitomycin C, the anthracyclines doxorubicin and epirubicin, cisplatin and etoposide. More recently the oral 5-FU prodrugs such as UFT and capecitabine, the taxane drugs, irinotecan and gemcitabine all feature in new phase II studies. Biological agents such as EGFR monoclonal antibodies represent a new potential means of improving outcomes.

There are early randomised clinical trials of palliative chemotherapy vs. best supportive care which clearly show improved survival (8–12 months chemotherapy vs. 3–5 months best supportive care).[95–97]

The FAM regimen (5-FU, doxorubicin and mitomycin) initially seemed to have a high response rate of 40%.[98] However, in the setting of a randomised trial by the North Central Cancer Treatment Group, it seemed to be no better than 5-FU alone.[99] In an attempt to modulate the activity of 5-FU within the FAM regimen, high-dose methotrexate was given 1 hour before the 5-FU in the FAMTX regimen (fluorouracil, doxorubicin and methotrexate). Klein produced impressive results in a study of 100 patients.[100] The response rate was 58%, with a complete remission rate of 12%. There were only 3% treatment-related deaths and a long-term survival rate of 6%. The response rate seen in subsequent studies was slightly lower but still confirmed acceptable toxicity. This regimen has now been tested against other combinations. A randomised EORTC trial[101] with 208 evaluable patients demonstrated its superiority against FAM. Median survival was better (42 weeks vs. 29 weeks; $P = 0.004$) with 41% and 9% of the FAMTX patients alive at 1 and 2 years respectively, compared with 22% and 0% for FAM patients. The EAP regimen (etoposide, doxorubicin and cisplatin) was found to have similar survivals, similar overall response rates but lower complete remission rates and was significantly more toxic.[102] A recent EORTC trial[103] has compared three regimens: FAMTX, ELF (etoposide, leucovorin and bolus 5-FU) and FUP (infusional 5-FU and cisplatin) in 399 randomised patients. There was no significant difference in median survivals between the regimens. The response rates were lower than in some previous trials (ELF 9%, FUP 20%, FAMTX 12%) but this trial had tight objective response criteria and required measurable disease. The conclusion is that they all produce modest response with comparable survival and toxicity.

The ECF regimen developed at The Royal Marsden Hospital was shown to have high activity against advanced oesophagogastric cancer.[13] It has become widely used in the UK and is well tolerated. Its status as the current gold standard was confirmed in a multicentre randomised trial of ECF against FAMTX.[104] A total of 274 patients with adenocarcinoma or undifferentiated carcinoma of the oesophagus, oesophagogastric junction or stomach were treated.

Patients were predominantly of good performance status with a median age of 60 years. The overall objective response rate was 45% in the ECF arm and 21% in the FAMTX arm ($P = 0.0002$). The response of locally advanced disease to ECF has previously been shown to be higher than in metastatic disease.[13] This was confirmed in both arms of the trial (56% ECF vs. 23% FAMTX). Of the 121 patients receiving ECF, 10 were able to undergo a resection due to improved status, six of whom

remain disease free. There were three cases of histological pCR. Only 5% of patients had progression whilst on either chemotherapy regimen.

The 2-year survival figures and median survival were 14% and 8.7 months for ECF and 5% and 6.1 months for FAMTX respectively ($P = 0.03$)

The ECF results have opened up a grey area in locally advanced gastric and junctional cancer management. Whilst a patient may not be operable, or it may be deemed inadvisable to operate due to the extent of disease at presentation, it may be possible to consider a potentially curative resection in some cases after chemotherapy. The intent of treatment may therefore need to be revisited by close reassessment after chemotherapy. This emphasises the need for teamwork between the surgeon and oncologist within a multidisciplinary setting.

In a study from Leeds[105] of advanced upper gastrointestinal cancer patients, oral UFT and leucovorin were substituted for the PVI 5-FU in ECF in an attempt to create a more practical, acceptable and cheaper alternative (the ECU regimen) without the need for central lines and pumps. In this dose-escalation pilot study 30 patients were treated. Toxicity was acceptable. Of 20 assessable patients, nine of the 15 with gastro-oesophageal cancer had an objective response and two of these were complete radiological responses.

The NCRI REAL2 trial[23] was designed to address some practical problems that surrounded delivery of the gold standard ECF regime. Infusional 5-FU has problems associated with Hickman lines, particularly thrombosis and infection. Cisplatin causes renal toxicity and requires prehydration and inpatient admission for higher doses. It tested the toxicity and response rates of oxaliplatin as a substitute for cisplatin, and of capecitabine (an oral fluoropyrimidine) as a substitute for infusional 5-FU in a randomised 2 × 2 study based on statistics of non-inferiority against ECF.

The REAL2 results demonstrated that oxaliplatin can be substituted for cisplatin with less renal toxicity and neutropenia and that capecitabine is a valid substitution for 5-FU. Although a secondary end-point, there was a significant improvement in median survival for the EOX (epirubicin–oxaliplatin–capecitabine) regimen compared to the ECF regime (11.2 months vs. 9.9 months). There was no significant difference in responses rates between regimens and a response rate of 40.7% in the ECF arm.

The EOX regimen has been taken forward as the control arm in the next REAL3 study with the addition of panitumumab (an EGFR antibody) in the investigational arm. Other attempts to improve treatment outcomes using the addition of docetaxel to cisplatin and 5-FU have uncovered high potential toxicities with neutropenia, treatment withdrawal rates of nearly 50% due to grade 3 and 4 toxicity and no improvement in response rates or survival, raising a question as to whether a plateau has been nearly reached with conventional approaches to chemotherapy.[106] New biological agents possibly bring new distinctions between different agents even within antibodies to the same receptor and very different response rates of gastric and gastro-esophageal/oesophageal cancers.[107] This emphasises the need for good tissue collection and analysis in parallel with clinical studies.

The selection of patients who are likely to benefit from palliative chemotherapy may be helped by the development of prognostic scoring methods. One study[108] has demonstrated that performance status, liver metastases, peritoneal metastases and alkaline phosphatase can be used to separate different risk groups. Problems in the literature with myelosuppression, and in particular toxic deaths, may be avoided by the use of growth factors to reduce the incidence of neutropenic sepsis. Many of the problems of severe emesis have already been improved by the use of 5-HT$_3$ antiemetic drugs.

Second-line chemotherapy using taxanes and irinotecan has been reported, with some evidence of worthwhile activity. In practice, however, great care will need to be taken in the selection of suitable patients, and such treatment should really only be undertaken within the context of a trial.

The success in palliative chemotherapy has brought about problems and patterns of recurrence which have not been common before. Brain metastases and bone metastases are increasingly seen. Palliative radiotherapy can be helpful in controlling symptoms.

Palliative radiotherapy

External beam radiotherapy

The whole literature surrounding radiotherapy in a palliative setting is poor. Nonetheless, the role of radiotherapy is important. There are many instances where patients have local symptoms from metastatic disease. With a high proportion of patients presenting with T3N1 disease it is not surprising that many will fail despite more complex and aggressive therapy. The pattern of metastases seems already to be changing in that patients are living to get metastases in brain, bone and skin as well as recurrent nodal masses. These clinical problems are amenable to short fractionated radiotherapy, which provides good symptomatic relief.

The role of external beam radiotherapy to treat dysphagia has changed with the ready availability of oesophageal stents. Radiotherapy can be very effective in relieving dysphagia but it can take weeks to accomplish this, and it can even temporarily worsen symptoms with radiation oesophagitis. The role of radiotherapy following successful stent placement is unproven. A UK trial has been proposed, largely to explore the possibility of improvements in survival and symptom-free survival. The attraction is in achieving a measure of local disease control and in treating the mediastinum. There is also an intermediate group of patients with good performance status and relatively localised disease who are clearly not appropriate for potentially curative treatment. Some short CRT regimes or primary chemotherapy with consolidation radiotherapy have been used, with some suggestion of improved results. This group of patients deserves greater study to optimise palliation.

There is a major difference between the fractionation regimens used in the USA and in the UK. 'Palliative' doses of 40–60 Gy in 4–6 weeks are quoted in the US literature. These are in the radical dose range and are felt to be inappropriate for UK practice, where doses of 20–30 Gy in 1 or 2 weeks are more likely to be used. These can be combined with brachytherapy. Good resolution of tumour and symptom relief in a majority of patients has been reported.[109] Often, however, whichever palliative technique is used first, other modalities have a role for patients with longer survival, to maintain swallowing.

Brachytherapy

Brachytherapy involves the placement of a high-dose-rate radioactive source, usually iridium-192, down the oesophagus in proximity to the tumour. The aim is to get direct tumour cell kill, thereby relieving dysphagia, or in the case of its use as a boost to external beam radiotherapy, to achieve an increased dose to the tumour with minimal dose to surrounding normal tissues. It does not require a general anaesthetic and can be done as a day-case procedure. Occasionally placement of a nasogastric guide tube is required under endoscopic vision. Pagliero and Rowlands[110] describe a single dose of 15 Gy with a response rate of about 60% measured at 6 weeks from treatment. It can be repeated in cases of symptomatic relapse.

The optimum dose of brachytherapy has been addressed in a randomised trial using three schedules.[111] Three doses and schedules were tested in 172 patients with advanced oesophageal cancer These were 12 Gy/two fractions (A), 16 Gy/two fractions (B) and 18 Gy/three fractions (C).

Patients were assessed for relief of dysphagia and survival. Dose and tumour length were found to be significant for survival on multivariate analysis.

Brachytherapy dose had a significant effect on tumour control. Overall survival for the whole group was 19.4% at 1 year.

The survival by group, although not statistically significant, suggests a trend towards better outcomes with the higher dose schedules of brachytherapy (at 12 months: A = 9.8%, B = 22.5%, C = 35.3%).[111]

There are good published guidelines[112] for the use of brachytherapy, taking into the account the potential wide range of applications for this technique.

A randomised multicentre trial[113] with 209 patients has shown that single-dose brachytherapy gave better long-term relief of dysphagia than metal stent placement with equivalent costs. The time to symptom relief was, however, worse for brachytherapy but there were fewer complications.

Future strategies

In order to achieve the best outcomes for patients, assessment, staging and treatment need to be closely coordinated and integrated in a multidisciplinary setting. Poor outcomes from single-modality therapy and increasing evidence of the value of a selective use of multiple modalities will be powerful drivers towards higher quality and more centralised services. Site specialist clinicians and support services can only meet demands for quality assurance in all possible modalities of treatment with appropriate resources and infrastructure. The essential role of high-quality radiology, including EUS, and expert pathology cannot be underestimated. The routine use of PET, both as diagnostic tool to pick up early metastatic disease, but also to predict response to non-surgical treatment, seems likely to become a key decision-making tool. Support services such as specialist nursing and dietetic services are particularly important in this area of disease management.

If the lessons from past trials are to be learned, namely the poor and variable results in control arm treatments, attention will have to be paid to rigorous quality assurance within each area of defined treatment. This will aid the process of new high-quality research trials aiming to develop new treatment strategies.

As chemoradiotherapy emerges as an alternative to radical surgery, particularly in squamous carcinoma, accurately predicting and defining those patients who will achieve good remission prospectively is important, as is the identification of patients who require salvage surgery. New molecular markers may be important tools for the future.

The need for quick assessment by site specialist teams, able to offer a full range of treatments, ranging from complex combined modality therapy all the way through to quick and efficient palliative care, is only likely to be achieved by teamwork and some degree of reorganisation. Ultimately, a greater improved understanding of the epidemiology of these diseases will be necessary to allow the identification of disease at a far earlier stage. The current presentation with predominantly nodal and advanced stage disease is likely to limit the improvements that are possible with existing treatments.

The need for continued randomised trials is important. Major centres with high-quality assurance and good research support can recruit sufficient patients to answer major questions that are important to improve the outcome for these diseases.

Key points

- Chemotherapy and radiotherapy have a major role, integrated with surgery, in the treatment of oesophageal and gastric cancer. Poor outcomes from single-modality therapy and increasing evidence of the value of a selective use of multiple modalities are powerful drivers towards higher quality and more centralised services.
- Effective staging is essential as surgery alone is now indicated only for early-stage disease.
- The benefit of preoperative radiotherapy in oesophageal cancer seems to be small.
- Preoperative chemotherapy has been demonstrated to improve survival and is accepted in the UK as a standard of care in oesophageal cancer. Cisplatin–5-FU combinations seem to be active in both squamous carcinoma and adenocarcinoma.

- Postoperative radiotherapy has a possible role in selected cases of oesophageal cancer (e.g. pathological stage III squamous cell carcinoma). The justification is less clear for adenocarcinoma outside the context of a clinical trial.
- An updated Cochrane review of 11 randomised trials concludes that there was a 21% increase in survival at 3 years with neoadjuvant chemotherapy prior to oesophageal resection, but that statistical significance was not reached until 5 years.
- There is good evidence that pCR rates are significantly higher with chemoradiotherapy (CRT) than with radiotherapy or chemotherapy given alone. CRT achieves enhanced local therapy coupled with a systemic benefit.
- The current approach in the UK is to concentrate on preoperative chemotherapy rather than CRT for adenocarcinoma. At present preoperative CRT should only be considered within the context of a clinical trial.
- Surgery remains a gold standard for local treatment against which new approaches to potentially curative treatment must be compared.
- Definitive CRT does provide an alternative to surgery in localised oesophageal cancer.
- In squamous carcinoma there is good evidence that a policy of primary CRT is a sustainable strategy (with or without surgical salvage) with equivalent results to surgery.
- The overall local control rate for definitive CRT is 70% in upper-third squamous cancers, for which it is presently the treatment of choice.
- The ability to predict which patients will respond to chemotherapy or CRT would allow greater certainty in a primary non-surgical approach.
- Better outcomes in gastric cancer can be achieved for all but early-stage tumours with the addition of chemotherapy to surgery (MAGIC).
- The American Intergroup postoperative CRT study has been reported to show a significant benefit to survival following gastric resection. However, it is possible that the CRT is only making up for less than adequate surgery and may not translate into routine practice where appropriate radical surgery is undertaken.
- Chemotherapy and radiotherapy have a major role in the palliative treatment of oesophageal and gastric cancer.
- The UK ECF regimen shows high activity against advanced oesophagogastric cancer but new derivatives such as EOX will be easier to deliver.
- The selection of patients who are likely to benefit from palliative chemotherapy may be helped by the development of prognostic scoring methods.

References

1. Bartels HE, Stein HJ, Siewert JR. Preoperative risk analysis and postoperative mortality of oesophagectomy for resectable oesophageal cancer. Br J Surg 1998; 85:840–4.

2. Nigro ND, Seydel HG, Considine B et al. Combined preoperative radiation and chemotherapy for squamous cell carcinoma of the anal canal. Cancer 1983; 51:1826–9.

3. Northover JM. Epidermoid cancer of the anus – the surgeon retreats. J R Soc Med 1991; 84:389–90.

4. Swedish Rectal Cancer Trial. Improved survival with preoperative radiotherapy in resectable rectal cancer. N Engl J Med 1997; 336:980–7.

5. Gignoux M, Roussel A, Paillot B et al. The value of preoperative radiotherapy in esophageal cancer: results of the EORTC. World J Surg 1987; 11:426–32.

6. Nygaard K, Hagen S, Hansen HS et al. Pre-operative radiotherapy prolongs survival in operable esophageal carcinoma: a randomized, multicentre study of pre-operative radiotherapy and chemotherapy. The Second Scandinavian Trial in esophageal cancer. World J Surg 1992; 16:1104–10.

7. Arnott SJ, Duncan W, Kerr GR et al. Low-dose preoperative radiotherapy for carcinoma of the oesophagus: results of a randomized clinical trial. Radiother Oncol 1992; 24:108–13.

8. Arnott SJ, Duncan W, Gignoux M et al. Preoperative radiotherapy in esophageal carcinoma: A meta-analysis using individual patient data (Oesophageal Cancer Collaborative Group). Int J Radiat Oncol Biol Phys 1998; 41:579–83.

9. Teniere P, Hay J, Fingethut A et al. Postoperative radiation therapy does not increase survival after curative resection for squamous carcinoma of the middle and lower oesophagus as shown by a multi-center controlled trial. Surg Gynaecol Obstet 1991; 173:123–30.

10. Fok M, Sham JST, Choy D et al. Postoperative radiotherapy for carcinoma of the esophagus: a prospective randomized controlled trial. Surgery 1993; 113:138–47.

11. Xiao ZF, Yang ZY, Liang J et al. Value of radiotherapy after radical surgery for esophageal carcinoma: a report of 495 patients. Ann Thorac Surg 2003; 75:331–6.

12. Schlag PM. Randomized trial of preoperative chemotherapy of squamous cell cancer of the esophagus. Arch Surg 1992; 127:1446–50.

13. Bamias A, Hill ME, Cunningham D et al. Epirubicin, cisplatin and protracted venous infusion of 5-fluorouracil for esophagogastric adenocarcinoma. Cancer 1996; 77:1978–85.

14. Andreyev HJN, Norman AR, Cunningham D et al. Squamous oesophageal cancer can be downstaged using protracted venous infusion of 5-fluorouracil with epirubicin and cisplatin (ECF). Eur J Cancer 1995; 31A:2209–14.

15. Roth JA, Pass HI, Flanagan MM et al. Randomized clinical trial of preoperative and postoperative adjuvant chemotherapy with cisplatin, vindesine and bleomycin for carcinoma of the esophagus. J Thorac Cardiovasc Surg 1988; 96:242–8.

16. Bhansali MS, Vaidya JS, Bhatt RG et al. Chemotherapy for carcinoma of the oesophagus: a comparison of evidence from meta-analyses of randomized trials and of historical control studies. Ann Oncol 1996; 7:355–9.

17. Kok TC, Lanschot JV, Siersema PD et al. for the Rotterdam Esophageal Tumor Study Group. Neoadjuvant chemotherapy in operable esophageal squamous cell cancer: final report of a phase III multicenter randomized controlled trial. Proc Am Soc Clin Oncol 1997; 16:A277.

18. Kelsen DP, Ginsberg R, Pajak TF et al. Chemotherapy followed by surgery compared with surgery alone for localized esophageal cancer. N Engl J Med 1998; 339:1979–84.

19. Medical Research Council Oesophageal Cancer Working Party. Surgical resection with or without preoperative chemotherapy in oesophageal cancer: a randomised controlled trial. Lancet 2002; 359:1727–33.

20. Allum WH, Fogaty PJ, Stenning SP et al. Long term results of the MRC OEO2 randomized trial of sur-gery with or without preoperative chemotherapy in resectable esophageal cancer. Proc ASCO GI Cancer Symp 2008; Abstr. 9.

21. Malthaner R, Fenlon D. Preoperative chemo-therapy for resectable thoracic esophageal cancer (Cochrane review). In: The Cochrane Library, Issue 2. Chichester: John Wiley, 2004.

22. Cunningham D, Allum WH, Stenning SP et al. Perioperative chemotherapy versus surgery alone for resectable gastroesophageal cancer. N Engl J Med 2006; 355:11–20.

23. Cunningham D, Starling N, Rao S et al. Capecitabine and oxaliplatin for advanced esophagogastric cancer. N Engl J Med 2008; 358:36–46.

24. Geh IJ, Crellin AM, Glynne-Jones R. A review of the role of preoperative (neoadjuvant) chemoradio-therapy in oesophageal carcinoma. Br J Surg 2001; 88:338–56.

25. Urba SG, Orringer MB, Perez-Tamayo C et al. Con-current preoperative chemotherapy and radiation therapy in localized esophageal adenocarcinoma. Cancer 1992; 69:285–91.

26. Bosset JF, Gignoux M, Triboulet JP et al. Chemoradiotherapy followed by surgery compared with surgery alone in squamous-cell cancer of the esophagus. N Engl J Med 1997; 337:161–7.

27. MacKean J, Burmeister BH, Lamb DS et al. Concurrent chemoradiation for oesophageal cancer: factors influencing myelotoxicity. Aust Radio 1996; 40:424–9.

28. Minsky BD, Neuberg D, Kelsen DP et al. Final report of Intergroup trial 0122 (ECOG PE-289, RTOG 90-12): phase II trial of neoadjuvant chemotherapy plus concurrent chemotherapy and high-dose radiation for squamous cell carcinoma of the esophagus. Int J Radiat Oncol Biol Phys 1999; 43:517–23.

29. Bartels HE, Stein HJ, Siewert JR. Tracheobronchial lesions following oesophagectomy: prevalence, pre-disposing factors and outcome. Br J Surg 1998; 85:403–6.

30. Mandard AM, Dalibard F, Mandard JC et al. Pathologic assessment of tumor regression after preoperative chemoradiotherapy of esophageal carcinoma. Cancer 1994; 73:2680–6.

31. Forastiere AA, Orringer MB, Perez-Tamayo C et al. Preoperative chemoradiation followed by transhi-atal esophagectomy for carcinoma of the esopha-gus: final report. J Clin Oncol 1993; 11:1118–23.

32. Smithers BM, Devitt P, Jamieson GG et al. A combined modality approach to the management of oesopha-geal cancer. Eur J Surg Oncol 1997; 23:219–23.

33. Vogel SB, Mendenhall WM, Sombeck MD et al. Downstaging of esophageal cancer after preopera-tive radiation and chemotherapy. Ann Surg 1995; 221:685–95.

34. Bates BA, Detterbeck FC, Bernard SA et al. Con-current radiation therapy and chemotherapy

followed by esophagectomy for localized esophageal carcinoma. J Clin Oncol 1996; 14:156–63.

35. Triboulet JP, Amrouni H, Guillem P et al. Long-term results of resected esophageal cancer with complete remission to pre-operative chemoradiation. Ann Chir 1998; 52:503–8.

36. Reynolds JV, Muldoon C, Hollywood D et al. Long-term outcomes following neoadjuvant chemoradiotherapy for oesophageal cancer. Ann Surg 2007; 245:707–16.

37. Le Prise E, Etienne PL, Meunier B et al. A randomized study of chemotherapy, radiation therapy, and surgery versus surgery for localized squamous cell carcinoma of the esophagus. Cancer 1994; 73:1779–84.

38. Apinop C, Puttisak P, Preecha N. A prospective study of combined therapy in esophageal cancer. Hepatogastroenterology 1994; 41:391–3.

39. Walsh TN, Noonan N, Hollywood D et al. A comparison of multimodal therapy and surgery for esophageal adenocarcinoma. N Engl J Med 1996; 335:462–7.

40. Urba S, Orringer M, Turrisi A et al. A randomized trial comparing surgery (S) to preoperative concomitant chemoradiation plus surgery in patients (pts) with resectable esophageal cancer (CA): updated analysis. Proc Am Soc Clin Oncol 1997; 16:277.

41. Burmeister BH, Smithers BM, Fitzgerald L et al. A randomised phase III trial of preoperative chemoradiation followed by surgery (CR-S) versus surgery alone (S) for localized resectable cancer of the esophagus. Proc Am Soc Clin Oncol 2002; 21:518.

42. Macdonald JS, Smalley S, Benedetti J et al. SWOG; ECOG; RTOG; CALGB; NCCTG. Postoperative combined radiation and chemotherapy improves disease-free survival (DFS) and overall survival (OS) in resected adenocarcinoma of the stomach and GE junction. Results of Intergroup Study INT-0116 (SWOG 9008). Proc Am Soc Clin Oncol 2000; 19:A1.

43. Tepper J, Krasna MJ, Niedzwiecki D et al. Phase III trial of trimodality therapy with cisplatin; fluorouracil, radiotherapy, and surgery compared with surgery alone for esophageal cancer: CALGB 9781. J Clin Oncol 2008; 26:1086–92.

44. Geh JI, Bond SJ, Bentzen SM et al. Stystematic overview of preoperative (neoadjuvant) chemoradiotherapy trials in oesophageal cancer: evidence of a radiation and chemotherapy dose response. Radiother Oncol 2006; 78:236–44.

45. Gebski V, Burmeister B, Foo K et al. Survival benefits from neoadjuvant chemoradiotherapy or chemotherapy in oesophageal carcinoma: a meta-analysis. Lancet Oncol 2007; 8:226–34.

46. Earlam R, Cunha-Melo JR. Oesophageal squamous cell carcinoma I. A critical review of radiotherapy. Br J Surg 1980; 67:457–61.

47. Sykes AJ, Burt PA, Slevin NJ et al. Radical radiotherapy for carcinoma of the oesophagus: an effective alternative to surgery. Radiother Oncol 1998; 48:15–21.

48. Kawashima M, Kagami Y, Toita T et al. Prospective trial of radiotherapy for patients 80 years of age or older with squamous cell carcinoma of the esophagus. Int J Radiat Oncol Biol Phys 2006; 64:1112–21.

49. Araujo CM, Souhami L, Gil RA et al. A randomized trial comparing radiation therapy versus concomitant radiation therapy and chemotherapy in carcinoma of the thoracic esophagus. Cancer 1991; 67(9):2258–61.

50. Coia LR, Engstrom PF, Paul AR et al. Long-term results of infusional 5-FU, mitomycin-C, and radiation as primary management of esophageal cancer. Int J Radiat Oncol Biol Phys 1991; 20:29–36.

51. Al-Sarraf M, Martz K, Herskovic A et al. Progress report of combined chemoradiotherapy versus radiotherapy alone in patients with esophageal cancer: an Intergroup study. J Clin Oncol 1997; 15:277–84.

52. Minsky BD, Neuberg D, Kelsen DP et al. Neoadjuvant chemotherapy plus high-dose radiation for squamous cell carcinoma of the esophagus: a preliminary analysis of the phase II Intergroup Trial 0122. J Clin Oncol 1996; 14(1):149–55.

53. Gaspar LE, Qian C, Kocha WI et al. A phase I/II study of external beam radiation, brachytherapy and concurrent chemotherapy in localized cancer of the esophagus (RTOG 92-07): preliminary toxicity report. Int J Radiat Oncol Biol Phys 1997; 37(3):593–9.

54. Coia LR, Soffen EM, Schultheiss TE et al. Swallowing function in patients with esophageal cancer treated with concurrent radiation and chemotherapy. Cancer 1993; 71:281–6.

55. O'Rourke IC, Tiver K, Bull C et al. Swallowing performance after radiation therapy for carcinoma of the esophagus. Cancer 1988; 61:2022–6.

56. Ribiero U, Finklestein SD, Safatle-Ribiero A et al. P53 sequence predicts treatment response and outcome of patients with esophageal carcinoma. Cancer 1998; 83:7–18.

57. Yamamoto M, Tsujinaka T, Shiozaki H et al. Metallothionein expression correlates with the pathological response of patients with esophageal cancer undergoing preoperative chemoradiation therapy. Oncology 1999; 56:332–7.

58. Beardsmore DM, Verbeke CS, Davies CL et al. Apoptotic and proliferative indexes in esophageal cancer: predictors of response to neoadjuvant therapy apoptosis and proliferation in esophageal cancer. J Gastrointest Surg 2003; 7:77–87.

59. Jones DR, Parker LA, Detterbeck FC et al. Inadequacy of computed tomography in assessing patients with esophageal carcinoma after induction chemoradiotherapy. Cancer 1999; 85:1026–32.

60. Lim JTW, Truong PT, Berthelet E et al. Endoscopic response predicts for survival and organ preserva-

tion after primary chemoradiotherapy for esophageal cancer. Int J Radiat Oncol Biol Phys 2003; 57:1328–35.

61. Giovannini M, Seitz JF, Thomas P et al. Endoscopic ultrasonography for assessment of the response to combined radiation therapy and chemotherapy in patients with esophageal cancer. Endoscopy 1997; 29:4–9.

62. Mallery S, DeCamp M, Bueno R et al. Pretreatment staging by endoscopic ultrasonography does not predict complete response to neoadjuvant chemoradiation in patients with esophageal carcinoma. Cancer 1999; 86:764–9.

63. Wieder HA, Brucher B, Zimmermann F et al. Time course of tumour metabolic activity during chemoradiotherapy of esophageal squamous cell carcinoma and response to treatment. J Clin Oncol 2004; 22:900–8.

64. Raoul JL, Le Prise E, Meunier B et al. Neoadjuvant chemotherapy and hyperfractionated radiotherapy with concurrent low-dose chemotherapy for squamous cell esophageal carcinoma. Int J Radiat Biol Phys 1998; 42:29–34.

65. Crellin AM, Sebag-Montefiore D, Martin I et al. Preoperative chemotherapy and radiotherapy, plus excision (CARE): a phase II study in esophageal cancer. Proc Am Soc Clin Oncol 2000; 19:A1128.

66. Denham JW, Steigler A, Kilmurray J et al. Relapse patterns after chemo-radiation for carcinoma of the oesophagus. Clin Oncol 2003; 15:98–108.

67. Thomas E, Crellin A, Harris K et al. The role of endoscopic ultrasound (EUS) in planning radiotherapy target volumes for oesophageal cancer. Radiother Oncol 2004; 73:149–51.

68. Leong T, Everitt C, Yuen K et al. A prospective study to evaluate the impact of FDG-PET on CT-based radiotherapy treatment planning for oesophageal cancer. Radiother Oncol 2006; 78:254–61.

69. Bonner JA, Harari PM, Giralt JL et al. Radiotherapy plus cetuximab for squamous-cell carcinoma of the head and neck. N Engl J Med 2006; 354:567–78.

70. Chan A, Wong A. Is combined chemotherapy and radiation therapy equally effective as surgical resection in localized esophageal carcinoma? Int J Radiat Oncol Biol Phys 1999; 45(2):265–70.

71. Murakami M, Kuroda Y, Nakajima T et al. Comparison between chemoradiation protocol intended for organ preservation and conventional surgery for clinical T1–T2 esophageal carcinoma. Int J Radiat Oncol Biol Phys 1999; 45(2):277–84.

72. Wilson KS, Lim JT. Primary chemotherapy–radiotherapy and selective oesophagectomy for oesophageal cancer: goal of cure with organ preservation. Radiother Oncol 2000; 54:129–34.

73. Bedenne L, Michel P, Bouche O et al. Chemoradiation Followed by Surgery Compared with Chemoradiation Alone in Squamous Cancer of the Esophagus: FFCD 9102. J Clin Oncol 2007; 25:1160–8.

74. Stahl M, Wilke H, Lehmann N et al. Long-term results of a phase III study investigating chemoradiation with and without surgery in locally advanced squamous cell carcinoma (LA-SCC) of the esophagus. J Clin Oncol 2008; 26(Suppl):Abstr. 4530.

75. Gardner-Thorpe J, Hardwick R, Dwerryhouse SJ. Salvage oesophagectomy after local failure of definitive chemoradiotherapy. Br J Surg 2007; 94:1059–66.

76. Hudson E, Powell J, Mukherjee S et al. Small cell oesophageal carcinoma: an institutional experience and review of the literature. Br J Cancer 2007; 96:708–11.

77. Ku GY, Minsky BD, Rusch VW et al. Small-cell carcinoma of the esophagus and gastresophageal junction: review of the Memorial Sloan-Kettering experience. Ann Oncol 2008; 19:533–7.

78. Douglass HO, Stabelein DM, Bruckner HM et al. Controlled trial of adjuvant chemotherapy following curative resection for gastric cancer. The Gastrointestinal Tumour Study Group. Cancer 1982; 49:1116–22.

79. Engstrom PF, Laqvin PT, Douglass HO et al. Postoperative adjuvant 5-fluorouracil and methyl-CCNU therapy for gastric cancer patients. Eastern Cooperative Oncology Group study. Cancer 1985; 55:1868–73.

80. Higgins GA, Amadeo JH, Smith DE et al. Efficacy of prolonged intermittent therapy with combined 5-FU and methyl-CCNU following resection for gastric carcinoma. A Veterans Administration Surgical Oncology Group report. Cancer 1983; 52:1105–12.

81. Cunningham D, Soukop M, McArdle CS et al. Advanced gastric cancer: experience in Scotland using FAM. Br J Surg 1984; 71:673–6.

82. Coombes RC, Schein PS, Chilvers CE et al. A randomized trial comparing adjuvant 5-fluorouracil, doxorubicin and mitomycin C with no treatment in operable gastric cancer. International Collaborative Cancer Group. J Clin Oncol 1990; 8:1362–9.

83. Hallissey MT, Dunn JA, Ward LC et al. The second British Stomach Cancer Group trial of adjuvant radiotherapy or chemotherapy in resectable gastric cancer: five year follow-up. Lancet 1994; 343:1309–12.

84. Hattori T, Inokuchi K, Taguchi T et al. Postoperative adjuvant chemotherapy for gastric cancer: the second report. Analysis of data on 2873 patients followed for 5 years. Jpn J Surg 1986; 16:175–80.

85. Nakajima T, Nashimoto A, Kitamura M et al. Adjuvant mitomycin and fluorouracil followed by oral uracil plus tegafur in serosa-negative gastric cancer: a randomised trial. Gastric Cancer Surgical Study Group. Lancet 1999; 354(9175):273–7.

86. Circera L, Balil A, Batiste-Alentorn et al. Randomized clinical trial of adjuvant mitomycin plus tegafur in patients with resected stage III gastric cancer. J Clin Oncol 1999; 17:3810–15.

87. Hermans J, Bonenkamp JJ, Ban MC et al. Adjuvant therapy after curative resection for gastric cancer: a meta-analysis of randomized trials. J Clin Oncol 1993; 11:1441–7.

88. Earle CC, Maroun JA. Adjuvant chemotherapy after curative resection for gastric cancer in non-Asian patients: revisiting a meta-analysis of randomised trials. Eur J Cancer 1999; 35(7):1059–64.

89. Mari E, Floriani I, Tinazzi A et al. Efficacy of adjuvant chemotherapy after curative resection for gastric cancer: a meta-analysis of published randomised trials. A study of the GISCAD (Gruppo Italiano per lo Studio dei Carcinomi della Apparato Digerente). Ann Oncol 2000; 11(7):837–43.

90. Hagiwara A, Takahashi T, Kojima O et al. Prophylaxis with carbon-adsorbed mitomycin against peritoneal recurrence of gastric cancer. Lancet 1992; 339(8794): 629–31.

91. Rosen HR, Jatzko G, Repse S et al. Adjuvant intraperitoneal chemotherapy with carbon-adsorbed mitomycin in patients with gastric cancer: results of a randomized multicenter trial of the Austrian Working Group for Surgical Oncology. J Clin Oncol 1998; 16(8):2733–8.

92. Hundahl SA, Macdonald JS, Benedetti J et al. for the Southwest Oncology Group and the Gastric Intergroup. Surgical treatment variation in a prospective randomized trial of chemoradiotherapy in gastric cancer: the effect of undertreatment. Ann Surg Oncol 2002; 9(3):278–86.

93. Bleiberg H, Jacob JH, Bedenne L et al. A randomized phase II trial of 5-fluorouracil (5FU) and cisplatin (DDP) versus DDP alone in advanced esophageal cancer. Proc Soc Clin Oncol 1991; 10:A447.

94. Zhang X Shen L, Li J et al. A phase II trial of paclitaxel and cisplatin in patients with advanced squamous-cell carcinoma of the esophagus. Am J Clin Oncol 2008; 31:29–33.

95. Murad A, Santiago F, Petroianu A et al. Modified therapy with 5-fluorouracil, doxorubicin, and methotrexate in advanced gastric cancer. Cancer 1993; 72:37–41.

96. Pyrhonen S, Kuitunen T, Nvandoto P et al. Randomised comparison of fluorouracil, epidoxorubicin and methotrexate (FEMTX) plus supportive care with supportive care alone in patients with non-resectable gastric cancer. Br J Cancer 1995; 71:587–91.

97. Glimelius B, Ekstrom K, Hoffman K et al. Randomized comparison between chemotherapy plus best supportive care with best supportive care in advanced gastric cancer. Ann Oncol 1997; 8:163–8.

98. Macdonald J, Schein P, Woolley P et al. 5-Fluorouracil, doxorubicin and mitomycin (FAM) combination chemotherapy for advanced gastric cancer. Ann Intern Med 1980; 93:533–6.

99. Cullinan S, Moertel C, Fleming T et al. A comparison of three chemotherapeutic regimens in the treatment of advanced pancreatic and gastric cancer. JAMA 1985; 253:2061–7.

100. Klein HO. Long term results with FAMTX (5-fluorouracil, Adriamycin, methotrexate) in advanced gastric cancer. Cancer Res 1989; 9:1025.

101. Wils JA, Klein HO, Wegener DJT et al. Sequential high-dose methotrexate and fluorouracil combined with doxorubicin: a step ahead in the treatment of advanced gastric cancer. A trial of the European Organisation for Research and Treatment of Cancer Gastrointestinal Tract Cooperative Group. J Clin Oncol 1991; 9:827.

102. Kelsen D, Atiq O, Saltz L et al. FAMTX versus etoposide doxorubicin and cisplatin: a random assignment in gastric cancer. J Clin Oncol 1992; 10:541–8.

103. Vanhoefer U, Rougier P, Wilke H et al. Final results of a randomized phase III trial of sequential high-dose methotrexate, fluorouracil, and doxorubicin versus etoposide, leucovorin, and fluorouracil versus infusional fluorouracil and cisplatin in advanced gastric cancer: a trial of the European Organization for Research and Treatment of Cancer Gastrointestinal Tract Cooperative Group. J Clin Oncol 2000; 18:2648–57.

104. Webb A, Cunningham D, Scarffe JH et al. Randomized trial comparing epirubicin, cisplatin and fluorouracil versus fluorouracil, doxorubicin, and methotrexate in advanced esophagogastric cancer. J Clin Oncol 1997; 15:261–7.

105. Seymour MT, Dent JT, Papamichael D et al. Epirubicin, cisplatin and oral UFT with leucovorin (ECU): a phase I–II study in patients with advanced upper gastrointestinal tract cancer. Ann Oncol 1999; 10(11):1329–33.

106. Van Cutsem E, Moiseyenko V, Tjulandin S et al. Phase III study of docetaxel and cisplatin plus fluorouracil compared with cisplatin and fluorouracil as first line therapy for advanced gastric cancer: a report of the V325 study group. J Clin Oncol 2006; 24:4991–7.

107. Dragovich T, McCoy S, Fenoglio-Preiser C et al. Phase II trial of erlotinib in gastroesophageal junction and gastric adenocarcinomas: SWOG 0127. J Clin Oncol 2006; 24:4922–7.

108. Chau I, Norman A, Cunningham D et al. Multivariate prognostic factor analysis in locally advanced and metastatic esophago-gastric cancer – pooled analysis from three multicenter, randomized, controlled trials using individual patient data. J Clin Oncol 2004; 22:2395–403.

109. Dawes PJDK, Clague MB, Dean EM. Combined external beam and intracavitary radiotherapy for carcinoma of the oesophagus. Brachytherapy 2. Proceedings of the 5th International Selectron User's Meeting 1988. Nucleotron International, 1989; pp. 442–4.

110. Pagliero KM, Rowlands CG. The place of brachytherapy in the treatment of carcinoma of the oesophagus. Brachytherapy HDR and LDR. Proceedings of a brachytherapy meeting: remote afterloading; state of the art. Nucleotron Corporation, 1990; pp. 44–51.

111. Sur RK, Donde B, Levin VC et al. Fractionated high dose rate brachytherapy in palliation of advanced esophageal cancer. Int J Radiat Oncol Biol Phys 1998; 40(2):447–53.

112. Gaspar LE, Nag S, Hersokic A et al. American Brachytherapy Society (ABS) consensus guidelines for brachytherapy of esophageal cancer. Int J Radiat Oncol Biol Phys 1997; 38(1):127–32.

113. Homs MY, Steyerberg EW, Eijkenboom WM et al. Single-dose brachytherapy verus metal stent placement for the palliation of dysphagia from oesophageal cancer: multicentre randomized trial. Lancet 2004; 364:1497–504.

10

Palliative treatments of carcinoma of the oesophagus and stomach

Jane M. Blazeby
Derek Alderson

Despite improvements in the detection of oesophageal and gastric cancer the majority of Western patients present with advanced disease that is not amenable to cure. Treatment is therefore palliative in intent and aims to lessen symptoms and lengthen survival with minimum risks until death occurs. This chapter concentrates on treatment modalities used for the palliation of oesophageal and gastric cancer.

Epidemiology and survival

Accurate information about the proportion of patients with oesophageal and gastric cancer who are treated with palliative intent is difficult to obtain. This largely reflects variations in the selection of patients for curative or palliative treatment. The proportions of patients therefore reported as potentially curable varies because of uncertainties in the numbers of patients in the denominator. Series of oesophagectomies published from the East or West report resection rates varying between 13% and 92%.[1] In the Western world, resection rates are about 25%, based upon population studies from Sweden and the UK.[2,3] Patients with oesophageal cancer selected for palliative treatment generally have a median survival of less than 8 months and few survive beyond 1 year. Although evidence is emerging to show possible survival benefits for palliative chemotherapy or radiotherapy, few well-designed randomised trials have directly compared different modes of palliative treatment, and evidence to compare palliative chemotherapy with best supportive care is lacking.[4] Treatment tailored to the general status of the patient and their type of tumour is therefore still recommended.[5]

There is little evidence to show that any single or combination of palliative treatment modality changes survival for patients not amenable to potentially curative treatment for oesophageal cancer. Future trials comparing palliative treatment modalities should assess survival and health-related quality of life using validated measures.

The resection rate for patients with gastric cancer is greater than that for oesophageal cancer, because distal gastrectomy is widely employed to overcome gastric outlet obstruction in patients with advanced disease with either curative or palliative intent.[6] Whether distal gastrectomy remains the best palliative treatment for distal gastric cancer is still not clear as experience develops with endoscopic stenting.[7] The role of palliative chemotherapy to extend survival and reduce symptoms is also increasing.[8] Despite this improvements in the treatment of advanced gastric cancer overall outcomes are poor. Median survival is only 6–8 months.

Evidence that chemotherapy improves survival in advanced gastric cancer in comparison to best supportive care is increasing. Palliative surgery for gastric outlet obstruction relieves symptoms in patients with reasonable prognoses and good performance status, but stenting may offer acceptable palliation of symptoms without the need for major surgery in patients with a relatively short life expectancy.

Disease stage, age and general performance status influence outcomes and survival, although the effect of age may be largely due to more comorbidity in older patients.[9,10] Another predictor of mortality is the length of the oesophageal tumour, mainly because this increases the likelihood of nodal involvement with large tumours.[11] All these factors need to be taken into consideration when planning treatment.

Patient selection and multidisciplinary teams

Since the introduction of the National Health Service Cancer plan in the UK in 2000, treatment decisions for patients with cancer are mandated to be made within the context of a multidisciplinary team.[12] Guidelines for the constitution and processes for upper gastrointestinal multidisciplinary teams have been published and national peer review processes audit team working.[12,13] Teams consist of core members, specialist nurses, gastroenterologists, oncologists, pathologists, radiologists, administrators, palliative medicine experts and surgeons. Additional members may include cytologists, dieticians and researchers from clinical trials unit. The aim of the team is to review available evidence for each new patient and make optimal treatment decisions. Evidence includes information about the cell type, disease stage, patient comorbidity and choice, and expert discussion of best available treatments. Although team working has been widely implemented across the UK and it is recommended by some continental European centres, in North America a similar role of 'tumour boards' is not mandatory within cancer care.[14] Currently evidence to support team working is sparse, based upon longitudinal or retrospective case series. It is also uncertain how to best evaluate the quality of multidisciplinary teams because outcomes are dependent upon so many variables. It has been suggested that monitoring implementation of team decisions further evaluates team working. In one centre it has been shown that 15% (95% CI 10–20%) of team decisions change after the meeting.[15] The most common reason cited for changing team decisions was lack of available information about patient choice and comorbidity. Team working is an area that is likely to develop over the next decade; professionals may need training in team-working skills and the infrastructure to support these processes is required.

After establishing a diagnosis, new patients require careful assessment to decide whether treatment is directed towards attempting a cure, or if palliation of symptoms is more appropriate. Careful patient selection has been shown to significantly influence results. Principal factors to consider are: type and stage of the tumour; physical and psychological well-being of the patient; and knowledge of patient preferences. Decisions should be considered in the knowledge of treatment outcomes, including impact on patients' health-related quality of life. **Figures 10.1** and **10.2** illustrate pathways that can be used to select patients for palliative treatment.

 Multidisciplinary cancer teams are a mandatory part of cancer care in the UK. The opportunity to elicit multiprofessional expertise in treatment decision-making is likely to benefit patient outcomes, but currently evidence to support this hypothesis is lacking. In the UK, selecting patients for palliative or potentially curative treatment is made within the context of a multidisciplinary team meeting and full expert review of tumour type and stage, patient comorbidity and wishes is required to make these decisions.

Fitness for treatment

The place of oesophagectomy in many older patients is often easily settled because of general debilitation or multiple coexistent medical problems. Age in itself does not preclude octogenarians from surgery, but most series of older patients are carefully selected. In general, patients who are not fit enough for oesophagectomy are also unable to tolerate a radical course of radiotherapy or definitive chemoradiation. On the whole, surgery for gastric tumours is tolerated better than oesophageal

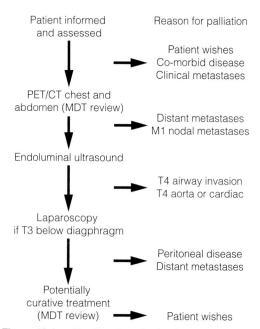

Figure 10.1 • Algorithm for selection for palliative or curative treatment of oesophageal and junctional tumours. CT, computed tomography; MDT, multidisciplinary team; PET, positron emission tomography.

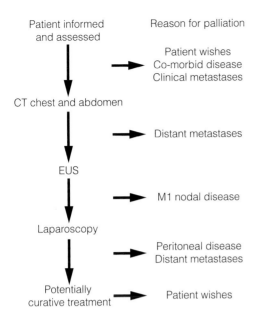

Figure 10.2 • Algorithm for selection for palliative or curative treatment for cancers of the gastric body or antrum. CT, computed tomography; EUS, endoscopic ultrasound.

surgery by the elderly population, but patients still require careful preoperative assessment before undergoing major resection. Anaesthetic assessment for surgery is considered in more detail in Chapter 4.

Staging investigations

Accurate tumour staging plays a crucial part in any therapeutic protocol, enabling patients to be assigned appropriately to treatments with either curative or palliative intent. Clear evidence of haematogenous tumour spread or irresectability directs patients with oesophageal cancer to palliative treatment. Despite advances in staging procedures, no single investigation is perfect and a small percentage of patients still require exploratory surgery to determine resectability. Palliative resection or bypass surgery to ameliorate bleeding or obstruction may be indicated for some patients with gastric cancer even in the presence of haematogenous tumour spread. The decision to proceed with palliative surgery requires careful consideration as many patients rapidly deteriorate in this situation.

Patient preferences and information provision

Information about the diagnosis and prognosis of oesophageal and gastric cancer should be offered to all patients and it is essential that a nurse specialist

is involved in this process whenever possible. The volume and type of information required will vary between individuals, although evidence from studies of patients' information needs performed in other disease sites generally show that patients wish to have as much information as possible and prefer the information to be provided by a health professional, as well as in other forms such as a booklet or CD-ROM.[16] It is necessary to inform patients of the potential treatment benefits and risks and to elicit their preferences. All clinicians will be faced with patients who demand every small chance of cure, despite its risks, and others who wish to receive minimal, dignified intervention. Communicating outcomes, providing adequate information and listening to patients' views is necessary so patients and their family have access to as much information and support as they require.

Symptoms and signs of advanced oesophageal and gastric cancer

Tumours of the oesophagus and gastric cardia

Dysphagia is the predominant symptom for most patients with tumours of the oesophagus, oesophagogastric junction or proximal stomach. The progressive nature of malignant dysphagia is usually apparent. Initial difficulties in swallowing solid food may cause bolus obstruction and odynophagia. Solid food intake gradually reduces and patients finally are unable to swallow even saliva. Complete dysphagia may lead to aspiration pneumonia. Less than 5% of patients with oesophageal cancer develop an aero-digestive fistula, but this is generally associated with locally advanced disease and a poor prognosis. Oesophageal tumours may also present with vomiting, haematemesis or gastro-oesophageal reflux. Many patients present with symptoms of advanced disease including fatigue, anorexia, upper abdominal pain caused by ascites or liver metastases, and constipation. Rapid weight loss frequently occurs because of cancer cachexia exacerbated by poor oral intake. Hoarseness caused by tumour infiltration of the recurrent laryngeal nerves may be the result of advanced local disease or mediastinal recurrence after oesophagectomy.

Tumours of the gastric body and antrum

Gastric cancer commonly has an insidious presentation and some patients have few symptoms. Slow blood loss may eventually result in symptoms of anaemia. Haematemesis is a rare first presentation. Vague upper gastrointestinal problems, such as epigastric discomfort, early satiety and gastro-oesophageal reflux, are common. Tumours of the distal stomach cause outlet obstruction and patients describe epigastric fullness, reflux and nausea, finally leading to effortless vomiting. The presence of an epigastric mass, supraclavicular lymphadenopathy, jaundice, ascites or pleural effusions all reflect advanced disease. Less commonly bony pain and symptoms of increased intracranial pressure are seen related to metastatic spread. Symptoms of oesophageal and gastric cancer are listed in Box 10.1.

The provision of rapid relief of dysphagia or gastric obstruction for patients with advanced oesophageal and gastric malignancies is the initial priority of palliative treatment for patients who are symptomatic. When patients with disease not amenable to cure have minimal symptoms related to the primary tumour, the main aim of palliative treatment is to extend survival and maintain or improve health-related quality of life. Many patients undergoing palliative treatment will also need dietary advice. Appropriate end-of-life care should be considered.

Box 10.1 • Symptoms of oesophageal and gastric cancer

Oesophageal cancer
Dysphagia
Odynophagia
Reflux
Chest pain
Haematemesis
Cough
Dyspnoea
Hoarseness

Gastric cancer
Dysphagia
Epigastric fullness/discomfort
Effortless vomiting
Haematemesis
Nausea
Reflux
Symptoms of anaemia

Metastatic disease
Upper abdominal pain
Epigastric fullness/discomfort
Anorexia
Bone pain
Constipation
Dyspnoea
Cough
Weight loss
Fatigue

Palliative treatments for cancer of the oesophagus and gastric cardia

A variety of approaches are available for the palliation of advanced tumours of the oesophagus and gastric cardia. In the past, surgery was considered to be the best palliation of malignant dysphagia and there are still a few advocates of this approach. Although palliative surgery may relieve dysphagia, there is evidence that it simultaneously reduced many other aspects of health. In particular, after oesophagectomy patients suffer a major deterioration in physical, role and social well-being, and increased pain, fatigue and dyspnoea.[17] Generally patients undergoing palliative surgery do not have sufficient time to recover from the operation before they experience symptoms of metastatic disease. Historically, palliative resection was also associated with high perioperative mortality and morbidity rates. The important issue is whether palliative resection provides better relief of symptoms than non-operative measures, as there is currently no high-quality evidence to show that palliative surgery extends survival. This is an area where further research is needed and some propose that minimally invasive surgery may be suitable for the palliation of oesophageal cancer. The following section concentrates on non-resectional palliative methods for treating oesophageal or oesophagogastric junctional cancer. It is divided into five categories:

1. Endoscopic methods of relieving luminal obstruction.
2. Chemotherapy, radiotherapy or chemoradiotherapy.
3. Management of aero-digestive fistulas.
4. Management of recurrent laryngeal nerve palsy.
5. Management of chronic bleeding.

The endoscopic relief of luminal obstruction

Malignant dysphagia may be relieved by stent insertion, tumour ablation with photothermal or photodynamic therapy, or by the injection of cytotoxic substances. Many modalities are complementary. No one method or combination is greatly superior to the rest in terms of relief of dysphagia, although some evidence is emerging to show better long-term relief of dysphagia with single-dose brachytherapy compared to metal stent placement.[18] Historically, dilatation was advocated for the palliation of malignant dysphagia and rigid plastic tubes were inserted following this. Because of the short-lived benefits of dilatation alone and the associated risks of perforation, its use nowadays is reduced to that of a preliminary measure before definitive management of dysphagia. Minimal oesophageal dilatation may be performed to allow insertion of a self-expanding metal stent or to place a brachytherapy bougie. Guidelines on the use of dilatation in clinical practice recommend careful preparation, polyvinyl wire-guided bougies or hydrostatic balloons.[19] Strictures with severe narrowing and angulation are best negotiated under X-ray screening.

A tissue diagnosis is desirable prior to dilatation of a malignant stricture and wherever possible oesophageal dilatation should be undertaken as a planned procedure with informed consent. It should be undertaken by experienced endoscopists with contrast radiology available if necessary.

The majority of randomised trials evaluating palliative treatments for dysphagia have been small and single-centred, and therefore may have lacked power to detect differences between treatment arms. Table 10.1 summarises the randomised controlled trials published before the end of 2007 evaluating interventions of the palliation of malignant dysphagia. This table only includes trials that randomised more than a total of 40 patients.

Intubation

Intubation is probably the most widely used form of palliation of malignant dysphagia at present and allows rapid relief of dysphagia with associated low morbidity. Prostheses may be placed endoscopically, radiologically or surgically at laparotomy, although there is little place for open insertion of a prosthesis when a tumour is unexpectedly found to be irresectable because endoscopic insertion is safer and has fewer complications. Over the past two decades self-expanding metal stents (SEMS) have superseded rigid plastic prostheses. This has been based upon ease of insertion and evidence that SEMS are associated with less morbidity.[20,21] One of the largest and best-designed studies that aimed to evaluate the cost-effectiveness and effectiveness of SEMS compared to conventional modalities (rigid intubation with a plastic stent) in patients with inoperable oesophageal cancer found no difference in costs, but rigid tubes were associated with worse quality of swallowing and increased late morbidity.[22]

It is evidence from this large study, numerous small trials and clinical experience of the benefits of SEMS that led to them becoming the standard method for intubating malignant oesophageal or oesophagogastric tumours.

Self-expanding metal stents (SEMS)

Metal stents were first used to palliate malignant dysphagia in the early 1990s and since this development, tube design has varied to offset drawbacks inherent to construction and placement. Stents are made from a compressible, flexible metal mesh, which expands after deployment to full size over 24–48 hours. The stents rapidly relieve dysphagia and have a large internal luminal diameter (16–25 mm). Early disadvantages of tumour ingrowth and stent migration have been largely overcome by newer materials and designs. Stents are expensive (approximately £800 each). Current design developments are centred upon using expandable plastic rather than metal to reduce the manufacturing costs.[23] Several studies have also investigated the addition of a valve in the distal part of the stent to reduce acid reflux.[24]

Method of insertion

Self-expanding metal stents may be inserted endoscopically or radiologically. There are several designs with very similar delivery devices. The Ultraflex Esophageal Stent (Boston Scientific Inc.) is made of an alloy of titanium and nickel and has a shape 'memory' as well as superelastic behaviour. It is loaded in a small-diameter delivery catheter, constrained in a compressed form by a double plastic membrane. During expansion the stent shrinks by approximately one-third. It is available either uncovered or partially covered. The design incorporates a proximal flare for secure placement and to reduce the possibility of food entrapment. The conical 'Flamingo' Wallstent is designed to reduce problems with migration, and the proximal and distal 1.5 cm of the stent remain uncovered. It may be recovered during deployment and repositioned, provided less than 50% of the endoprosthesis has been released. The Gianturco Z stent also uses stainless steel and it is entirely coated with a polyethylene film. It has long wire hooks at its midportion to facilitate anchoring. Unlike the Ultraflex and Wallstents it undergoes very little shortening upon release. A 'windsock' design to reduce the possibility of gastro-oesophageal reflux is available. Other stents are variations on these basic designs. Comparative studies show that reintervention rates for tumour ingrowth are higher with uncovered than covered stents. Other comparative studies of SEMS show conflicting results and although these trials may have design weaknesses, there is currently no good evidence that one design is superior to another in terms of morbidity or relief of dysphagia.

Contraindications to metal stent placement are tumours requiring stent placement within 2 cm of the upper oesophageal sphincter. This is not recommended because of concerns about proximal

Table 10.1 • Prospective randomised controlled trials of endoscopic palliation of malignant dysphagia (*n* > 40)

Authors	n	Group 1	Group 2	Dysphagia	Clinical outcomes	Health-related quality of life*
Knyrim et al., 1993[20]	42	Cook plastic tube	SEMS: uncovered Wallstent	No difference	Morbidity and hospital stay worse in Group 1	Not assessed
Lightdale et al., 1995[27]	218	Nd:YAG laser	Photodynamic therapy + argon pumped dye laser	No difference	Perforations more common in Group 1	Not assessed
Heier et al., 1995[28]	42	Nd:YAG laser	Photodynamic therapy	No difference	Better performance status at 1 month in Group 2	Not assessed
Adam et al., 1997[47]	60	SEMS either: covered Wallstent or uncovered Ultraflex	Nd:YAG laser	Worse in Group 2	Stent migration worse in Group 1, covered Wallstent	Not assessed
Sargeant et al., 1997[48]	67	Nd:YAG laser	Nd:YAG laser and external beam radiotherapy	Longer treatment intervals in Group 2	No difference	Not assessed
Siersema et al., 1998[21]	75	Medoc plastic Celestin tube	SEMS: covered Gianturco	No difference	Morbidity and hospital stay worse in Group 1	Not assessed
Carazzone et al., 1999[33]	47	Nd:YAG laser	98% intratumoral ethanol injection	No difference	More pain in Group 2	Not assessed
Dallal et al., 2001[49]	65	Nd:YAG laser	SEMS: uncovered Ultraflex	No difference	Morbidity similar, survival better Group 1	Significant HRQOL deterioration in stent group at 1 month

Study	N	Intervention 1	Intervention 2	Dysphagia/swallowing	Morbidity/complications	Pain
Siersema et al., 2001[50]	100	SEMS: covered Wallstent	SEMS: covered Ultraflex Or Gianturco Z stent	No difference	No difference	Not assessed
Vakil et al., 2001[51]	62	SEMS: covered	SEMS: uncovered	No difference	Fewer reinterventions in covered SEMS group	Not assessed
O'Donnell et al., 2002[52]	50	Cook plastic tube	SEMS: covered Wallstent	No difference	No difference	No difference
Sabharwal et al., 2003[53]	53	SEMS: covered Wallstent	SEMS: covered Ultraflex	No difference	No difference	Not assessed
Homs et al., 2004[18,35]	209	SEMS: covered Ultraflex	Brachytherapy	SEMS better short-term relief. Brachytherapy better long-term relief	Morbidity higher with SEMS	In favour of brachytherapy
Shenfine et al., 2005[22]	217	SEMS (then randomised to 18- or 24-mm-diameter stent)	Standard treatment (then randomised to plastic tube or no tube treatment)	Worse quality swallowing with plastic tubes	Survival advantage in standard group randomised to no tube treatment	18-mm stents less pain reported than with 24-mm SEMS
Conio et al., 2007[23]	101	Self-expandable plastic stent	SEMS: covered Ultraflex	No difference	Morbidity higher with expandable plastic stents	Not assessed
Power et al., 2007[24]	49	SEMS: covered Ultraflex	SEMS: covered Ultraflex with an antireflux valve	Better passage of soft food at 2 months with standard SEMS	Similar outcomes, but less reflux with antireflux valve	No difference

Note: 30-day mortality rates were similar in all of the above trials.

HRQOL, health-related quality of life; Nd:YAG, neodymium ytrium–aluminium–garnet laser; SEMS, self-expanding metal stent.

*Health-related quality-of-life results in article reported from a valid multidimensional questionnaire.

migration, laryngeal compression, intractable pain and a globus sensation. Relative contraindications to stent placement are more dependent on operator expertise, but these include: total luminal obstruction; non-circumferential tumour growth prohibiting proper anchoring of the prosthesis; almost horizontal orientation of the malignant lumen; prior chemoradiation; and multiangulated lesions, particularly with tumours at the gastro-oesophageal junction. All of these situations render endoscopic intubation hazardous.

Preparation

Endoscopic prosthesis insertion is usually possible under intravenous sedation, although some endoscopists continue to use general anaesthesia. Routine monitoring is required with intravenous sedation, as is continual attention to the airway. Saliva and regurgitated fluids should be constantly removed to prevent aspiration during the procedure.

Endoscopic insertion with fluoroscopy

After endoscopic assessment and measurement of the tumour, a guidewire is passed into the stomach (after successful negotiation of the tumour with the endoscope or under fluoroscopic control). Occasionally dilatation may be required to a minimum of 10 mm before passage of the delivery system over the guidewire. The proximal and distal extents of the tumour may be marked with radio-opaque skin markers or the tumour limitations injected with contrast. The slim delivery device is advanced over the guidewire until the radio-opaque markers of the compressed stent are correctly aligned with the tumour. Once in position the stent is deployed. It is possible to reposition some of the stents after partial deployment. The guidewire and delivery device are then carefully removed under fluoroscopic guidance. After release of the stent, the endoscope may be reinserted to check the final position. Immediate balloon dilatation is recommended to improve expansion and prevent early migration, but may still be performed up to several days after stent insertion.

Radiological insertion

Morphological imaging of the malignant stricture with oral contrast is performed prior to stent insertion. This assesses length and position of the tumour. A fine steerable catheter is then negotiated over a guidewire through the stricture to the stomach and skin markers aligned. The proximal and distal ends of the tumour are marked (similar to endoscopic positioning). Balloon dilatation to 10–15 mm may be performed if the stricture is very narrow. The stent insertion device is than passed safely and positioned radiographically over the guidewire and released according to the type of stent.

Postoperative management

After stent insertion the patient must be instructed to sit upright. Oral fluids are usually allowed the same day unless there is concern about complications or symptoms or signs of perforation. Clinical and radiological examination may be performed to exclude perforation before oral fluids are commenced. Patients should receive written dietary information with advice to chew food carefully and drink regularly during and after meals. A daily intake of 10 mL hydrogen peroxide (20 vol.) is sometimes recommended.

Complications

Even in experienced hands, intubation with SEMS has a procedure-related mortality of about 1–2% and early complication rates of between 0% and 30%. Complications are listed in Box 10.2.

1. Malposition of the stent may require insertion of a second or even third stent (if the tumour is long). This may overlap the malpositioned stent to adequately cover the tumour.
2. Incomplete stent expansion and early dysphagia may require balloon dilatation, if no improvement is seen within 48 hours.
3. Early stent migration. This occurs in about 1% of patients and is more prone in stents placed at the oesophagogastric junction than in stents with both ends anchored within the oesophagus. Endoscopic retrieval may be performed safely, especially with the newer devices. Stents that have migrated into the stomach may also be safely left as they rarely obstruct the pyloric channel or cause intestinal perforation.

Box 10.2 • Complications of stent insertion

Early complications
Malposition/migration
Incomplete expansion
Oesophageal perforation
Upper gastrointestinal bleeding
Aspiration pneumonia
Pain

Late complications
Migration
Tumour ingrowth or overgrowth
Aspiration pneumonia
Pain
Reflux
Late perforation and fistulation
Disintegration of prosthesis
Stent torsion
Bleeding

4. Oesophageal perforation is the most serious complication and is more likely if the stricture has been dilated before stent insertion, there has been prior use of radiotherapy and/or chemotherapy, if the tumour is sharply angulated or if it extensively encases the oesophagus. Rapid development of subcutaneous emphysema, severe pain, radiological evidence of pneumomediastinum, air under the diaphragm or a pleural effusion should all raise suspicion. The extent of the leak is confirmed by contrast radiography. The most appropriate form of therapy depends on the time of detection and the extent of the leak. If recognised at endoscopy, the insertion of the prosthesis itself may seal off the perforation and prevent mediastinitis. Alternatively, the procedure may be abandoned and conservative treatment undertaken. This involves administration of broad-spectrum antibiotics, cessation of oral intake and feeding either parenterally or by jejunostomy. An intercostal drain may need to be inserted if there is evidence of pleural contamination. Specific management of this serious complication is covered in detail in Chapter 19.

5. Severe upper gastrointestinal haemorrhage occasionally occurs. This is difficult to treat, and only supportive measures may be possible.

Late complications

Long-term problems occur in at least 20% of patients and are most frequently related to eating. Problems often require hospital admission, further endoscopic manoeuvres and occasionally replacement of the prosthesis.

1. Prostheses may block because of tumour overgrowth at either end of the stent or tumour ingrowth through the metallic stent latticework if an uncovered design is used. This leads to recurrent dysphagia and occurs in 5–30% of patients. Tumour ingrowth is best managed with laser, argon-beam coagulation or photodynamic therapy. Overgrowth at either end of the stent may be successfully treated with placement of a second stent.

2. Food bolus obstruction occurs in metallic stents despite their wide diameter. Spontaneous resolution can occur or endoscopy may be required to displace the impacted food bolus into the stomach.

3. Reflux of gastric acid occurs in all patients whenever the tube crosses the gastro-oesophageal junction. It may lead to oesophagitis and occasionally benign stricture formation above the tube. This can be controlled by conservative measures, dilatation and acid suppression therapy. The use of a stent with an antireflux valve may reduce reflux symptoms.

4. Pressure necrosis and late oesophageal perforation leading to mediastinal fistulation has been reported.

5. Stents can fracture or twist leading to serious morbidity. These are rare problems as most patients do not live long enough. Operative removal of these tubes is only very occasionally required.

6. Eating difficulties exist due to incomplete relief of dysphagia. Once a prosthesis is in place all food must pass through a tube with a fixed diameter. Patients therefore need appropriate nutritional support and advice.

Manufacturers continue to develop new designs to decrease the risk of migration, increase the ease of insertion and enable stents to be repositioned or extracted. A new self-expanding plastic stent (SEPS) prosthesis has been evaluated but may lead to particular problems of stent migration. However, it is likely that future developments will overcome these issues.[23] Despite the associated morbidity with stent insertion, the immediate relief of dysphagia in one endoscopy session has made intubation an attractively simple palliative treatment, particularly for patients with poor performance status whose life expectancy is short.

Laser treatment

Laser therapy as a treatment for palliation of malignant dysphagia is diminishing. This is because it is time-consuming and requires repeated hospital visits. Where patients are sufficiently fit enough for multiple hospital treatments, patients may be offered palliative chemotherapy or brachytherapy. Laser treatment is useful for temporary relief of dysphagia before surgery or definitive palliation and is useful for overgrowth or ingrowth of tumour in patients with oesophageal stents. Laser therapy may also be valuable for tumours of the cervical oesophagus (where a stent is contraindicated). The principles of tumour ablation with laser treatment are similar to those used in other techniques such as argon-beam coagulation. Successful recanalisation and relief of dysphagia may be achieved after a mean of two treatment sessions, although most patients will continue to manage only semisolid or liquid foods. The mean dysphagia-free interval after laser treatment varies from 4 to 16 weeks. Repeated recanalisations can be performed with a laser or argon beam as many times as necessary.

The most popular type of laser in Britain is the non-contact neodymium yttrium–aluminium–garnet (Nd:YAG) laser. Laser energy is conveyed through a single monofibre, which is enclosed in a Teflon sheath. At an irradiation distance of 5–10 mm, multiple pulses for a duration of about 0.5–1 s are given. It causes tissue necrosis with eventual vaporisation, depending on the power used, the duration of application, the distance between the fibre tip and target, the aim of the application and the colour of the tissue. Coaxial gas (usually CO_2 or NO_2) is administered around the quartz fibre, to cool the probe tip and clear debris. Gas is removed with the suction channel of the endoscope. A nasogastric tube next to the endoscope can be used to vent the oesophagus. The low-power contact Nd:YAG system uses coaxial water to cool the tip, remove debris and reduce adherence of the contact probe. This employs a sapphire tip, which acts like a hot knife. Lower power settings theoretically mean that the chances of perforation by excessive laser energy are reduced. Tissue damage only occurs up to 0.5 mm beyond the treatment site. Each laser treatment session may recanalise the whole or part of the stricture. Some recommend routine endoscopic review at 48–72 hours, when oedema has subsided and accurate assessment of the overall effect can be made. The destroyed tumour may then be evacuated with forceps, polyp graspers, lavage or pushed distally with the endoscope. Others administer treatment as dictated by clinical response.

Endoscopic technique

Laser treatment is usually carried out with intravenous sedation, although some centres use a rigid endoscope, general anaesthesia and endotracheal intubation. Those in favour of a rigid scope believe its advantages are that it allows better suction of fluid, smoke and debris, with improved visualisation of the tumour. If a malignant stricture is negotiable, the laser is first applied to the distal end of the tumour. The scope is then withdrawn in a circular fashion into the more proximal tumour. If complete obstruction is encountered, tumours can be vaporised in the antegrade direction or first dilated to allow passage of the endoscope. Antegrade therapy may be more dangerous because information about the luminal axis is lacking, and the area first treated rapidly becomes oedematous, thus impairing visualisation and access more distally.

Early complications

The incidence of major complications and mortality (which is in the region of 1–5%) is usually lower for laser destruction than endoscopic intubation (with

Box 10.3 • Complications of laser treatment

Early complications
Pain
Perforation
Pneumatoperitoneum
Pneumomediastinum
Gastric distension
Bleeding
Aspiration pneumonia

Late complications
Repeated hospital admissions
Tumour recurrence
Benign strictures
Functional swallowing problems

plastic stents). Few studies have compared laser treatment with metal stents (Table 10.1). Early complications after laser treatment are listed in Box 10.3.

1. Chest pain may result from extensive mucosal burning. It is common but not severe.
2. Oesophageal perforation is less common following laser recanalisation than intubation with a rigid endoprosthesis. The risk is about 5% and is said to be related to predilatation rather than a direct complication of the laser treatment.
3. A benign pneumatoperitoneum or pneumomediastinum is sometimes detected by chest X-ray after laser treatment. This is thought to be related to jets of coaxial gas passing through abnormal, often necrotic, tumour tissue. Patients rarely have symptoms. Contrast studies do not show a leak and patients usually make an uneventful recovery.
4. Gastric distension as a result of carbon dioxide infusion can be quite uncomfortable despite adequate decompression. The pain is visceral in nature and may be confused with chest pain from excessive mucosal burning.
5. Haemorrhage after laser treatment is rare, occurring in about 1%.

Late complications

Late complications frequently occur following laser destruction and require repeated endoscopic treatment.

1. The main problem is tumour recurrence. Patients require about monthly treatment sessions. It is perceived by the medical profession that this is burdensome and disruptive, but there have been few studies that have objectively measured

patients' views about this matter. Some may feel that continued hospital contact contributes to their sense of well-being.

2. Delayed laser-associated benign strictures can occur in up to 20% of patients. They require repeated dilatation and occasionally stent insertion.

3. Persistent dysphagia for solids. Laser treatment may recanalise 90% of all stenoses, but a wide luminal diameter does not necessarily equate to normal swallowing. Distal tumours may cause 'pseudoachalasia' that impairs swallowing. Residual intramural tumour may cause impaired oesophageal body motility and together with progressive cachexia may make it impossible for some patients to take solid foods again.

Combination laser treatment

In view of the varied responses with laser treatment alone, means of improving the efficacy of laser treatment by increasing the period between laser therapy and symptomatic relapse have been explored through combination treatments. Laser therapy can be combined with external- or internal-beam radiotherapy to prolong the interval between treatments, although the patient must attend for radiotherapy, which does increase hospital attendance. Intraluminal radiotherapy is useful for treating mural invasion following laser debulking of the tumour.

Thermal recanalisation or stenting?

Laser therapy is rapid, safe and effective, and may have superior relief of dysphagia compared to rigid intubation. It may be preferable for non-circumferential, polypoid or exophytic tumours, and stents may be preferable for circumferential obstructing tumours. The main drawback of laser palliation is the need for the patient to attend hospital on a regular basis and the capital cost of the equipment. Laser treatment has nothing to offer patients with an extrinsic lesion causing oesophageal compression, or those with a fistula or diffuse subepithelial tumour. It is therefore increasingly viewed as a complementary rather than competing palliative treatment, to deal with tube overgrowth or ingrowth or local recurrence after surgery.

Argon-beam plasma coagulation

High-frequency diathermy electrocoagulation has become widely used for surgical haemostasis and to ablate tumour tissue. The argon-beam coagulator utilises a jet of ionised argon gas to conduct high-frequency electrical energy to the tumour. This is readily applied through an endoscope. Once the surface of the tumour has been coagulated and dried, the electrical current passes through to an adjacent

area. Unlike laser light, the argon beam will arc to the nearest point of contact. The depth of extension is minimal (2–3 mm) and this reduces the risk of perforation. The gas flow is high, which means that regular aspiration is required to prevent gastric distension. It is not expensive and operator confidence is high given the low risk of perforation. Because of these pragmatic features it has largely replaced laser reatment as a primary debulking treatment.[25] As with laser treatment, it is time-consuming and there is a need for repeated treatments.

Photodynamic therapy

Photodynamic therapy (PDT) is an investigational treatment that modifies conventional laser treatment. It uses a selective technique that targets tumour tissues and limits damage to adjacent tissue. It essentially has three elements: light, a photosensitising drug (a haematoporphyrin derivative) and oxygen. The drug acting as a photosensitiser is injected intravenously 3–4 days before irradiation of the tumour. Laser light (administered endoscopically) then activates the drug within the tissue. Once stimulated, the photosensitiser interacts with oxygen to create a highly reactive oxygen species that is cytotoxic. Retention of the photosensitiser is longer in dysplastic or frankly neoplastic than normal tissues, at a ratio of about 2:1. Damage to normal tissues heals by regeneration.[26]

Clinical indications

The role of PDT in palliative treatments is yet to be determined and is likely to be small. It may be used to treat patients with small mucosal tumours (uT1, N0) who are unfit or who do not wish to undergo major surgery (see Chapter 6), or it can be used on larger inoperable lesions where other treatments have failed. Two prospective randomised studies have compared PDT with laser therapy.[27,28] Perforations were more common after laser treatment alone, although relief of dysphagia was similar in both groups. PDT seemed to have a longer duration of response than laser therapy.

Complications

A number of specific complications have been recognised. The activated photosensitiser creates an iatrogenic porphyria, which may persist for up to 6 weeks after injection of the drug and leads to skin photosensitivity. Patients are advised to avoid sunlight. Perforation and fistulas may occur as well as oesophagitis leading to stricture formation. PDT has yet to enter widespread clinical use, partly because of cost. New photosensitisers with shorter durations of action may make the treatment more acceptable. At present, there are no data to support PDT as first-line palliative treatment, but it may be considered for high oesophageal tumours, for salvage treatment if stents have migrated or for stent over/ingrowth.

Bipolar electrocoagulation

Bipolar electrocoagulation (BICAP) is another thermal endoscopic treatment that has been used to relieve dysphagia.[29] Usually 2–4 mm of coagulation occurs at the tumour surface and one or two treatment sessions are required to treat the entire tumour. Although dysphagia may be partially relieved, problems with perforation, fistula formation, strictures and bleeding have occurred, and the technique has never been widely used.

Chemically induced tumour necrosis

The use of intralesional injection of alcohol (usually ethanol) to induce tumour necrosis is a simple and readily available palliative treatment, suitable for exophytic tumours and tumours in the proximal oesophagus.[30,31] It may also be used to control haemorrhage from bleeding tumours.

Endoscopic technique

Patients require intravenous sedation and flexible endoscopy. A sclerotherapy needle is used to inject 0.5- to 1-mL aliquots of alcohol into the protuberant part of the tumour. Endoscopic observation of the tumour blanching and swelling confirms needle position. In patients with long tumours it is best to start injections distally so that induced oedema does not impede the passage of the endoscope. There is no limit to the total volume injected in one session (1–36 mL have been reported). Dilatation is needed if the endoscope is unable to traverse the stricture. Several treatment sessions may be required to improve swallowing but it usually occurs within a week.

Outcome

An improvement in dysphagia score is reported in most patients after treatment with absolute alcohol, although it may be made temporarily worse because of initial tumour oedema and swelling. Retrosternal chest pain and a low-grade pyrexia may occur. Perforation and fistula formation have been reported.[32] The pattern of necrosis may be unpredictable and the main disadvantage is the need for repetitive treatments.

Injection of chemicals to relieve malignant dysphagia has all the hallmarks of a good technique, being safe, inexpensive and readily available. The technique is less precise than laser treatment because it is difficult to be sure where the alcohol is going once it enters the tissue. One prospective trial compared laser treatment with ethanol injections.[33] Significantly more pain was experienced by those being treated by ethanol but dysphagia and other complications were similar in both groups. Despite these reports the use of ethanol has not become widespread and its place may be as an adjunct to more conventional methods for relieving dysphagia. Like thermal methods for recanalisation, it cannot be used for patients with aero-digestive fistula.

External beam or intracavity radiotherapy

External beam radiotherapy

The aim of palliative radiotherapy is to recanalise the oesophagus and inhibit local tumour progression. It may be delivered by external beam or an intraluminal source (brachytherapy). External beam radiotherapy is widely used. It is straightforward to plan and does not require admission to hospital. Regimens are based on 30–60 Gy in 10 or more fractions given over a 5- to 6-week period. Initially swallowing may deteriorate because of radiation-induced oedema and swelling of the tumour. For patients whose nutrition is at risk prior to treatment, a form of nutritional support may first be required (endoscopic recanalisation or enteral feeding by gastrostomy, jejunostomy or nasogastric tube).

Complications

Side-effects are common and often serious, particularly if initial treatment seems successful: pulmonary fibrosis, fistula and benign stricture formation have all been described. Data from the 1970s show that acceptable palliation of dysphagia occurs with external beam radiotherapy in less than 40% of patients. Problems with recurrent dysphagia as a result of cicatricial narrowing of the oesophagus also occurs.[34] As a single modality it has probably been superseded by intracavity irradiation or combination treatment.

Brachytherapy (intracavitary irradiation)

The development of the Selectron (Nucleotron, Zeersum, the Netherlands) remote control afterloading machine has generated considerable interest in recent years because it places the radiotherapy source close to the tumour and maximises the tumour radiation dose. It is a simple and safe procedure, and there is no radiation exposure to staff. The brachytherapy applicator, only 8 mm in diameter, is passed over an endoscopically placed guidewire and positioned in the tumour by fluoroscopy. This is immobilised at the mouth or nose. The patient is then transferred to a protected treatment room and connected to the Selectron machine. A microprocessor controls the pneumatic transfer of caesium-137 pellets down a flexible tube inserted into the applicator. The optimal dose is unknown and varies from 15 to 20 Gy to a depth of 1 cm in single or multiple fractions. Treatment may be repeated on alternate days leaving the nasogastric tube in situ or replacing it as necessary, although it is usually given as a single-dose fraction of 10–15 Gy. It is necessary to precisely map the tumour by endoscopy, fluoroscopy or computed tomography and planning aims to incorporate a few centimetres of normal oesophagus at either end. The great merit of brachytherapy is that the radiation dose is highest to the tumour while adjacent normal tissues are relatively spared. It can be used in combination with other treatments.

Relief of dysphagia and patient reported outcomes

One well-designed large randomised trial has been reported that compared single-dose brachytherapy (12 Gy) with SEMS (Ultraflex covered stent) in patients not suitable for curative treatment.[18,35] The main end-point of this trial was dysphagia. Results showed that SEMS provided better short-term relief of dysphagia but associated increased morbidity. Longer-lasting relief of dysphagia was achieved in the brachytherapy group. Survival was similar in both arms (median survival 155 days (95% CI 127–183 days) after brachytherapy and 145 days (95% CI 103–187 days) after stent placement), but morbidity was significantly higher after stent insertion than after brachytherapy. Major complications included perforation, haemorrhage and fistula formation. Major haemorrhage occurred more significantly after metal stent insertion. Other complications include the development of post-irradiation strictures or tracheo-oesophageal fistula. This trial also included a robust assessment of health-related quality of life and costs. Health-related quality-of-life differences between treatments were initially small but increased over time. Indeed, for emotional, cognitive and social function, differences in effect over time were statistically significant and differences were also seen in the dysphagia scale.[34] There were ony minor differences in costs between the two treatments. The authors of the trial concluded that brachytherapy should be the primary treatment for palliation of dysphagia from oesophageal cancer.

Intracavity irradiation (brachytherapy) with a single dose appears to be a good palliative treatment of malignant dysphagia. High-quality randomised evidence including patient reported outcome measures support this approach.[18,34,36] Changes in the delivery of radiotherapy services may be necessary if this is to be widely adopted in the UK. Selecting patients for this treatment is important and some frail patients will still require immediate relief of dysphagia with a single admission for placement of an SEMS. Otherwise for patients who require palliation of malignant dysphagia brachytherapy is recommended.

Palliative chemotherapy or combination chemoradiotherapy for oesophageal cancer

The role of palliative chemotherapy for oeophageal cancer remains ill defined. The aim of treatment is to control local and distant tumour to improve quality of life and prolong survival. A recent Cochrane systematic review found limited evidence evaluating palliative chemotherapy compared with best supportive care.[4] Indeed, only two randomised controlled trials with a total of 42 patients compared chemotherapy with best supportive care for metastatic oesophageal cancer. The median survival in the intervention group was 6 months. In the five randomised trials that compared different chemotherapeutic regimes in 1242 participants, no consistent benefit to any specific chemotherapy regimen was observed and it was not possible to perform a formal pooled analysis.[4] It is possible that combination chemoradiotherapy may improve response rates and survival, although evidence is also limited. There is also a lack of evidence to support the role of second-line chemotherapy for the palliation of oesophageal cancer. Patients suitable for palliative chemotherapy often require attention for nutritional needs. If the initial course of chemotherapy can be tolerated and a response achieved, it is possible that relief of dysphagia will occur and last for some months before further progression is experienced. Trials comparing palliative treatment modalities that are in preparation will include an assessment of survival and health-related quality of life.

Aero-digestive fistulas

Aero-digestive fistulas cause paroxysmal coughing fits, aspiration and, if untreated, eventually death from recurrent chest infections. They occur in about 5% of patients with oesophageal cancer, either because of spontaneous necrosis of the tumour and/or local nodes through the oesophageal wall into the bronchial tree, or as a result of treatment. These fistulas are difficult to treat and life expectancy is usually short. The creation of a cervical oesophagostomy and gastrostomy may relieve symptoms but is not usually appropriate. Palliative bypass surgery with stomach or colon for interposition is highly invasive and is also not generally recommended because of the poor general health and prognosis of patients in these situations. Endoscopic insertion of a prosthesis is the treatment of choice, although results following the use of rigid prostheses have not been encouraging, despite the availability of modified cuffed prostheses. The use of covered metal stents to seal aero-digestive fistulas seems to be a more promising development, although no randomised trials have been performed.[37] Fistulas close to the cricopharyngeus are particularly difficult to manage. In this situation simultaneous tracheal and oesophageal stenting may be performed. The possibility that an oesophageal prosthesis may cause significant airway compression should always be considered for tumours in the upper half of the oesophagus and particularly when a fistula of the airway is known or suspected. Preliminary bronchoscopy may clarify this and indicate that tracheal stenting may be preferable to oesophageal stenting, or at least should be performed before oesophageal stenting. Tracheal stenting may also be necessary before commencing chemoradiation treatment for T4 tumours close to, but not actually invading, the airway.[38] At present the role of chemotherapy or radiotherapy in this regard needs further evaluation. The endoscopic placement of fibrin tissue glue may be worthwhile where stenting is not achievable.

Recurrent laryngeal nerve palsy

Recurrent laryngeal nerve palsy caused by tumour infiltration results in eating difficulties, a weak voice, poor cough and repeated chest infections because of aspiration pneumonia. Patients are usually hoarse and complain of swallowing difficulties in the oropharynygeal phase. Coughing and a sensation of choking are typical on consuming solids and liquids. The diagnosis is confirmed by laryngoscopy. Endoscopy may be required to exclude other problems contributing to dysphagia. Aspiration can be confirmed during the pharyngeal phase of swallowing on barium studies. The left nerve is more commonly involved because of its intrathoracic course. Teflon injection to re-establish glottic competence should help swallowing, speech and problems with coughing. In a series of 15 patients, all improved except one, who developed stridor and required emergency tracheostomy.[39] Recurrent laryngeal nerve damage at the time of oesophagectomy usually causes a temporary paralysis that resolves within 6 weeks.

Bleeding

Bleeding from inoperable oesophageal and cardia tumours causes problems with refractory anaemia and occasionally acute upper gastrointestinal haemorrhage. It is often difficult to deal with because of the advanced nature of the tumour and it may be a terminal event. Symptoms may be controlled endoscopically using laser energy, adrenaline injection or electrocoagulation. External-beam radiotherapy is also said to reduce bleeding and extend the interval between blood transfusions, although there is no evidence for this practice.

Palliative treatments of tumours of the gastric body and antrum

Patients in whom potentially curative radical surgery for gastric cancer is not appropriate often require palliation of symptoms. Many with advanced disease may be asymptomatic but even for patients with obstructive symptoms or bleeding, palliative chemotherapy is recommended for symptom relief. There are also situations where problems with gastric outlet obstruction or bleeding are severe and palliative surgery or endoscopic therapy is necessary. The role of palliative chemotherapy or radiotherapy, and the management of gastric outflow obstruction and chronic and acute gastric bleeding, will be discussed separately.

Chemotherapy for advanced gastric cancer

Systemic chemotherapy is the main treatment option for patients with inoperable gastric tumours. A recent systematic review and meta-analysis of aggregate data of phase 2 and 3 clinical trials on first-line chemotherapy in advanced gastric cancer has summarised current knowledge.[8] Palliative chemotherapy offers survival benefits compared with best supportive care (hazard ratio 0.83, 95% CI 0.74–0.93). Combination three-drug chemotherapy also has survival advantages compared to 5-flourouracil/cisplatin-containing regimens with or without anthracyclines (hazard ratio 0.77, 95% CI 0.62–0.95). Epirubicin, cisplatin and 5-fluorouracil (as a continuous infusion, rather than as bolus) therefore is recommended to achieve best survival results and minimise rates of toxicity. The recent development and licensing of an oral form of 5-fluorouracil (capecitabine) may allow the prolonged continuous use of this drug without the problems associated with a long-term central venous line. Irrespective of the positive impact of any of the presently available palliative chemotherapies for gastric cancer, the median survival is only 7–10 months in most large clinical trials. Full, frank and kind discussion with patients considering palliative treatments is therefore recommended. The main drawbacks of chemotherapy are the potential complications. Toxicities include haematological problems, thrombovenous embolism and infective complications. During treatment itself, generic aspects of quality of life deteriorate (physical, role function) but symptoms are relieved (dysphagia, eating restrictions). Patients with a good baseline performance status usually tolerate temporary problems well. Patients require information to help them cope with treatments and to meet information needs, and this will include data about treatment advantages (survival) and disadvantages (morbidity and temporary negative impact on quality of life).

 Palliative combination (three-drug) chemotherapy is recommended for patients with advanced gastric cancer. There is evidence that this extends survival compared with best supportive care, and combination treatment is better than single-drug regimens. Median life expectancy is 7–10 months. Patients require realistic information about expected survival benefits, toxicity and impact on quality of life before undergoing this type of treatment, and further studies comparing novel therapies should include robust assessment of patient experience and detailed assessment of health-related quality of life.

Gastric outlet obstruction

Obstruction associated with cancer of the gastric corpus or antrum can be difficult to manage. Many of these extend proximally to involve extensive segments of the stomach, resulting in interference with both reservoir function and emptying. Resection of the primary tumour may provide symptomatic relief and generally is a better guarantee of success than bypass surgery. The problem is that many patients with incurable distal gastric cancer with obstruction are nutritionally depleted and frail. Surgery may therefore be best avoided, as patients never sufficiently recover from surgery to benefit from it during their remaining time alive (median survival 6 months). There are also differing opinions about the type of palliative gastrectomy that should be performed in this situation (subtotal or total). In the Western world, where morbidity associated with total gastrectomy is high, it is not generally recommended for palliative purposes. The role of gastric resection in linitis plastica remains controversial. It probably has little to offer for those patients who additionally have peritoneal or liver metastasis or contiguous organ involvement, where life expectancy is very poor at around only 4 months. Patients with linitis plastica who have disease limited to the stomach or regional lymph nodes may, however, survive beyond 12 months and thus be appropriately palliated by total gastrectomy. In the authors' unit palliative total gastrectomy is rarely performed. It is best restricted to patients who are generally fit, but where severe bleeding prevents the patient from leaving the hospital. Wherever possible, endoscopic palliative treatment of obstructive symptoms or palliative chemotherapy are offered to these patients.

Patients with non-resectable distal lesions may undergo gastrojejunostomy. The loop of jejunum is anastomosed close to the greater curve of the stomach. There is little consensus regarding anterior or posterior loops. The latter may theoretically be more prone to recurrent obstruction due to proximity to the tumour. The Devine exclusion bypass operation for inoperable antral tumours was thought to increase survival by preventing recurrent tumour obstructing the gastrojejunostomy.[40] There is some evidence that laparoscopic gastrojejunostomy for palliation of incurable gastric outlet obstruction causes less morbidity than standard open surgery. A systematic review of the role of stents versus gastrojejunostomy for the palliation of gastric outlet obstruction suggested that stent placement may be associated with more favourable results in patients with a relatively short life expectancy.[7] The review recommended that gastrojejunostomy was the recommended palliative treatment in patients with a better prognosis.

Metal stents can be more successfully placed across recurrent tumours at oesophagojejunal anastomoses and in recurrent peritoneal disease causing high small-bowel obstruction following total gastrectomy. Recanalisation of the gastric outlet with laser coagulation has not been used successfully. The insertion of nasogastric tubes, percutaneous endoscopically placed feeding tubes and jejunostomies enables nutrition to be delivered to patients with inoperable tumours. These manoeuvres alone, however, fail to palliate most of the patient's symptoms. Many believe that such palliation merely perpetuates suffering except in situations where they are used as an adjunct to recanalisation. They may be indicated to provide preliminary nutritional support in patients selected for palliative chemotherapy.

 Duodenal stents may be used as first-line treatment in patients with a poor prognosis requiring palliation of gastric outlet obstruction. Fitter patients with longer life expectancy may benefit more from surgical gastrojejunostomy. High-quality evidence with large clinical trials is required to compare these treatment modalities.

Chronic bleeding

Surgery remains a useful therapeutic manoeuvre to palliate the symptoms and problems of chronic blood loss from gastric tumours. Laser therapy can successfully achieve haemostasis in bleeding gastric malignancies and there are increasing reports of argon-beam coagulation to limit bleeding from gastric tumours.[41] Both methods require repeated hospital admissions. Radiotherapy may also be used to control chronic bleeding from gastric tumours, although there are no published data to support this practice.

Summary

The number of therapeutic options available for the palliation of patients with oesophageal and gastric cancer has increased significantly over the past decade. No single treatment completely relieves all symptoms without side-effects and median life expectancy for patients with either tumour type is only between 6 and 12 months. Common clinical situations such as the management of fistulas, high oesophageal tumours and bleeding inoperable gastric lesions continue to present formidable management problems. The introduction of self-expanding metal stents, argon-beam coagulation, brachytherapy, chemotherapy and combination treatments offers new hope, although evidence of significant survival benefits or improvements in quality of life with new treatments have yet to be realised. The increasing centralisation of cancer services in order to provide high-technology specialised care may improve outcomes and increase recruitment into national randomised trials that focus on palliative treatments. There are still many patients who present with advanced disease who are severely debilitated and have a limited life expectancy. Such patients need to be identified early to prevent travelling long distances to a centre with specialised endoscopic facilities only to find that treatment has to be performed more than once. Genuine efforts should be made to see if patients with very short survival times (less than 4 weeks) can be identified and perhaps spared unnecessarily aggressive attempts at palliation.

There remains a need to define outcomes for patients with inoperable malignancies of the upper gastrointestinal tract. Although it would be useful to standardise dysphagia scores and improve audit, in the palliative setting the most important outcome should be patients' assessment of benefits of treatment. The use of self-report quality-of-life questionnaires in clinical practice will provide such data, although at present these are mainly research tools.[42–44] The role of the specialist upper gastrointestinal nurse to support patients undergoing palliative treatment and to provide nutritional support is increasing, and links between palliative care and upper gastrointesintal cancer teams need to be well established and used.[45,46]

The selection of palliation for patients with advanced disease is difficult. Every patient is unique with regard to tumour histology, stricture location, clinical stage, premorbid state and emotional requirements. Choosing one technique over another must be justifiable on the grounds of treatment efficacy, ease of application, overall adaptability to other therapeutic areas and patient acceptance, while minimising both complications and cost. Skilled multidisciplinary teams with a thorough understanding of all the available palliative treatments are needed and close liaison with palliative care services is essential to minimise suffering.

Key points

- Patients with oesophageal cancer selected for palliative treatment have a median survival of less than 8 months and few survive beyond 1 year. There is little evidence to show that any single or combination of palliative treatment modalities changes survival for patients with incurable oesophageal cancer.
- The median survival for patients with gastric cancer undergoing palliative treatment is poor; 50% of patients die within 6 months of diagnosis and the remainder within 2 years. Combination three-drug palliative chemotherapy increases survival compared with best supportive care, and it is recommended for patients with sufficient performance status and desire to undergo this intervention.
- Palliative treatment decisions should be taken in the context of a multidisciplinary team meetings and subsequently be shared with the patient. Patients require information that is imparted kindly but truthfully and it should include data about likely survival benefits and impact of treatment of symptom relief and quality of life.
- Accurate tumour staging and assessment of patient comorbidity and choice plays a critical part in any therapeutic protocol, enabling patients to be assigned appropriately to treatments with either curative or palliative intent.
- Surgery has a limited role to play in palliative treatments of cancer of the oesophagus and stomach. Subtotal gastrectomy may be useful to palliate outlet obstruction in patients with a reasonable prognosis and it will allow them to undergo palliative chemotherapy. The role of

palliative total gastrectomy is very limited to patients with advanced disease causing intractable dysphagia or bleeding. It is possible that death will occur from disease recurrence before the benefits of surgery are realised.

- Single-dose brachytherapy provides better long-term relief of dysphagia than self-expanding metal stents (SEMS). There is no longer a role for intubation with rigid plastic prostheses and SEMS have become the standard method for intubating malignant oesophageal or oesophagogastric tumours.

- Laser therapy is particularly useful for oesophageal tumours with an exophytic component. Argon-beam coagulation provides similar palliation and is a more cost-effective, readily available local treatment.

- Laser treatment may be preferable for non-circumferential, polypoid or exophytic tumours, while intubation is preferable in sclerotic stenosing tumours.

- Injection of chemicals to relieve malignant dysphagia has all the hallmarks of a good technique, being safe, inexpensive and readily available. The technique is less precise than laser treatment because it is difficult to be sure where the alcohol is going once it enters the tissue.

- Palliative chemotherapy has an increasingly important role to play in advanced oesophageal cancer and tumours of the oesophagogastric junction, but currently evidence to routinely support its role is lacking.

- The main drawbacks of palliative chemotherapy for gastric cancer are the potential complications and reduction in quality of life. Patients with a good baseline performance status, however, usually tolerate temporary problems well.

- The selection of palliation for patients with advanced disease is difficult and requires skilled motivated input from multidisciplinary teams with a thorough understanding of all the available palliative treatments and awareness of the patient's individual needs.

References

1. Muller JM, Erasmi H, Stelzner M et al. Surgical therapy of oesophageal carcinoma. Br J Surg 1990; 77:845–57.

2. Rouvelas I, Zeng W, Lindblad M et al. Survival after surgery for oesophageal cancer: a population-based study. Lancet Oncol 2005; 6:864–70.

3. Al-Sarira AA, David G, Willmott S et al. Oesophagectomy practice and outcomes in England. Br J Surg 2007; 94:585–91.

4. Homs MY, Gaast A, Siersema PD et al. Chemotherapy for metastatic carcinoma of the esophagus and gastro-esophageal junction. Cochrane Database Syst Rev 2006; CD004063.

5. Allum WH, Griffin SM, Watson A et al. Guidelines for the management of oesophageal and gastric cancer. Gut 2002; 50(Suppl 5):v1–23.

6. McCulloch P, Ward J, Tekkis PP. Mortality and morbidity in gastro-oesophageal cancer surgery: initial results of ASCOT multicentre prospective cohort study. BMJ 2003; 327:756–61.

7. Jeurnink SM, van Eijck CH, Steyerberg EW et al. Stent versus gastrojejunostomy for the palliation of gastric outlet obstruction: a systematic review. BMC Gastroenterol 2007; 7:18.

8. Wagner AD, Grothe W, Haerting J et al. Chemotherapy in advanced gastric cancer: a systematic review and meta-analysis based on aggregate data. J Clin Oncol 2006; 24:2903–9.

9. Blazeby JM, Brookes ST, Alderson D. The prognostic value of quality of life scores during treatment for oesophageal cancer. Gut 2001; 49:227–30.

10. Bartels HE, Stein HJ, Siewert JR. Preoperative risk analysis and postoperative mortality of oesophagectomy for resectable oesophageal cancer. Br J Surg 1998; 85:840–4.

11. Eloubeidi MA, Desmond R, Arguedas MR et al. Prognostic factors for the survival of patients with esophageal carcinoma in the U.S.: the importance of tumor length and lymph node status. Cancer 2002; 95:1434–43.

12. The NHS cancer plan. London: Department of Health, 2000.

13. Executive NHS. Improving outcomes in upper gastro-intestinal cancers. The Manual, 2001.

14. Fleissig A, Jenkins V, Catt S et al. Multidisciplinary teams in cancer care: are they effective in the UK? Lancet Oncol 2006; 7:935–43.

15. Blazeby JM, Wilson L, Metcalfe C et al. Analysis of clinical decision-making in multi-disciplinary cancer teams. Ann Oncol 2006; 17:457–60.

16. Rutten LJ, Arora NK, Bakos AD et al. Information needs and sources of information among cancer patients: a systematic review of research (1980–2003). Patient Educ Couns 2005; 57:250–61.

17. Blazeby JM, Farndon JR, Donovan JL et al. A prospective longitudinal study examining the quality of life of patients with esophageal cancer. Cancer 2000; 88:1781–7.

18. Homs MY, Steyerberg EW, Eijkenboom WM et al. Single-dose brachytherapy versus metal stent placement for the palliation of dysphagia from oesophageal cancer: multicentre randomised trial. Lancet 2004; 364:1497–504 (Abstract).

19. Riley SA, Attwood SEA. Guidelines on the use of oesophageal dilation in clinical practice. Gut 2004; 53:i1–6.

20. Knyrim K, Wagner HJ, Bethge N et al. A controlled trial of an expansile metal stent for palliation of oesophageal obstruction due to inoperable cancer. N Engl J Med 1993; 329:1302–7.

21. Siersema PD, Hop WCJ, Dees J et al. Coated self-expanding metal stents versus latex prostheses for esophagogastric cancer with special reference to prior radiation and chemotherapy: a controlled, prospective study. Gastrointest Endosc 1998; 47:113–20.

22. Shenfine J, McNamee P, Steen N et al. A pragmatic randomised controlled trial of the cost-effectiveness of palliative therapies for patients with inoperable oesophageal cancer. Health Technol Assess 2005; 9:1–136 (Abstract).

23. Conio M, Repici A, Battaglia G et al. A randomized prospective comparison of self-expandable plastic stents and partially covered self-expandable metal stents in the palliation of malignant esophageal dysphagia. Am J Gastroenterol 2007; 102:2667–77.

24. Power C, Byrne PJ, Lim K et al. Superiority of anti-reflux stent compared with conventional stents in the palliative management of patients with cancer of the lower esophagus and esophago-gastric junction: results of a randomized clinical trial. Dis Esophagus 2007; 20:466–70.

25. Manner H, May A, Rabenstein T et al. Prospective evaluation of a new high-power argon plasma coagulation system (hp-APC) in therapeutic gastrointestinal endoscopy. Scand J Gastroenterol 2007; 42:397–405.

26. Barr H, Dix AJ, Kendall C et al. Review article: the potential role for photodynamic therapy in the management of upper gastrointestinal disease. Aliment Pharmacol Ther 2001; 15:311–21.

27. Lightdale CJ, Heier SK, Marcon NE et al. Photodynamic therapy with porfimer sodium versus thermal ablation therapy with Nd:YAG laser for palliation of esophageal cancer: a multicentre randomised trial. Gastrointest Endosc 1995; 42:507–12.

28. Heier SK, Rothman KA, Heier LM et al. Photodynamic therapy for obstructing esophageal cancer: light dosimetry and randomised comparison with Nd:YAG laser therapy. Gastroenterology 1995; 109:63–72.

29. Jensen DM, Machicado G, Randall G et al. Comparison of low power YAG laser and BICAP tumour probe for palliation of oesophageal cancer strictures. Gastroenterology 1988; 94:1263–70.

30. Nwokolo CU, Payne-James JJ, Silk DBA et al. Palliation of malignant dysphagia by ethanol induced tumour necrosis. Gut 1994; 35:299–303.

31. Payne-James JJ, Spiller RC, Misiewicz JJ et al. Use of ethanol-induced tumour necrosis to palliate dysphagia in patients with oesophagogastric cancer. Gastrointest Endosc 1990; 36:43–6.

32. Chung SCS, Leong HT, Choi CYC et al. Palliation of malignant oesophageal obstruction by endoscopic alcohol injection. Endoscopy 1994; 26:275–7.

33. Carazzone A, Bonavina L, Segalin A et al. Endoscopic palliation of oesophageal cancer: results of a prospective comparison of Nd:YAG laser and ethanol injection. Eur J Surg 1999; 165:351–6.

34. Earlam R, Cunha-Melo JR. Oesophageal squamous cell carcinoma: II. A critical view of radiotherapy. Br J Surg 1980; 67:457–61.

35. Homs MY, Essink-Bot ML, Borsboom GJ et al. Quality of life after palliative treatment for oesophageal carcinoma – a prospective comparison between stent placement and single dose brachytherapy. Eur J Cancer 2004; 40:1862–71.

36. Polinder S, Homs MYV, Siersema PD et al. for the Dutch SIREC Study Group. Cost study of metal stent placement vs. single-dose brachytherapy in the palliative treatment of oesophageal cancer. Br J Cancer 2004; 90:2067–72.

37. Cook TA, Dehn TCB. Use of covered expandable metal stents in the treatment of oesophageal carcinoma and tracheo-oesophageal fistula. Br J Surg 1996; 83:1417–18.

38. Ellul JPM, Morgan R, Gold D et al. Parallel self-expanding covered metal stents in the trachea and oesophagus for the palliation of complex high tracheo-oesophageal fistula. Br J Surg 1996; 83:1767–8.

39. Griffin SM, Chung SCS, van Hasselt CA et al. Late swallowing and aspiration problems after oesophagectomy for cancer: malignant infiltration of the recurrent laryngeal nerves and its management. Surgery 1992; 112:533–5.

40. Kwok SPY, Chung SCS, Griffin SM et al. Devine exclusion for unresectable carcinoma of the stomach. Br J Surg 1991; 78:684–5.

41. Heindorff H, Wojdemann M, Bisgaard T et al. Endoscopic palliation of inoperable cancer of the oesophagus or cardia by argon electrocoagulation. Scand J Gastroenterol 1998; 33:21–3.

42. Blazeby JM, Conroy T, Bottomley A et al. Clinical and psychometric validation of a questionnaire module, the EORTC QLQ-STO 22, to assess quality of life in patients with gastric cancer. Eur J Cancer 2004; 40:2260–8.

43. Lagergren P, Fayers P, Conroy T et al. Clinical and psychometric validation of a questionnaire module, the EORTC QLQ-OG25, to assess health-related quality of life in patients with cancer of the oesophagus, the oesophago-gastric junction and the stomach. Eur J Cancer 2007; 43:2066–73.

44. Blazeby JM, Conroy T, Hammerlid E et al. Clinical and psychometric validation of an EORTC questionnaire module, the EORTC QLQ-OES18, to assess quality of life in patients with oesophageal cancer. Eur J Cancer 2003; 39:1384–94.

45. Nicklin J, Blazeby J. Anorexia in patients dying from oesophageal and gastric cancers. Gastrointest Nursing 2003; 1:35–9.

46. Irving M. Oesophageal cancer and the role of the nurse specialist. Nursing Times 2002; 98:38–40.

47. Adam A, Ellul J, Watkinson AF et al. Palliation of inoperable oesophageal carcinoma: a prospective randomised trial of laser therapy and stent placement. Radiology 1997; 202:344–8.

48. Sargeant IR, Tobias JS, Blackman G et al. Radiotherapy enhances laser palliation of malignant dysphagia: a randomised study. Gut 1997; 40:362–9.

49. Dallal HJ, Smith GD, Grieve DC et al. A randomized trial of thermal ablative therapy versus expandable metal stents in the palliative treatment of patients with esophageal carcinoma. Gastrointest Endosc 2001; 54:549–57.

50. Siersema PD, Hop WC, van Blankenstein M et al. A comparison of 3 types of covered metal stents for the palliation of patients with dysphagia caused by esophagogastric carcinoma: a prospective, randomized study. Gastrointest Endosc 2001; 54:145–53.

51. Vakil N, Morris AI, Marcon N et al. A prospective, randomized, controlled trial of covered expandable metal stents in the palliation of malignant esophageal obstruction at the gastroesophageal junction. Am J Gastroenterol 2001; 96:1791–6.

52. O'Donnell CA, Fullarton GM, Watt E et al. Randomized clinical trial comparing self-expanding metallic stents with plastic endoprostheses in the palliation of oesophageal cancer. Br J Surg 2002; 89:985–92.

53. Sabharwal T, Hamady MS, Chui S et al. A randomised prospective comparison of the flamingo wallstent and ultraflex stent for palliation of dysphagia associated with lower third oesophageal carcinoma. Gut 2003; 52:922–6.

11

Other oesophageal and gastric neoplasms

Richard H. Hardwick

Introduction

This chapter will cover a group of rarer upper gastrointestinal tumours whose treatment has changed greatly in the past decade; some are often cured by surgery alone while others are managed almost exclusively by chemotherapy. By far the largest group are the gastrointestinal stromal tumours (GISTs), and better understanding of the pathologophysiology of these interesting tumours has occurred simultaneously with the introduction of effective medical treatment in the form of imatinib (Glivec®, Novartis Pharma AG, Basel, Switzerland). A large part of this chapter will therefore cover the presentation, diagnosis and management of upper GISTs. The importance of accurate histological diagnosis of gastric tumours cannot be overemphasised; the treatment and prognosis of gastric lymphoma is very different from adenocarcinoma and this will be covered in its own section along with gastric carcinoid. In the final section on 'rareties' we will look briefly at leiomyomas, leiomyosarcomas and small-cell tumours of the oesophagus.

Gastrointestinal stromal tumours (GISTs)

Pathophysiology

GISTs are soft-tissue sarcomas of mesenchymal origin that arise in the gastrointestinal tract; they are rare, representing 0.1–3% of all gut tumours and 5% of all soft-tissue sarcomas.[1] Historically, these tumours were considered to be of smooth muscle origin and were generally regarded as leiomyomas (benign) or leiomyosarcomas (malignant). Electron microscopy and immunohistochemical studies indicated, however, that only a minority of stromal tumours have the typical features of smooth muscle, with some having a more neural appearance and others appearing undifferentiated.[2] 'Gastrointestinal stromal tumour' was subsequently introduced as being a more appropriate term for these neoplasms, with the variable histological features (smooth muscle, neural or undifferentiated) considered to be of little clinical relevance. Gastrointestinal autonomic nerve tumour was also introduced to describe sarcomas with ultrastructural evidence of autonomic nervous system differentiation;[3] these tumours are now recognised as a variant of GISTs.[4] The discovery of CD34 expression in many GISTs suggested that they were a specific entity,[5] distinct from smooth muscle tumours. It was also observed that GISTs and the interstitial cells of Cajal express the receptor tyrosine kinase KIT (CD117).[6] This has led to the now widely accepted classification of mesenchymal tumours of the gastrointestinal (GI) tract into GISTs, true smooth muscle tumours and, far less frequently, true Schwann cell tumours.[7]

Incidence and malignant potential

Studies using diagnostic markers including CD117 immunoreactivity have shown that GISTs are under-diagnosed.[6] The morphological spectrum of GISTs was also wider than previously recognised. The estimated annual incidence of GISTs is around 15 per million,[8] which equates to approximately 900 new cases per year in the UK. A true measure of the incidence, prevalence and ratio of 'benign' to 'malignant' GISTs may not be possible as these tumours appear to possess varying degrees of malignant potential. The size of the tumour, the symptoms at diagnosis, the organ of origin (small-bowel GISTs have the worst prognosis) and mitotic count seem to be the most important factors when assessing prognosis.[9]

 A scheme for defining the risk of aggressive behaviour in GIST based on tumour size and mitotic count has been proposed[10] (Fig. 11.1). Most GISTs <2 cm have negligible mitotic activity (usually <5 per 50 high-power fields), and are considered very low or low risk in all sites when completely removed. Large tumours have a much poorer prognosis, even after apparently complete resection (Fig. 11.2).[11]

Patient demographics and anatomical distribution

No marked sex difference is apparent for GISTs. Two larger series of malignant gastrointestinal sarcomas did, however, demonstrate a slight male predominance.[11,12] The age distribution appears to be unimodal with a median age at presentation of 58 years (range 16–94). The peak incidence in men occurs in the fifth decade, slightly before that in women, where it peaks in the sixth decade. The median age at presentation appears constant in several series, ranging from 58 to 61 years.[13] Only 1–2% of GISTs present in patients before 30 years of age.[11]

Most GISTs arise in the stomach or small intestine, and infrequently in the oesophagus, mesentery, omentum, colon or rectum[12,14] (Table 11.1). Approximately 10–30% of GISTs are overtly malignant at presentation;[15] the principal sites of metastasis are the liver and the peritoneal cavity and spread to lymph nodes is very rare.[11]

Presentation

The symptoms of GISTs are non-specific and depend on the size and location of the lesion. Small GISTs (2 cm or less) are usually asymptomatic and are detected during investigations or surgical procedures for unrelated disease. The vast majority of these are of low risk for malignancy.[16] In many cases

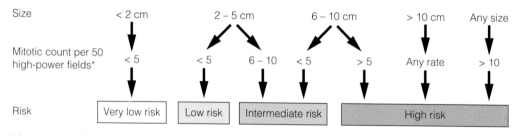

Figure 11.1 • Algorithm based on the consensus approach for assessing the risk of malignancy of GIST reached at the National Institutes of Health workshop.[10] *A high-power field approximates to 0.2 mm².

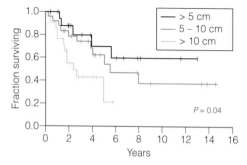

Figure 11.2 • Disease-specific survival after resection of primary GIST based on tumour size.[11] Eighty patients underwent gross resection of primary GISTs. Patients with tumours >10 cm (n = 27) had significantly worse survival than those with tumours between 6 and 10 cm (n = 30) or ≤5 cm (n = 23).

Table 11.1 • Anatomical site of GISTs

Site	Percentage
Stomach	60–70%
Small intestine	20–30%
Oesophagus, mesentery, omentum, colon or rectum	10%

the mucosa is normal so that endoscopic biopsies are unremarkable. Incidental discovery accounts for approximately one-third of cases.[17]

The most common symptom is GI bleeding, which is present in approximately 50% of patients[18] (Table 11.2). In addition, systemic symptoms such as fever, night sweats and weight loss are common in GIST and rare in other sarcomas. Patients with larger tumours may experience abdominal discomfort or develop a palpable mass.[19] GISTs are often clinically silent until they reach a large size, bleed or rupture. Symptomatic oesophageal GISTs, although rare, typically present with dysphagia, while gastric and small-intestinal GISTs often present with vague symptoms leading to their eventual detection by gastroscopy or radiology. Most duodenal GISTs occur in the second part of the duodenum where they push or infiltrate into the pancreas.[20]

Investigation

Approximately 60% of GISTs are submucosal and grow towards the lumen where, if in the proximal GI tract, they may be visualised endoscopically as smooth submucosal projections. If a small

submucosal mass is seen as an incidental finding at the time of endoscopy, an endoscopic ultrasound (EUS) should be the first investigation as a significant proportion will be due to extrinsic impression from normal adjacent structures, e.g. gallbladder in the antrum, spleen in the proximal stomach and caudate lobe in the body. If this is the case, no further investigation is required. For larger palpable masses, or where the patients present with haemorrhage, abdominal pain or obstruction, computed tomography (CT) is usually the first investigation after endoscopy to assess both the primary and to look for metastases.[21]

Endoscopic ultrasound (EUS)

The classical features are of a hypoechoic mass contiguous with the fourth (muscularis propria) or second (muscularis mucosae) layers of the normal gut wall, both of which are hypoechoic (**Fig. 11.3**a,b). The EUS features most predictive of 'benign' tumours are regular margins, tumour size ≤30 mm and a homogeneous echo pattern. Larger tumours with irregular extraluminal margins and cystic spaces are more likely to behave aggressively.[22,23]

To further aid diagnostic accuracy it is possible to use a linear array EUS scope through which needle aspirates and core biopsies can be taken without breaching surgical resection planes. EUS with fine-needle aspiration (FNA) in experienced hands has a diagnostic accuracy of up to 97% for GIST lesions,[24] is becoming more widely available and should be considered in the diagnostic work-up of a possible GIST lesion if the result could change clinical management.

Table 11.2 • Symptoms of GIST at diagnosis[18]

Symptoms	Incidence (%)
Abdominal pain	20–50
Gastrointestinal bleeding	50
Gastrointestinal obstruction	10–30
Asymptomatic	20

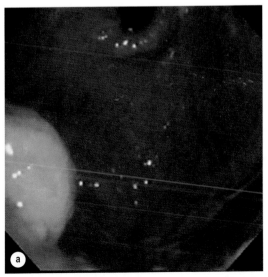
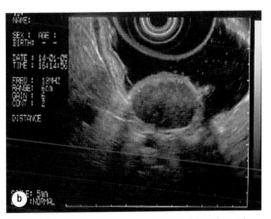

Figure 11.3 • (a) Endoscopic view of a small incidental gastric GIST. **(b)** A 12 MHz EUS image of the incidental gastric GIST seen in (a), showing the lesion arising from the muscularis propria.

CT scanning

GIST imaging by CT typically shows an extralumi-nal mass, often with central necrosis, arising from the digestive tract wall.[17] Small tumours typically appear as sharply margined, smooth-walled, homo-geneous, soft-tissue masses with moderate con-trast enhancement.[25] Large tumours tend to have mucosal ulceration, central necrosis and cavitation, and heterogeneous enhancement following i.v. con-trast.[25] As well as defining the presence and nature of a mass, if possible, the likely organ of origin should be defined. Multiplanar reconstruction can assist this, particularly with large masses. Negative oral contrast (e.g. tap water) and intravenous contrast for the assessment of gastric GISTs are recommended. CT of chest, abdomen and pelvis is recommended for staging of GIST, with the exception of small incidental tumours or when a patient presents as an emergency requiring urgent surgery. With regards to assessing treatment response, traditional CT criteria (RECIST criteria) have been shown to be inaccurate for measuring GIST response to imatinib and the Choi criteria are recommended (10% reduction in size and 15% reduction in density).[26]

Magnetic resonance imaging (MRI)

In general, MRI offers no additional information regarding the intralesional tissue characterisation of primary GISTs. However, MRI provides excellent soft-tissue contrast resolution and direct multipla-nar imaging, which can help delineate the relation-ships of the tumour and adjacent organs and is useful in anorectal disease.[25]

Positron emission tomography (PET)

PET scanning using a standard fluorodeoxyglucose (FDG)-PET technique has proven extremely useful in the prediction of tumour response to the tyrosine kinase inhibitor imatinib (Glivec, Norvartis Pharma AG) now used in the treatment of unresectable and metastatic malignant GISTs.[27] Glucose uptake of the tumours decreases within a few hours to days of the start of treatment, which can be verified with FDG-PET.[16] The PET scan can be utilised to distinguish between tumour progression and increase in volume due to intratumoral bleeding. PET scan responses have also been demonstrated to predict subsequent tumour volume reductions found on CT or MRI.[28]

GIST syndromes

Families have been reported with single-base 'gain of function' mutation in the kinase domain of *KIT*. The resultant effect is the development of multiple GISTs in the small bowel. Diffuse hyperplasia of spindle-shaped cells within the myenteric plexus at sites unaffected by GIST formation was also noted.[29,30] The association of three uncommon neoplasms – gastric GIST, func-tioning extra-adrenal paraganglionoma and pulmo-

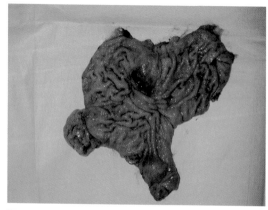

Figure 11.4 • Specimen from completion gastrectomy for bleeding GIST (ulcer clearly visible) in a 34-year-old woman with Carney's triad.

nary chondroma – was first reported in 1977 and has been recognised as 'Carney's triad' since (**Fig. 11.4**).[31] A subsequent review of 79 cases demonstrated that, unlike isolated sporadic GIST, where no significant sex difference was noted,[32] 85% were female.[32] Twenty-two per cent of the patients had all three tumours; the remainder had two of the three, usually the gastric and pulmonary lesions. Adrenocortical adenoma has since been identified as a new constituent of the disor-der. The presence of two of the three main tumours is considered sufficient for the syndrome.

Treatment and prognosis (Box 11.1)

A chest, abdominal and pelvic CT should be included in the preoperative assessment for all patients. If the tumour is located in the right or left upper quadrant then the patient should have an endocrine assess-ment to exclude a large functioning adrenal tumour. Male patients (under the age of 40 years) presenting with large centrally placed retroperitoneal tumours should have α-fetoprotein and β-human chorionic gonadotrophin levels measured to exclude non-seminomatous germ-cell tumour.

Percutaneous (ultrasound or CT) or laparoscopi-cally guided biopsies should not be used in resectable disease due to the risk of tumour rupture or seed-ing, unless it may result in a change of treatment.[16]

The main goal of GIST management is com-plete macroscopic and microscopic removal of the tumour – that is, R0 resection.[33] Complete excision offers a good chance of cure and must be attempted whenever possible; the presence of a positive resection margin or tumour rupture leads to a significant reduction in survival.[34] In one study, only 11% of patients died of recurrent disease after R0 resection compared with 75% of those in whom the resection was R1 or R2, with a median follow-up of 2.2 years.[13]

Locoregional disease

Principles of surgery

A wide local resection with macroscopic and microscopic removal of the entire tumour is recommended (R0)

The surgeon should aim to preserve function, but not at the expense of an R0 resection

Extended lymphadenectomy is normally not required

Some small tumours may be resected laparoscopically

Where adjacent organs are involved, en bloc resection is recommended whenever possible – input from other specialist surgeons should be considered prior to embarking on a resection

Endoscopic resection is not recommended

Unresectable and/or metastatic disease

Conventional cytotoxic chemotherapy and radiotherapy are not recommended

Imatinib should be used as treatment for unresectable and/or metastatic GISTs

The recommended starting dose of imatinib is 400 mg/day

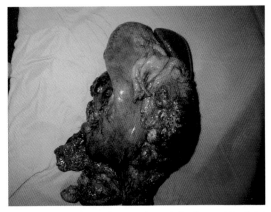

Figure 11.5 • Operative specimen following en bloc total gastrectomy, splenectomy and distal pancreatectomy for locally advanced GIST.

Laparoscopy may be considered in the staging of large lesions to exclude peritoneal metastases but an exploratory laparotomy is usually required to decide whether a large primary tumour is technically resectable or not.

At all sites the extent of resection is therefore dictated by the size of the tumour and its location in relation to, or invasion of, adjacent structures (**Fig. 11.5**). Oesophagectomy is the standard procedure for oesophageal GISTs but these are very rare and submucosal lesions in the oesophagus are much more likely to be leiomyomas. EUS-FNA core biopsy from these lesions is recommended to make a preoperative diagnosis so that surgical planning is appropriate.[24] Oesophageal GISTs and leiomyosarcomas require an oesophagectomy whereas leiomyomas can safely be enucleated without removing the oesophagus.

In the stomach, R0 resection may involve a partial, subtotal or total gastrectomy, although 'wedge' excision and 'sleeve' resections are also frequently performed to preserve as much stomach as possible. Small gastric lesions lend themselves well to laparoscopic resection (**Fig. 11.6**a–c). Resection of GIST tumours arising at the gastro-oesophageal junction create particular problems as a poor quality of life may result from simple excision with anastomosis of stomach to oesophagus. Alternatively, reconstruction using a short jejunal interposition should be considered for these patients, the Merendino procedure (**Fig. 11.7**),[35] as it results in a better quality of life compared to an oesophagogastric anastomosis.[36]

The most important factors are that the tumour is not ruptured and that negative resection margins are obtained. Simple enucleation of the tumour is inadequate as these lesions do not possess a true capsule. Direct invasion of adjacent structures occurs in 10–15% of GISTs and surgery in such cases should include en bloc resection of involved adjacent organs.[11,13] Nodal metastases are extremely rare and routine extended lymph node dissection is therefore unjustified.[37]

As very few studies address the issue of GISTs found incidentally, there are no clear data to support one definitive management plan over another. In their study of 39 GISTs, which included 16 identified incidentally, Ludwig and Traverso concluded that as a consequence of the frequency of serious complications in symptomatic patients, complete excision should also be recommended for asymptomatic patients.[38] However, the UK guidelines for the management of GISTs recommend that small asymptomatic incidental lesions can be treated conservatively, particularly if serial examination shows no change in size over 1–2 years.[39] However, there are no long-term studies of the natural history of these lesions and surgeons should explain these uncertainties to their patients and discuss the pros and cons of resection before proceeding to surgery. In patients of borderline fitness for resection, or those who decline surgery at initial presentation, monitoring the lesion with EUS and/or CT for evidence of enlargement is acceptable so long as the results of surveillance influence the final management.

Unresectable or metastatic disease

The treatment of patients with unresectable and metastatic GISTs has been transformed recently. Prior to the introduction of imatinib mesylate, patients with advanced GISTs faced severe morbidity and short life expectancy. Untreated, the

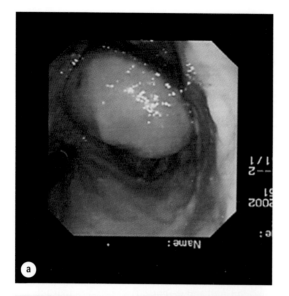

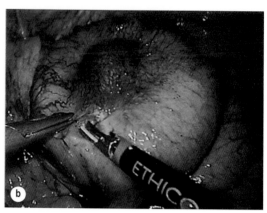

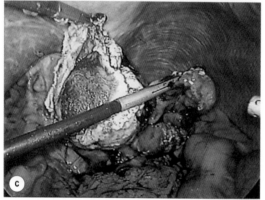

Figure 11.6 • (a) Endoscopic view of a moderate-sized gastric fundal GIST. **(b)** Laparoscopic image of the lesion seen in (a). **(c)** Completed harmonic scalpel dissection of the gastric GIST in (a) prior to removal of specimen in a retrieval bag and closure of the resulting gastric defect with a linear EndoGIA stapler.

median overall survival for unresectable or metastatic disease is around 12 months (ranging from 2 to 20 months).[40] Conventional chemotherapy and radiotherapy are ineffective in patients with metastatic GISTs.[41] Imatinib is a receptor tyrosine kinase inhibitor that inhibits the constitutively activated tyrosine kinases of ABL (including the stable transfection product fusion kinase BCR-ABL seen in chronic myeloid leukaemia), platelet-derived growth factor receptor (PDGFR) and KIT. The drug is administered orally and its use, dosage and side-effect profile are well established following use in the treatment of chronic myeloid leukaemia. It has very little effect on normal cells, where the kinase is not active. Experiments on human tumour cell lines dependent upon the KIT pathway demonstrate that imatinib blocks the kinase activity of KIT, arrests proliferation and causes apoptotic cell death.[42] Imatinib is generally well tolerated, although most patients experience some mild or moderate adverse events. Serious adverse events occur in around 20%

of patients, the most serious of which is life-threatening tumour haemorrhage in approximately 5%.

Early phase I studies of imatinib (then coded ST1571) took the oncology world by storm.[43] Never before had response rates of 80–90% been seen in metastatic sarcomas and a new era of 'smart' compounds was born. Over 50% of patients with metastatic or unresectable GISTs will survive more than 5 years if treated with imatinib.

 In a randomised controlled trial of 147 patients with metastatic or unresectable GISTs the median survival was 54 months regardless whether the 400 or 600 mg dose regimen of imatinib was used.[44] A larger phase III trial recruited 746 patients and compared 400 mg with 800 mg imatinib and again found no difference in survival between the two doses, but 33% of patients on the lower dose who progressed appeared

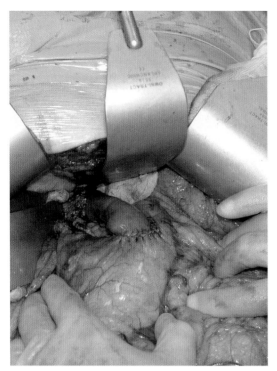

Figure 11.7 • Completed Merendino procedure showing distal anastomosis between the jejunal interposition and the stomach.

to stabilise when transferred to the higher dose.[45] Similar results were obtained from an even larger randomised trial involving 946 patients, although a longer progression-free survival was seen for patients on the higher dose of imatinib.[46]

Although 80% of GISTs respond to imatinib, 20% demonstrate initial resistance to the drug and, of those that respond initially, some will develop late resistance.[47]

Surgery has a limited role in metastatic disease except when patients present with low-volume liver metastases; about a third of such patients may be cured by hepatic resection.[48] In selected patients with large incurable tumours surgery may play a limited role in palliation of symptoms but whether to operate is best decided by a multidisciplinary team who have expertise in GIST management.[49] Downsizing of unresectable primary tumours and hepatic metastasis following treatment with imatinib can render lesions resectable, but long-term survival is uncommon, particularly if imatinib resistance has developed.[50] Randomised studies in the USA and Europe are now under way to assess the value of neoadjuvant imatinib for unresectable GISTs which might be rendered resectable (and potentially curable) and adjuvant imatinib for resectable GISTs with a high risk of recurrence.

Gastric lymphoma

Primary gastric lymphoma is rare, accounting for about 5% of gastric tumours, but is one of the commonest sites for 'extranodal' lymphoma.[51] It is twice as common in men than women and median age of diagnosis is 60–65 years,[52,53] except in human immunodeficiency virus (HIV)-infected patients who develop the disease earlier.[54] It often presents with the same non-specific signs of dyspepsia and vague epigastric discomfort seen in both benign peptic ulceration and gastric adenocarcinoma. However, it may take longer than epithelial cancer to grow and cause persistent pain and weight loss. Diagnosis is by endoscopy and biopsy. It is essential that patients who fulfil the National Institute for Clinical Excellence (NICE) criteria for urgent upper GI endoscopy are referred and that the endoscopist performs a thorough investigation and takes adequate diagnostic biopsies.[55] If the biopsies are non-diagnostic they should be repeated immediately; accurate histological diagnosis is essential as the treatment and prognosis of gastric lymphoma are very different from adenocarcinoma.

Staging

Once a diagnosis of gastric lymphoma is made the patient should undergo a CT scan of chest, abdomen and pelvis, and an endoluminal ultrasound (EUS) as this is the most accurate way of assessing depth of invasion and regional node involvement,[56,57] and a bone marrow aspirate to look for distant spread of the disease. Many staging systems have been employed over the years but the most clinically useful is the modified Blackledge system[58] (Table 11.3).

Classification

Low-grade MALT lymphomas arise from the mucosa-associated lymphoid tissue, and behave in an indolent fashion. The WHO classifies MALT as extranodal marginal zone B-cell lymphomas and they are a form of non-Hodgkin's lymphoma.[55,59,60] Men and women are equally affected and they account for about 4% of all gastric tumours and 50% of gastric lymphomas.[61,62]

 Low-grade gastric MALT lymphomas are associated with *Helicobacter pylori* (HP) infection and early tumours will often regress with HP eradication therapy.[55,63] More advanced lesions that involve the full thickness of the stomach wall and have spread to local lymph nodes are much less likely to regress with HP eradication.[64]

Table 11.3 • Modified Blackledge system for staging gastrointestinal lymphoma[58]

Stage I	Tumour confined to GI tract without serosal penetration: single primary or multiple non-contiguous lesions
Stage II	Tumour extends into abdomen nodes from the primary: II$_1$: local nodes (regional gastric) II$_2$: distant nodes (para-aortic or intercaval)
Stage II$_E$	Perforation of the serosa with involvement of adjacent structures: e.g. stage II$_E$ (pancreas) or stage II$_E$ (colon) Also patients who present with perforated tumours and peritonitis
Stage IV	Disseminated extranodal disease (lung, bone marrow, etc.) or supradiaphragmatic nodal involvement

Histopathologically they can be difficult to differentiate from chronic gastritis and experienced pathologists will look for lymphoepithelial lesions which are diagnostic.[65] Treatment of stage I disease is with HP eradication and 6-monthly endoscopic biopsy for 2 years. More advanced tumours, those that persist after HP eradication or those that recur are treated with chlorambucil and rituximab, and those with large-cell transformation require CHOP chemotherapy (cyclophosphamide, doxorubicin, vincristine and prednisolone) and rituximab.[66,67] Surgery is very rarely indicated for low-grade MALT lymphomas.

High-grade MALT lymphoma and diffuse B-cell lymphomas do not regress with HP eradication. Histologically they consist of sheets of destructive blast cells, do not contain lymphoepitheial lesions and have frequent mitoses and apoptotic bodies.[68] They may resemble diffuse carcinomas, sarcomas, T-cell lymphomas and even metastatic melanoma.

A randomised controlled trial of treatment with CHOP alone versus CHOP and rituximab showed improved 5-year survival from 63% to 76%.[69] A large randomised trial involving 589 patients with diffuse B-cell gastric lymphoma compared four treatment arms: surgery alone, surgery with radiotherapy, surgery with CHOP and CHOP alone. Aviles et al. found that CHOP alone gave the best 10-year survival rates and had the lowest morbidity.[70]

Surgery therefore has a limited role in the modern management of gastric lymphoma.[71] It is used for resection of locoregional disease if medical treatment fails or in the emergency setting for bleeding or perforation.

Carcinoid

Gastric carcinoid tumours are rare and make up just under 2% of all gastric neoplasms and there is some evidence that the incidence has been rising over the past two to three decades.[72] The appendix is the commonest site for carcinoid tumours (48%), followed by the rectum (17%) and the ileum (12%); the stomach only accounts for 9%.[73,74] Carcinoids are neuroendocrine tumours, have characteristic histological and ultrastructural features and contain chromogranin A (CgA).[74] They were first described in 1907 by Oberndorfer, who named them *karzinoide*, meaning 'carcinoma-like', in recognition of their more benign behaviour compared to adenocarcinomas.[75] Gastric carcinoids arise from histamine-containing enterochromaffin-like (ECL) cells that are found in the fundus and body of the stomach. Gastric acid is produced by parietal cells when they are stimulated by gastrin directly (secreted by the G cells in the gastric antrum) or by histamine released locally by ECL cells when these are stimulated by gastrin. Negative feedback is provided by D cells, which release somatostatin (SST) when stimulated by rising luminal H$^+$ concentrations; SST binds to G cells and ECL cells and inhibits the production of gastrin and histamine respectively, hence reducing stimulation to parietal cells to produce acid. In patients with chronic atrophic gastritis the lack of acid production by parietal cells results in decreased SST levels, with excess production of gastrin and an overstimulation of ECL cells. As gastrin is trophic to ECL cells this can lead to ECL hyperplasia, dysplasia and eventually carcinoid tumour.

Presentation, classification and treatment

Gastric carcinoids are often discovered incidentally during upper GI endoscopy. Alternatively, they may present with bleeding (iron deficiency anaemia or frank GI blood loss), abdominal pain or dyspepsia. Rarely they present late with metastatic disease and symptoms from the release of bioactive substances. Atypical carcinoid syndrome is due to histamine release and presents with a patchy cutaneous flush, oedema, watering eyes, bronchoconstriction and headaches, whereas classical carcinoid syndrome presents with cutaneous flushing, bronchospasm and diarrhoea, and is probably due to circulating serotonin and tachykinins.[76] Diagnosis is made by histology of endoscopic biopsies and the argyrophil reaction with the presence of CgA mRNA or protein.[77] Raised plasma CgA is a very sensitive and specific test for diagnosing metastatic carcinoid in patients with suspected carcinoid syndrome.[74] Initial staging is by EUS and CT. Gastric carcinoid tumours express somatostatin-2 receptors and these will bind the synthetic octapeptide, octreotide; radiolabelled octrotide is used in the OctreoScan™.

In a prospective study Gibril et al.[78] found the OctreoScan test to have a positive and negative predictive value of 63% and 97% respectively for the detection of gastric carcinoid and its use should be considered in all patients with carcinoid tumours.

Gastric carcinoids are classified according to their behaviour and are rare under the age of 50 years.[79] Type I tumours are the commonest (75%), arise in patients with chronic atrophic gastritis (often those with pernicious anaemia) and are commoner in women than men (3:1). They are usually small, well-differentiated polypoid lesions that behave in a benign fashion, but when larger (1–2 cm) can occasionally metastasise to regional lymph nodes. Small lesions (<1 cm) can be removed by endoscopic mucosal resection, although long-term follow-up for this treatment is lacking.

The gold-standard treatment for a lesion under 2 cm in diameter is local surgical resection and antrectomy as this reduces gastrin levels.[80] Background ECL hyperplasia will often regress after antrectomy. Surgery may be open or laparoscopic depending upon local preference and experience. Patients should have endoscopic surveillance after surgery and the prognosis is excellent, with >90% 5-year survival.

Type II gastric carcinoids are rare (8%) and occur in patients with a gastrinoma as part of the autosomal dominant disorder multiple endocrine neoplasia syndrome type 1 (MEN-1). They have an intermediate behaviour between type I and type III carcinoids, with a 10–30% risk of metastasising. For early lesions the treatment is the same as for type I tumours, although great care should be taken to find and remove the gastrinoma whenever possible. Prognosis is again good, with about 70% 5-year survival, but the MEN-1 syndrome dictates outcomes more than the carcinoid tumour.[81]

Type III lesions constitute 21% of gastric carcinoids and are much more aggressive.[82] They usually present as a large ulcerating solitary mass, sometimes with liver metastases, and are not associated with atrophic gastritis, MEN-1 or

hypergastrinaemia. Treatment for non-metastatic type III tumours is by gastrectomy, usually total, with clearance of the local lymph nodes (D2 resection).[83] Local resection is not recommened for these tumours. Survival is around 50% at 5 years.[84]

For patients with symptomatic metastatic carcinoid the initial treatment of choice is with somatostatin analogues such as octreotide or lanreotide, which is longer acting.[81] Phase II trials of the monoclonal antibody bevacizumab[85] have shown promise and phase III studies are now awaited.

Rarities

Leiomyomas are benign smooth muscle tumours of the upper GI tract, are usually located in the oesophagus and may be very large at presentation.[86] They may present as an incidental submucosal swelling found at endoscopy or with dysphagia or, rarely, with GI bleeding. Similar lesions found in the stomach are nearly always GISTs. Incidental leiomyomas of the oesophagus can be treated conservatively, although an EUS to confirm the diagnosis is recommended and a follow-up EUS examination 1–2 years later will provide reassurance that the lesion is not growing. Symptomatic leiomyomas can be excised by dividing the muscularis propria and enucleating the lesion without disrupting the mucosa. This is usually done now using minimally invasive techniques (thoracoscopically).[87] Leiomyosarcomas look exactly like their benign counterparts but behave differently. A large submucosal lesion in the oesophagus (>2 cm) or one that is enlarging rapidly should be treated as potentially malignant. EUS-guided fine-needle or core biopsy of such a lesion is now possible and should be attempted if leiomyosarcoma is suspected.[88] If confirmed or doubt continues after biopsy a formal oesophagectomy is recommended as long-term survival is dependent upon achieving an R0 resection.[89]

Small-cell carcinoma of the oesophagus is thankfully rare. It has an even worse prognosis than squamous or adenocarcinoma. As with most oesophageal tumours it presents late and has already spread to locoregional nodes and haematogenously when diagnosed.[90] Even radical surgery with three-field lymph node resection results in 5-year survival of less than 10%. Treatment should therefore be by chemotherapy as this will occasionally result in a cure and, if it does not, provides moderately good palliation with less morbidity than radical surgery. There are no randomised studies of treatment but much has been extrapolated from experience with small-cell tumours of the lung.

Key points

- Complete surgical resection (R0) of gastric GISTs is often curative and is the treatment of choice whenever possible.
- Surgeons should aim to achieve an R0 resection for GISTs with as minimal negative impact on a patient's quality of life as possible.
- Patients having high-risk GISTs (large lesions with high mitotic counts) may in the future benefit from adjuvant or even neoadjuvant imatinib, but the results of randomised controlled trials are awaited.
- Metastatic and unresectable GISTs should be treated with 400 mg imatinib daily in the first instance and their overall care managed by a multidisciplinary team.
- Type I gastric carcinoids can safely be treated with minimal surgery (including endoscopic resection) and have a good prognosis, whereas type III carcinoid tumours require a gastrectomy and nodal resection and have a poorer prognosis.
- Low-grade B-cell gastric MALT lymphoma is caused by *Helicobacter pylori* (HP) and will often regress after HP eradication therapy.
- Surgery has a limited role in the treatment of gastric lymphoma and primary treatment is usually with chemotherapy.
- Submucosal lesions in the oesophagus are usually leiomyomas and, if symptomatic, can be enucleated thoracoscopically.

References

1. Rossi CR, Mocellin S, Mencarelli R et al. Gastrointestinal stromal tumors: from a surgical to a molecular approach. Int J Cancer 2003; 107(2):171–6.

2. Mazur MT, Clark HB. Gastric stromal tumors. Reappraisal of histogenesis. Am J Surg Pathol 1983; 7(6):507–19.

3. Walker P, Dvorak AM. Gastrointestinal autonomic nerve (GAN) tumor. Ultrastructural evidence for a newly recognized entity. Arch Pathol Lab Med 1986; 110(4):309–16.

4. Lee JR, Joshi V, Griffin JW Jr. et al. Gastrointestinal autonomic nerve tumor: immunohistochemical and molecular identity with gastrointestinal stromal tumor. Am J Surg Pathol 2001; 25(8):979–87.

5. Romert P, Mikkelsen HB. c-kit immunoreactive interstitial cells of Cajal in the human small and large intestine. Histochem Cell Biol 1998; 109(3):195–202.

6. Kindblom LG, Remotti HE, Aldenborg F et al. Gastrointestinal pacemaker cell tumor (GIPACT): gastrointestinal stromal tumors show phenotypic characteristics of the interstitial cells of Cajal. Am J Pathol 1998; 152(5):1259–69.

7. Joensuu H, Kindblom LG. Gastrointestinal stromal tumors – a review. Acta Orthop Scand 2004; 75(311):62–71.

8. Nilsson B, Bumming P, Meis-Kindblom JM et al. Gastrointestinal stromal tumors: the incidence, prevalence, clinical course, and prognostication in the preimatinib mesylate era – a population-based study in western Sweden. Cancer 2005; 103(4):821–9.

9. Hassan I, You YN, Shyyan R et al. Surgically managed gastrointestinal stromal tumors: a comparative and prognostic analysis. Ann Surg Oncol 2008; 15(1):52–9.

10. Fletcher CD, Berman JJ, Corless C et al. Diagnosis of gastrointestinal stromal tumors: a consensus approach. Human Pathol 2002; 33(5):459–65.

11. DeMatteo RP, Lewis JJ, Leung D et al. Two hundred gastrointestinal stromal tumors: recurrence patterns and prognostic factors for survival. Ann Surg 2000; 231(1):51–8.

12. Emory TS, Sobin LH, Lukes L et al. Prognosis of gastrointestinal smooth-muscle (stromal) tumors: dependence on anatomic site. Am J Surg Pathol 1999; 23(1):82–7.

13. Langer C, Gunawan B, Schuler P et al. Prognostic factors influencing surgical management and outcome of gastrointestinal stromal tumours. Br J Surg 2003; 90(3):332–9.

14. Lee YT. Leiomyosarcoma of the gastro-intestinal tract: general pattern of metastasis and recurrence. Cancer Treat Rev 1983; 10(2):91–101.

15. Miettinen M, El-Rifai W, Sobin HL et al. Evaluation of malignancy and prognosis of gastrointestinal stromal tumors: a review. Human Pathol 2002; 33(5):478–83.

16. Connolly EM, Gaffney E, Reynolds JV. Gastrointestinal stromal tumours. Br J Surg 2003; 90(10):1178–86.

17. Bucher P, Villiger P, Egger JF et al. Management of gastrointestinal stromal tumors: from diagnosis to treatment. Swiss Med Wkly 2004; 134(11–12):145–53.

18. Lehnert T. Gastrointestinal sarcoma (GIST) – a review of surgical management. Ann Chir Gynaecol 1998; 87(4):297–305.

19. DeMatteo RP. The GIST of targeted cancer therapy: a tumor (gastrointestinal stromal tumor), a mutated gene (c-kit), and a molecular inhibitor (STI571). Ann Surg Oncol 2002; 9(9):831–9.

20. Berman J, O'Leary TJ. Gastrointestinal stromal tumor workshop. Human Pathol 2001; 32(6):578–82.

21. Joensuu H, Fletcher C, Dimitrijevic S et al. Management of malignant gastrointestinal stromal tumours. Lancet Oncol 2002; 3(11):655–64.

22. Palazzo L, Landi B, Cellier C et al. Endosonographic features predictive of benign and malignant gastrointestinal stromal cell tumours. Gut 2000; 46(1):88–92.

23. Chak A, Canto MI, Rosch T et al. Endosonographic differentiation of benign and malignant stromal cell tumors. Gastrointest Endosc 1997; 45(6):468–73.

24. Akahoshi K, Sumida Y, Matsui N et al. Preoperative diagnosis of gastrointestinal stromal tumor by endoscopic ultrasound-guided fine needle aspiration. World J Gastroenterol 2007; 13(14):2077–82.

25. Lau S, Tam KF, Kam CK et al. Imaging of gastrointestinal stromal tumour (GIST). Clin Radiol 2004; 59(6):487–98.

26. Benjamin RS, Choi H, Macapinlac HA et al. We should desist using RECIST, at least in GIST. J Clin Oncol 2007; 25(13):1760–4.

27. Antoch G, Kanja J, Bauer S et al. Comparison of PET, CT, and dual-modality PET/CT imaging for monitoring of imatinib (STI571) therapy in patients with gastrointestinal stromal tumors. J Nucl Med 2004; 45(3):357–65.

28. Stroobants S, Goeminne J, Seegers M et al. 18FDG-Positron emission tomography for the early prediction of response in advanced soft tissue sarcoma treated with imatinib mesylate (Glivec). Eur J Cancer 2003; 39(14):2012–20.

29. Isozaki K, Terris B, Belghiti J et al. Germline-activating mutation in the kinase domain of KIT gene in familial gastrointestinal stromal tumors. Am J Pathol 2000; 157(5):1581–5.

30. O'Brien P, Kapusta L, Dardick I et al. Multiple familial gastrointestinal autonomic nerve tumors and small intestinal neuronal dysplasia. Am J Surg Pathol 1999; 23(2):198–204.

31. Carney JA, Sheps SG, Go VL et al. The triad of gastric leiomyosarcoma, functioning extra-adrenal paraganglioma and pulmonary chondroma. N Engl J Med 1977; 296(26):1517–18.

32. Carney JA. Gastric stromal sarcoma, pulmonary chondroma, and extra-adrenal paraganglioma (Carney Triad): natural history, adrenocortical component, and possible familial occurrence. Mayo Clin Proc 1999; 74(6):543–52.

33. Demetri GD, Benjamin RS, Blanke CD et al. NCCN Task Force report: management of patients with gastrointestinal stromal tumor (GIST) – update of the NCCN clinical practice guidelines. J Natl Compr Cancer Network 2007; 5(Suppl 2):S1–29; quiz S30.

34. Ng EH, Pollock RE, Romsdahl MM. Prognostic implications of patterns of failure for gastrointestinal leiomyosarcomas. Cancer 1992; 69(6):1334–41.

35. Merendino KA, Thomas GI. The jejunal interposition operation for substitution of the esophago-gastric sphincter; present status. Surgery 1958; 44(6):1112–15.

36. Stein HJ, Feith M, Mueller J et al. Limited resection for early adenocarcinoma in Barrett's esophagus. Ann Surg 2000; 232(6):733–42.

37. Dematteo RP, Heinrich MC, El-Rifai WM et al. Clinical management of gastrointestinal stromal tumors: before and after STI-571. Human Pathol 2002; 33(5):466–77.

38. Ludwig DJ, Traverso LW. Gut stromal tumors and their clinical behavior. Am J Surg 1997; 173(5):390–4.

39. UK GIST Consensus Group. Guidelines for the management of gastrointestinal stromal tumours (GISTs), 2005. Available from www.augis.org

40. Katz SC, DeMatteo RP. Gastrointestinal stromal tumors and leiomyosarcomas. J Surg Oncol 2008; 97(4):350–9.

41. Van Glabbeke M, van Oosterom AT, Oosterhuis JW et al. Prognostic factors for the outcome of chemotherapy in advanced soft tissue sarcoma: an analysis of 2,185 patients treated with anthracycline-containing first-line regimens – a European Organization for Research and Treatment of Cancer Soft Tissue and Bone Sarcoma Group Study. J Clin Oncol 1999; 17(1):150–7.

42. Tuveson DA, Willis NA, Jacks T et al. STI571 inactivation of the gastrointestinal stromal tumor c-KIT oncoprotein: biological and clinical implications. Oncogene 2001; 20(36):5054–8.

43. Van Oosterom AT, Judson I, Verweij J et al. Safety and efficacy of imatinib (STI571) in metastatic gastrointestinal stromal tumours: a phase I study. Lancet 2001; 358(9291):1421–3.

44. Blanke CD, Demetri GD, von Mehren M et al. Long-term results from a randomized phase II trial of standard- versus higher-dose imatinib mesylate for patients with unresectable or metastatic gastrointestinal stromal tumors expressing KIT. J Clin Oncol 2008; 26(4):620–5.

A randomised study of 400 mg vs. 600 mg imatinib in unresectable or metastatic GIST. No difference was found in median survival between the two groups.

45. Blanke CD, Rankin C, Demetri GD et al. Phase III randomized, intergroup trial assessing imatinib mesylate at two dose levels in patients with unresectable or metastatic gastrointestinal stromal tumors expressing the kit receptor tyrosine kinase: S0033. J Clin Oncol 2008; 26(4):626–32.

A phase III randomised study involving 746 patients comparing imatinib dosage in advanced GISTs: 800 mg seemed no better than 400 mg but was useful in stabilising about a third of patients who progressed on the lower dose.

46. Verweij J, Casali PG, Zalcberg J et al. Progression-free survival in gastrointestinal stromal tumours with high-dose imatinib: randomised trial. Lancet 2004; 364(9440):1127–34.

Another randomised study (946 patients) comparing 800 mg with 400 mg imatinib found some small improvement in progression-free survival for the higher dose.

47. Van Glabbeke M, Verweij J, Casali PG et al. Initial and late resistance to imatinib in advanced gastrointestinal stromal tumors are predicted by different prognostic factors: a European Organisation for Research and Treatment of Cancer–Italian Sarcoma Group–Australasian Gastrointestinal Trials Group study. J Clin Oncol 2005; 23(24):5795–804.

48. DeMatteo RP, Shah A, Fong Y et al. Results of hepatic resection for sarcoma metastatic to liver. Ann Surg 2001; 234(4):540–7.

49. Barnes G, Bulusu VR, Hardwick RH et al. A review of the surgical management of metastatic gastrointestinal stromal tumours (GISTs) on imatinib mesylate (Glivec). Int J Surg (Lond, Engl) 2005; 3(3):206–12.

50. Sym SJ, Ryu MH, Lee JL et al. Surgical intervention following imatinib treatment in patients with advanced gastrointestinal stromal tumors (GISTs). J Surg Oncol 2008; 98(1):27–33.

51. Sandler RS. Has primary gastric lymphoma become more common? J Clin Gastroenterol 1984; 6(2):101–7.

52. Cogliatti SB, Schmid U, Schumacher U et al. Primary B-cell gastric lymphoma: a clinicopathological study of 145 patients. Gastroenterology 1991; 101(5):1159–70.

53. Weingrad DN, Decosse JJ, Sherlock P et al. Primary gastrointestinal lymphoma: a 30-year review. Cancer 1982; 49(6):1258–65.

54. Imrie KR, Sawka CA, Kutas G et al. HIV-associated lymphoma of the gastrointestinal tract: the University of Toronto AIDS–Lymphoma Study Group experience. Leuk Lymph 1995; 16(3–4):343–9.

55. Stolte M. Helicobacter pylori gastritis and gastric MALT-lymphoma. Lancet 1992; 339(8795):745–6.

56. Caletti G, Fusaroli P, Togliani T et al. Endosonography in gastric lymphoma and large gastric folds. Eur J Ultrasound 2000; 11(1):31–40.

57. Yucel C, Ozdemir H, Isik S. Role of endosonography in the evaluation of gastric malignancies. J Ultrasound Med 1999; 18(4):283–8.

58. Rohatiner A, d'Amore F, Coiffier B et al. Report on a workshop convened to discuss the pathological and staging classifications of gastrointestinal tract lymphoma. Ann Oncol 1994; 5(5):397–400.

59. Isaacson P, Wright DH. Extranodal malignant lymphoma arising from mucosa-associated lymphoid tissue. Cancer 1984; 53(11):2515–24.

60. Parsonnet J, Hansen S, Rodriguez L et al. Helicobacter pylori infection and gastric lymphoma. N Engl J Med 1994; 330(18):1267–71.

61. Shimm DS, Dosoretz DE, Anderson T et al. Primary gastric lymphoma. An analysis with emphasis on prognostic factors and radiation therapy. Cancer 1983; 52(11):2044–8.

62. Sutherland AG, Kennedy M, Anderson DN et al. Gastric lymphoma in Grampian Region: presentation, treatment and outcome. J R Coll Surg Edinb 1996; 41(3):143–7.

63. Pinotti G, Zucca E, Roggero E et al. Clinical features, treatment and outcome in a series of 93 patients with low-grade gastric MALT lymphoma. Leuk Lymph 1997; 26(5–6):527–37.

64. Montalban C, Manzanal A, Boixeda D et al. Treatment of low-grade gastric MALT lymphoma with Helicobacter pylori eradication. Lancet 1995; 345(8952):798–9.

65. Chan JK. Gastrointestinal lymphomas: an overview with emphasis on new findings and diagnostic problems. Semin Diagnost Pathol 1996; 13(4):260–96.

66. Raderer M, Chott A, Drach J et al. Chemotherapy for management of localised high-grade gastric B-cell lymphoma: how much is necessary? Ann Oncol 2002; 13(7):1094–8.

67. Wohrer S, Puspok A, Drach J et al. Rituximab, cyclophosphamide, doxorubicin, vincristine and prednisone (R-CHOP) for treatment of early-stage gastric diffuse large B-cell lymphoma. Ann Oncol 2004; 15(7):1086–90.

68. Hiyama T, Haruma K, Kitadai Y et al. Clinicopathological features of gastric mucosa-associated lymphoid tissue lymphoma: a comparison with diffuse large B-cell lymphoma without a mucosa-associated lymphoid tissue lymphoma component. J Gastroenterol Hepatol 2001; 16(7):734–9.

69. Coiffier B, Lepage E, Briere J et al. CHOP chemotherapy plus rituximab compared with CHOP alone in elderly patients with diffuse large-B-cell lymphoma. N Engl J Med 2002; 346(4):235–42.

A randomised study investigating the value of rituximab when added to standard chemotherapy for treating gastric lymphoma.

70. Aviles A, Nambo MJ, Neri N et al. The role of surgery in primary gastric lymphoma: results of a controlled clinical trial. Ann Surg 2004; 240(1):44–50.

A large and important study randomising 589 patients to four treatment arms. Surgery did not improve survival and CHOP chemotherapy came out on top.

71. Popescu RA, Wotherspoon AC, Cunningham D et al. Surgery plus chemotherapy or chemotherapy alone for primary intermediate- and high-grade gastric non-Hodgkin's lymphoma: the Royal Marsden Hospital experience. Eur J Cancer 1999; 35(6):928–34.

72. Hodgson N, Koniaris LG, Livingstone AS et al. Gastric carcinoids: a temporal increase with proton pump introduction. Surg Endosc 2005; 19(12):1610–12.

73. Berge T, Linell F. Carcinoid tumours. Frequency in a defined population during a 12-year period. Acta Pathol Microbiol Scand 1976; 84(4):322–30.

74. Kidd M, Modlin IM, Mane SM et al. RT–PCR detection of chromogranin A: a new standard in the identification of neuroendocrine tumor disease. Ann Surg 2006; 243(2):273–80.

75. Oberndorfer S. Karzinoid tumoren des dunndarms. Frankf Z Pathol 1907; 1:237–40.

76. Conlon JM, Deacon CF, Richter G et al. Circulating tachykinins (substance P, neurokinin A, neuropeptide K) and the carcinoid flush. Scand J Gastroenterol 1987; 22(1):97–105.

77. Nobels FR, Kwekkeboom DJ, Coopmans W et al. Chromogranin A as serum marker for neuroendocrine neoplasia: comparison with neuron-specific enolase and the alpha-subunit of glycoprotein hormones. J Clin Endocrinol Metab 1997; 82(8):2622–8.

78. Gibril F, Reynolds JC, Lubensky IA et al. Ability of somatostatin receptor scintigraphy to identify patients with gastric carcinoids: a prospective study. J Nucl Med 2000; 41(10):1646–56.

   A blinded prospective study of 162 patients with Zollinger–Ellison syndrome comparing the results of radionuclear studies with gastric biopsies looking for gastric carcinoid tumours.

79. Modlin IM, Kidd M, Latich I et al. Current status of gastrointestinal carcinoids. Gastroenterology 2005; 128(6):1717–51.

80. Dakin GF, Warner RR, Pomp A et al. Presentation, treatment, and outcome of type 1 gastric carcinoid tumors. J Surg Oncol 2006; 93(5):368–72.

81. Modlin IM, Latich I, Kidd M et al. Therapeutic options for gastrointestinal carcinoids. Clin Gastroenterol Hepatol 2006; 4(5):526–47.

82. Rindi G. Clinicopathologic aspects of gastric neuroendocrine tumors. Am J Surg Pathol 1995; 19(Suppl 1):S20–9.

83. Modlin IM, Kidd M, Lye KD. Biology and management of gastric carcinoid tumours: a review. Eur J Surg (Acta Chir) 2002; 168(12):669–83.

84. Modlin IM, Lye KD, Kidd M. A 50-year analysis of 562 gastric carcinoids: small tumor or larger problem? Am J Gastroenterol 2004; 99(1):23–32.

85. Yao JC, Phan A, Hoff PM et al. Targeting vascular endothelial growth factor in advanced carcinoid tumor: a random assignment phase II study of depot octreotide with bevacizumab and pegylated interferon alpha-2b. J Clin Oncol 2008; 26(8):1316–23.

86. Pompeo E, Francioni F, Pappalardo G et al. Giant leiomyoma of the oesophagus and cardia. Diagnostic and therapeutic considerations: case report and literature review. Scand Cardiovasc J 1997; 31(6):361–4.

87. Roviaro GC, Maciocco M, Varoli F et al. Videothoracoscopic treatment of oesophageal leiomyoma. Thorax 1998; 53(3):190–2.

88. Stelow EB, Jones DR, Shami VM. Esophageal leiomyosarcoma diagnosed by endoscopic ultrasound-guided fine-needle aspiration. Diagnost Cytopathol 2007; 35(3):167–70.

89. Rocco G, Trastek VF, Deschamps C et al. Leiomyosarcoma of the esophagus: results of surgical treatment. Ann Thorac Surg 1998; 66(3):894–6; discussion 897.

90. Yun JP, Zhang MF, Hou JH et al. Primary small cell carcinoma of the esophagus: clinicopathological and immunohistochemical features of 21 cases. BMC Cancer 2007; 7:38.

12

Pathophysiology and investigation of gastro-oesophageal reflux disease

Rami R. Sweis
Abraham J. Botha

Introduction

Gastro-oesophageal reflux disease (GORD) occurs when gastric contents pass into the oesophagus resulting in symptoms and/or mucosal damage.[1] It is one of the most common health problems afflicting modern Western societies. Its treatment accounts for the biggest single pharmaceutical expenditure in the UK's National Health Service (NHS). GORD is probably responsible for the increasing incidence of oesophageal adenocarcinoma, as this cancer arises in a columnar-lined oesophagus consequent to severe reflux disease.[2] Motility disorders of the oesophagus are much less frequent, but they can cause similar symptoms to GORD (see Chapter 16). Understanding the pathophysiology of GORD and its investigation is therefore very important.

The clinical problem

Everybody has daily gastro-oesophageal reflux (GOR) manifested by physiological burping. Prolonged pH monitoring in asymptomatic subjects has shown short-lived, postprandial episodes of GOR, which are presumably normal.[3,4] After overindulgence reflux symptoms and even vomiting may be considered normal protective mechanisms. Pathological GOR or GORD is defined as chronic acid and/or bile reflux causing unacceptable symptoms or demonstrable pathology. Determining the true incidence of GORD is made difficult because many people regard heartburn/indigestion as normal and are content to treat themselves with antacids

without seeking medical attention.[5] Furthermore, not all patients with typical reflux symptoms of heartburn and acid regurgitation have oesophagitis.

 Two studies of patients with reflux symptoms disclosed a normal oesophagus on endoscopy in 32% and 38% of subjects.[6,7]

At the other end of the scale oesophagitis is now the commonest finding in upper gastrointestinal endoscopic examinations,[8] yet several studies have shown that up to 20% of patients with endoscopic oesophagitis and/or Barrett's never experience heartburn.[9]

A clinical diagnosis of GORD can be made in patients who have heartburn responding to proton pump inhibitors, and/or oesophagitis or Barrett's metaplasia found at endoscopy. Additional symptoms often encountered by patients with typical GORD are regurgitation (so-called volume reflux) and intermittent dysphagia.

The atypical presentations of GORD can be more difficult to diagnose. GORD can contribute significantly to upper aerodigestive disease such as voice change, throat clearing, sore mouth, dental decay, pharyngitis, tonsillitis and sinusitis. It is also a causative factor in lower respiratory disease such as chronic coughing and asthma. Diagnosing GOR that reaches the proximal oesophagus can be difficult and even when GORD is diagnosed in patients with atypical symptoms, it may be impossible to prove a causal link between GORD and these symptoms and/or pathology.[1]

- Endoscopy
- Histology
- Barium radiology
- 24-hour pH study/Bravo
- Manometry (standard, high resolution)
- Bilitec probe (bile reflux)
- Multichannel intraluminal impedance:
  - MII–pH (impedance + pH sensors)
  - MII–EM (impedance + manometric sensors)
  - MII–EM–pH

Equally challenging are patients who have typical or atypical GORD symptoms in addition to other functional digestive symptoms such as functional dyspepsia or the bloating and/or changes in bowel habit associated with irritable bowel disease.

In view of this difficulty in establishing a diagnosis of GORD, a range of additional diagnostic tests can be performed (Box 12.1).

 Twenty-four-hour ambulatory pH monitoring in the lower oesophagus is usually regarded as the gold standard.[10]

Even this method can, however, reveal normal pH profiles in symptomatic patients,[11] and in up to 25% of subjects with endoscopic oesophagitis.[12] Furthermore, tolerability of the catheter can be a problem[13] (see Investigations).

GORD has a multifactorial aetiology and understanding its pathophysiology is important both for diagnosis and treatment.

Normal adult oesophageal anatomy

The oesophagus is a muscular tube approximately 25 cm long connecting the pharynx in the neck to the stomach in the abdomen. It is subdivided into three anatomical segments on the basis of position rather than function (cervical, thoracic and abdominal). The cervical oesophagus is a direct continuation of the pharynx, commencing at the cricopharyngeal muscle and is about 5 cm in length. The thoracic oesophagus is about 18 cm long, starting at the thoracic inlet at T1 and ending where the oesophagus passes through the hiatal opening of the diaphragm at T10. The abdominal oesophagus is of variable length due to the variable frequency of a hiatus hernia, but is usually only about 1–2 cm in length.

The body of the oesophagus is composed of an outer longitudinal and inner circular layer of muscle, though the longitudinal muscle does spiral slightly down the oesophagus. Though functioning as a single unit, the muscle is unique in being composed of both striated and smooth muscle. At its proximal end (including the cricopharyngeal sphincter) it is entirely striated muscle. Over the next 4–5 cm it is a mixture of both muscle types, with smooth muscle becoming more common distally. The middle and lower oesophagus is composed entirely of smooth muscle. This muscular tube is lined by non-keratinised stratified squamous epithelium down to the gastro-oesophageal junction, where it abruptly changes to glandular mucosa at the endoscopic z-line. Deep to the mucosa and the muscularis mucosa, but superficial to the circular muscle, lie the connective tissue, blood vessels, nerves and glands that form the submucosa.

The nerve supply of the oesophagus is predominantly vagal, either from the recurrent laryngeal nerves to the upper oesophagus or the vagus proper to the main bulk of the oesophageal body. Sympathetic supply comes from cell bodies in the middle cervical ganglion supplying the upper part of the oesophagus and from the upper four thoracic ganglia of the sympathetic trunk to the rest of the oesophagus.

The upper oesophageal sphincter is formed by the lower part of the inferior constrictor of the pharynx, cricopharyngeus and the upper part of the circular muscle of the oesophagus. This sphincter is closed at rest, with a high resting pressure of about 100 mmHg in an anteroposterior direction (less in the lateral direction) protecting the airway from reflux of gastric contents.

Oesophageal motility and GORD

During swallowing, the upper oesophageal sphincter relaxes and the bolus of saliva, liquid or food is pushed from the pharynx into the upper oesophagus. It is then transported to the stomach within 5–10 seconds. Normal oesophageal transport occurs through two mechanisms. Primary (or swallow-initiated) peristalsis is centrally mediated, originates in the pharynx and progresses aborally to the stomach (**Fig. 12.1**). If food were to remain in the oesophagus, distending its lumen, then local neural reflexes would induce secondary (or non-swallow-initiated) peristaltic activity to clear it.[14] Tertiary contractions (non-peristaltic) are not often seen in normal subjects during short-term radiological or manometric investigations, but are more commonly observed during 24-hour manometry investigations.

Oesophageal peristalsis depends primarily upon the interaction of myogenic and intrinsic and external neural factors. The electrical activity of the circular muscle appears to be different from the longitudinal muscle as, instead of depolarisation after stimulation, the circular muscle initially hyperpolarises.[15]

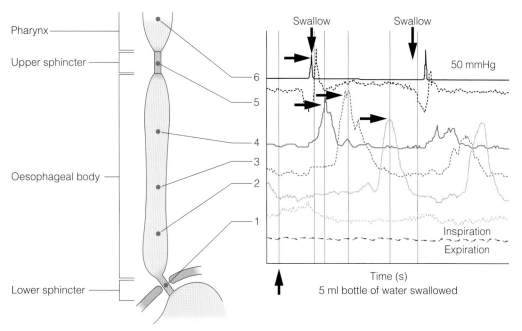

Figure 12.1 • A standard six-sensor manometry trace of normal oesophageal peristalsis. Reproduced from Anggiansah A, Marshal R. Use of the oesophageal laboratory, 1st edn. Oxford: Isis Medical Media, 2000. With permission from Isis Medical Media.

The resulting time delay allows the longitudinal muscle to contract first, thus providing form and rigidity to the oesophagus during bolus transport. Inherent myogenic properties are necessary for the occurrence of muscle contraction, but central and local neural controls are required for coordination of peristalsis. Peripherally, neural control is mediated via the vagus nerve, which links to the intrinsic neurones of the myenteric plexus between the inner and outer muscle layers. Neural mechanisms for afferent input to the central nervous system from the oesophagus are also present. In humans, there is a sensitive system located in the oesophageal body for the detection of volume changes in the oesophageal lumen. There is also evidence for the existence of acidity receptors, which may produce a centrally mediated peristaltic clearance wave.[16] While the function of afferent nerves from the oesophagus is poorly understood, they probably have an important controlling or modulating effect on normal peristalsis since the vagus is composed largely of sensory fibres. For instance, dry swallows often fail to generate a peristaltic sequence, whereas wet swallows are almost always followed by a propagated contraction of longer duration and greater amplitude.[17] The temperature of the swallowed bolus also affects oesophageal peristalsis, with warm substances producing stronger contractions, while the rapid ingestion of ice-cream leads to complete absence of distal oesophageal activity.[18]

Numerous oesophageal body motility abnormalities are associated with GORD, the most common being ineffective peristalsis and hypomotility. What is not clear is whether the dysmotility develops as a consequence of GORD, whether it causes GORD, or whether the dysmotility contributes to the symptoms and pathology of GORD.

Olsen and Schlegel reported a study of oesophageal motility in 50 patients with oesophagitis. Normal peristaltic activity was found in only 28%, 32% had motor incoordination, 37% low-amplitude peristalsis and 8% complete motor failure. As the degree of oesophagitis became more severe, so the proportion of patients with motor abnormalities increased.[19] Kahrilas et al. also found that patients with GOR had peristaltic dysfunction (failed primary peristalsis or hypotensive peristalsis) that became more prevalent with increasing oesophagitis.

 Twenty-five per cent of patients with mild oesophagitis had peristaltic dysfunction, and this rate increased to 48% in patients with severe oesophagitis.[20]

In patients with strictures secondary to GOR, aperistalsis and non-specific motor abnormalities may occur in up to 64% of patients compared with 32% of subjects with GOR but no stricture.[21]

231

Patients with Barrett's oesophagus have more severe oesophageal dysmotility than those with other forms of reflux disease or healthy controls.[22]

In addition, oesophageal sensitivity to acid is reduced.[1] This combination of motor and sensory dysfunction is linked to increased severity of acid exposure,[13] in particular highly prolonged reflux events that predispose to mucosal damage.[23] Moreover, Barrett segment length (and the risk of complications) is associated with the severity of oesophageal dysmotility and acid exposure.[22]

The case for dysmotility developing secondary to acid-induced mucosal damage has been made by investigators who found improvements in peristalsis following successful antireflux surgery.[24] Cytokines present in reflux oesophagitis (e.g. interleukin (IL)-1β, IL-6, IL-8 (Th1)) inhibit oesophageal muscle contractility in vitro.[25] Others have found no improvement in oesophageal clearance times or peristaltic behaviour following healing of oesophagitis after surgery.[26,27] This could mean that reflux-induced oesophageal myoneuronal damage is irreversible. The alternative argument, that primary oesophageal dysmotility is associated with GORD, has been made by Eriksen et al. who, using 24-hour pH monitoring and solid egg bolus transit times, found no correlation between delayed transit times (found in GOR patients) and severity of oesophagitis,[28] a point made earlier by Maddern and Jamieson.[29]

No causal link has been found between the symptoms of heartburn and dysphagia, and oesophageal dysmotility. Heartburn is rather caused by a direct action of acid on oesophageal pain receptors.[30]

It is well known that patients with reflux disease experience intermittent dysphagia in the absence of a mechanical cause. It would seem logical that a motor abnormality would result in abnormalities in food bolus transport thereby causing dysphagia. However, doubt has been cast on the validity of manometrically determined motor abnormalities in reflux disease. Several studies showed little correlation between motility and dysphagia after antireflux surgery.[31] Indeed, while dysphagia and motility abnormalities occur in patients with reflux disease in similar proportions, there is no correlation between the two groups – patients with dysphagia are just as likely to have normal or abnormal motility.[32]

In addition to transporting swallowed boluses down the oesophagus, peristalsis is also very important in clearing refluxed gastric contents. This oesophageal clearance also occurs by both the primary and secondary mechanisms. Kahrilas et al. have shown the importance of orderly peristalsis in acid clearance by using combined videofluoroscopic and manometric recordings in patients with non-obstructive dysphagia or heartburn. A single normal peristaltic wave resulted in 100% clearance of a barium bolus from the oesophagus. A peristaltic amplitude of >20 mmHg was required to clear barium from the distal oesophagus, though lower pressures were required in the proximal oesophagus.[33]

Booth et al. introduced the standard acid clearance test.[34] They found that patients with GOR required more swallows to clear the acid than asymptomatic subjects. However, this test is neither specific nor sensitive, as 47% of the patients with GOR had a normal result while subjects with oesophageal motor disorders but no acid reflux had an abnormal result.[35]

Barham et al. suggested that the prolonged mean duration of reflux episodes was taken to reflect a problem with the acid clearance ability of the oesophagus.[36] DeMeester et al. found different patterns of acid reflux in controls and patients with GORD. Patients with oesophagitis were more likely to experience prolonged reflux episodes at night (supine refluxers) compared with shorter daytime episodes (upright refluxers). They suggested that poor oesophageal clearance during sleep would account for greater oesophageal damage.[4] Further work has reinforced this idea of the importance of delayed acid clearance in recumbent sleeping patients in the development of oesophagitis.[37] The supine position is said to be important for two reasons the effect of gravity and a reduction in oesophageal peristalsis at night. Acid clearance times during a standard acid clearance test are longer when carried out lying down compared with sitting up (and even longer if the head is tilted down).[38] Sleeping with the head of the bed elevated results in improvement in nocturnal acid clearance[39] and healing of microscopic oesophagitis,[35] suggesting that gravity plays an important role in helping to clear acid from the oesophagus. Peristaltic frequency (primary and secondary) is greatly reduced during sleep[40] and this by itself is claimed to lead to prolonged acid clearance times in both controls and patients with oesophagitis.[41]

Oesophagitis patients therefore have twin risks in that they experience more acid reflux at night when the oesophagus is unprotected by frequent peristalsis, and in some there is decreased acid clearance ability.[42]

The antireflux barrier

In the resting state, most of the oesophagus lies in the slightly negative-pressure environment of the thorax (−5 mmHg compared with atmospheric pressure). This is in contrast to its lower end, which, for about 1–2 cm, having passed through the diaphragmatic hiatus, lies in the slightly positive-pressure (+5 mmHg) environment of the abdomen. Thus the oesophagus and the stomach are the only parts of the gastrointestinal tract where bowel in continuity is contained within cavities of opposing pressure. The pressure gradient across the diaphragm, if unopposed, ought to lead to the free flow of gastric contents back into the oesophagus (located in the relative vacuum of the thorax). That this does not usually occur is dependent upon the antireflux barrier at the gastro-oesophageal junction (see Box 12.2).

This antireflux barrier has four components, i.e. sling and clasp fibres of the gastric cardia, diaphragmatic crura, intra-abdominal oesophageal compression and the lower oesophageal sphincter.

Sling and clasp fibres of the gastric cardia

It is thought that the cardio-oesophageal angle is held in its acute position by contraction of oblique gastric sling fibres in the muscular coat of the stomach and that this disappears in cadavers.[43] The oblique angle of entry of the oesophagus into the stomach was said to cause a 'flap-like' mechanism, so preventing reflux. This mechanism is not essential in preventing reflux because the flap-valve angle disappears in a sliding hiatus hernia, yet the presence of a hernia is not always associated with acid reflux. In addition, the gastric sling fibres, which form a cone-like constriction at the cardiac notch, lie at a level below that of a radiologically defined barrier to instilled barium.[44]

Diaphragmatic crura

The right pillar of the crus of the diaphragm probably contributes to the measured lower oesophageal sphincter (LOS) pressure when there is no sliding

hiatus hernia present and may partly explain the marked longitudinal and radial asymmetry of the LOS.[45] Respiratory-induced pressure oscillations are readily seen during manometric measurement of the LOS,[46] and amplitudes are related to inspiratory depth.[47] Diaphragmatic contractions in humans have been shown by one group to augment LOS tone and this enhancing effect was maximal during deep, sustained inspiration when the gastro-oesophageal pressure gradient was greatest.[48] This diaphragmatic pinch-cock may work by buttressing the LOS when the greatest gastro-oesophageal pressure gradients occur (deep inspiration, coughing, straining, straight-leg raising and so on).

Distal oesophageal compression

The phreno-oesophageal ligament is a prolongation of the endoabdominal fascia from the under surface of the diaphragm. At the lower margin of the hiatus it decussates into upper and lower leaves. The lower leaf is an ill-defined, loose collection of fibroelastic fibres, which is absent in many cases.[49] The upper layer is a strong, consistent and well-defined membrane that inserts into the oesophagus and is attached to the submucosa and intramuscular septae of the lower oesophageal wall by fascicles of fibroelastic tissue. This anatomical arrangement anchors the oesophagogastric junction within the abdomen to prevent herniation through the hiatus, thereby maintaining a portion of the oesophagus within the positive-pressure environment of the abdomen.

The height of insertion of the phreno-oesophageal ligament determines the length of the oesophagus that is maintained within the positive-pressure environment of the abdomen. This factor would also apply in patients with sliding hiatus hernias who, despite having a portion of the stomach within the anatomical chest, still retain a segment of the oesophagus within an envelope of endoabdominal fascia. Rises in abdominal pressure will still be transmitted to the lower part of the oesophagus, leaving no net gradient across the gastro-oesophageal junction, thus preventing acid reflux.[50]

The LOS length and the length of the sphincter exposed to intra-abdominal pressure are said by some groups to be important for the prevention of reflux precipitated by increases in intragastric pressure.[51] DeMeester et al. have found that, in the clinical situation, a low basal LOS pressure (<5 mmHg) and/or a short intra-abdominal sphincter length (<1 cm) resulted in a 90% incidence of abnormal GOR. A short LOS is thought to be particularly relevant in the observed increased severity of GORD with age and in the recumbent position.[13]

Box 12.2 • Natural barriers to gastro-oesophageal reflux

Lower oesophageal sphincter
- Basal tone
- Adaptive pressure changes
- Transient LOS relaxation

External mechanical factors
- Flap-valve mechanism:
  - cardio-oesophageal angle
  - diaphragmatic pinchcock
  - mucosal rosette
- Distal oesophageal compression:
  - phreno-oesophageal ligament
  - transmitted abdominal pressure

Lower oesophageal sphincter

Although an LOS cannot be demonstrated anatomically, manometric studies have shown the presence of a high-pressure zone (HPZ) in the lower oesophagus that behaves like a physiological sphincter, i.e. it has a basal tone, but relaxes during swallowing, belching and vomiting. This physiological LOS, responsible for the control of acid reflux, extends over the terminal 1–4 cm of the oesophagus and has marked axial and radial asymmetry, with the highest pressures recorded in the posterior and right posterior directions.[45,52]

The pressure in the LOS varies in the same individual on separate occasions[53] and there are also marked diurnal variations in basal LOS pressure in relation to posture,[54] meals[55] and the migrating motor complex.[56] The pressure gradient across the diaphragm can increase significantly during activities such as abdominal compression, bending, straining and coughing, which produce a rise in intra-abdominal pressure, and sniffing, hiccoughing and deep breathing, which produce a drop in intrathoracic pressure. Several studies have shown an LOS pressure rise in response to these activities. This pressure rise may occur by a reflex-mediated increase in sphincter tone, a change in extrinsic mechanical factors or perhaps a simple transmission of abdominal pressure to the sphincter.

The regulation of LOS pressure depends on the interplay of myogenic, neural and humoral factors. In humans, resting LOS pressure is reduced by atropine and vagal interruption, suggesting that the neural component is dominant.[57] This LOS innervation is by both excitatory and inhibitory autonomic nerves, with the cell bodies of the inhibitory nerves located in the enteric nervous system. Preganglionic vagal fibres originate in the dorsal motor nucleus of the vagus. These vagal fibres synapse on the myenteric ganglionic cell bodies,[58] where the transmitter is acetylcholine. Acetylcholine exerts its effects on the postganglionic neurone by both nicotinic and muscarinic receptors, but recent evidence indicates that nitric oxide may be the non-adrenergic, non-cholinergic transmitter between the nerves and the muscle of the LOS.

The concept of transient lower oesophageal sphincter relaxation (TLOSR) was introduced by Dent following the development of a sleeve manometry device in 1976.[59] Appropriate or physiological TLOSRs follow primary or secondary peristaltic swallows or as a response to gastric distension and bloating resulting in a belch[1] (**Fig. 12.2**). These relaxations usually occur within 5 seconds (from resting pressure to maximal relaxation) and last between 5 and 40 seconds.[60] In studies of asymptomatic patients TLOSRs resulted in reflux episodes. The frequency of TLOSRs were increased after eating,[55,61] and were higher in the sitting position when compared with lying down.[62] In these studies, approximately 50% of TLOSRs led to a reflux episode.[63,64]

 Inappropriate TLOSRs have been shown to be the dominant cause of reflux in symptomatic patients.

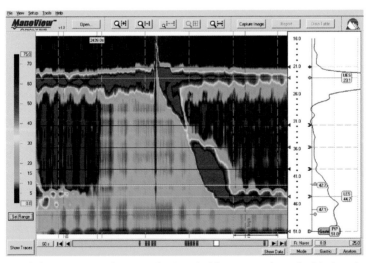

Figure 12.2 • High-resolution manometry demonstrating transient lower oesophageal sphincter relaxation (TLOSR). The upper oesophageal sphincter is demonstrated by the upper red and yellow zone, and the LOS by the lower red and yellow zone. On relaxation of the lower oesophageal sphincter a common cavity is created between the stomach and oesophagus – demonstrated by the light blue zone on the spatiotemporal plot (centre). These events are observed also on the axial pressure plot (right). The event is terminated and oesophagus cleared by primary peristalsis with intra-oesophageal pressure returning to baseline levels. Images acquired by 36-channel SSI Manoscan 360. Reproduced from Fox MR, Bredenoord AJ. Oesophageal high-resolution manometry: moving from research into clinical practice. Gut 2008; 57(3):405–23. With permission from BMJ Publishing Group Ltd.

The proportion of reflux episodes due to TLOSRs varies with the experimental study and the severity of reflux disease. As the disease becomes more severe a greater proportion of reflux episodes are caused by spontaneous reflux across a low-pressure sphincter. Even in this situation, however, TLOSRs remain the dominant reflux mechanism. The cause of inappropriate TLOSRs has been the subject of much debate. While some have felt that some relaxations were due to failed peristalsis, others believe that TLOSRs are a variant of the belch reflex and were primarily a response to gastric distension.[62] Certainly the frequency of TLOSRs increases with gastric distension by gas or by balloons, both in controls and reflux patients. Belching occurs through a relaxed sphincter with a manometric pattern very similar to that seen in the TLOSR of a reflux episode. In addition, in ambulant patients, many reflux episodes seem to be precipitated by belching.[65,66] Studies have shown that TLOSRs are the result of a vagally mediated reflex that is triggered by mechanoreceptors located in the proximal stomach.[67]

Patients with mild to moderate GORD do not necessarily just have increased TLOSR frequency,[68] and not all TLOSRs are associated with reflux.[69]

 Although a hiatus hernia is not always present or required for the diagnosis of GORD,[70] the structural integrity and function of the gastro-oesophageal junction are of great importance in the pathophysiology of GORD.

As the anatomical changes of the hiatus hernia progress, the likelihood of reflux during TLOSR increases, as does the volume of the refluxate. However, in many patients the LOS function is maintained despite their hiatus hernias and they do not have GORD. This is in contrast to those patients with no hiatus hernia but defective LOS who could have quite severe oesophagitis.[71]

Sliding hiatus hernia

 While it is known that the majority of patients with hiatus hernia are asymptomatic, many patients with GORD have a hernia.

A previous multicentre study found the endoscopic prevalence of hiatus hernias to be 5.8%, while in patients with oesophagitis this rate rose to 32%.[54] A radiological study of patients with oesophagitis found the incidence to be as high as 90%.[72] Ambulatory oesophageal pH monitoring has demonstrated both increased frequency of reflux and prolonged oesophageal acid exposure in patients with hiatus hernia compared with those without.[72] This is because postprandial acid-rich gastric contents reside unimpeded in the hernia pocket above the diaphragmatic crura.[48] From here it refluxes into the oesophagus upon LOS relaxation or with small increases of intra-abdominal pressure, such as on straining or even deep breathing[1] (**Fig. 12.3**).

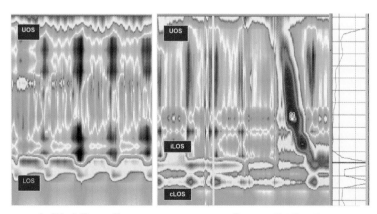

Initial Baseline   Same Patient

Figure 12.3 • High-resolution manometry showing a single high-pressure zone in the lower oesophagus crossing the diaphragm on the left (LOS). In this spatiotemporal plot higher pressures are presented in the yellow–red spectrum and lower pressures in the green–blue spectrum. On the right there is separation of the lower oesophageal high-pressure zone (iLOS) and the high-pressure zone created by the diaphragmatic crura (cLOS) suggestive of a transient hiatus hernia. The longitudinal red and yellow zone on the right demonstrates the propagation of a peristaltic wave down the oesophagus. LOS, lower oesophageal sphincter; cLOS, crural LOS; iLOS, intrinsic LOS; UOS, upper oesophageal sphincter. Reproduced from Fox MR, Bredenoord AJ. Oesophageal high-resolution manometry: moving from research into clinical practice. Gut 2008; 57(3):405–23. With permission from BMJ Publishing Group Ltd.

Saliva

Although oesophageal peristalsis is the most important mechanism to clear refluxed acid, the neutralising ability of saliva provides additional protection. Helm et al. found that 95% of an acid bolus was cleared by the initial primary or secondary peristaltic wave. Neutralisation of residual acid occurred in a stepwise fashion with each subsequent swallow.[73] Stimulation of salivation shortened the time required for acid clearance, whereas aspiration of saliva from the mouth abolished acid clearance.[74] The rate of production of saliva is directly related to and determines swallowing frequency,[75] which in the resting awake state is about once per minute.[40] Resting salivary flow in normal adults is 0.44 mL/min with a pH of 7.02 ± 0.05,[76] and is capable of neutralising small amounts of acid over several minutes due mainly to its bicarbonate content. At night, saliva production virtually ceases, as does primary oesophageal peristalsis.[40]

Oesophageal submucosal glands can secrete bicarbonate,[77] and theoretically the amount of bicarbonate secreted would be able to neutralise sufficient residual acid from an episode of reflux to raise pH from 2.5 to almost 7. This additional defence mechanism may be important at night when peristalsis and saliva production are greatly reduced.

Gastric function

As the source of most of the refluxate that produces oesophageal damage, the stomach ought to be a major contributor to the pathophysiology of acid reflux disease either with excessive acid production or with abnormalities of gastric emptying. Conditions that cause mechanical gastric outlet obstruction (benign or malignant causes) can indeed result in severe oesophagitis. Delayed gastric emptying (gastroparesis) has also been reported in some patients with GORD and this may be secondary to conditions such as diabetes.[78] In the majority of acid reflux patients, however, no abnormalities in gastric emptying can be determined and the significance of delayed gastric emptying in the pathogenesis of GORD is unclear.

Acid hypersecretion found in Zollinger–Ellison syndrome is associated with a high rate of oesophagitis.[79] While studies have shown hypersecretion in some patients with GORD,[80] as well as differences in basal and peak acid outputs, the majority show little difference in acid secretory levels compared with control subjects.

Helicobacter pylori infection of the distal stomach (antral gastritis) increases gastric acid production and eradication of the infection results in a reduced risk of gastric ulceration as well as acid reflux. However, proximal gastric involvement may be associated with atrophic gastritis and results in decreased acid production. In this case eradication of *H. pylori* worsens reflux severity. Realistically and in clinical practice, however, studies have found little effect of *H. pylori* eradication on GORD.[1] Current guidelines promote the eradication of *H. pylori* regardless of GORD due to its increased risk on peptic ulceration and gastric cancer.

The pylorus

The pylorus is the anatomical and physiological sphincter that regulates gastric emptying and prevents duodenogastric reflux.

There is no doubt that duodenal contents reflux into the stomach as a normal physiological process. From here they can pass into the oesophagus during episodes of gastro-oesophageal reflux. It is thought that the bile and pancreatic juice reflux contribute to the development of oesophagitis, metaplasia and dysplasia.[81] In general the greater the duration of acid reflux, the greater the amount of bile reflux,[82] but the concentrations of refluxed bile acids are unlikely to be cytotoxic.[83] Acid reflux is clearly the most important factor as reflux symptoms and oesophageal inflammation can be eradicated with potent acid suppressive therapy. While this acid suppression alone will not reverse the metaplastic epithelium, mucosal injury of the Barrett's with laser or argon-gas coagulation returns the epithelium to a squamous phenotype despite continuing 'bile reflux'.[84]

Methods of investigation

The oesophagus is the easiest part of the gastrointestinal tract to investigate because of its accessibility. Consequently many techniques have been developed over the years to study structure and function. Some tests are widely used in clinical practice (barium radiology and flexible endoscopy), while others are predominantly research tools (oesophageal aspiration studies). Some of the modern techniques used to investigate the oesophagus are described below but a detailed description of individual methodologies is beyond the scope of this chapter.

Endoscopy

Flexible endoscopy is often the first line of investigation in patients with symptoms that may involve the oesophagus. In addition to visual examination of the mucosa, histological and cytological specimens can be obtained and therapeutic procedures such as stricture dilatation, oesophageal stent insertion and arresting haemorrhage can be performed. Not only can endoscopy detect mucosal abnormalities, it could also point towards the presence of an oesophageal motility abnormality. For example, a dilated oesophagus containing food debris with a tight but passable lower oesophageal sphincter may suggest achalasia. An oesophageal diverticulum might suggest a motility abnormality. For the most part, however, the endoscope is a poor method of investigating motility problems as it detects mucosal structural problems rather than muscular functional abnormalities.

Radiology

It can be used for both acid reflux disease and certain motility problems. A simple chest X-ray may show lung changes that would support a history of aspiration or reveal the presence of a large hiatus hernia.

Contrast radiology plays an important part in the investigation of oesophageal problems, detecting anatomical, mucosal and functional abnormalities.

A double-contrast barium study can reveal the mucosal abnormalities of oesophageal inflammation and strictures. It will demonstrate the presence of webs, rings, diverticula and hiatus hernias, along with the presence or absence of normal propagating contractions. As such it may reveal the classical motility abnormalities of achalasia or diffuse oesophageal spasm ('corkscrew' appearance). However, the diagnoses such as achalasia and diffuse oesophageal spasm are often missed. While endoscopy has overtaken radiology in the investigation of reflux disease, radiology still retains an important role in the investigation of patients with motility abnormalities. Techniques such as videofluoroscopy combined with solid and liquid bolus swallows can help in the diagnosis of pharyngeal and upper oesophageal motility disorders.

pH studies

The development of miniaturised pH catheters, digital recording devices and computer analysis software has allowed prolonged (24-hour) ambulatory pH recordings to become widely available in clinical practice. Not only does the equipment record acid reflux episodes as they occur, it also allows a correlation between patient symptoms and those episodes to be made using an event marker (**Fig. 12.4**). Computerised software then analyses the recording to produce tables of standard variables that can be compared with known control values. With prolonged recordings of frequent reflux episodes several measures have become standard. These include the total number of reflux episodes, the number lasting more than 5 minutes and the total acid reflux time (as a percentage of the total recording time). The latter is robust and the single most reproducible diagnostic marker for GORD, and, in most centres, an oesophageal pH of <4, recorded 5 cm above a manometrically defined LOS, should be present for less than 5% of a 24-hour period in normal individuals.[84A] If the recording is further divided

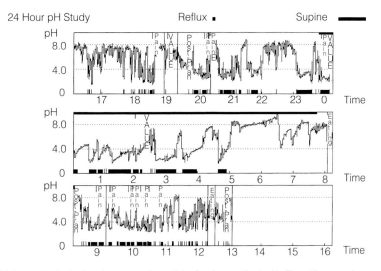

Figure 12.4 • A 24-hour pH study showing excessive acid reflux in a patient with Barrett's oesophagus. Note the correlation of the patient's pain with acid in the oesophagus.

into daytime, night-time and postprandial periods a large number of values are possible. As there is a wide spectrum of severity of acid reflux disease, with day-to-day variation, the recorded variables have to be referenced to known control values. One such system that is widely used is the revised Johnson–DeMeester score, which tries to produce a score based on the above variables (from control subjects) above which acid reflux is likely (Tables 12.1 and 12.2). This is a convenient, clinically validated system for assessing the severity of reflux disease, based on the number of reflux episodes and duration of acid exposure in the upright and supine positions (weighted towards the percentage time of supine oesophageal pH exposure).[3]

In addition, consideration has to be given to the symptom (event) marker so that the patient's typical symptoms can be correlated with what is happening in the oesophagus at the moment of the symptoms. For example, a patient may still be considered to suffer from acid reflux disease if every typical symptom is correlated in time with acid in the oesophagus despite an overall oesophageal pH time within the normal range. At the other extreme a patient

with no correlation of their symptoms with acid in the oesophagus and with pH study variables above the normal range does not necessarily have acid reflux disease.

Three symptom-association analyses are in routine use for clinical reporting and research to define the temporal relationship between reflux and symptoms.[85] These are usually incorporated into commercial ambulatory pH software. By convention, recordings are made within a 2–minute time window just prior the onset of each symptom.

Symptom Index (SI) describes the proportion of patient symptoms that are related to reflux:

$$SI = (\text{number of reflux – related symptom episodes} / \text{Total number of symptom episodes}) \times 100$$

A symptom association of $\geq 50\%$ is considered to be positive. This is a very common and simple tool used and automatically calculated by the dedicated software that comes with the pH recording systems. One study looking at SI as a predictor of response to therapy showed that in a group of patients with symptoms of heartburn and regurgitation and evidence of physiological oesophageal acid exposure,

Table 12.1 • Findings of pH study conducted on patient illustrated in Fig. 12.4

	Total	Upright	Supine	Eating	Postprandial	Fasting
Duration (h)	20:48	12:50	7:58	0:55	2:30	0:00
No. of reflux episodes	123	106	17	1	19	–
Time below pH 4.0 (min)	426:34	228:19	198:15	0:03	53:17	–
Time below pH 4.0 (%)	34.1	29.6	41.4	0.1	35.5	–
No. of episodes >5 min	24	15	9	0	4	–
Longest reflux (min)	42:27	27:15	42:27	0:03	12:16	–

Table 12.2 • Scores according to Johnson and DeMeester for pH <4 for findings in Table 12.1 (study of patient illustrated in Fig. 12.4)

Component	Patient value	Normal values	Score
Total time (%)	34.1	4.45	24.96
Upright time (%)	29.6	8.42	12.64
Supine time (%)	41.4	3.45	41.77
No. of episodes	123	46.90	9.08
No. >5 min	24	3.45	20.62
Longest episode	42:27	19.80	5.54
Composite score			**114.61**
A normal composite score is <14.72			

those who showed most improvement to the addition of a proton-pump inhibitor were those with a positive SI.[86] One important shortfall, however, is that it does not take into account the number of reflux episodes, rather it only describes the association between reflux and symptoms.

Symptom Sensitivity Index (SSI)[87] is a simple parameter that is also easy to understand and to manually calculate, which takes into account the number of reflux episodes:

SSI = (number of symptom – associated reflux episodes / Total number of reflux episodes) × 100

SSI is considered to be positive with a value of ≥10%. However, one shortcoming is that it does not take into account the total number of symptom episodes.

The **Symptom Association Probability (SAP)**[88] is a statistical function which calculates the probability that the relationship observed between reflux and symptoms is not brought on by chance. Generally, it is performed by dividing the 24-hour period into 2-minute segments and determining whether or not a symptom occurred 2 minutes prior to every episode of reflux recorded. The results are then collated and analysed via a 2 × 2 contingency table. By statistical convention an SAP of ≥95% is considered positive. One study showed that independently SAP is a good predictor to the success of antireflux surgery.[89] Although SAP uses all parameters to provide a better insight into the relationship between symptoms and reflux, it is difficult to calculate, and it is important to note that it is only a statistical test for association. Even though a statistically significant association is shown it does not necessarily imply a causal relationship between the two parameters.[85]

The result of a pH study should be taken into consideration with the clinical history, endoscopy and radiology findings and response to acid suppression with a proton-pump inhibitor.

For those with incomplete or poor response to acid suppression or atypical symptoms (globus sensation, chest pain, cough) with non-diagnostic endoscopy, ambulatory pH monitoring can help not only to achieve a diagnosis, but also to establish the temporal relationship between reflux and symptoms. This information can then be used to consider an appropriate method of management and indeed help with the decision for antireflux surgery. Patients with a positive relationship between reflux and symptoms are more likely to respond to conservative or surgical management.[85]

While the precise details of the technique of pH studies are beyond the scope of this chapter, a few important points are worth mentioning. In order to produce standardised and reproducible results most studies are carried out in an agreed way.

- Indications for 24-hour pH monitoring include: classic symptoms of oesophageal reflux (which may or may not be refractory to antacids), atypical symptoms (globus, chest pain, chronic cough) and dysphagia, or those with a suspected motility disorder as it is almost always combined with manometry.[90]

- The pH probe is positioned so that it lies 5 cm above the top of the LOS. If the probe is positioned too low it will slip into the stomach on the upward movement of the lower oesophagus and will then result in excessive acid reflux times. Conversely if the probe is too high then acid reflux times will be underestimated. As different subjects have different distances from the tip of the nose (where the probe is secured) to the LOS, a guess of the distance cannot be used. The only reliable way to accurately place a pH probe is to determine the position of the LOS by manometry.

- An acid reflux episode, as recorded by a pH probe, starts when the oesophageal pH drops below 4 and ends when it rises above 5 (or 4 in some laboratories).

- Proximal oesophageal acid reflux that may result in chronic cough, hoarseness and dental erosions can be investigated by placing pH sensors at multiple levels above the LOS. Furthermore, if there is doubt regarding the reading obtained, it is possible to have two pH sensors at 5 and 10 cm above the LOS in order to avoid a false-positive reading of the tip of the catheter dipping into the stomach.

- Using the number of reflux episodes that last more than 5 minutes to imply poor clearance and hence poor motility is inaccurate. Long-lasting reflux episodes on a pH study are just as likely to be due to multiple superimposed reflux episodes than to poor clearance of a single reflux event.[36] Assuming pH rises above 7.5 are due to alkaline reflux is also inaccurate.[83]

- pH monitoring is usually performed with the patients off acid suppression therapy in order to elucidate the severity and content of their reflux. Alternatively, patients could be tested while on antacids or other medication if their symptoms are refractory to therapy.[90]

- Completion of a diary sheet to record symptoms, activities and ingested food types is also important. Several foods and drinks are acidic and may be inaccurately recorded as a reflux episode if not eliminated from the analysis. The alternative is to restrict the patient to particular neutral foodstuffs, but this then becomes increasingly less of a physiological outpatient ambulatory study. Patients should eat and drink the 'normal' foods that would result in a typical day of reflux symptoms.

- At the completion of the study the quantity and type of symptoms experienced should also be recorded to help in the analysis of the data.

- Instruction to the patient on the use of the event marker and to document in a diary what symptom was being recorded is also important, particularly if the event marker can be pressed accidentally.

A criticism of prolonged catheter-based pH recording is that the catheter itself may inhibit normal daily activities including eating. Between 5% and 10% of patients are intolerant.[13] This in turn may lead to an underestimation of the patient's usual degree of oesophageal acidification. In order to overcome this, implantable capsule pH recording systems have been developed that can be placed endoscopically and fixed to the oesophageal wall. It must be acknowledged, however, that precise placement of such a device requires the same considerations given to the placement of a pH catheter as detailed above.

Wireless pH monitoring

Limitations to standard 24-hour pH monitoring are nasal and pharyngeal discomfort with gagging, nausea and vomiting reported by some patients. It is also socially embarrassing and can result in a modified diet and lifestyle that may not be representative of normal daily life and thus reduce reflux provoking activities.[91] Furthermore there is significant day-to-day variation with the total percentage of time pH is <4/24 hours over 2 consecutive days varying by up to 3.2–fold.[92] Studies have shown that the 24-hour catheter test has a reproducibility of only 70–80%.[85] In patients with non-diagnostic findings on endoscopy, failure to tolerate naso-oesophageal catheter or inconclusive results due to technical failure prevents a definitive measurement of oesophageal pH and an assessment of symptom association with reflux episodes. This will therefore hinder diagnosis and management.

The Bravo® pH system (Medtronic, Shoreview, MN, USA) is an innovative, endoscopically placed, catheter-free pH monitoring system (**Fig. 12.5**). A radiotelemetric capsule is attached to oesophageal mucosa 6 cm above the z-line identified at endoscopy using a specially designed transoral delivery device. This is because the HPZ has been found

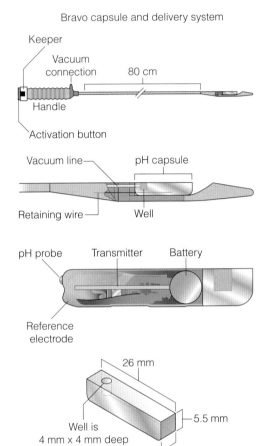

Figure 12.5 • Bravo® delivery system and capsule. The delivery system is inserted in the same way as a nasogastric tube, although it is usually delivered orally. Markings on the side depict the distance from the incisors. The capsule is deployed 6 cm above the anatomical z-line (or 5 cm above the proximal LOS high-pressure zone). The delivery system is then retracted and the receiver is synchronised. It remains attached to the patient (via belt clip or shoulder pouch) for 48 hours at least. Capsules all fall off inevitably within 10 days (usually 5–7). Complications requiring early removal are almost unheard of. Reprinted by permission from Macmillan Publishers Ltd: Pandolfino JE, Richter JE, Ours T et al. Ambulatory oesophageal pH monitoring using a wireless system. AM J Gastroenterol 2003; 98 (4): 740–9, copyright 2003.

to be approximately 1–1.5 cm above the squamo-columnar junction identified at endoscopy.[93] Oesophageal pH data are then transmitted to a portable receiver attached to the patient's belt for 48 hours. Prolonged measurement, up to 96 hours, increases diagnostic reproducibility and sensitivity, especially in patients with intermittent symptoms.[94] Moreover, the Bravo® system is better tolerated than catheter-based pH measurement and is preferred by unselected patients referred for pH investigation.[93,95] The major disadvantage of the Bravo® system is higher costs. As a result recent UK guidelines state that 'catheter-free oesophageal pH monitoring is particularly suitable for patients who do not tolerate nasal intubation'.[96]

Manometry

As the main function of the oesophagus is the transport of food and drink into the stomach, manometry ought to be a useful technique for studying disorders of this organ. 'The ideal manometric system would acquire continuous, high-fidelity pressure data from the pharynx to the stomach with circumferential sensitivity. The equipment should be cheap. The procedure should be quick and easy to perform and analyse. Presentation of pressure data should not only display oesophageal contractility but also provide an accurate assessment of the forces that drive bolus movement, and identify (or exclude) abnormal oesophageal function as the cause of a patient's symptoms.[97]

Manometry is required for the diagnosis of those with suspected motility disorders, particularly for those under consideration for surgery (e.g. antireflux or myotomy). Fundoplication has been performed on patients with achalasia after being mistaken for GORD with reflux-like symptoms and odynophagia. Odynophagia and oesophageal pain in achalasia are due to fermentation of bacteria in food residue, which results in lactic acid production. It can be difficult to differentiate this from reflux and pain due to oesophagitis.[90]

Standard manometry

Standard static manometry measures the circumferential contraction, pressure-wave duration and peristaltic velocity of oesophageal swallows, therefore providing information regarding the peristaltic and non-peristaltic activity down the oesophagus. Furthermore it is used to assess the LOS function and position as well as to facilitate placement of the pH catheter probe thereafter (see above).[90]

The normal swallow (as assessed by standard manometry)

A normal swallow of 5 mL of fluid starts with the contraction of the pharynx to propel the bolus towards the upper oesophageal sphincter, which quickly relaxes. A propagated peristaltic wave helps the bolus progress down the oesophagus and the relaxation of the LOS permits the bolus to successfully pass through the sphincter and into the stomach. Contraction amplitude (mmHg) is measured from the mean intra-oesophageal baseline pressure to the peak of the contraction wave. Normal amplitude values range from 30 mmHg in the proximal oesophagus to as high as 180 mmHg distally. Contraction duration is usually up to 6 seconds and is measured from the onset of the major upstroke to the end of the pressure wave. Peristaltic velocity is normally approximately 5 cm/s in the body of the oesophagus.[90]

Static manometry recordings can be obtained from catheters containing solid-state pressure transducers or water-perfused channels. The manometry catheter is passed into the stomach and then slowly withdrawn 1 cm at a time so that the pressure ports pass through the lower oesophageal sphincter. This allows the baseline sphincter pressure (above resting gastric pressure) to be measured along with estimations of sphincter length. The values of several pressure ports can be averaged out to give a mean sphincter pressure and sphincter length. Next the pressure ports are positioned in the oesophageal body, a minimum of three sensors placed 5 cm apart. Motility is assessed by the use of the standard ten wet swallow test. Like the pH study, control data are used to compare the findings from patients, including such parameters as the number of peristaltic contractions that occur in response to the wet swallows, the amplitude and velocity of the contractions, and the occurrence of abnormal contractions such as simultaneous or non-propagated waves. A further procedure that can be added to the standard study using a water-perfused catheter assembly is measurement of LOS relaxation. This has to be performed with a sleeve device that straddles the LOS, allowing up and down movement of the LOS relative to the catheter. Sleeve devices provide better accuracy in measuring sphincter pressures and relaxation as they allow for axial movement of the sphincter and provide the location of the maximum pressure within the LOS which it straddles. As the catheter needed is water perfused, these studies almost always have to be performed with patients immobile in the laboratory. While LOS function is of prime importance in the pathogenesis of acid reflux disease, its clinical measurement is of limited value (outside of research studies) as detection of GORD is by other methods and treatment ignores LOS behaviour.

The standard motility study is extensively used in physiology laboratories but could be criticised as being unphysiological. In a 24-hour period there are between 1000 and 2000 peristaltic swallows along with many other contraction types. Several meals and drinks are consumed and many pressure events occur. If motility abnormalities occur, particularly if they are intermittent, they may be missed on a study measuring just ten water swallows. This procedure can be used to diagnose specific disorders such as achalasia, diffuse oesophageal spasm and nutcracker oesophagus. Other motility disorders are not so easily recognised and are described as ineffective motility.

Standard manometry has several downfalls. Firstly, symptoms are rarely triggered by small-volume water swallows of fasted patients. Patients with GORD usually complain of symptoms postprandially and with manoeuvres that compromise the reflux barrier. Secondly, with only five to eight pressure sensors the ability of standard manometry to predict effective bolus transport is limited by poor spatial resolution. Segmental or focal abnormalities within the oesophagus (wide transition zone, focal hyper- or hypoperistalsis, segmental spasm) will be missed. Thirdly, the LOS anatomy is poorly appreciated, especially in the context of a hiatus hernia or very weak LOS. Furthermore the catheter does not take into account oesophageal shortening, which may shift the LOS above the sleeve device giving the false impression of LOS relaxation. Nevertheless, it is readily available, inexpensive and, for now, the most commonly used method for the measurement of motor function and motility disorders of the oesophagus.[98]

High-resolution manometry (HRM)

The cause of swallowing problems and other oesophageal symptoms remains uncertain in some patients despite conventional investigation. HRM can detect focal oesophageal dysmotility and measure the oesophagogastric pressure gradient that drives bolus transport, factors that have been linked to improved diagnostic accuracy.

The fundamentals of HRM were first established in the early 1990s by Clouse and Staiano,[99,100] who developed a model by which a functional image of the oesophageal anatomy was generated from multiple pressure sensors on a catheter. This information was reconstructed into a three-dimensional topographic plot using time, distance down the oesophagus and pressure amplitude as its axes. With the advent of micromanometric water-perfused assemblies,[25,101] and later solid-state catheter assemblies,[102,103] up to 36 sensors could be used, hence improving the image resolution dramatically. The 3D plot is superimposed onto a 2D image and the pressure changes are depicted by colour (**Fig. 12.6**). These data can be analysed in real time as a spatiotemporal plot that reveals the segmental neurofunctional anatomy of oesophageal peristalsis as well as the intraluminal pressure gradient operating on the bolus, the force that directs the move-

ment of food and fluid towards the stomach. These features improve the ability to predict bolus transport from pressure recordings compared to conventional manometry[98] (**Fig. 12.7**).

The pattern of oesophageal peristalsis and gastro-oesophageal junction function depicted by HRM shows whether or not the peristalsis is normal. The intrabolus pressure gradient defines whether this peristalsis will result in effective oesophageal clearance. These features improve the ability of HRM to identify abnormalities of the oesophagus as a function of disturbed bolus transport. In addition HRM can assess LOS dysfunction that may predispose to GORD.

Such features are unique to HRM and are important as symptoms and mucosal damage are more likely to occur due to a disturbance of bolus transport and poor clearance of refluxate rather than abnormal function as described by standard manometry.[98]

An 'e-sleeve', which electronically emulates the sleeve device of standard manometry, can be applied in order to provide stable LOS function during analysis. This facilitates the positioning of the catheter and removes the need for the time-consuming pull-through of standard manometry.

Normal values have been established for peristalsis and the gastro-oesophageal junction for water swallows.[103,104] Although small volumes of liquid swallows have conventionally been used in standard manometry, HRM facilitates the assessment of the dynamics of swallows with the use of different food consistency (solids) and volumes (e.g. multiple repeated swallows of large volumes of fluids).[97] These activities provide a more physiological assessment of swallow and can act as a stressor to the oesophagus, therefore allowing it to work harder and in turn improve the sensitivity of investigation for functional and structural pathology (strictures, rumination, achalasia).[97,105,106] Advantages and disadvantages of standard manometry vs. HRM can be seen in Table 12.3.

Measurement of duodenogastric oesophageal reflux

Although acid is responsible for the majority of oesophageal symptoms, these symptoms can occur without acid being detected in the refluxate, especially in Barrett's treated with acid suppression therapy. While many believe that duodenogastric oesophageal reflux may contribute to the pathophysiology of reflux disease, the paucity of convincing clinical evidence and the lack of effective treatment (excluding surgery), in combination with the eradication of inflammation and symptoms with acid suppression alone, makes the routine investigation of bile reflux unnecessary. In the past a rise in oesophageal pH above 8 and aspiration

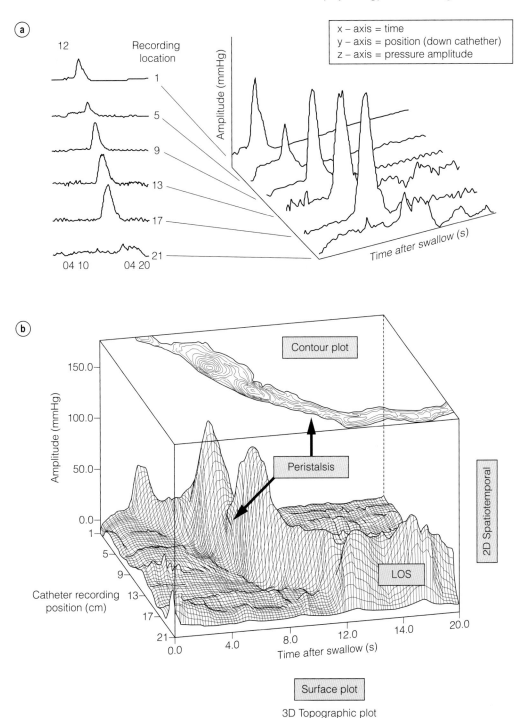

Figure 12.6 • **(a)** Early 1990s (Clouse and Staiano) foundations of HRM laid: time, catheter position and average pressure were reconstructed into pseudo-3D 'topographic plots' that demonstrated the functional anatomy of the oesophagus. **(b)** Topographic display of normal oesophageal pressure data. The pseudo-3D surface plot displays the characteristic peaks and troughs of the peristaltic pressure wave proceeding from the proximal oesophagus (background), until it merges with the LOS after-contraction (foreground). The contour plot of the same swallow superimposed at the top of the figure demonstrates how 3D data are represented using concentric rings at 10-mmHg intervals to indicate increasing amplitudes. Reproduced from Clouse RE, Staiano A, Bickston SJ et al. Characteristics of the propagating pressure wave in the oesophagus. Dig Dis Sci 1996; 41(12):2369–76. Used with permission from The American Physiological Society.

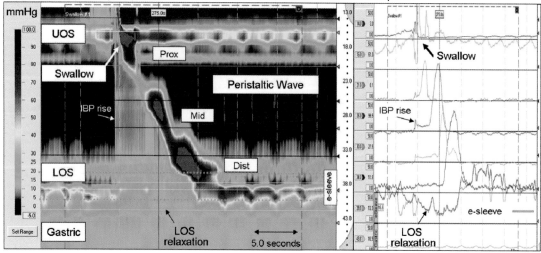

Figure 12.7 • High-resolution manometry depicts oesophageal pressure activity from the pharynx to the stomach via pressure sensors spaced at <2 cm intervals apart. Recordings can be analysed and presented either as line plots (similar to conventional manometry) or spatiotemporal plots. The spatiotemporal plot presents the same information as the line plots. Time is on the *x*-axis, distance from the nares is on the *y*-axis and pressure amplitude on the *z*-axis (each pressure is assigned a colour (legend left)). The segmental functional anatomy of the oesophagus is clearly demonstrated. The synchronous relaxation of the UOS and LOS (deglutitive inhibition) is obvious, as is the increasing pressure and duration of the peristaltic wave as it passes distally. The virtual 'e-sleeve' application provides a summary measurement of LOS pressure and relaxation (bold brown line plot). Similar to a conventional sleeve sensor, the maximum pressure over a 6-cm distance is displayed. Images acquired by 36-channel SSI Manoscan 360. Reproduced from Fox MR, Bredenoord AJ. Oesophageal high-resolution manometry: moving from research into clinical practice. Gut 2008; 57(3):405–23. With permission from BMJ Publishing Group Ltd.

Table 12.3 • Comparison between standard and high-resolution manometry

	Conventional pull-through manometry	Conventional sleeve manometry	High-resolution manometry
Costs	Inexpensive	Inexpensive	Expensive
Execution	Relatively elaborate and time consuming	Relatively elaborate and time consuming	Relatively simple and fast
Interpretation	Requires experience	Requires experience	Relatively easy
Measuring LOS function and relaxation	Limited	Yes	Yes
Measuring UOS function and relaxation	No	Limited	Yes

LOS, lower oesophageal sphincter; UOS, upper oesophageal sphincter.
Reproduced from Fox MR, Bredenoord AJ. Oesophageal high-resolution manometry: moving from research into clinical practice. Gut 2008; 57(3):405–23. With permission from BMJ Publishing Group Ltd.

studies were the only methods available for detecting duodenogastric reflux. However, pH rises above 8 have been shown to be too unreliable to detect alkaline reflux,[83] and aspiration studies too cumbersome and uncomfortable to be clinically useful.[103] The measurement of bile reflux with the Bilitec 2000 recorder (Synectics, Stockholm, Sweden) is performed in a similar way as an ambulatory pH recording. It uses spectrophotometry to detect the absorbance spectrum of bilirubin as an indirect measure of bile salt reflux. It showed that bile reflux is only responsible for a minority of symptoms.[107] One study showed that in their group of patients with GORD only 7% had a positive SAP for bile reflux using Bilitec 2000, which they calculated as being only 2% greater than that which would have been found by chance.[108] Technical limitations to the bilirubin absorbance technique, such as the distortion of its signal–response relationship in an acidic environment, make its usefulness very limited.[109]

Oesophageal impedance measurement

Multiple intraluminal impedance (MII) is a fairly new technique and was first introduced in 1991 to detect the flow of gas and liquid through a hollow lumen[110] (**Fig. 12.8**). Impedance is the opposition to current flow, an inverse measurement of electrical conductance of the contents within a lumen. Impedance varies with bolus conductivity. Liquid bolus has high conductivity and low impedance while air has low conductivity and high impedance. Therefore the arrival of a liquid bolus will result in a rapid voltage drop of over 50% from the nadir and the successful clearance of the bolus results in a rapid rise of the voltage back up to baseline. One electrode will detect bolus movement through the lumen; multiple electrodes will determine the direction. Impedance therefore can be used to:

1. determine the direction of bolus movement (antegrade in normal swallow, retrograde in reflux);
2. determine the success of bolus transit or escape;

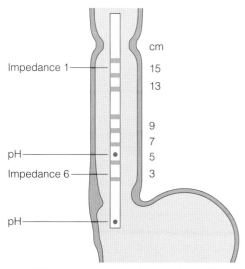

Figure 12.8 • Example of impedance catheter. This one has six impedance sensors and two pH sensors. Reprinted by permission from Macmillan Publishers Ltd: Sifrim D, Blondeau K. Technology insight: the role of impedance testing for esophageal disorders. Nat Clin Pract Gastroenterol Hepatol 2006; 3(4):210–19, copyright 2006.

3. calculate the velocity of propagation of the bolus;
4. differentiate between liquid and gas;
5. determine the proximal extent of reflux within the oesophagus;
6. determine superimposed reflux (also known as re-reflux), which occurs when more than one reflux episode occurs during the same period of pH drop.

Manometry and reflux studies often fail to establish the physiologic basis of oesophageal symptoms or guide therapy. Oesophageal symptoms are often related to disturbed bolus transport rather than acid reflux.[111] Also, non-acid reflux can be a cause of persistent symptoms despite effective acid suppression.[112] At present, only barium videofluoroscopy can assess the efficiency of bolus transport; however, this test is limited by radiation exposure and lack of ambulatory data. MII can follow bolus transport and detect reflux with no radiation risk and can be used in an ambulatory manner similar to pH manometry. Studies have shown MII to be a reproducible method of assessing GORD.[113] MII is often combined with other investigation modalities such as pH monitoring in order to improve detection of pathology. Impedance–pH (MII–pH) can be used to determine whether the antegrade movement of the refluxate is acidic (pH < 4), weakly acidic (pH 4–7) or weakly alkaline (pH > 7).[114] This is an improvement on isolated ambulatory pH monitoring and can be used over a 24-hour period in a similar manner. The indications for its use are the same as that for 24-hour pH monitoring. As it can detect non-acid reflux, MII–pH is considered the most sensitive method for reflux detection.[115] This is especially important in the detection of postprandial reflux, which is often non-acidic, and in reflux while on acid-reducing therapy, as therapeutic inhibition of acid does not alter the mechanism or frequency of reflux episodes but can still lead to mucosal damage. Another use of MII–pH is for those patients who are on maximal acid suppression therapy but continue to have reflux symptoms (considered to be up to 1 in 4). In this group of patients MII–pH, used to ascertain SI positivity, can increase the detection rate for pathological reflux from 11% to 48%.[112] MII–pH has been shown to improve the association of symptoms with reflux by 10–20% in GORD,[116] which may help to stratify those who could benefit from surgical antireflux therapy.[112]

Acknowledgement

We would like to thank Dr Angela Anggiansah, Director of the Oesophageal Laboratory at Guy's & St Thomas' Hospitals NHS Foundation Trust, for advice regarding the laboratory investigations.

Key points

- Manometric studies have shown the presence of a high-pressure zone that behaves like a physiological sphincter (relaxing to allow swallowing, belching and vomiting) extending over the terminal 1–4 cm of the oesophagus.
- The regulation of lower oesophageal sphincter (LOS) pressure depends on the interplay of myogenically, neurally and humorally mediated factors.
- Transient lower oesophageal sphincter relaxation (TLOSR) can be appropriate when it follows primary or secondary peristaltic swallows, or inappropriate when relaxation occurs spontaneously or after a non-propagated pharyngeal swallow.
- TLOSRs have been shown to be the dominant cause of reflux in symptomatic patients.
- GOR is more likely to occur across a deficient LOS in the presence of a hiatus hernia. In addition, oesophageal acid clearance may be impaired in patients with a sliding hiatus hernia.
- Twenty-four-hour ambulatory pH monitoring is usually nominated as the gold standard in establishing a diagnosis of GORD. Wireless pH monitoring can increase diagnostic reproducibility and sensitivity, especially in patients with intermittent symptoms. It remains, however, more costly and usually requires endoscopic placement.
- Prolonged pH monitoring has shown that even asymptomatic subjects have episodes of GOR, which are mainly short-lived and occur postprandially. However, normal pH profiles may be seen in symptomatic patients and in up to 25% of subjects with endoscopic oesophagitis.
- Some patients with GOR have oesophageal motor abnormalities and the prevalence of these abnormalities increases with the severity of oesophagitis. Whether the motor dysfunction is the primary abnormality or whether it develops secondary to reflux-induced oesophageal inflammation is yet to be established.
- Regardless of its suggested effects on stomach acidity, current guidelines promote the eradication of *H. pylori* regardless of GORD due to its increased risk on peptic ulceration and gastric cancer.
- The total acid reflux time (as a percentage of the total recording time) is the single most useful and reproducible measurement in a pH study. An oesophageal pH of <4, recorded 5 cm above a manometrically defined LOS, should be present for less than 5% of a 24-hour period in normal individuals.
- The DeMeester score is a convenient, clinically validated system for assessing the severity of reflux disease. It is based on the number of reflux episodes and duration of acid exposure in the upright and supine positions. A score of ≤14.72 is considered normal.
- The symptom-association analyses that are most commonly used are:
    (i). Symptom Index (SI) – the proportion of patient symptoms that are related to reflux.
    (ii). Symptom Association Probability (SAP) – statistical function that calculates the probability that the relationship observed between reflux and symptoms is not brought on by chance.
- The result of a pH study should be taken into consideration with the clinical history, endoscopy and radiology findings and response to acid suppression with a proton-pump inhibitor.
- Standard manometry is a static test that measures the contraction amplitude, duration of pressure wave, velocity of peristalsis as well as LOS function and position. It is also required to identify the correct position for pH catheter tip placement. It is especially useful for patients with dysphagia or when a motility disorder is suspected.
- High-resolution manometry uses multiple pressure-recording sensors down the length of the oesophagus to acquire pressure data that are reconstructed by a computer into a visually intuitive spatiotemporal plot in real time. It is used to detect focal dysmotility, measure the oesophagogastric pressure gradient that predicts bolus transport, and depict the LOS function and anatomy in great detail.
- Multiple intraluminal impedance (MII) is a tool used to follow bolus transit and detect reflux in those with maximal acid suppression therapy, postprandial non-acid reflux and bolus escape in those with dysmotility. There is no radiation risk. It can be used in an ambulatory manner similar to pH manometry. MII catheters can be combined with pH and manometry sensors for additional information.

References

1. Fox M, Forgacs I. Gastro-oesophageal reflux disease. BMJ 2006; 332(7533):88–93.

2. Lagergren J, Bergstrom R, Lindgren A et al. Symptomatic gastroesophageal reflux as a risk factor for oesophageal adenocarcinoma. N Engl J Med 1999; 340(11):825–31.

3. Johnson LF, DeMeester TR. Twenty-four-hour pH monitoring of the distal oesophagus. A quantitative measure of gastroesophageal reflux. Am J Gastroenterol 1974; 62(4):325–32.

4. DeMeester TR, Johnson LF, Joseph GJ et al. Patterns of gastroesophageal reflux in health and disease. Ann Surg 1976; 184(4):459–70.

5. Graham DY, Smith JL, Patterson DJ. Why do apparently healthy people use antacid tablets. Am J Gastroenterol 1983; 78(5):257–60.

6. Johansson KE, Ask P, Boeryd B et al. Oesophagitis, signs of reflux, and gastric acid secretion in patients with symptoms of gastro-oesophageal reflux disease. Scand J Gastroenterol 1986; 21(7):837–47.

7. Fuchs KH, DeMeester TR, Albertucci M. Specificity and sensitivity of objective diagnosis of gastroesophageal reflux disease. Surgery 1987; 102(4):575–80.

8. Stoker DL, Williams JG, Leicester RG et al. Oesophagitis – a five year review. Gut 1988; 29:A1450.

9. Sloan S, Rademaker AW, Kahrilas PJ. Determinants of gastroesophageal junction incompetence: hiatal hernia, lower oesophageal sphincter, or both. Ann Intern Med 1992; 117(12):977–82.

10. Gotley D, Cooper M. The investigation of gastro-oesophageal reflux. Surg Res Comm 1987; 2:1–17.

11. Johnsson F, Joelsson B. Reproducibility of ambulatory oesophageal pH monitoring. Gut 1988; 29(7):886–9.

12. Johnsson F, Joelsson B, Gudmundsson K et al. Symptoms and endoscopic findings in the diagnosis of gastroesophageal reflux disease. Scand J Gastroenterol 1987; 22(6):714–18.

13. Lee J, Anggiansah A, Anggiansah R et al. Effects of age on the gastroesophageal junction, oesophageal motility, and reflux disease. Clin Gastroenterol Hepatol 2007; 5(12):1392–8.

14. Castell D. Anatomy and physiology of the oesophagus and its sphincters. In: Castell DO, Richter JE, Dalton CB (eds) Esophageal motility testing. New York: Elsevier Science, 1987; pp. 13–27.

15. Sugarbaker DJ, Rattan S, Goyal RK. Mechanical and electrical activity of oesophageal smooth muscle during peristalsis. Am J Physiol 1984; 246 (2, Pt 1):G145–50.

16. Madsen T, Wallin L, Boesby S et al. Oesophageal peristalsis in normal subjects. Influence of pH and volume during imitated gastro-oesophageal reflux. Scand J Gastroenterol 1983; 18(4):513–18.

17. Hollis JB, Castell DO. Effect of dry swallows and wet swallows of different volumes on oesophageal peristalsis. J Appl Physiol 1975; 38(6):1161–4.

18. Winship DH, Viegas de Andrade SR, Zboralske FF. Influence of bolus temperature on human oesophageal motor function. J Clin Invest 1970; 49(2):243–50.

19. Olsen AM, Schlegel JF. Motility disturbances caused by esophagitis. J Thorac Cardiovasc Surg 1965; 50(5):607–12.

20. Kahrilas PJ, Dodds WJ, Hogan WJ et al. Esophageal peristaltic dysfunction in peptic esophagitis. Gastroenterology 1986; 91(4):897–904.

21. Ahtaridis G, Snape WJ Jr, Cohen S. Clinical and manometric findings in benign peptic strictures of the oesophagus. Dig Dis Sci 1979; 24(11):858–61.

22. Shah AK, Wolfsen HC, Hemminger LL et al. Changes in oesophageal motility after porfimer sodium photodynamic therapy for Barrett's dysplasia and mucosal carcinoma. Dis Esophagus 2006; 19(5):335–9.

23. Jones MP, Sloan SS, Jovanovic B et al. Impaired egress rather than increased access: an important independent predictor of erosive oesophagitis. Neurogastroenterol Motil 2002; 14(6):625–31.

24. Escandell AO, De Haro LFM, Paricio PP et al. Surgery improves defective oesophageal peristalsis in patients with gastro-oesophageal reflux. Br J Surg 1991; 78:1095–7.

25. Reider F, Cheng L, Harnett KM et al. Gastroesophageal reflux disease-associated esophagitis induces endogenous cytokine production leading to motor abnormalities. Gastroenterology 2007; 132: 154–65.

26. Eckardt VF. Does healing of esophagitis improve oesophageal motor function. Dig Dis Sci 1988; 33(2):161–5.

27. Baldi F, Ferrarini F, Longanesi A et al. Oesophageal function before, during, and after healing of erosive oesophagitis. Gut 1988; 29(2):157–60.

28. Eriksen CA, Sadek SA, Cranford C et al. Reflux oesophagitis and oesophageal transit: evidence for a primary oesophageal motor disorder. Gut 1988; 29(4):448–52.

29. Maddern GJ, Jamieson GG. Oesophageal emptying in patients with gastro-oesophageal reflux. Br J Surg 1986; 73(8):615–17.

30. Richter JE, Johns DN, Wu WC et al. Are oesophageal motility abnormalities produced during the intraesophageal acid perfusion test. JAMA 1985; 253(13):1914–17.

31. Baigrie RJ, Watson DI, Myers JC et al. Outcome of laparoscopic Nissen fundoplication in patients with disordered preoperative peristalsis. Gut 1997; 40(3):381–5.

32. Anthony A, Barham CP, Mills AE et al. Nonobstructive dysphagia in patients with gastro-oesophageal reflux disease – is manometry helpful? Br J Surg 2000; 87(Suppl 1):32.

33. Kahrilas PJ, Dodds WJ, Hogan WJ. Effect of peristaltic dysfunction on oesophageal volume clearance. Gastroenterology 1988; 94(1):73–80.

34. Booth DJ, Kemmerer WT, Skinner DB. Acid clearing from the distal oesophagus. Arch Surg 1968; 96(5):731–4.

35. Stanciu C, Bennett JR. Oesophageal acid clearing: one factor in the production of reflux oesophagitis. Gut 1974; 15(11):852–7.

36. Barham CP, Gotley DC, Mills A et al. Oesophageal acid clearance in patients with severe reflux oesophagitis. Br J Surg 1995; 82(3):333–7.

37. Little AG, DeMeester TR, Kirchner PT et al. Pathogenesis of esophagitis in patients with gastroesophageal reflux. Surgery 1980; 88(1):101–7.

38. Kjellen G, Tibbling L. Influence of body position, dry and water swallows, smoking, and alcohol on oesophageal acid clearing. Scand J Gastroenterol 1978; 13(3):283–8.

39. Johnson LF, DeMeester TR. Evaluation of elevation of the head of the bed, bethanechol, and antacid form tablets on gastroesophageal reflux. Dig Dis Sci 1981; 26(8):673–80.

40. Lichter I, Muir RC. The pattern of swallowing during sleep. Electroenceph Clin Neurophysiol 1975; 38(4):427–32.

41. Orr WC, Robinson MG, Johnson LF. Acid clearance during sleep in the pathogenesis of reflux esophagitis. Dig Dis Sci 1981; 26(5):423–7.

42. Kruse-Anderson S, Wallin L, Madsen T. Acid gastro-oesophageal reflux and oesophageal pressure activity during postprandial and nocturnal periods. A study in subjects with and without pathologic acid gastro-oesophageal reflux. Scand J Gastroenterol 1987; 22(8):926–30.

43. Atkinson M, Summerling M. The competence of the cardia after cardiomyotomy. Gastroenterologia 1954; 92:123–34.

44. Clark MD, Rinaldo JA Jr., Eyler WR. Correlation of manometric and radiologic data from the esophagogastric area. Radiology 1970; 94(2):261–70.

45. Kaye M, Showater J. Manometric configuration of the lower oesophageal sphincter in normal human subjects. Gastroenterology 1971; 61:213–23.

46. Winans CS. Alteration of lower oesophageal sphincter characteristics with respiration and proximal oesophageal balloon distention. Gastroenterology 1972; 62(3):380–8.

47. Welch RW, Gray JE. Influence of respiration on recordings of lower oesophageal sphincter pressure in humans. Gastroenterology 1982; 83(3):590–4.

48. Mittal RK, Rochester DF, McCallum RW. Effect of the diaphragmatic contraction on lower oesoph-ageal sphincter pressure in man. Gut 1987; 28(12):1564–8.

49. Bombeck CT, Dillard DH, Nyhus LM. Muscular anatomy of the gastroesophageal junction and role of phrenoesophageal ligament; autopsy study of sphincter mechanism. Ann Surg 1966; 164(4):643–54.

50. De Caestecker J, Heading R. The pathophysiology of reflux. In: Hennessy TPJ, Cuschieri A, Bennett JR (eds) Reflux oesophagitis. London: Butterworth, 1989: pp. 1–36.

51. Joelsson BE, DeMeester TR, Skinner DB et al. The role of the oesophageal body in the antireflux mechanism. Surgery 1982; 92(2):417–24.

52. Bemelman W, Van Der Hulst V, Dijkhuis T et al. The lower oesophageal sphincter shown by a computerized representation. Scand J Gastroenterol 1990; 25:601–8.

53. Goodall RJ, Hay DJ, Temple JG. Assessment of the rapid pullthrough technique in oesophageal manometry. Gut 1980; 21(2):169–73.

54. Baldi F, Ferrarini F, Labate A et al. Prevalence of esophagitis in patients undergoing routine upper endoscopy: a multicenter survey in Italy. In: DeMeester TR, Skinner DB (eds) Esophageal disorders: pathophysiology and therapy. New York: Raven Press, 1985: pp. 213–19.

55. Dent J, Dodds WJ, Friedman RH et al. Mechanism of gastroesophageal reflux in recumbent asymptomatic human subjects. J Clin Invest 1980; 65(2):256–67.

56. Dent J, Dodds WJ, Sekiguchi T et al. Interdigestive phasic contractions of the human lower oesophageal sphincter. Gastroenterology 1983; 84(3):453–60.

57. Rattan S, Goyal RK. Neural control of the lower oesophageal sphincter: influence of the vagus nerves. J Clin Invest 1974; 54(4):899–906.

58. Gonella J, Niel JP, Roman C. Vagal control of lower oesophageal sphincter motility in the cat. J Physiol 1977; 273(3):647–64.

59. Dent J. A new technique for continuous sphincter pressure measurement. Gastroenterology 1976; 71(2):263–7.

60. Mittal RK, McCallum RW. Characteristics of transient lower oesophageal sphincter relaxation in humans. Am J Physiol 1987; 252 (5, Pt 1):G636–41.

61. Freidin N, Mittal RK, McCallum RW. Does body posture affect the incidence and mechanism of gastro-oesophageal reflux? Gut 1991; 32(2):133–6.

62. Wyman JB, Dent J, Heddle R et al. Control of belching by the lower oesophageal sphincter. Gut 1990; 31(6):639–46.

63. Dodds WJ, Dent J, Hogan WJ et al. Mechanisms of gastroesophageal reflux in patients with reflux esophagitis. N Engl J Med 1982; 307(25):1547–52.

64. Dent J, Holloway RH, Toouli J et al. Mechanisms of lower oesophageal sphincter incompetence in

patients with symptomatic gastrooesophageal reflux. Gut 1988; 29(8):1020–8.

65. Barham CP, Gotley DC, Mills A et al. Precipitating causes of acid reflux episodes in ambulant patients with gastro-oesophageal reflux disease. Gut 1995; 36(4):505–10.

66. Barham CP, Gotley DC, Miller R et al. Pressure events surrounding oesophageal acid reflux episodes and acid clearance in ambulant healthy volunteers. Gut 1993; 34(4):444–9.

67. Penagini R, Carmagnola S, Cantu P et al. Mechanoreceptors of the proximal stomach: role in triggering transient lower oesophageal sphincter relaxation. Gastroenterology 2004; 126(1):49–56.

68. Cameron AJ, Lagergren J, Henriksson C et al. Gastroesophageal reflux disease in monozygotic and dizygotic twins. Gastroenterology 2002; 122(1):55–9.

69. Bredenoord AJ, Weusten BL, Timmer R et al. Gastro-oesophageal reflux of liquids and gas during transient lower oesophageal sphincter relaxations. Neurogastroenterol Motil 2006; 18(10):888–93.

70. Allison PR. Reflux esophagitis, sliding hiatal hernia, and the anatomy of repair. Surg Gynecol Obstet 1951; 92(4):419–31.

71. Cohen S, Harris LD. Does hiatus hernia affect competence of the gastroesophageal sphincter. N Engl J Med 1971; 284(19):1053–6.

72. Ott DJ, Wu WC, Gelfand DW. Reflux esophagitis revisited: prospective analysis of radiologic accuracy. Gastrointest Radiol 1981; 6(1):1–7.

73. Helm JF, Dodds WJ, Riedel DR et al. Determinants of oesophageal acid clearance in normal subjects. Gastroenterology 1983; 85(3):607–12.

74. Helm JF, Dodds WJ, Pelc LR et al. Effect of oesophageal emptying and saliva on clearance of acid from the oesophagus. N Engl J Med 1984; 310(5):284–8.

75. Kapila YV, Dodds WJ, Helm JF et al. Relationship between swallow rate and salivary flow. Dig Dis Sci 1984; 29(6):528–33.

76. Helm JF, Dodds WJ, Hogan WJ et al. Acid neutralizing capacity of human saliva. Gastroenterology 1982; 83(1, Pt 1):69–74.

77. Meyers RL, Orlando RC. In vivo bicarbonate secretion by human oesophagus. Gastroenterology 1992; 103(4):1174–8.

78. Dubois A. Pathophysiology of gastroesophageal reflux disease: role of gastric factors. In: Castell DO (ed.) The esophagus. Boston, MA: Little, Brown, 1992; pp. 479–92.

79. Miller LS, Vinayek R, Frucht H et al. Reflux esophagitis in patients with Zollinger–Ellison syndrome. Gastroenterology 1990; 98(2):341–6.

80. Barlow AP, DeMeester TR, Ball CS et al. The significance of the gastric secretory state in gastroesophageal reflux disease. Arch Surg 1989; 124(8):937–40.

81. Nehra D, Howell P, Williams CP et al. Toxic bile acids in gastro-oesophageal reflux disease: influence of gastric acidity. Gut 1999; 44(5):598–602.

82. Marshall RE, Anggiansah A, Owen WA et al. The temporal relationship between oesophageal bile reflux and pH in gastro-oesophageal reflux disease. Eur J Gastroenterol Hepatol 1998; 10(5):385–92.

83. Gotley DC, Appleton GV, Cooper MJ. Bile acids and trypsin are unimportant in alkaline oesophageal reflux. J Clin Gastroenterol 1992; 14(1):2–7.

84. Barham CP, Jones RL, Biddlestone LR et al. Photothermal laser ablation of Barrett's oesophagus: endoscopic and histological evidence of squamous re-epithelialisation. Gut 1997; 41(3):281–4.

84A. Bodger K, Trudgill N. Guidelines for oesophageal manometry and pH monitoring. BSG Guidelines in Gastroenterology 2006; 1–11.

85. Bredenoord AJ, Weusten BL, Smout AJ. Symptom association analysis in ambulatory gastro-oesophageal reflux monitoring. Gut 2005; 54(12):1810–17.

86. Watson RG, Tham TC, Johnston BT et al. Double blind cross-over placebo controlled study of omeprazole in the treatment of patients with reflux symptoms and physiological levels of acid reflux – the "sensitive oesophagus". Gut 1997; 40(5):587–90.

87. Breumelhof R, Smout AJ. The symptom sensitivity index: a valuable additional parameter in 24-hour oesophageal pH recording. Am J Gastroenterol 1991; 86(2):160–4.

88. Weusten BL, Roelofs JM, Akkermans LM et al. The symptom-association probability: an improved method for symptom analysis of 24-hour oesophageal pH data. Gastroenterology 1994; 107(6):1741–5.

89. Diaz S, Aymerich R, Clouse R et al. The symptom association probability (SAP) is superior to the symptom index (SI) for attributing symptoms to gastroesophageal reflux: validation using outcome from laparoscopic antireflux surgery (LARS). Gastroenterology 2002; 122:A75.

90. Anggiansah A, Marshal R. Use of the oesophageal laboratory, 1st edn. Oxford: Isis Medical Media, 2000.

91. Wong WM, Bautista J, Dekel R et al. Feasibility and tolerability of transnasal/per-oral placement of the wireless pH capsule vs. traditional 24-h oesophageal pH monitoring – a randomized trial. Aliment Pharmacol Ther 2005; 21(2):155–63.

92. Wiener GJ, Morgan TM, Copper JB et al. Ambulatory 24-hour oesophageal pH monitoring. Reproducibility and variability of pH parameters. Dig Dis Sci 1988; 33(9):1127–33.

93. Pandolfino JE, Richter JE, Ours T et al. Ambulatory oesophageal pH monitoring using a wireless system. Am J Gastroenterol 2003; 98(4):740–9.

94. Scarpulla G, Camilleri S, Galante P et al. The impact of prolonged pH measurements on the diag-

nosis of gastroesophageal reflux disease: 4-day wireless pH studies. Am J Gastroenterol 2007; 102(12):2642–7.

95. Ward EM, Devault KR, Bouras EP et al. Successful oesophageal pH monitoring with a catheter-free system. Aliment Pharmacol Ther 2004; 19(4):449–54.

96. Catheterless Oesophageal pH Monitoring. NICE, July 2006.

97. Fox MR, Bredenoord AJ. Oesophageal high-resolution manometry: moving from research into clinical practice. Gut 2008; 57(3):405–23.

98. Fox M, Hebbard G, Janiak P et al. High-resolution manometry predicts the success of oesophageal bolus transport and identifies clinically important abnormalities not detected by conventional manometry. Neurogastroenterol Motil 2004; 16(5):533–42.

99. Clouse R, Staiano A. Topography of the oesophageal peristaltic pressure wave. Am J Physiol Gastrointest Liver Physiol 1991; 261:G677–84.

100. Clouse RE, Staiano A. Topography of normal and high-amplitude oesophageal peristalsis. Am J Physiol 1993; 265(6, Pt 1):G1098–107.

101. Andrews JM, Nathan H, Malbert CH et al. Validation of a novel luminal flow velocimeter with video fluoroscopy and manometry in the human oesophagus. Am J Physiol 1999; 276 (4, Pt 1):G886–94.

102. Pandolfino JE, Shi G, Zhang Q et al. Measuring EGJ opening patterns using high resolution intraluminal impedance. Neurogastroenterol Motil 2005; 17(2):200–6.

103. Ghosh SK, Pandolfino JE, Zhang Q et al. Quantifying oesophageal peristalsis with high-resolution manometry: a study of 75 asymptomatic volunteers. Am J Physiol Gastrointest Liver Physiol 2006; 290(5):G988–97.

104. Pandolfino JE, El-Serag HB, Zhang Q et al. Obesity: a challenge to esophagogastric junction integrity. Gastroenterology 2006; 130(3):639–49.

105. Fox M. Multiple rapid swallowing in idiopathic achalasia: from conventional to high resolution manometry. Neurogastroenterol Motil 2007; 19(9):780–1; author reply 782.

106. Fox M, Young A, Anggiansah R et al. A 22 year old man with persistent regurgitation and vomiting: case outcome. BMJ 2006; 333(7559):133; discussion 134–7.

107. Marshall RE, Anggiansah A, Owen WA et al. The relationship between acid and bile reflux and symptoms in gastro-oesophageal reflux disease. Gut 1997; 40(2):182–7.

108. Koek GH, Tack J, Sifrim D et al. The role of acid and duodenal gastroesophageal reflux in symptomatic GERD. Am J Gastroenterol 2001; 96(7):2033–40.

109. Vaezi MF, Lacamera RG, Richter JE. Validation studies of Bilitec 2000: an ambulatory duodenogastric reflux monitoring system. Am J Physiol 1994; 267(6, Pt 1):G1050–7.

110. Silny J. Intraluminal multiple electric impedance procedure for measurement of gastrointestinal motility. J Gastrointest Motil 1991; 3:151–62.

111. Bernhard A, Pohl D, Fried M et al. Influence of bolus consistency and position on esophageal high-resolution manometry findings. Dig Dis Sci 2008; 53(5):1198–205.

112. Mainie I, Tutuian R, Agrawal A et al. Combined multichannel intraluminal impedance-pH monitoring to select patients with persistent gastro-oesophageal reflux for laparoscopic Nissen fundoplication. Br J Surg 2006; 93(12):1483–7.

113. Bredenoord AJ. Impedance–pH monitoring: new standard for measuring gastro-oesophageal reflux. Neurogastroenterol Motil 2008; 20(5):434–9.

114. Sifrim D, Castell D, Dent J et al. Gastro-oesophageal reflux monitoring: review and consensus report on detection and definitions of acid, non-acid, and gas reflux. Gut 2004; 53(7):1024–31.

115. Shay S, Richter J. Direct comparison of impedance, manometry, and pH probe in detecting reflux before and after a meal. Dig Dis Sci 2005; 50(9):1584–90.

116. Bredenoord AJ, Weusten BL, Curvers WL et al. Determinants of perception of heartburn and regurgitation. Gut 2006; 55(3):313–18.

13

Treatment of gastro-oesophageal reflux disease

David I. Watson

Introduction

Gastro-oesophageal reflux is a common problem, affecting between 10% and 40% of the population of most Western countries.[1,2] Whether its incidence is increasing is unclear. What is certainly increasing is the treatment of the condition and this has led to a dramatic rise in the overall cost of medical therapy in many countries over the last two decades. In addition there is also good evidence that the incidence of distal oesophageal adenocarcinoma is increasing,[3] and this provides circumstantial evidence that complications of gastro-oesophageal reflux (e.g. the development of Barrett's oesophagus) are increasing also.

Gastro-oesophageal reflux disease is caused by excessive reflux of gastric contents, which contain acid and sometimes bile and pancreatic secretions, into the oesophageal lumen. Pathological reflux leads to symptoms such as heartburn, upper abdominal pain and the regurgitation of gastric contents into the oropharynx. Gastro-oesophageal reflux is associated with a range of contributing factors, and a multifactorial aetiology is likely. First is hiatus herniation, which is found in approximately half of the patients who undergo surgical treatment.[4,5] This results in widening of the angle of His, effacement of the lower oesophageal sphincter and loss of the assistance of positive intra-abdominal pressure acting on the lower oesophagus. Second is the reduced lower oesophageal sphincter pressure, which is often found, although in many patients with reflux the resting lower oesophageal sphincter pressure is normal. Reflux in these patients results from an excessive number of transient lower oesophageal sphincter relaxation events.[6] Other factors that might contribute to the genesis of reflux include abnormal oesophageal peristalsis (which causes poor clearance of refluxed fluid) and delayed gastric emptying.

The treatment of reflux is usually incremental, commencing with various levels of medical measures, surgery being reserved for patients with more severe disease, who either fail to respond adequately to medical treatment or who do not wish to take lifelong medication. Non-operative therapy treats the effects of reflux, as the underlying reflux problem is not corrected, and therapy for most patients must be continued indefinitely.[7] Surgical procedures, however, aim to be curative, preventing reflux by reconstructing an antireflux valve at the gastro-oesophageal junction.[6,8] In the past, surgery has tended to be reserved for patients with complicated reflux disease or those with very severe symptoms. However, since the introduction of laparoscopic surgical approaches some surgeons advocate utilising surgery at earlier stages in the course of reflux disease. In the future, if effective endoscopic (transoral) antireflux procedures can be developed, then early curative therapy may have a greater role.

Medical treatment

Simple measures

A variety of simple measures can be helpful for the management of patients who experience mild symptoms. These include simple antacids, the avoidance of precipitating factors such as spicy foods, and the avoidance of alcohol. Additional measures include weight loss (when appropriate), avoiding cigarette smoking, modification of the timing and quantity of meals (e.g. avoiding going to bed with a full stomach), and raising the bed head. Unfortunately, these measures are rarely effective for patients with moderate to severe disease, and most patients who present for surgery cannot be adequately treated with these measures.

H$_2$-receptor antagonists

The first effective non-operative treatment for reflux was the development of medications that reduced the production of acid by the stomach. The histamine type 2 (H$_2$)-receptor antagonists sometimes relieve mild to moderate reflux symptoms. When first used in the 1970s they revolutionised the medical approach to duodenal ulcer disease. However, they were much less effective for reflux disease and few patients achieve complete relief of reflux symptoms with these medications.[9] Even so, in milder forms of the disease they can reduce symptoms. When medications are ceased, however, symptoms usually return and treatment has to be recommenced. With the current widespread availability of proton-pump inhibitors, H$_2$-receptor antagonists are now only occasionally used as first-line medical therapy.

Proton-pump inhibitors

Proton-pump inhibitors (omeprazole, lanzoprazole and pantoprazole) were introduced into clinical practice in the late 1980s,[7] along with rabeprazole and esomeprazole more recently. Proton-pump inhibitors are much more effective for the relief of symptoms and achieve better healing of oesophagitis than H$_2$-receptor antagonists. However, patients with worse oesophagitis such as Savary Miller grade 2 or 3 have a higher failure rate with these medications,[10] and in addition many patients who initially achieve good symptom control go on to develop 'breakthrough' symptoms at a later date, usually requiring an increased dose of medication to maintain symptom control. It is presumed that failure is due to inadequate acid suppression, although in some cases the presence of bile or duodenal fluid in the refluxate may play a role. In patients who respond well to proton-pump inhibitors, symptoms usually recur rapidly (sometimes in less than 24 hours) following cessation of medication, and for this reason lifelong medical treatment is likely to be required, unless surgery is performed.[7] The long-term use of proton-pump inhibitors has not been shown to cause any adverse outcome to date. One study has shown, however, that long-term use can be associated with the development of atrophic gastritis with intestinal metaplasia in patients with concurrent *Helicobacter pylori* infection.[11] Long-term use can also be associated with parietal cell hyperplasia.[12] This latter phenomenon may be the reason why symptoms recur rapidly in some patients on cessation of therapy, and may be another reason why some patients require escalating dosages of proton-pump inhibitors to control their symptoms.

Prokinetic agents

Cisapride is the only prokinetic agent that has been shown to be better than placebo for the treatment of reflux.[13] It acts by accelerating oesophageal and gastric emptying, thereby improving acid clearance from the distal oesophagus, and emptying gastric contents more quickly. Its therapeutic benefit is similar to that of the H$_2$-receptor antagonists. Hence, its clinical role has been limited since proton-pump inhibitors became widely available, and more recently an incidence of cardiac arrhythmias led to its withdrawal in many parts of the world.

Surgical treatment

The principle underlying the surgical management of gastro-oesophageal reflux disease is the creation of a mechanical antireflux barrier between the oesophagus and stomach. This works independently of the composition of the refluxate. Whilst medical therapy is effective in relieving symptoms for many patients with acid reflux, only surgery achieves effective control of duodeno-gastro-oesophageal reflux.

Selection criteria for surgery

As a general rule, all patients who undergo anti-reflux surgery should have objective evidence of reflux. This may be the demonstration of erosive oesophagitis on endoscopy or an abnormal amount of acid reflux demonstrated by 24-hour pH monitoring. Neither of these tests are sufficiently reliable to base all preoperative decisions on their outcome,[14] as a number of patients with troublesome reflux will have either a normal 24-hour pH study or no evidence of oesophagitis at endoscopy (and, very occasionally, both). For this reason the tests have to be interpreted in the light of the patient's clinical presentation, and a final recommendation for surgery must be based on all available clinical and objective information.[14]

Patients selected for surgery fall into two general groups: (1) patients who have failed to respond (or have responded only partially) to medical therapy; (2) patients whose symptoms are fully controlled by medications, but who do not wish to continue with medication throughout their lives. The latter group are more likely to be younger patients who face decades of acid suppression to alleviate their symptoms. In the first group, the response to surgery is usually more certain if the patient has had a good response to acid suppression in the past, or at least has had some symptom relief from medication. In patients who have had no response to proton-pump inhibitors, their symptoms are often due to something other than reflux, despite concurrent objective evidence of reflux (which can be asymptomatic). Such patients will not benefit from antireflux surgery.

Failure of medical treatment can be defined as continuing symptoms of reflux while on an adequate dose of acid suppression. In most countries this means at least a standard dose of a proton-pump inhibitor for a minimum period of 3 months. Proton-pump inhibitors are more effective for the control of the symptom of heartburn than volume regurgitation, and it is the latter symptom that is often the dominant problem in patients who have failed on medical therapy.

A further classification of patients who undergo surgery for gastro-oesophageal reflux disease can be made into two groups: (1) patients who have complicated reflux disease; and (2) patients who have straightforward disease without complications.

Patients with complicated reflux disease

Reflux with stricture formation

The treatment of peptic oesophageal strictures has been greatly altered since proton-pump inhibitors became available, and this is one area where the role of surgery seems to have lessened.[15] In the past, surgery was the only effective treatment for strictures, and when the stricture was densely fibrotic this even meant resection of the oesophagus. Fortunately, it is now unusual to see patients with such advanced strictures. Strictures in young and fit patients are usually best treated by antireflux surgery and dilatation. However, many patients who develop strictures are elderly or infirm and the use of proton-pump inhibitors with dilatation is usually effective in this group.

Reflux with respiratory complications

When gastro-oesophageal regurgitation spills over into the respiratory tree, this can cause chronic respiratory illness, such as recurrent pneumonia, asthma or bronchiectasis. This is a firm indication for antireflux surgery, as the predominant action of proton-pump inhibitors is to block acid secretion and the volume of reflux is not greatly altered. Such problems as halitosis, chronic cough, chronic laryngitis, chronic pharyngitis, chronic sinusitis and loss of enamel on teeth are sometimes attributed to gastro-oesophageal reflux. Whilst there is little doubt that on occasions such problems do arise in refluxing patients, these problems in isolation are not reliable indications for surgery. As acid is usually the damaging agent, antireflux surgery is probably not advisable unless proton-pump inhibition unequivocally reverses the problem.

Columnar-lined (Barrett's) oesophagus

At present it remains an open question whether Barrett's oesophagus alone is an indication for antireflux surgery. There is little argument that patients with Barrett's oesophagus who have reflux symptoms should be selected for surgery on the basis of their symptoms and their response to medications. It should not simply be because they have a columnar-lined oesophagus.[16] There is some experimental evidence to suggest that continuing reflux may be deleterious in regard to malignant change in oesophageal mucosa,[17] and one prospective randomised trial has suggested that antireflux surgery gives superior results to drug therapy in this patient group.[17] However, proton-pump inhibitors were only introduced into the medical arm of that trial in its later years.

There is emerging evidence that abolition of symptoms with proton-pump inhibition does not equate to 'normalising' the pH profile in a patient's oesophagus.[18] Since antireflux surgery does usually abolish acid reflux, this may become a further reason to recommend surgery in patients with Barrett's oesophagus. There is limited evidence to support the contention that either surgical or medical treatment of reflux in patients with Barrett's oesophagus consistently leads to regression of the columnar lining.[19] A report from Gurski et al.[20] suggests that although fundoplication is not followed by a reduction in the length of Barrett's oesophagus, it can be followed by 'histological' regression. In 68% of patients in this study with low-grade dysplasia, there was regression to non-dysplastic Barrett's mucosa. Further studies have also shown that a combination of medical or surgical therapy with argon-beam plasma coagulation or photodynamic therapy ablation of the columnar lining achieves complete or near complete reversion to squamous mucosa.[21,22]

 Longer-term follow-up from a randomised trial of ablation vs. surveillance in patients with Barrett's oesophagus who had a undergone a fundoplication showed a reduction in the length of Barrett's oesophagus in both study groups, although to a greater extent following ablative therapy.[23]

Unfortunately, ablation therapies have not yet been proven to reduce the risk of subsequent progression to cancer.

Patients with uncomplicated reflux disease

Medical therapy, in the form of proton-pump inhibitors, is so effective today that only a minority of patients do not get substantial or complete relief of their symptoms using these agents. Despite this, patients continue to present for antireflux surgery in large numbers for reasons already discussed. An additional factor that has emerged is the rising incidence of adenocarcinoma of the cardia associated with gastro-oesophageal reflux disease.[3] Whether antireflux surgery is more effective than long-term proton-pump inhibition at preventing the development of columnar-lined oesophagus and subsequently carcinoma of the lower oesophagus is controversial. If duodenal fluid has a role in the pathogenesis of adenocarcinoma of the oesophagus, then antireflux surgery would be preferable to acid suppression alone in patients with Barrett's oesophagus, and of course it may also prevent the development of Barrett's oesophagus in the first place. However, this hypothesis has yet to be adequately tested and at present there is insufficient evidence to support a position that antireflux surgery should be performed to prevent subsequent malignant transformation.

Medical versus surgical therapy

The issue of the most appropriate treatment for gastro-oesophageal reflux disease has been the subject of disagreement between surgeons and gastro-enterologists. Whilst most would agree that a single management strategy is unlikely to be appropriate for all patients, there is a need for better comparative data for medical vs. surgical therapy. Seven randomised trials[17,24–31] have been reported that have investigated this issue, although five of these were completed or commenced before the availability of both laparoscopic antireflux surgery or proton-pump inhibitor medication.

In 1992 Spechler[25] reported a study in which 247 patients (predominantly men) were randomised to either continuous medical therapy with an H_2 blocker, medical therapy for symptoms only or an open Nissen fundoplication. Overall patient satisfaction was highest following surgery at 1 and 2 years follow-up. However, neither the surgical approach nor the medical treatment investigated in this study would now be regarded as optimal. The longer-term outcomes from this study were published in 2001, with median follow-up of approximately 7 years and with proton-pump inhibitors now used for the medically treated patients.[32] Unfortunately, follow-up was not complete and only 37 surgical patients were available for late follow-up, with 23% of the original surgical group unable to be found or unwilling to participate in follow-up, and 32% died during follow-up. The later results did, however, show reasonable outcomes in both the medically and surgically treated groups. However, 62% of the surgical patients consumed antireflux medications at late follow-up, although when these medications were ceased in both the study groups the surgical group

had significantly less reflux symptoms than the medical group, suggesting that most of the surgical patients did not actually need the medications!

In 1996 Ortiz et al.[17] reported a randomised study of 59 patients with Barrett's oesophagus. Twenty-seven patients had the best medical treatment available and 32 underwent a short Nissen fundoplication. Satisfactory symptomatic control was achieved in 24 and 29 patients respectively. However, there was significantly better improvement in the follow-up endoscopy findings in the surgical group. Since proton-pump inhibitors were only used in the last few years of the study, this trial becomes of historical relevance. Parrilla et al.[26] performed a similar trial that randomised 101 patients with Barrett's oesophagus. Medical therapy was initially an H_2 blocker and later a proton-pump inhibitor. A satisfactory clinical outcome was achieved at 5 years follow-up in 91% of each group, although medical treatment was associated with a poorer endoscopic outcome. Progression to dysplasia was similar in both groups.

In 2000 Lundell et al.[27,28] reported a trial of proton-pump inhibitor medication vs. open antireflux surgery. This study only enrolled patients who had complete symptom control with a proton-pump inhibitor at the commencement of the trial, and all patients with uncontrolled symptoms were excluded. Hence, the surgical group excluded the patients who represent the majority of those currently selected for surgery, i.e. patients with a poor response to a proton-pump inhibitor. Three hundred and ten patients were randomised, and antireflux surgery achieved a better outcome at up to 3 years follow-up. A later report of 7 years follow-up in 228 patients confirmed that surgery still achieved better reflux control than medication, although dysphagia and various wind-related side-effects were more common after fundoplication.[33]

Rhodes et al. reported the first randomised trial to compare proton-pump inhibitor medication with laparoscopic Nissen fundoplication; 217 patients were enrolled. Surgery was followed by less oesophageal acid exposure 3 months after treatment, and better symptom control at 12 months.[29,30,34] A similar study from Anvari et al. enrolled 104 patients into a trial of proton-pump inhibitor therapy vs. laparoscopic Nissen fundoplication.[31] Eighty-three patients were followed to 12 months and control of reflux was better in the patients who underwent surgery.

It could be contended from the results all of these trials that the majority of patients who have gastro-oesophageal reflux sufficient to require treatment with a proton-pump inhibitor should at least be offered the opportunity to undergo surgical correction of their reflux irrespective of whether their symptoms are well controlled by medication or not. Certainly, the clinical trials all support an ongoing and important role for surgery in the treatment of reflux, and potentially a wider role in the future management of reflux.

Pros and cons of antireflux surgery

Advantages
The advantages of surgery are clear. The operation is the only treatment that actually cures the problem, i.e. stopping gastric contents from refluxing into the oesophagus. Hence patients treated by surgery can usually eat whatever foods they choose, they can lie down flat and bend over without reflux occurring, and importantly they do not need to take any tablets.

Disadvantages
The first disadvantage is the morbidity associated with the operation (see discussion of complications). Whilst laparoscopic surgery has meant that the pain of the open operation has been greatly reduced, most patients have some difficulty in swallowing in the immediate postoperative period, although in the great majority this is only temporary.[35] The time taken to get better is quite variable, and often several months are required.[5] Furthermore, the great majority of patients feel full quickly after eating even small meals, and this often leads to some postoperative weight loss.[5] In the patients who are overweight at the time of surgery (the majority!) this is sometimes seen as an advantage. This restriction on meal size also usually disappears over a few months.

Because fundoplication produces a one-way valve, swallowed air that has passed into the stomach usually cannot pass back through the valve. Thus, patients have to be forewarned that they will not be able to belch effectively after the operation and so should be cautious about drinking gassy drinks.[36] This applies particularly to patients who undergo a Nissen (total) fundoplication. For similar reasons, patients will usually be unable to vomit after the procedure, and should be informed of this. As swallowed gas cannot be belched effectively, the great majority of patients are aware of increased passage of wind after the procedure.[37] Although patients who undergo a partial fundoplication (particularly anterior) have a lower incidence of these problems,[4] difficulties can still occur. Despite these possible disadvantages, the overwhelming majority of patients claim that the disadvantages are far outweighed by the advantages of the operation.[4,35,38] To date it has not been possible to predict preoperatively those patients who will develop problems following surgery.

Preoperative investigations

Apart from the assessment of each patient's general suitability for surgery by determining comorbidities, some specific investigations should be performed before undertaking antireflux surgery.

Endoscopy
Endoscopy is essential. It enables oesophagitis to be documented (confirming reflux disease), strictures to be dilated, and other gastro-oesophageal pathology to be excluded, documented and treated. The position of the squamocolumnar junction and the presence and size of any hiatus hernia is also assessed. The presence of a large hiatus hernia is not a contraindication to a laparoscopic approach, although the surgery is technically more difficult.[39,40]

Manometry

 Manometry is used to exclude primary motility disorders such as achalasia. It is also able to document the adequacy of oesophageal peristalsis.[14] The presence of weak peristaltic amplitudes or poor propagation of peristalsis is not a contraindication to antireflux surgery. Although many surgeons recommend a tailored approach to patient selection by choosing a partial fundoplication in patients with poor peristalsis,[41,42] there is no strong evidence to support this.[43,44] Evidence from four randomised trials[45–48] has shown good results following the Nissen procedure in patients with poor peristalsis, suggesting that tailoring with a posterior partial fundoplication is not necessary. Nevertheless, common sense suggests that a partial fundoplication procedure is probably safer in patients with a true adynamic oesophagus and especially in patients with systemic scleroderma, in whom we would use an anterior partial fundoplication.[49]

Oesophageal pH monitoring
While many surgeons advocate the routine assessment of patients with 24-hour ambulatory pH monitoring before antireflux surgery, we use a selective approach. This test is not sufficiently accurate to be regarded as the 'gold standard' for the investigation of reflux, and if an abnormal pH profile is used to select patients for surgery, up to 20% of patients who have oesophagitis and typical reflux symptoms will be excluded unnecessarily from antireflux surgery. Hence, we apply this investigation in patients with endoscopy-negative reflux disease and in patients with atypical symptoms.[14] The test's ability to clarify whether symptoms are associated with reflux events is useful for the assessment of these patients.

Other investigations

The role of bile reflux monitoring remains undefined in gastro-oesophageal reflux disease, although in the future the measurement of bile reflux may be helpful in patients who fail to respond to acid suppression. Currently, this is measured using either 'Bilitec' or intraluminal impedance monitoring. 'Bilitec' measures intraoesophageal bilirubin as an indirect marker of duodeno-oesophageal reflux, whereas intraluminal impedance monitoring measures 'volume' reflux.

Operations available

To the non-surgeon, it might seem that there is a bewildering array of operations available for the treatment of reflux. In fact, the fundoplication introduced by Rudolf Nissen in 1956, or some variant of it, is overwhelmingly the most popular antireflux operation in the world today. Total fundoplications, such as the Nissen, or partial fundoplications, whether anterior or posterior, probably all work in a similar fashion,[8,50] and that fashion may be as much mechanical as physiological, as it has been demonstrated that these procedures are effective not only when placed in the chest in vivo,[51] but also on the benchtop, i.e. ex vivo.[8] The principles of fundoplication are to mobilise the lower oesophagus and to wrap the fundus of the stomach, either partially or totally, around the oesophagus. When the oesophageal hiatus is enlarged, it is narrowed by sutures to prevent paraoesophageal herniation postoperatively and also to prevent the wrap being pulled up into the chest (although the fundoplication will work in the chest, other complications such as gastric ulceration and gastric obstruction sometimes occur in this situation). Complications of reflux such as fibrotic stricturing with shortened oesophagus are seen rarely compared to the past. In the circumstance of true oesophageal shortening, an oesophageal lengthening (Collis) procedure can be undertaken to provide a long enough oesophagus to reach the abdomen. The upper lesser curvature of the stomach is used to produce the new oesophagus and the stomach is then wrapped around this. However, in our experience the Collis procedure is now not indicated or required.

Mechanisms of action of antireflux operations

The mechanisms of action of an antireflux operation are not completely clear. Some of the proposed mechanisms include:

1. The creation of a floppy valve by maintaining close apposition between the abdominal oesophagus and the gastric fundus. As intragastric pressure rises the intra-abdominal oesophagus is compressed by the adjacent fundus.
2. Exaggeration of the flap valve at the angle of His.
3. Increase in the basal pressure generated by the lower oesophageal sphincter.
4. Reduction in the triggering of transient lower oesophageal sphincter relaxations.
5. Reduction in the capacity of the gastric fundus, thereby speeding proximal and total gastric emptying.
6. Prevention of effacement of the lower oesophagus (which effectively weakens the lower sphincter).

Since the procedures seem to work, even ex vivo,[8] it seems likely that the first two mechanisms account for the efficacy of the majority of antireflux procedures. The increase in lower oesophageal sphincter pressure following surgery is not important, and in some partial fundoplication procedures there is very little increase in pressure, yet reflux is well controlled.[4,52] The trend towards increasingly looser and shorter total fundoplications or greater use of partial fundoplication procedures suggests that there is no such thing as a fundoplication that is 'too loose'.

Techniques of antireflux surgery

A range of different antireflux operations are currently performed and all have their advocates. No one procedure currently yields perfect results, i.e. 100% cure of reflux and no side-effects. Despite this, published reports can be found that support every known procedure, and it is probably better to consider results from randomised trials when assessing the merits of these procedural variants (see below) rather than relying on uncontrolled outcomes reported by advocates of a single procedure. It should also be recognised that the experience of the operating surgeon is of great importance for achieving a good postoperative outcome.[53] Variability can be reduced, but not eliminated, by detailed technical descriptions and effective surgical training. The arrival of laparoscopic antireflux surgery has also changed the way in which the vast majority of antireflux surgery is now performed. Over the last 15 years this approach has become standard for primary antireflux surgery, making surgery more acceptable to patients and their physicians.

Nissen fundoplication (**Figs 13.1** and **13.2**)

This is probably the most commonly performed antireflux operation worldwide. Nissen originally

Treatment of gastro-oesophageal reflux disease

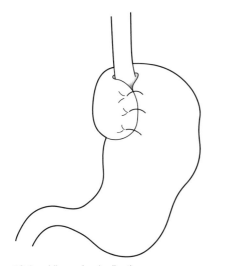

Figure 13.1 • Nissen fundoplication.

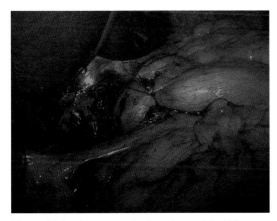

Figure 13.2 • Laparoscopic view of completed Nissen fundoplication.

outcome. Most surgeons now agree that calibration of the wrap with a large (52 Fr) intraoesophageal bougie, and shortening the fundoplication to 1–2 cm in length, achieves a better outcome.[55,56] Furthermore, whilst the need for routine hiatal repair was uncertain in the era of open surgery, most surgeons routinely include this step during laparoscopic antireflux surgery. Omission of this step is associated with a higher incidence of postoperative hiatal herniation.[57] The hepatic branch of the vagus nerve is usually preserved during this procedure.

Controversy still exists about the need to divide the short gastric vessels to achieve full fundal mobilisation. The so-called floppy Nissen procedure described by Donahue and Bombeck[58] relies on extensive fundal mobilisation. On the other hand, the modification of the Nissen fundoplication using the anterior fundal wall alone, also first described by Nissen and Rossetti,[54,59] does not require short gastric vessel division to construct the fundoplication. This simplifies the dissection, although more judgement and experience may be required to select the correct piece of stomach to use for the construction of a sufficiently loose fundoplication. Both procedures have their advocates, and good results (90% good or excellent long-term outcome) have been reported for both variants.[55,59] Nevertheless, strong opinions are held about whether the short gastric vessels should be divided or not, and this controversy has been heightened by the introduction of laparoscopic fundoplication.

Posterior partial fundoplication (**Fig. 13.3**)

A variety of fundoplication operations have been described in which the fundus is wrapped partially round the back of the oesophagus, with the aim of

described a procedure that entailed mobilisation of the oesophagus from the diaphragmatic hiatus, reduction of any hiatus hernia into the abdominal cavity, preservation of the vagus nerves and mobilisation of the posterior gastric fundus around behind the oesophagus, without dividing the short gastric vessels, and suturing of the posterior fundus to the anterior wall of the fundus using non-absorbable sutures, thereby achieving a complete wrap of stomach around the intra-abdominal oesophagus.[54] The original fundoplication was 5 cm in length and an oesophageal bougie was not used to calibrate the wrap.

 Because this procedure was associated with an incidence of persistent postoperative dysphagia, gas bloat syndrome and an inability to belch, the procedure has been progressively modified in an attempt to improve long-term

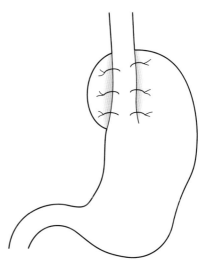

Figure 13.3 • Posterior partial fundoplication.

reduction of the possible side-effects of total fundoplication due to overcompetence of the cardia, i.e. dysphagia and gas-related problems. Toupet described a posterior partial fundoplication in which the fundus is passed behind the oesophagus and sutured to the left lateral and right lateral walls of the oesophagus, as well as to the right diaphragmatic pillar, creating a 270° posterior fundoplication.[60] A very similar procedure was described by Lind et al.[61] This entails a 300° posterior fundoplication, which is constructed by suturing the fundus to the oesophagus at the left and right lateral positions, and additionally anteriorly on the left, leaving a 60° arc of oesophageal wall uncovered. The hiatus is repaired if necessary.

Anterior partial fundoplication

Several anterior fundoplication procedures have been described, and all purport to reduce the incidence of dysphagia and other side-effects. The Belsey Mark IV procedure (popular in thoracic practice) entails a 240° anterior partial fundoplication that is usually performed through a left thoracotomy approach.[62] The distal oesophagus is mobilised, sutured to the gastric fundus and sutured to the diaphragm. Any hiatus hernia is repaired, and the anterior two-thirds of the abdominal oesophagus is covered by the fundoplication The open thoracic access required is associated with significant morbidity, and for this reason it has fallen from favour since the arrival of laparoscopic antireflux surgery. A minimally invasive thoracoscopic approach was described 10 years ago,[63] although clinical outcomes have never been reported, and this procedure is now rarely performed.

The Dor procedure is an anterior hemifundoplication that involves suturing of the fundus to the left and right sides of the oesophagus.[64] The Dor procedure is commonly used in combination with an abdominal cardiomyotomy for achalasia as it is unlikely to cause dysphagia, and it may reduce the risk of gastro-oesophageal reflux following cardiomyotomy.

A 120° anterior fundoplication has also been described.[52] This entails reduction of any hiatus hernia, posterior hiatal repair, suture of the posterior oesophagus to the hiatal pillars posteriorly, suture of the fundus to the diaphragm to accentuate the angle of His, and creation of an anterior partial fundoplication by suturing the fundus to the oesophagus on the right anterolateral aspect. Satisfactory medium-term reflux control following open surgery has been reported for this procedure, and a low incidence of gas-related problems. However, published laparoscopic experience is limited.[65]

We have reported the results from prospective randomised trials of laparoscopic 180° anterior partial fundoplication and laparoscopic 90° anterior partial fundoplication vs. a Nissen procedure[4,66-68] (see below). The anterior 180° partial fundoplication procedure entails hiatal repair, suture of the distal oesophagus to the hiatus posteriorly and construction of an anterior fundoplication that is sutured to the oesophagus and the hiatal rim on the right and anteriorly (**Figs 13.4** and **13.5**). The anterior 90° partial fundoplication procedure entails hiatal repair, posterior oesophagopexy, narrowing of the angle of His, and construction of a limited anterior fundoplication that covers the left anterolateral aspect of the oesophagus (**Fig. 13.6**). These variants of anterior fundoplication show promise.

Other antireflux procedures

Hill procedure

Hill described a procedure that is often regarded as a gastropexy rather than a fundoplication.[69] However, it also plicates the cardia and when examined endoscopically the intragastric appearances are similar to a fundoplication. The procedure entails suturing the anterior and posterior phreno-oesophageal bundles to the pre-aortic fascia and the median arcuate ligament. Whilst excellent results have been reported by Hill et al.,[69,70] it has not been applied widely because most surgeons have difficulty understanding the anatomical principles and, in particular, the so-called phreno-oesophageal bundles are not clear structures. Hill also emphasises the need for intraoperative manometry. This is not widely available, limiting the dissemination of his technique.

Collis procedure (**Fig. 13.7**)

The Collis procedure is useful for patients whose oesophagogastric junction cannot be reduced below the diaphragm.[71] However, this situation is

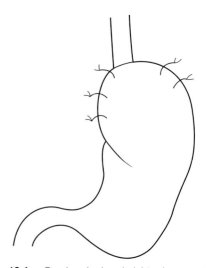

Figure 13.4 • One-hundred-and-eighty-degree anterior partial fundoplication performed by the transabdominal route.

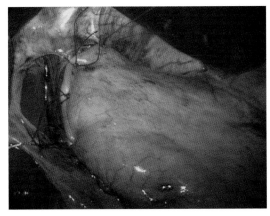

Figure 13.5 • Laparoscopic view of completed 180° anterior partial fundoplication.

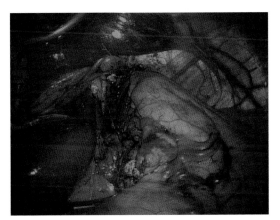

Figure 13.6 • Laparoscopic view of completed anterior partial fundoplication. This particular fundoplication was fashioned as a 90° wrap, leaving an area of exposed oesophagus on the right side.

very rare in current practice. The Collis procedure entails the construction of a tube of gastric lesser curve to recreate an abdominal length of oesophagus, around which a fundoplication can then be constructed to help with oesophageal shortening. It is often constructed by using a circular end-to-end stapler to create a transgastric window; a linear cutting stapler is used from this hole up to the angle of His to construct the neo-oesophagus. Laparoscopic and thoracoscopic techniques for this procedure have been described, although longer-term outcomes are not available.[72–74] A disadvantage of this procedure is that the gastric tube does not have peristaltic activity and furthermore it can secrete acid. This leads to a poorer overall success rate for this procedure, although some of this could be due to the end-stage nature of the reflux disease that led to the choice of this procedure in the first place.

Angelchik prosthesis

Perhaps the most interesting thing about this prosthesis is that it actually controlled reflux and induced a rethink about the pathophysiology of reflux. It may work by preventing proximal gastric distension, which in turn mitigates against transient lower oesophageal sphincter relaxation, or effacement and weakening of the lower oesophageal sphincter, or both mechanisms.[75] The procedure involved the placement of a gel-filled silastic prosthesis around the gastro-oesophageal junction but has now been consigned to surgical history, as long-term follow-up revealed an unacceptably high rate of surgical revision, particularly for troublesome dysphagia as well as migration of the prosthesis into the mediastinum and even into the lumen of the gastrointestinal tract.[76,77]

Figure 13.7 • Collis gastroplasty, with subsequent Nissen fundoplication.

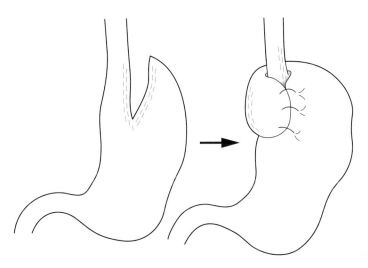

Complete or partial fundoplication?

Because fundoplication is associated with an incidence of postoperative dysphagia, gas bloat and other gas-related symptoms such as increased flatulence, the relative merits of the Nissen fundoplication procedure vs. various partial fundoplication variants have been debated for many years. The introduction of laparoscopic approaches has only served to heighten this controversy. On the one hand, the Nissen procedure produces an overcompetent gastro-oesophageal junction, which is the cause of some of the problems with dysphagia and gas bloat. On the other hand, it has been suggested that partial fundoplications reduce the risk of overcompetence, but perhaps at the expense of a less durable antireflux repair.

Several prospective randomised trials of Nissen vs. a partial fundoplication have been performed. Most studies have investigated a posterior partial fundoplication, and data are more limited for the other procedures. DeMeester et al.[78] had the distinction of reporting the first randomised study in the field of surgery for reflux disease in 1974. Their trial randomised 45 patients to undergo either a Nissen, Hill or a Belsey procedure, and they followed up their patients for 6 months following surgery. The dysphagia and recurrent reflux rates were similar for all three procedures. However, the number of patients was too small to allow a meaningful comparison to be made.

Nissen versus posterior fundoplication

Eight randomised trials have compared a Nissen with a posterior partial fundoplication. Some of the early trials were relatively small and underpowered to identify differences in outcome, and they contribute little to the pool of evidence.[46,79–81]

Lundell et al. reported the outcomes of the first large trial of Nissen vs. a posterior (Toupet) partial fundoplication; 137 patients were enrolled. The early outcomes at 6 months follow-up were similar.[82] At 5 years follow-up[83] reflux control and dysphagia rates were also similar, although flatulence was commoner after Nissen fundoplication at 2 and 3 years but not at 4 or 5 years follow-up. Re-operation was more common following Nissen fundoplication, with one patient in the posterior fundoplication group undergoing further surgery for severe gas bloat symptoms and five of the Nissen group undergoing reoperation for postoperative paraoesophageal herniation. A reanalysis of the data from this trial[45] sought to answer the question of whether a tailored approach to antireflux surgery should be applied. There were no demonstrable disadvantages for the Nissen procedure in those patients who had manometrically abnormal

peristalsis before surgery. In 2002, a median follow-up of 11.5 years was reported.[84] The procedures remained equivalent for reflux control (88% following total fundoplication and 92% after posterior partial) and late dysphagia, although the posterior fundoplication was associated with significantly less postprandial fullness and flatulence at late follow-up.

Zornig et al.[85] reported a trial that enrolled 200 patients to either total fundoplication with division of the short gastric vessels vs. posterior fundoplication. One hundred patients had normal preoperative oesophageal motility and 100 had 'abnormal' motility. At 4 months follow-up an overall good outcome was obtained in about 90% of patients in each group, and reflux control was equivalent. Short-term dysphagia was less common following posterior partial fundoplication, and no correlation was seen between preoperative oesophageal motility and outcome, providing no support for the selective application of a partial fundoplication in patients with abnormal preoperative motility. The 2-year follow-up outcomes were similar.[48] Eighty-five percent of each group was satisfied with their clinical outcome, and dysphagia remained significantly more common after Nissen fundoplication (19 vs. 8 patients).

A study from Guérin et al.[86] enrolled 140 patients. At 3 years follow-up 118 patients were evaluated and no outcome differences could be identified. Similarly, Booth et al.[47] enrolled 127 patients in a trial of Nissen vs. Toupet fundoplication. They showed no differences in reflux control 1 year after surgery, although dysphagia was more common following Nissen fundoplication. A subgroup analysis did not reveal any differences between patients with or without poor preoperative oesophageal motility.

If one combines all the data of the Nissen vs. posterior fundoplication trials together, the available evidence supports the view that side-effects are less common following a posterior partial fundoplication, particularly for wind-related problems. The hypothesis that dysphagia is less of a problem following a posterior partial fundoplication has only been substantiated by two of the larger trials.

Nissen versus anterior fundoplication

In 1999 we reported the first prospective randomised trial to compare a Nissen fundoplication with an anterior partial fundoplication technique.[4] Both procedures were performed laparoscopically. This study enrolled 107 patients to undergo either a Nissen or anterior partial fundoplication. The partial fundoplication variant entailed a 180°

fundoplication that was anchored to the right hiatal pillar and the oesophageal wall (Figs 13.4 and 13.5). Whilst no overall outcome differences between the two procedures were demonstrated at 1 and 3 months follow-up, at 6 months patients who underwent an anterior fundoplication were less likely to experience dysphagia for solid food, were less likely to be troubled by excessive passage of flatus, were more likely to be able to belch normally, and the overall outcome was better. The outcomes at 5 years confirmed the results of the initial report.[66] Reflux control was slightly better after total fundoplication, but this was offset by significantly less dysphagia, less epigastric bloating and better preservation of belching, resulting in a greater proportion of patients reporting a good or excellent overall outcome at 5 years after an anterior fundoplication (94% vs. 86%).

Baigrie et al. reported 2-year follow-up from a similar study in which 161 patients underwent either a Nissen or anterior 180° partial fundoplication.[87] This trial demonstrated equivalent control of reflux symptoms and less dysphagia following anterior 180° partial fundoplication, although the incidence of re-operation for recurrent reflux was higher after anterior fundoplication.

Two further trials have compared a laparoscopic anterior 90° partial fundoplication with a Nissen fundoplication. In the first of these, 112 patients were enrolled in a multicentre randomised trial that was conducted in seven cities in Australia and New Zealand.[67] Side-effects were significantly less common following anterior 90° partial fundoplication, although this was offset by a slightly higher incidence of recurrent reflux. Satisfaction with the overall outcome was better after anterior fundoplication. Improvements in quality of life were also more likely following anterior fundoplication.[88] Similar outcomes were reported from a parallel single-centre randomised trial that enrolled 79 patients.[68]

In another recently reported trial, Hagedorn et al.[89–91] randomised 95 patients to undergo either a laparoscopic posterior (Toupet) or anterior 120° partial fundoplication. Their results showed better reflux control following posterior partial fundoplication. Unfortunately the clinical and objective outcomes following anterior 120° fundoplication were much worse than the outcomes from other randomised and non-randomised studies. The average exposure time to acid (pH <4) was 5.6% following anterior fundoplication in this study. In other studies this figure has been reported to be between 2.5% and 2.7%,[4,67] suggesting that the procedure performed in the study of Hagedorn et al. was less effective and therefore different to the procedures performed in other studies.

Currently, the overall results from the five anterior fundoplication trials suggest that these variants do achieve satisfactory control of reflux, a reduced incidence of post-fundoplication dysphagia and other side-effects, and a good overall clinical outcome. However, the reduced incidence of troublesome side-effects might, to some extent, be offset by a higher risk of recurrent reflux. Nevertheless, excellent long-term outcomes have been reported following anterior 180° partial fundoplication, with approximately 85% of patients highly satisfied with the clinical outcome at 5–11 years follow-up.[92]

The controversy of division/no division of short gastric vessels

Until the 1990s the issue of division vs. non-division of the short gastric vessels was rarely discussed. However, following anecdotal reports of increased problems with postoperative dysphagia following laparoscopic Nissen fundoplication without division of the short gastric vessels,[93,94] this aspect of surgical technique became a much debated topic. Routine division of the short gastric vessels during fundoplication, to achieve full fundal mobilisation and thereby ensure a loose fundoplication, is thought by some to be an essential step during laparoscopic (and open) Nissen fundoplication.[55,56] This opinion was popularised by the publication of studies that compared experience with division of the short gastric vessels with historical experience with a Nissen fundoplication performed without dividing these vessels.[44,45,95] However, other uncontrolled studies of Nissen fundoplication either with or without division of the short gastric vessels confuse the issue further, as good results have been reported whether these vessels were divided or not.[43,56]

Four randomised trials have been reported that investigate this aspect of technique. Luostarinen et al.[96–98] reported the outcome of a small trial of division vs. no division of the short gastric vessels during open total fundoplication. Fifty patients were entered into this trial and a later report[98] described outcomes following a median 3-year follow-up period. Both procedures effectively corrected endoscopic oesophagitis. However, there was a trend towards a higher incidence of disruption of the fundoplication (5 vs. 2) and reflux symptoms (6 vs. 1) in patients whose short gastric vessels were divided, and furthermore 9 of 26 patients who underwent vessel division developed a postoperative sliding hiatus hernia, compared to only 1 of 24 patients whose vessels were kept intact. The likelihood of long-term dysphagia or gas-related symptoms was not influenced by mobilising the gastric fundus in this trial.

In 1997 we reported a randomised trial that enrolled 102 patients undergoing a laparoscopic Nissen fundoplication to have a procedure either with or without division of the short gastric blood vessels.[5] No difference in overall outcome was demonstrated at short-term follow-up of 6 months and the trial failed to show that dividing the short gastric vessels during laparoscopic Nissen fundoplication reduced the incidence or severity of early postoperative dysphagia. Nor was there any significant difference in lower oesophageal sphincter pressure, oesophageal emptying time or barium meal X-ray appearances. At 5 years follow-up,[99] both procedures were equally durable in terms of reflux control and the incidence of postoperative dysphagia. However, at 5 years division of the short gastric vessels was associated with a significant increase in the incidence of flatulence and upper abdominal bloating, and greater difficulties with belching. A more recent report of 10 years follow-up from this trial showed no significant outcome differences, and the overall clinical success rate at 10 years was 85–90%.[100]

Blomqvist et al.[101] reported the outcome of a similar trial that enrolled 99 patients. At 12 months follow-up, this study also showed that dividing the short gastric vessels did not result in any improvement in short-term outcome. In a study of 56 patients from Chrysos et al.,[102] reflux control and postoperative dysphagia in the first postoperative year were not influenced by division of the short gastric vessels. However, as with our trial, they also demonstrated an increased incidence of bloating symptoms after division of the short gastric vessels. These trials have not been performed in open surgery.

The belief that dividing the short gastric vessels will improve the outcome following laparoscopic total fundoplication is not supported by the results of any published trials. Furthermore, dividing the vessels increases the complexity of the procedure and actually produced a poorer outcome in two of the four trials due to an increase in the incidence of wind-related sequelae.

Laparoscopic antireflux surgery

Results and complications following laparoscopic fundoplication

Laparoscopic Nissen fundoplication was first reported in 1991[103,104] and rapidly established itself as the procedure of choice for reflux disease, with the vast majority of antireflux procedures now being performed this way. The results of several large series with long-term clinical follow-up have

now been published.[105,106] These confirm that laparoscopic Nissen fundoplication is effective, and that 10 years after surgery it achieves an excellent clinical outcome in more than 85–90% of patients. Furthermore, with even longer follow-up, it is likely that this procedure will be as durable as open fundoplication, where a 70–80% success rate can be expected at up to 25 years follow-up.[107]

However, several complications unique to the laparoscopic approach have been described[108] (see below). Dysphagia could be more common following laparoscopic fundoplication, although this may be due to the more intense nature of the prospective follow-up applied in many centres. Furthermore, in our experience dysphagia has been less of a problem after fundoplication than it was before surgery, with a reduction in the incidence from approximately 30% before surgery to less than 10% at 12 months following surgery,[4,5] and for the majority of these patients dysphagia has not been troublesome in the long term.

Up to 10% of patients are dissatisfied. Some of this dissatisfaction is because of a complication of the original surgery. In our experience this has usually been either the development of a paraoesophageal hernia or because of continuing troublesome dysphagia (with either the wrap or the hiatus being too tight). Some patients are dissatisfied, however, even though their reflux has been cured and they have not had any complications.[109] This is usually because they do not like the flatulence that can follow the procedure. It is also important to recognise that there is a learning curve associated with this form of surgery, and we have demonstrated that the first 20 patients in an individual surgeon's experience are associated with a higher complication rate, and as experience increases the re-operation rates fall to below 5%.[53] There are no specific contraindications to the laparoscopic approach, and the repair of giant hiatal hernias and re-operative antireflux surgery are both feasible (although technically more demanding).

There are some differences between the management of patients during and after laparoscopic and open fundoplication procedures. Laparoscopic surgery may increase the risk of thromboembolic complications (see below) and therefore prophylaxis for deep vein thrombosis is mandatory. Other differences are primarily due to the accelerated recovery following laparoscopic surgery. Our practice is to avoid the use of a nasogastric tube, commence oral intake within 6 hours of surgery, and to arrange a barium meal X-ray the day after surgery to check the postoperative anatomy at a time when problems are easily corrected. Since implementing this approach, a similar strategy has been applied to patients undergoing open surgery (usually revision procedures), and this has facilitated a quicker recovery in some of these patients too.

Laparoscopic versus open antireflux surgery

Non-randomised comparisons between open and laparoscopic fundoplication generally showed that laparoscopic surgery required more operating time than the equivalent open surgical procedure,[110,111] that the incidence of postoperative complications was reduced, the length of postoperative hospital stay was shortened by 3–7 days, patients returned to full physical function 6–27 days quicker, and overall hospital costs were reduced. The efficacy of reflux control appeared to be similar between the two approaches. Ten randomised controlled trials have been reported that compare a laparoscopic fundoplication with its open surgical equivalent.[112–126] Nine of these investigated a Nissen fundoplication and one recent study compared laparoscopic vs. open posterior partial fundoplication.[120] The early reports that described follow-up extending up to 12 months confirmed advantages for the laparoscopic approach, albeit less dramatic than the advantages expected from the results of non-randomised studies. More recently, longer-term outcomes from some studies have been reported.[121,123,125]

Early reports from smaller trials[113–115] that each enrolled 20–42 patients demonstrated equivalent short-term clinical outcomes, shortening of the postoperative stay by about 1 day (3 vs. 4 median), longer operating times (extended by approximately 30 minutes), and an overall reduction in the incidence of postoperative complications following laparoscopic Nissen fundoplication. The reduction in the length of the postoperative hospital stay by only 1 day was unexpected. This was achieved entirely by a shorter hospital stay following open fundoplication, suggesting that at least some of the apparent benefits of the laparoscopic approach could be due to a general change in management policy, and if any surgeon uses an open approach then there are probably significant gains to be made by encouraging earlier oral intake, avoiding nasogastric tubes and encouraging earlier discharge from hospital.

Chrysos et al.[116] reported 12 months follow-up for a trial that enrolled 106 patients. Both approaches achieved effective reflux control, post-fundoplication dysphagia was similar, and the laparoscopic approach was followed by less complications, a quicker recovery, and less symptoms of epigastric bloating and distension. Similar 12-month postoperative outcomes were demonstrated by Ackroyd et al.[126] in a trial that enrolled 99 patients.

Håkanson et al.[120] enrolled 192 patients into a trial of laparoscopic vs. open posterior partial fundoplication. Their results were similar to the trials of laparoscopic vs. open Nissen fundoplication. Early complications were more common after open

surgery, the length of the hospital stay was longer (5 vs. 3 days) and return to work was slower (42 vs. 28 days). However, this was offset by a higher incidence of early side-effects and recurrent reflux in the laparoscopic group. At 3 years follow-up, however, there were no outcome differences, satisfaction with the surgery was similar for the two groups, and the need for re-operative surgery of any sort was not influenced by the choice of technique.

Laine et al.[112] reported 110 patients randomised to undergo laparoscopic or open Nissen fundoplication. As with the other trials, hospital stay was halved from 6.4 to 3.2 days and patients returned to work quicker (37 vs. 15 days), but operating time was also prolonged by 31 minutes. A subsequent report from this group[125] described 11-year postoperative clinical and endoscopic follow-up in 86 patients. Whilst symptom control and side-effects were similar at late follow-up and 82% of the laparoscopic surgery group were satisfied with the late outcome, the incidence of wrap disruption at endoscopic assessment was significantly higher following open surgery (40% vs. 13%) and there were 10 incisional hernias, all following the open technique. Similar outcomes were reported by Nilsson et al. in a smaller trial that followed patients for 5 years.[124]

The study that created the most controversy in this area was published by Bais et al. in 2000.[117] This multicentre study initially enrolled 103 patients. The early (3 months) results of this trial showed a disadvantage for the laparoscopic approach and the trial was stopped early because of an excess of adverse end-points. The investigators were criticised for terminating the trial prematurely,[127–129] as it can be argued that the conclusions were misleading. The decision to stop the trial was based primarily on postoperative dysphagia within the first 3 months. Other studies have reported that most patients who undergo a Nissen fundoplication still have some dysphagia 3 months after surgery,[108,118] but that this dysphagia usually subsides as time passes. Hence, a follow-up period of 3 months is too short for the end-point of dysphagia to be adequately assessed. A subsequent report of 5-year follow-up from this trial[121] confirmed the validity of this critique. With further enrolment boosting the number of patients to 177, no differences in symptoms or subjective outcome could be demonstrated at late follow-up. In addition, 24-hour pH monitoring confirmed equivalent reflux control. Hence, the results of this trial also support the application of laparoscopic antireflux surgery.

 If the overall results of these trials are synthesised, it is clear that laparoscopic antireflux surgery has short-term advantages over the open approach in terms of reduced overall morbidity and quicker recovery. In addition, control of reflux and risk of side-effects at late follow-up (up to 11 years) is not influenced by the choice of a laparoscopic approach. For these reasons the laparoscopic approach in expert hands offers advantages over the open approach, and it has effectively superseded the open approach for most clinical situations.

Complications of laparoscopic antireflux surgery

As experience with laparoscopic approaches for antireflux surgery has grown, complications unique to the laparoscopic approach have emerged (Box 13.1). These include postoperative paraoesophageal hiatus hernia, re-operation for dysphagia, and gastrointestinal perforation. Nevertheless, the risk of complications should be balanced against the advantages of the laparoscopic approach, as it is likely that the overall complication rate is reduced following laparoscopic surgery.[108] The likelihood of complications can be influenced by a number of factors, including surgeon experience and expertise, operative technique, and perioperative care. Furthermore, the final outcome of some complications can be moderated significantly by applying appropriate early management strategies.

Complications that are more common following laparoscopic antireflux surgery

Paraoesophageal hiatus hernia

Paraoesophageal hiatus herniation was thought to be an uncommon finding following open fundoplication, presenting usually in the late follow-up period, although its frequency was probably underestimated in the past. Most large series of laparoscopic procedures report the occurrence of paraoesophageal herniation following surgery (**Fig. 13.8**), particularly in the immediate postoperative period.[57,137,149] The incidence of this complication ranges up to 7% in published reports,[57,108] and it seems that this is exacerbated by some factors inherent in the laparoscopic approach. These include a tendency to extend laparoscopic oesophageal dissection further into the thorax than during open surgery, an increased risk of breaching the left pleural membrane[150] and the effect of reduced postoperative pain. Loss of the left pleural barrier can allow the stomach to slide more easily into the left hemithorax, and less pain permits more abdominal force to be transmitted to the hiatal area during coughing, vomiting or other forms of exertion in the initial postoperative period, pushing the stomach into the thorax, as the normal anatomical barriers have been disrupted by surgical dissection. Early resumption of heavy physical work also has been associated with acute herniation. Strategies are available that can reduce the likelihood of herniation. Routine hiatal repair has been shown to reduce the incidence by approximately 80%.[57] In addition, excessive strain on the hiatal repair during the early postoperative period should be avoided by the routine use of antiemetics, and advising patients to avoid excessive lifting or straining for about 1 month following surgery.

Box 13.1 • Unique or common complications following laparoscopic antireflux surgery

- Pneumothorax[130,131]
- Pneumomediastinum[132,133]
- Pulmonary embolism[134,135]
- Injury to major vessels[136]
- Paraoesophageal hiatus hernia[57,135,137]
- Hiatal stenosis[138]
- Mesenteric thrombosis[139,140]
- Bilobed stomach[134]
- Oesophageal perforation[135,141–144]
- Gastric perforation[134,135,141]
- Duodenal perforation[145]
- Bowel perforation[144]
- Cardiac laceration and tamponade[146,147]
- Pleuropericarditis[148]
- Necrotising fasciitis[149]

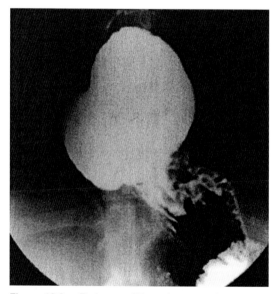

Figure 13.8 • Barium meal X-ray demonstrating a large paraoesophageal hiatus hernia 3 months after laparoscopic fundoplication.

Dysphagia

The debate in the laparoscopic era is whether dysphagia is more likely to occur following laparoscopic antireflux surgery. Nearly all patients, including those who undergo a partial fundoplication, experience dysphagia requiring dietary modification in the first weeks to months following laparoscopic surgery. However, it is dysphagia that is severe enough to need further surgery that is of most concern. Early severe dysphagia requiring surgical revision has been reported in a number of series.[138,151,152] Conversion of a Nissen fundoplication to a partial fundoplication has been performed for troublesome dysphagia following both open and laparoscopic techniques, usually with success.[152,153]

More common with the laparoscopic approach, however, is the problem of a tight oesophageal diaphragmatic hiatus causing dysphagia[138,153] (**Figs 13.9** and **13.10**). Two factors may cause this problem: over-tightening of the hiatus during hiatal repair and excessive perihiatal scar tissue formation. Most surgeons use an intraoesophageal bougie to distend the oesophagus, to assist with calibration of the hiatal closure. However, this will not always prevent over-tightening from occurring. If a problem does arise in the immediate postoperative period, it can usually be corrected by early laparoscopic reintervention with release of one or more hiatal sutures. Later narrowing of the oesophageal

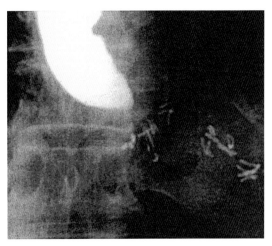

Figure 13.10 • Day 2 postoperative barium meal in a patient with total dysphagia following Nissen fundoplication due to a tight oesophageal hiatus. The problem was corrected by widening the hiatus and removing the hiatal repair sutures.

hiatus due to postoperative scar tissue formation in the second and third postoperative weeks, even in patients not undergoing initial hiatal repair, has also been described. In our experience, endoscopic dilatation with standard bougies usually only provides temporary relief of symptoms rather than a long-term solution. Correction of this problem often requires widening of the diaphragmatic hiatus. This can be achieved by a laparoscopic approach, with anterolateral division of the hiatal ring and adjacent diaphragm until the hiatus is sufficiently loose. An alternative strategy, which is sometimes successful, is pneumatic balloon dilatation (using a 30-mm-diameter balloon).

Pulmonary embolism

Pulmonary embolism was more common in some of the early reports of laparoscopic Nissen fundoplication[134] and in particular following conversion of cases to open surgery, suggesting that prolonged operating times might be an important aetiological factor. In addition, several mechanical factors inherent in the laparoscopic antireflux surgery environment create a scenario in which venous thrombosis is more likely. The combination of head-up tilt of the operating table, intra-abdominal insufflation of gas under pressure and elevation of the legs in stirrups greatly reduces venous flow in the leg veins, potentially predisposing to deep venous thrombosis. This problem can be minimised by the routine use of vigorous antithromboembolism prophylaxis, including low-dose heparin, antiembolism stockings and mechanical compression of the calves.

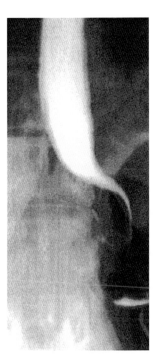

Figure 13.9 • Barium meal X-ray demonstrating usual appearance following laparoscopic Nissen fundoplication.

Complications unique to laparoscopic antireflux surgery

Bilobed stomach

A technical error that has been described during early experiences with laparoscopic Nissen fundoplication is the 'bilobed stomach'.[134] This problem occurs using too distal a piece of stomach to form a Nissen fundoplication, usually the gastric body rather than the fundus, resulting in a bilobular-shaped stomach (**Fig. 13.11**). Whilst most patients are asymptomatic, in extreme cases it is possible for the upper part of the stomach to become obstructed at the point of constriction in the gastric body, resulting in postprandial abdominal pain, which requires surgical revision (**Fig. 13.12**). Ensuring that the correct piece of stomach (the fundus) is used for construction of the fundoplication prevents this problem from arising.

Pneumothorax

Intraoperative pneumothorax occurs in up to 2% of patients due to injury to the left pleural membrane during retro-oesophageal dissection, particularly if dissection is directed too high within the mediastinum.[130] This is more likely to occur during dissection of a large hiatus hernia. Careful dissection behind the oesophagus, ensuring that the tips of instruments passed from right to left behind the oesophagus do not pass above the level of the

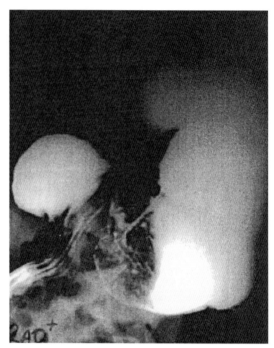

Figure 13.12 • Barium meal image of a more severe 'bilobed' stomach. This patient developed gastric obstruction and required surgical revision.

diaphragm, and experience with laparoscopic dissection at the hiatus reduce its likelihood. The occurrence of a pneumothorax does not usually require the placement of a chest drain, as CO_2 gas in the pleural cavity is rapidly reabsorbed at the completion of the procedure, allowing the lung to re-expand rapidly.

Vascular injury

Vascular injury to the inferior vena cava, the left hepatic vein and the abdominal aorta have all been reported.[136,154] This problem may be associated with aberrant anatomy, inexperience, the excessive use of monopolar diathermy cautery dissection, the incorrect application of ultrasonic shears, or a combination of several of these. Intraoperative bleeding more commonly follows inadvertent laceration of the left lobe of the liver by a laparoscopic liver retractor or other instrument and haemorrhage from poorly secured short gastric vessels during fundal mobilisation. A rare complication is cardiac tamponade. This has been reported twice,[146,147] once due to laceration of the right ventricle by a liver retractor and once due to an injury of the cardiac wall from a suture needle. Certainly the proximity of the heart, inferior vena cava and aorta to the distal oesophagus render potentially life-threatening injuries a distinct possibility if surgeons are unfamiliar with the hiatal anatomy as seen via the laparoscope. Nevertheless, the overall

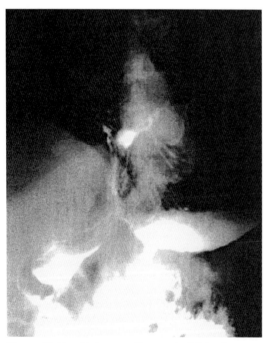

Figure 13.11 • Barium meal image of a 'bilobed' stomach. This patient continues to have an excellent clinical result at 7 years follow-up.

risk of perioperative haemorrhage during and after antireflux surgery is probably reduced by the laparoscopic approach, and the likelihood of splenectomy is significantly reduced by the laparoscopic approach.

Perforation of the upper gastrointestinal tract

Oesophageal and gastric perforation are specific risks, with an incidence of approximately 1% reported in most series.[37,108,145] Gastric perforation is usually an avulsion injury of the gastric cardia due to excessive traction by the surgical assistant. Perforation of the back wall of the oesophagus usually occurs during dissection of the posterior oesophagus. The anterior oesophageal wall is probably at greatest risk when a bougie is passed to calibrate the tightness of a Nissen fundoplication or the oesophageal hiatus. All these injuries can be repaired by sutures, placed either laparoscopically or by an open technique. Awareness that injury can occur enables surgeons to institute strategies that reduce the likelihood of their occurrence. Furthermore, injury is less likely with greater experience.

Mortality

Deaths have been reported following laparoscopic antireflux procedures. Causes include peritonitis secondary to duodenal perforation,[145] thrombosis of the superior mesenteric artery and the coeliac axis,[139] and infarction of the liver.[155] However, the overall mortality of laparoscopic antireflux surgery is probably less than 0.1%.

Avoiding complications following laparoscopic antireflux surgery and minimising their impact

To avoid or minimise complications following a laparoscopic antireflux procedure, a range of strategies should be considered and applied whenever possible. Surgeons should apply a surgical technique that will reduce the likelihood of an adverse outcome arising. Most agree that the oesophageal hiatus should be narrowed or reinforced with sutures, irrespective of whether a hiatus hernia is present or not.[57] However, as complications will occur in a small number of patients following any surgical procedure, a strategy should be sought that will minimise the impact of problems when they arise. One such strategy is to perform a barium swallow examination on the first or second postoperative day to confirm that the fundoplication is in the correct position and that the stomach is entirely intra-abdominal. If there is any uncertainty endoscopic examination may clarify the situation. If the appearances are not acceptable, or if other problems such as severe dysphagia or excessive pain occur, then laparoscopic re-exploration should be performed. Early laparoscopic reintervention is associated with minimal morbidity and

usually delays the patient's recovery by only a few days. Most complications requiring reintervention can be readily dealt with laparoscopically within a week of the original procedure.[35] Beyond this time, however, laparoscopic re-operation becomes difficult, and for this reason we have a relatively low threshold for laparoscopic re-exploration in the first postoperative week if early problems arise.

If complications become apparent at a later stage, laparoscopic re-operation is often still feasible if an experienced surgeon is available.[153] However, the likelihood of success is reduced in the intermediate period following the original procedure. Waiting, if possible, until scar tissue has matured (i.e. at least 3–6 months) simplifies subsequent laparoscopic dissection and increases the likelihood of completing the procedure laparoscopically.

Other randomised trials

Angelchik prosthesis and ligamentum teres cardiopexy

The Angelchik prosthesis was a failure of both antireflux therapy and its complications and has been abandoned. Janssen et al.[156] enrolled 20 patients in a randomised study of Nissen fundoplication vs. ligamentum teres cardiopexy. Although both procedures effectively corrected reflux for the first 3 months following surgery, by 12 months, 6 of the 10 patients who underwent the ligamentum teres repair required further surgery for recurrent reflux, and despite the small number of patients entered, the results of the ligamentum teres repair were so poor that continued use of this procedure can no longer be justified.

Antrectomy with Roux-en-Y duodenal diversion

Washer et al.[157] randomised 42 patients with 'severe reflux oesophagitis' (most with reflux strictures) to receive either a total fundoplication or an antrectomy with Roux-en-Y duodenal diversion. At an average of 5 years follow-up good to excellent results were achieved in 20 of 22 patients having an antrectomy and Roux-en-Y anastomosis, compared to 13 of 20 patients having a fundoplication. The study was originally reported in 1984, and since the advent of more effective medical treatment, the type of patients enrolled in this study are now seen less often.

Synthesis of the results from prospective randomised trials

The results of randomised trials can be assessed together to facilitate the development of guidelines

- Laparoscopic Nissen fundoplication is associated with less complications overall and a shorter convalescence than open Nissen fundoplication*
- The longer-term outcome following laparoscopic Nissen fundoplication is at least as good as the equivalent open surgical procedure*
- The Nissen fundoplication has a lower complication and re-operation rate than the Angelchik prosthesis*
- The Nissen fundoplication controls reflux better than the ligamentum teres cardiopexy
- Whether both vagus nerves are included or excluded from the wrap makes no difference
- Division of the short gastric blood vessels does not improve the outcome following Nissen fundoplication*
- The incidence of recurrent reflux is similar following posterior partial fundoplication and Nissen fundoplication*
- The incidence of dysphagia is probably less following posterior partial fundoplication compared to Nissen fundoplication*
- The incidence of dysphagia and 'gas-related' complications is reduced following anterior partial fundoplication*
- Partial fundoplications are associated with less wind-related problems than total fundoplication*

*Statement is supported by evidence from more than one randomised trial.

for antireflux surgery (Box 13.2). Some of these will meet with wide acceptance as they support the current body of thought of the international surgical community. However, others are controversial, as they do not support the opinions of the majority of experts in the field.

Most surgeons performing surgery for reflux agree that the laparoscopic approach has been a major advance in surgical technique for antireflux surgery and that this has led to surgery becoming a more attractive management option. Controversy, however, will be raised by conclusions drawn about division of the short gastric blood vessels, and the place of partial fundoplications in the surgeon's armamentarium.

The longer-term outcomes from published trials that have investigated division of the short gastric vessels clearly support the position that this manoeuvre is not necessary for the creation of a satisfactory Nissen fundoplication and that it could even increase the likelihood of some side-effects.

Evidence has now emerged from the larger trials of posterior vs. Nissen fundoplication that

demonstrates advantages for the posterior partial fundoplication technique. Whilst the combined data from the reported trials can be confusing, with most of the smaller trials showing no advantages for posterior partial fundoplication, the larger trials do support the proposition that this technique reduces the risk of gas-related side-effects and might reduce the risk of post-fundoplication dysphagia. However, the magnitude of these differences is probably less than for anterior partial vs. Nissen fundoplication. Four of five randomised trials support the anterior partial fundoplication approach, although poor results were reported in one study.[89] However, longer-term results for the anterior partial fundoplication techniques do confirm its efficacy as an antireflux procedure.[66,92]

The large caseload of many surgical units performing laparoscopic surgery for gastro-oesophageal reflux is now providing an impetus for further trials of antireflux surgery techniques, and these are contributing to the rapidly expanding evidence base from which future conclusions will be drawn.

Endoscopic therapies for reflux

Over recent years, endoscopic procedures for the treatment of reflux have emerged. These procedures have the potential to enable curative procedures for reflux to be performed without the abdominal wall incisions required for conventional or laparoscopic surgical access. Such approaches are likely to appeal to both patients and physicians, as they open the possibility of an even less invasive, curative procedure. These approaches can be broadly categorised into four types (Box 13.3). Three types of procedures aim to narrow the gastro-oesophageal junction. This is done by using either radiofrequency energy,[158] injection of an inert substance[95] or endoscopic suturing.[159] Since the early 2000s these procedures have been applied with enthusiasm in some centres, particularly in the USA. However, none of these treatments apply the established principles that underpin the efficacy of antireflux surgery (see 'Mechanism of action of antireflux operations' section above) and the clinical outcomes have predictably been disappointing.[160] More recently, however, techniques have been described that use a totally endoscopic (transoral) technique to construct an anterior partial fundoplication.[161,162] Because the latter approaches aim to fix the fundus of the stomach to a length of intra-abdominal oesophagus, first principles suggest that these approaches could be more successful.

Procedures that narrow the gastro-oesophageal junction

Radiofrequency
- Stretta procedure

Polymer injection
- Enteryx
- Gatekeeper
- PMMA (Plexiglas microspheres)

'Suturing'
- EndoCinch
- NDO Plicator

Procedures that aim to create a partial fundoplication
- EsophyX endoluminal fundoplication procedure
- Medigus SRS procedure

Radiofrequency

The Stretta procedure (Curon Medical, Sunnyvale, CA)[158] used a purpose-built device to apply radio-frequency energy to the muscular layer of the oeso-phageal wall at the gastro-eosophageal junction. The device comprises a 30-mm-diameter balloon, four 5.5-mm-long retractable stylet electrodes and a mucosal irrigation system. It was passed over an endoscopically placed guidewire and positioned at the gastro-oesophageal junction. The electrodes were deployed so that they puncture the oesophageal wall, and radiofrequency energy is applied to cauter-ise the oesophageal muscle. The Stretta procedure probably generates fibrosis in the muscle layer and this aims to tighten the gastro-oesophageal junction. In general, patients with high grades of ulcerative oesophagitis, Barrett's oesophagus and patients with a hiatus hernia >2 cm in length have been deemed to be unsuitable for this procedure, and the patients selected for treatment have had milder reflux.

Short-term follow-up of case series suggested that this procedure improves reflux symptoms and reduces acid exposure in the oesophagus. However, the magnitude of the reduction in acid exposure has been disappointing, and the US open-label study showed that most patients con-tinued to have abnormal reflux after treatment.[163] A subsequent randomised trial that compared the Stretta procedure with a sham endoscopy showed no differences at 6 months follow-up.[164] The trial demonstrated a large placebo effect in the sham controls, and this should be remembered when considering the outcomes of any antireflux ther-apy. The company that made the Stretta device closed in 2006, and this device is no longer avail-able for clinical use.

Polymer injection

Polymer injection (and similar procedures) aims to add bulk to the gastro-oesophageal junction, thereby narrowing it, to reduce reflux. The most popular of these procedures was Enteryx (Enteric Medical Technologies, Foster City, CA).[95] The procedure entailed endoscopic injection of 5–8 mL of a bioinert polymer into the plane between the circular and lon-gitudinal muscle of the distal oesophagus. Following injection, the polymer precipitated into a spongy mass, creating a ring of polymer just above the gas-tro-oesophageal junction. As with the Stretta pro-cedure, initial reports from uncontrolled case series suggested success rates of 70–80% at 12 months follow-up.[95] However, the results from a subsequent randomised sham-controlled trial were also unim-pressive, with no difference in acid exposure (11.2% vs. 12.7%) at 3 months follow-up. In addition, this trial also demonstrated a significant placebo effect, with 41% of the sham-treated patients able to cease proton-pump inhibitor medication, compared to 68% of the treated group.[165] Unfortunately, expe-rience in the USA was associated with some cata-strophic complications, including four deaths,[166,167] and the manufacturer has since withdrawn the proce-dure. A similar product, the Gatekeeper reflux repair system (Endonetics, San Diego, CA),[168] entailed the placement of six hydrogel prostheses into the sub-mucosa at the gastro-oesophageal junction. It too has been withdrawn from clinical use.

Endoscopic suturing

EndoCinch

The EndoCinch (Bard Endoscopic Technologies, Murray Hill, NJ) procedure entails the endoscopic placement of two 3-mm-deep sutures into adjoin-ing gastric mucosal folds immediately below the gastro-oesophageal junction, to create pleats to nar-row this region. The sutures are not deep enough to include the underlying muscle layer. Data from uncontrolled case series demonstrate improvements in symptoms and distal oesophageal acid exposure (15.4% to 8.7%).[169] However, as with the other endoscopic procedures, reflux is only cured in a minority of patients. Ninety per cent of sutures dis-appeared within 12 months and 80% of patients resumed proton-pump inhibitor medication in one study.[170] In a randomised sham-controlled trial, 40% of patients treated by EndoCinch were not taking medications at 3 months, compared to 5% following sham endoscopy,[171] and symptom scores improved more following the EndoCinch proce-dure. However, oesophageal acid exposure was sim-ilar in the treated and sham groups, and the results of this trial did not compare well with the outcomes for laparoscopic antireflux surgery.

NDO Plicator

The NDO Plicator (NDO Surgical, Mansfield, MA) represents the first attempt to perform a more 'surgical' procedure via a transoral approach. It uses a flexible overtube that can be retroflexed in the stomach. A screw device penetrates and retracts the gastro-oesophageal junction, and a full-thickness plication of the cardia is fashioned to narrow the gastro-oesophageal junction. This is secured with a pre-tied pledgeted suture. For the first time, a sham-controlled trial[172] actually showed a significant reduction in oesophageal acid exposure (measured by ambulatory pH monitoring) from 10% to 7% at 3 months following treatment. However, acid exposure was not restored to normal in most patients, and the degree of improvement was certainly inferior to the 0–2.5% expected following laparoscopic Nissen, posterior or anterior fundoplication.[4,82] At 3 months follow-up, 50% of patients were able to cease proton-pump inhibitor medication compared to 25% of the sham-treated patients. Again, these results are inferior to those of laparoscopic antireflux surgery and it is likely that this procedure does not create a true fundoplication.

Endoscopic fundoplication

EsophyX

Unlike the previous procedures, the EsophyX (Endogastric Solutions, Washington) procedure aims to construct an actual fundoplication.[162,172] This procedure requires general anaesthesia and two operators. A standard endoscope is passed through the device (**Figs 13.13** and **13.14**) and both are passed transorally into the stomach. The endoscope is retroflexed for vision and a screw device anchors tissue at the gastro-oesophageal junction to retract it caudally. A plastic arm (tissue mould) then compresses the fundus against the side of the oesophagus, and polypropylene fasteners are passed between the oesophagus and the gastric fundus to anchor these structures. Multiple fasteners are applied, with the procedure commencing on the greater curve aspect, and progressing radially

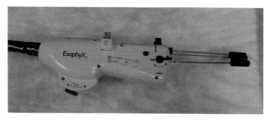

Figure 13.13 • Operating handle for the EsophyX device for endoluminal anterior partial fundoplication.

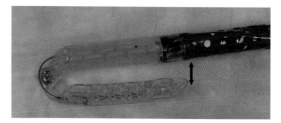

Figure 13.14 • Distal end of EsophyX device. The tip is sited within the stomach and the shaft in the distal oesophagus. The two components close together as indicated to allow the fasteners to be deployed.

towards the lesser curve to fashion a 200–300° anterior partial fundoplication.

Clinical experience with this procedure has been limited to a small number of centres in Europe. Only one clinical study has been published.[173] This paper described 12-month outcomes in 17 patients. Patients with circumferential ulcerative oesophagitis, Barrett's oesophagus, hiatus hernia ≥3 cm and body mass index >30 were excluded. The median procedure time was 123 minutes and the median number of fasteners used was 11. Most patients recovered uneventfully, although one was readmitted with abdominal pain and pneumoperitinoneum, and was managed conservatively. At 12 months, 14 (82%) patients were not using proton-pump inhibitor medication and were satisfied with the clinical outcome. Sixteen patients underwent postoperative pH monitoring. The median percentage time pH was less than 4 was 4.7%. Seven (44%) patients had a normal pH study and 9 (56%) continued to have abnormal acid reflux following the EsophyX procedure. The results from this study suggest that in some patients a fundoplication can be constructed. However, these short-term results are still inferior to those achieved by the equivalent laparoscopic anterior partial fundoplication,[4] and less than half of the patients had objective evidence that their reflux had been cured. Nevertheless, if the procedure can be improved so that a partial fundoplication can be reliably fashioned then it may well have a place in the treatment of some patients with gastro-oesophageal reflux disease.

Medigus

The Medigus SRS procedure (Medigus, Omer, Israel) is an alternative endoscopic approach for the construction of an anterior partial fundoplication.[161,174] It uses a purpose-built endoscope that contains stapling and ultrasound mechanisms. The tip of the endoscope retroflexes more acutely than a standard endoscope, enabling the tip of the endoscope to bend far enough to meet the side of the instrument (**Fig. 13.15**). The tip and side of the endoscope can be locked together to form two halves of

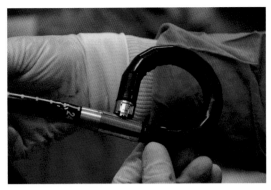

Figure 13.15 • Medigus device for endoluminal anterior partial fundoplication. The photograph shows the fully flexed end of the endoscope. The end of the device can be locked to the side, forming two halves of a stapler. The fundus of the stomach is stapled to the side of the oesophagus, 2–3 cm above the gastro-oesophageal junction.

a stapling device, and ultrasound is used to measure the gap between the tip and the side, to facilitate optimum staple formation. The selection criteria for this procedure are similar to those for the EsophyX procedure. The procedure is undertaken under general anaesthesia by a single operator. The stapling mechanism in the side of the endoscope is positioned approximately 2–3 cm above the gastro-oesophageal junction and the instrument is flexed to bring the fundus of the stomach to the side of the intra-abdominal oesophagus. The components of the instrument are locked together and a cluster of five titanium staples are fired, attaching the structures. The instrument is rotated and the process is undertaken two to three times to create an anterior partial fundoplication (**Fig. 13.16**). The fundoplication is similar to the fundoplication constructed by the EsophyX procedure, and the early outcomes for 13 patients are also similar. At short-term follow-up 92% were able to cease proton-pump inhibitor medication and 54% had a normal post-procedure 24-hour pH study (A. Shapira, personal communication).

Overview of endoscopic antireflux surgery

None of the initial endoscopic suturing, injection or radiofrequency-based approaches to the treatment of gastro-oesophageal reflux achieved outcomes that were comparable to those of a surgical fundoplication, and some of the procedures that were initially applied enthusiastically by the gastroenterological community have now been withdrawn from clinical use, either because

of safety concerns, lack of efficacy, or both. This is not surprising, as these procedures all ignored the principles that underpin antireflux surgery, i.e. accentuation of the angle of His, and maintaining a close anatomical relationship between the fundus of the stomach and the intra-abdominal oesophagus.

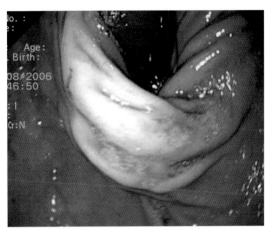

Figure 13.16 • Endoscopic view of completed endoscopic anterior partial fundoplication from initial clinical trials of the Medigus SRS endoscope.

The newer procedures that aim to perform an anterior partial fundoplication are based on more sound principles, and in the future they might offer an alternative to antireflux surgery in appropriately selected patients. However, until now the application of the endoscopic procedures has been limited to patients with milder forms of reflux disease, and all trials have specifically excluded patients in whom the risk of failure is more likely, i.e. more severe ulcerative oesophagitis or Barrett's oesophagus. Furthermore, a hiatus hernia cannot be repaired properly using an endoscopic approach, and for this reason patients with a hiatus hernia >2 cm in length have also been excluded. Hence, only a minority of the patients who currently undergo a laparoscopic fundoplication for reflux and none of the patients with a large hiatus hernia can be considered for endoscopic treatment. If an effective treatment becomes available, then perhaps up to 25–30% of the patients who currently undergo a laparoscopic procedure will be suitable for this procedure, although some patients who are satisfactorily managed with proton-pump inhibitor medication might consider endoscopic treatment to be a reasonable alternative to medication, and this could expand the indications for an antireflux procedure.

However, lessons should be learnt from the experience with failed endoscopic antireflux treatments (Enteryx and Stretta), and before any new endoscopic treatment is now made widely available it should first be evaluated in well-designed clinical trials. An appropriate procedure must be as effective as a conventional fundoplication, it should apply the same principles that underpin an effective antireflux operation and it should be equally safe or safer. Furthermore, surgeons will need to have an appropriate strategy to deal with patients who develop recurrent reflux. Any procedure that makes a subsequent laparoscopic fundoplication procedure more difficult or more dangerous will be a problem, particularly if there is a substantial risk of the primary endoscopic procedure failing.

Key points

- The treatment of reflux is usually incremental, commencing with various levels of medical measures. Surgery is reserved for patients with more severe disease, who either fail to respond adequately to medical treatment or who do not wish to take lifelong medication.
- It is apparent that a single management strategy is unlikely to be appropriate for all patients. Surgical therapy achieves better control of reflux in patients with moderate to severe reflux.
- Endoscopic findings and 24-hour pH studies have to be interpreted in the light of the patient's clinical presentation. A final recommendation for surgery must be based on all available clinical and objective information.
- It remains an open question whether Barrett's oesophagus alone is an indication for antireflux surgery. Patients with Barrett's should be selected for surgery on the basis of their reflux symptoms and their response to medications, not simply because they have a columnar-lined oesophagus.
- The overwhelming majority of patients claim that the disadvantages of an antireflux operation (temporary dysphagia, early fullness, increased flatulence, and inability to belch and vomit) are far outweighed by the advantages of the operation.
- Endoscopy is a mandatory prerequisite before recommending antireflux surgery.
- The presence of weak peristaltic amplitudes or poor propagation of peristalsis is not a contraindication to antireflux surgery. Many surgeons recommend a tailored approach to patient selection by choosing a partial fundoplication in patients with poor peristalsis – there is no strong evidence to support this.
- Twenty-four-hour ambulatory pH monitoring is not sufficiently accurate to select patients for surgery, as up to 20% of patients who have oesophagitis and typical reflux symptoms would be unnecessarily excluded from antireflux surgery.
- Total fundoplications and partial fundoplications (whether anterior or posterior) probably all work in a similar fashion. No one procedure currently yields perfect results, i.e. 100% cure of reflux and no side-effects.
- The available evidence appears to support the view that the main difference in outcome between total and posterior fundoplication is in the wind-related problems.
- Reflux control is slightly better after total compared with anterior fundoplication, but this is offset by significantly less dysphagia, less epigastric bloating and better preservation of belching, resulting in the proportion of patients reporting a good or excellent overall outcome at 5 years being greater following anterior fundoplication.
- The results of randomised trials of open vs. laparoscopic surgery confirm advantages for the laparoscopic approach, albeit less dramatic than the advantages expected from the results of non-randomised studies.
- Most large series of laparoscopic procedures report the occurrence of paraoesophageal herniation following surgery, particularly in the immediate postoperative period. Routine hiatal repair has been shown to reduce the incidence by approximately 80%.
- None of the currently reported endoscopic procedures achieve the level of reflux control associated with fundoplication.

References

1. Nebel OT, Fornes MF, Castell DO. Symptomatic gastroesophageal reflux: incidence and precipitating factors. Am J Dig Dis 1976; 21:953–6.

2. Thompson WE, Heaton KW. Heartburn and globus in apparently healthy people. Can Med Assoc J 1982; 126:46–8.

3. Lord RVN, Law MG, Ward RL et al. Rising incidence of oesophageal adenocarcinoma in men in Australia. J Gastroenterol Hepatol 1998; 13:356–62.

4. Watson DI, Jamieson GG, Pike GK et al. A prospective randomised double blind trial between laparoscopic Nissen fundoplication and anterior partial fundoplication. Br J Surg 1999; 86:123–30.

   The first published randomised trial to compare an anterior partial fundoplication with the Nissen procedure.

5. Watson DI, Pike GK, Baigrie RJ et al. Prospective double blind randomised trial of laparoscopic Nissen fundoplication with division and without division of short gastric vessels. Ann Surg 1997; 226:642–52.

   A randomised trial of 102 patients who underwent a total fundoplication with vs. without division of the short gastric vessels.

6. Ireland AC, Holloway RH, Toouli J et al. Mechanisms underlying the antireflux action of fundoplication. Gut 1993; 34:303–8.

7. Dent J. Australian clinical trials of omeprazole in the management of reflux oesophagitis. Digestion 1990; 47:69–71.

8. Watson DI, Mathew G, Pike GK et al. Comparison of anterior, posterior and total fundoplication using a viscera model. Dis Esoph 1997; 10:110–14.

9. Bate CM, Keeling PW, O'Morain C et al. Comparison of omeprazole and cimetidine in reflux oesophagitis: symptomatic, endoscopic, and histological evaluations. Gut 1990; 31:968–72.

10. Hetzel DJ, Dent J, Reed WD et al. Healing and relapse of severe peptic esophagitis after treatment with omeprazole. Gastroenterology 1998; 95:903–13.

11. Kuipers EJ, Lundell L, Klinkenberg-Knol EC et al. Atrophic gastritis and Helicobacter pylori infection in patients with reflux esophagitis treated with omeprazole or fundoplication. N Engl J Med 1996; 334:1018–22.

12. Driman DK, Wright C, Tougas G et al. Omeprazole produces parietal cell hypertrophy and hyperplasia in humans. Dig Dis Sci 1996; 41:2039–47.

13. Verlinden M. Review article: a role for gastrointestinal prokinetic agents in the treatment of reflux oesophagitis? Aliment Pharmacol Ther 1989; 3:113–31.

14. Waring JP, Hunter JG, Oddsdottir M et al. The preoperative evaluation of patients considered for laparoscopic antireflux surgery. Am J Gastroenterol 1995; 90:35–8.

15. Bischof G, Feil W, Riegler M et al. Peptic esophageal stricture: is surgery still necessary? Wei Klin Wochenschr 1996; 108:267–71.

16. Farrell TM, Smith CD, Metreveli RE et al. Fundoplication provides effective and durable symptom relief in patients with Barrett's esophagus. Am J Surg 1999; 178:18–21.

17. Ortiz EA, Martinez de Haro LF, Parrilla P et al. Conservative treatment versus antireflux surgery in Barrett's oesophagus: long-term results of a prospective study. Br J Surg 1996; 83:274–8.

18. Ortiz A, De Maro LT, Parrilla P et al. 24-h pH monitoring is necessary to assess acid reflux suppression in patients with Barrett's oesophagus undergoing treatment with proton pump inhibitors. Br J Surg 1999; 86:1472–4.

19. Sagar PM, Ackroyd R, Hosie KB et al. Regression and progression of Barrett's oesophagus after antireflux surgery. Br J Surg 1995; 82:806–10.

20. Gurski RR, Peters JH, Hagen JA et al. Barrett's esophagus can and does regress after antireflux surgery: a study of prevalence and predictive features. J Am Coll Surg 2003; 196:706–12.

21. Ackroyd R, Brown NJ, Davis MF et al. Photodynamic therapy for dysplastic Barrett's oesophagus: a prospective, double blind, randomised, placebo controlled trial. Gut 2000; 47:612–17.

22. Ackroyd R, Tam W, Schoeman M et al. Prospective randomised controlled trial of argon plasma coagulation ablation versus endoscopic surveillance of Barrett's oesophagus in patients following antireflux surgery. Gastrointest Endosc 2004; 59:1–7.

23. Bright T, Watson DI, Tam W et al. Randomized trial of argon plasma coagulation vs. endoscopic surveillance for Barrett's oesophagus following antireflux surgery – late results. Ann Surg 2007; 246:1016–20.

24. Behar J, Sheahan DG, Biancani P. Medical and surgical management of reflux oesophagitis, a 38-month report on a prospective clinical trial. N Engl J Med 1975; 293:263–8.

25. Spechler SJ. Comparison of medical and surgical therapy for complicated gastroesophageal reflux disease in veterans. N Engl J Med 1992; 326:786–92.

   The first large prospective randomised trial to compare medical with surgical therapy for gastro-oesophageal reflux.

26. Parrilla P, Martinez de Haro LF, Ortiz A et al. Long-term results of a randomized prospective study comparing medical and surgical treatment of Barrett's esophagus. Ann Surg 2003; 237:291–8.

27. Lundell L, Miettinen P, Myrvold HE et al. Continued (5-year) followup of a randomized clinical study

comparing antireflux surgery and omeprazole in gastroesophageal reflux disease. J Am Coll Surg 2001; 192:172–81.

A randomised trial of proton-pump inhibitor vs. open antireflux surgery.

28. Lundell L, Miettinen P, Myrvold HE et al. Long-term management of gastroesophageal reflux disease with omeprazole or open antireflux surgery: results of a prospective, randomized clinical trial. Eur J Gastro Hepatol 2000; 12:879–87.

29. Mehta S, Bennett J, Mahon D et al. Prospective trial of laparoscopic Nissen fundoplication versus proton pump inhibitor therapy for gastroesophageal reflux disease: seven-year follow-up. J Gastrointest Surg 2006; 10:1312–16.

30. Mahon D, Rhodes M, Decadt B et al. Randomized clinical trial of laparoscopic Nissen fundoplication compared with proton-pump inhibitors for treatment of chronic gastro-oesophageal reflux. Br J Surg 2005; 92:695–9.

The first randomised trial of proton-pump inhibitor vs. laparoscopic antireflux surgery.

31. Anvari M, Allen C, Marshall J et al. A randomized controlled trial of laparoscopic Nissen fundoplication versus proton pump inhibitors for treatment of patients with chronic gastroesophageal reflux disease: one-year follow-up. Surg Innov 2006; 13:238–49.

32. Spechler SJ, Lee E, Ahnen D et al. Long-term outcome of medical and surgical therapies for gastroesophageal reflux disease. Follow-up of a randomized controlled trial. JAMA 2001; 285:2331–8.

Longer-term follow-up from a randomised trial of medical vs. surgical therapy.

33. Lundell L, Miettinen P, Myrvold HE et al. Seven-year follow-up of a randomized clinical trial comparing proton-pump inhibition with surgical therapy for reflux oesophagitis. Br J Surg 2007; 94:198–203.

Longer-term follow-up from a randomised trial of medical vs. open surgical therapy.

34. Cookson R, Flood C, Koo B et al. Short-term cost effectiveness and long-term cost analysis comparing laparoscopic Nissen fundoplication with proton-pump inhibitor maintenance for gastro-oesophageal reflux disease. Br J Surg 2005; 92:700–6.

35. Watson DI, Jamieson GG, Baigrie RJ et al. Laparoscopic surgery for gastro-oesophageal reflux: beyond the learning curve. Br J Surg 1996; 83:1284–7.

36. Ackroyd R, Watson DI, Games PA. Fizzy drinks following laparoscopic Nissen fundoplication: a cautionary tale of explosive consequences. Aust NZ J Surg 1999; 69:887–8.

37. Gotley DC, Smithers BM, Rhodes M et al. Laparoscopic Nissen fundoplication – 200 consecutive cases. Gut 1996; 38:487–91.

38. Trus TL, Laycock WS, Branum G et al. Intermediate follow-up of laparoscopic antireflux surgery. Am J Surg 1996; 171:32–5.

39. Oddsdottir M, Franco AL, Laycock WS et al. Laparoscopic repair of paraesophageal hernia. New access, old technique. Surg Endosc 1995; 9:164–8.

40. Watson DI, Davies N, Devitt PG et al. Importance of dissection of the hernial sac in laparoscopic surgery for very large hiatus hernias. Arch Surg 1999; 134:1069–73.

41. Kauer WKH, Peters JH, DeMeester TR et al. A tailored approach to antireflux surgery. J Thorac Cardiovasc Surg 1995; 110:141–7.

42. Little AG. Gastro-oesophageal reflux and oesophageal motility diseases; who should perform antireflux surgery? Ann Chir Gynaecol 1995; 84:103–5.

43. Beckingham IJ, Cariem AK, Bornman PC et al. Oesophageal dysmotility is not associated with poor outcome after laparoscopic Nissen fundoplication. Br J Surg 1998; 85:1290–3.

44. Baigrie RJ, Watson DI, Myers JC et al. The outcome of laparoscopic Nissen fundoplication in patients with disordered pre-operative peristalsis. Gut 1997; 40:381–5.

45. Rydberg L, Ruth M, Abrahamsson H et al. Tailoring antireflux surgery: a randomized clinical trial. World J Surg 1999; 23:612–18.

46. Chrysos E, Tsiaoussis J, Zoras OJ et al. Laparoscopic surgery for gastroesophageal reflux disease patients with impaired esophageal peristalsis: total or partial fundoplication? J Am Coll Surg 2003; 197:8–15.

47. Booth MI, Stratford J, Jones L et al. Randomized clinical trial of laparoscopic total (Nissen) versus posterior partial (Toupet) fundoplication for gastro-oesophageal reflux disease based on preoperative oesophageal manometry. Br J Surg 2008; 95(1):57–63.

48. Strate U, Emmermann A, Fibbe C et al. Laparoscopic fundoplication: Nissen versus Toupet two-year outcome of a prospective randomized study of 200 patients regarding preoperative esophageal motility. Surg Endosc 2007; 22:21–30.

49. Watson DI, Jamieson GG, Bessell JR et al. Laparoscopic fundoplication in patients with an aperistaltic esophagus and gastroesophageal reflux. Dis Esoph 2006; 19:94–8.

50. Watson DI, Mathew G, Pike GK et al. Efficacy of anterior, posterior and total fundoplication in an experimental model. Br J Surg 1998; 85:1006–9.

51. Collard JM, De Koninck XJ, Otte JB et al. Intrathoracic Nissen fundoplication: long-term clinical and pH-monitoring evaluation. Ann Thorac Surg 1991; 51:34–8.

52. Watson A, Jenkinson LR, Ball CS et al. A more physiological alternative to total fundoplication for the surgical correction of resistant gastro-oesophageal reflux. Br J Surg 1991; 78:1088–94.

53. Watson DI, Baigrie RJ, Jamieson GG. A learning curve for laparoscopic fundoplication. Definable, avoidable, or a waste of time? Ann Surg 1996; 224:198–203.

54. Nissen R. Eine einfache operation zur beeinflussung der refluxoesophagitis. Schweiz Med Wochenschr 1956; 86:590–2.

55. DeMeester TR, Bonavina L, Albertucci M. Nissen fundoplication for gastroesophageal reflux disease. Evaluation of primary repair in 100 consecutive patients. Ann Surg 1986; 204:9–20.

56. DeMeester TR, Stein HJ. Minimizing the side effects of antireflux surgery. World J Surg 1992; 16:335–6.

57. Watson DI, Jamieson GG, Devitt PG et al. Paraoesophageal hiatus hernia: an important complication of laparoscopic Nissen fundoplication. Br J Surg 1995; 82:521–3.

58. Donahue PE, Bombeck CT. The modified Nissen fundoplication – reflux prevention without gas bloat. Chir Gastroent 1977; 11:15–27.

59. Rossetti M, Hell K. Fundoplication for the treatment of gastroesophageal reflux in hiatal hernia. World J Surg 1977; 1:439–44.

60. Toupet A. Technique d'oesophago-gastroplastie avec phrenogastropexie appliquee dans la cure radicale des hernies hiatales et comme complement de l'operation d'heller dans les cardiospasmes. Med Acad Chir 1963; 89:374–9.

61. Lind JF, Burns CM, MacDougal JT. 'Physiological' repair for hiatus hernia – manometric study. Arch Surg 1965; 91:233–7.

62. Belsey R. Mark IV repair of hiatal hernia by the trans thoracic approach. World J Surg 1977; 1:475–81.

63. Nguyen NT, Schauer PR, Hutson W et al. Preliminary results of thoracoscopic Belsey Mark IV antireflux procedure. Surg Laparosc Endosc 1998; 8:185–8.

64. Dor J, Himbert P, Paoli JM et al. Treatment of reflux by the so-called modified Heller–Nissen technic. Presse Med 1967; 75:2563–9.

65. Watson A, Spychal RT, Brown MG et al. Laparoscopic 'physiological' antireflux procedure: preliminary results of a prospective symptomatic and objective study. Br J Surg 1995; 82:651–6.

66. Ludemann R, Watson DI, Game PA et al. Laparoscopic total versus anterior 180 degree fundoplication – five year follow-up of a prospective randomized trial. Br J Surg 2005; 92:240–3.

    Longer-term follow-up from a randomised trial of anterior vs. Nissen fundoplication.

67. Watson DI, Jamieson GG, Lally C et al. Multicentre prospective double blind randomized trial of laparoscopic Nissen versus anterior 90 degree partial fundoplication. Arch Surg 2004; 139:1160–7.

    Early outcomes from a multicentre randomised trial of anterior 90° vs. Nissen fundoplication.

68. Spence GM, Watson DI, Jamieson GG et al. Single centre prospective randomized trial of laparoscopic Nissen versus anterior 90 degree partial fundoplication. J Gastrointest Surg 2006; 10:698–750.

69. Hill LD. An effective operation for hiatal hernia: an eight year appraisal. Ann Surg 1967; 166:681–92.

70. Aye RW, Hill LD, Kraemer SJM et al. Early results with the laparoscopic Hill repair. Am J Surg 1994; 167:542–6.

71. Jobe BA, Horvath KD, Swanstrom LL. Postoperative function following laparoscopic Collis gastroplasty for shortened esophagus. Arch Surg 1998; 133:867–74.

72. Swanstrom LL, Marcus DR, Galloway GQ. Laparoscopic Collis gastroplasty is the treatment of choice for the shortened esophagus. Am J Surg 1996; 171:477–81.

73. Johnson AB, Oddsdottir M, Hunter JG. Laparoscopic Collis gastroplasty and Nissen fundoplication. A new technique for the management of esophageal foreshortening. Surg Endosc 1998; 12:1055–60.

74. Falk GL, Harrison RI. Laparoscopic cut Collis gastroplasty: a novel technique. Dis Esoph 1998; 11:260–2.

75. Maddern GJ, Myers JC, McIntosh N et al. The effect of the Angelchik prosthesis on esophageal and gastric function. Arch Surg 1991; 126:1418–22.

76. Hill ADK, Walsh TN, Bolger CM et al. Randomized controlled trial comparing Nissen fundoplication and the Angelchik prosthesis. Br J Surg 1994; 81:72–4.

77. Kmiot WA, Kirby RM, Akinola D et al. Prospective randomized trial of Nissen fundoplication and the Angelchik prosthesis. Br J Surg 1991; 78:1181–4.

78. DeMeester TR, Johnson LF, Kent AH. Evaluation of current operations for the prevention of gastro-esophageal reflux. Ann Surg 1974; 180:511–25.

79. Thor KBA, Silander T. A long-term randomized prospective trial of the Nissen procedure versus a modified Toupet technique. Ann Surg 1989; 210:719–24.

80. Walker SJ, Holt S, Sanderson CJ et al. Comparison of Nissen total and Lind partial transabdominal fundoplication in the treatment of gastro-oesophageal reflux. Br J Surg 1992; 79:410–14.

81. Laws HL, Clements RH, Swillies CM. A randomized, prospective comparison of the Nissen versus the Toupet fundoplication for gastroesophageal reflux disease. Ann Surg 1997; 225:647–54.

82. Lundell L, Abrahamsson H, Ruth M et al. Lower esophageal sphincter characteristics and esophageal acid exposure following partial or 360° fundoplication: results of a prospective, randomized clinical study. World J Surg 1991; 15:115–21.

83. Lundell L, Abrahamsson H, Ruth M et al. Long-term results of a prospective randomized comparison of total fundic wrap (Nissen–Rossetti) or semifundoplication (Toupet) for gastro-oesophageal reflux. Br J Surg 1996; 83:830–5.

    Longer-term follow-up from a randomised trial of Nissen vs. posterior partial fundolication.

84. Hagedorn C, Lonroth H, Rydberg L et al. Long-term efficacy of total (Nissen–Rossetti) and posterior

partial (Toupet) fundoplication: results of a randomized clinical trial. J Gastrointest Surg 2002; 6:540–5.

85. Zornig C, Strate U, Fibbe C et al. Nissen vs. Toupet laparoscopic fundoplication. Surg Endosc 2002; 16:758–66.

86. Guérin E, Bétroune K, Closset J et al. Nissen versus Toupet fundoplication: results of a randomized and multicenter trial. Surg Endosc 2007; 21:1985–90.

87. Baigrie RJ, Cullis SN, Ndhluni AJ et al. Randomized double-blind trial of laparoscopic Nissen fundoplication versus anterior partial fundoplication. Br J Surg 2005; 92:819–23.

   A large randomised trial of anterior vs. Nissen fundoplication.

88. Woodcock SA, Watson DI, Lally C et al. Quality of life following laparoscopic anterior 90 degrees versus Nissen fundoplication: results from a multicenter randomized trial. World J Surg 2006; 30:1856–63.

89. Hagedorn C, Jonson C, Lonroth H et al. Efficacy of an anterior as compared with a posterior laparoscopic partial fundoplication: results of a randomized, controlled clinical trial. Ann Surg 2003; 238:189–96.

90. Engström C, Lönroth H, Mardani J et al. An anterior or posterior approach to partial fundoplication? Long-term results of a randomized trial. World J Surg 2007; 31:1221–5.

91. Engström C, Ruth M, Lönroth H et al. Manometric characteristics of the gastroesophageal junction after anterior versus posterior partial fundoplication. Dis Esoph 2005; 18:31–6.

92. Rice S, Watson DI, Lally CJ et al. Laparoscopic anterior 180-degree partial fundoplication – 5 year results and beyond. Arch Surg 2006; 141:271–5.

93. Hunter JG, Swanstrom L, Waring JP. Dysphagia after laparoscopic antireflux surgery. The impact of operative technique. Ann Surg 1996; 224:51–7.

94. Dallemagne B, Weerts JM, Jehaes C et al. Causes of failures of laparoscopic antireflux operations. Surg Endosc 1996; 10:305–10.

95. Johnson DA, Ganz R, Aisenberg J et al. Endoscopic implantation of enteryx for treatment of GERD: 12-month results of a prospective, multicenter trial. Am J Gastroenterol 2003; 98:1921–30.

96. Luostarinen M, Koskinen M, Reinikainen P et al. Two antireflux operations: floppy versus standard Nissen fundoplication. Ann Med 1995; 27:199–205.

97. Luostarinen MES, Koskinen MO, Isolauri JO. Effect of fundal mobilisation in Nissen–Rossetti fundoplication on oesophageal transit and dysphagia. Eur J Surg 1996; 162:37–42.

98. Luostarinen ME, Isolauri JO. Randomized trial to study the effect of fundic mobilization on long-term results of Nissen fundoplication. Br J Surg 1999; 86:614–18.

99. O'Boyle CJ, Watson DI, Jamieson GG et al. Division of short gastric vessels at laparoscopic Nissen fundoplication – a prospective double blind randomized trial with five year follow-up. Ann Surg 2002; 235:165–70.

100. Yang H, Watson DI, Lally CJ et al. Randomized trial of division versus non-division of the short gastric vessels during laparoscopic Nissen fundoplication – 10 year outcomes. Ann Surg 2008; 247:38–42.

   Long-term follow-up from a randomised trial of Nissen fundoplication with vs. without division of the short gastric blood vessels.

101. Blomqvist A, Dalenback J, Hagedorn C et al. Impact of complete gastric fundus mobilization on outcome after laparoscopic total fundoplication. J Gastrointest Surg 2000; 4:493–500.

102. Chrysos E, Tzortzinis A, Tsiaoussis J et al. Prospective randomized trial comparing Nissen to Nissen–Rossetti technique for laparoscopic fundoplication. Am J Surg 2001; 182:215–21.

103. Geagea T. Laparoscopic Nissen's fundoplication: preliminary report on ten cases. Surg Endosc 1991; 5:170–3.

104. Dallemagne B, Weerts JM, Jehaes C et al. Laparoscopic Nissen fundoplication: preliminary report. Surg Laparosc Endosc 1991; 1:138–43.

105. Kelly J, Watson DI, Chin K et al. Laparoscopic Nissen fundoplication – clinical outcomes at 10 years. J Am Coll Surg 2007; 205:570–5.

106. Cowgill SM, Gillman R, Kraemer E et al. Ten-year follow up after laparoscopic Nissen fundoplication for gastroesophageal reflux disease. Am Surg 2007; 73:748–52.

107. Luostarinen M, Isolauri J, Laitinen J et al. Fate of Nissen fundoplication after 20 years. A clinical, endoscopical, and functional analysis. Gut 1993; 34:1015–20.

108. Watson DI, Jamieson GG. Antireflux surgery in the laparoscopic era (Review). Br J Surg 1998; 85:1173–84.

109. Watson DI, Chan ASL, Myers JC et al. Illness behaviour influences the outcome of laparoscopic antireflux surgery. J Am Coll Surg 1997; 184:44–8.

110. Rattner DW, Brooks DC. Patient satisfaction following laparoscopic and open antireflux surgery. Arch Surg 1995; 130:289–94.

111. Peters JH, Heimbucher J, Kauer WKH et al. Clinical and physiological comparison of laparoscopic and open Nissen fundoplication. J Am Coll Surg 1995; 180:385–93.

112. Laine S, Rantala A, Gullichsen R et al. Laparoscopic vs conventional Nissen fundoplication. A prospective randomized study. Surg Endosc 1997; 11:441–4.

113. Franzen T, Anderberg B, Tibbling L et al. A report from a randomized study of open and laparoscopic 360° fundoplication. Surg Endosc 1996; 10:582 (Abstract).

114. Heikkinen T-J, Haukipuro K, Koivukangas P et al. Comparison of costs between laparoscopic and open Nissen fundoplication: a prospective randomized study with a 3-month follow-up. J Am Coll Surg 1999; 188:368–76.

115. Perttila J, Salo M, Ovaska J et al. Immune response after laparoscopic and conventional Nissen fundoplication. Eur J Surg 1999; 165:21–8.

116. Chrysos E, Tsiaoussis J, Athanasakis E et al. Laparoscopic vs open approach for Nissen fundoplication. Surg Endosc 2002; 16:1679–84.

117. Bais JE, Bartelsman JFWM, Bonjer HJ et al. Laparoscopic or conventional Nissen fundoplication for gastro-oesophageal reflux disease: randomised clinical trial. Lancet 2000; 355:170–4.

118. Luostarinen M, Vurtanen J, Koskinen M et al. Dysphagia and oesophageal clearance after laparoscopic versus open Nissen fundoplication. A randomized, prospective trial. Scand J Gastroenterol 2001; 36:565–71.

119. Nilsson G, Larsson S, Johnsson F. Randomized clinical trial of laparoscopic versus open fundoplication: blind evaluation of recovery and discharge period. Br J Surg 2000; 87:873–8.

120. Håkanson BS, Thor KB, Thorell A et al. Open vs laparoscopic partial posterior fundoplication. A prospective randomized trial. Surg Endosc 2007; 21:289–98.

121. Draaisma WA, Rijnhart-de Jong HG, Broeders IA et al. Five-year subjective and objective results of laparoscopic and conventional Nissen fundoplication: a randomized trial. Ann Surg 2006; 244:34–41.

   Long-term follow-up from a randomised trial of laparoscopic vs. open Nissen fundoplication.

122. Draaisma WA, Buskens E, Bais JE et al. Randomized clinical trial and follow-up study of cost-effectiveness of laparoscopic versus conventional Nissen fundoplication. Br J Surg 2006; 93:690–7.

123. Franzén T, Anderberg B, Wirén M et al. Long-term outcome is worse after laparoscopic than after conventional Nissen fundoplication. Scand J Gastroenterol 2005; 40:1261–8.

124. Nilsson G, Wenner J, Larsson S et al. Randomized clinical trial of laparoscopic versus open fundoplication for gastro-oesophageal reflux. Br J Surg 2004; 91:552–9.

125. Salminen PT, Hiekkanen HI, Rantala AP et al. Comparison of long-term outcome of laparoscopic and conventional Nissen fundoplication: a prospective randomized study with an 11-year follow-up. Ann Surg 2007; 246:201–6.

   Long-term follow-up from a randomised trial of laparoscopic vs. open Nissen fundoplication.

126. Ackroyd R, Watson DI, Majeed AW et al. Randomized clinical trial of laparoscopic versus open fundoplication for gastro-oesophageal reflux disease. Br J Surg 2004; 91:975–82.

127. Bloechle C, Mann O, Gawad KA et al. Gastro-oesophageal reflux disease. Lancet 2000; 356:69.

128. Gorecki PJ, Hinder RA. Gastro-oesophageal reflux disease. Lancet 2000; 356:70.

129. deBeaux AC, Watson DI, Jamieson GG. Gastro-oesophageal reflux disease. Lancet 2000; 356:71–2.

130. Watson DI, Mitchell PC, Game PA et al. Pneumothorax during laparoscopic dissection of the oesophageal hiatus. Aust NZ J Surg 1996; 66:711–12.

131. Reid DB, Winning T, Bell G. Pneumothorax during laparoscopic dissection of the diaphragmatic hiatus. Br J Surg 1993; 80:670.

132. Stallard N. Pneumomediastinum during laparoscopic Nissen fundoplication. Anaesthesia 1995; 50:667–8.

133. Overdijk LE, Rademaker BM, Ringers J et al. Laparoscopic fundoplication: a new technique with new complications? J Clin Anesth 1994; 6:321–23.

134. Jamieson GG, Watson DI, Britten-Jones R et al. Laparoscopic Nissen fundoplication. Ann Surg 1994; 220:137–45.

135. Munro W, Brancatisano R, Adams IP et al. Complications of laparoscopic fundoplication: the first 100 patients. Surg Laparosc Endosc 1996; 6:421–3.

136. Baigrie RJ, Watson DI, Game PA et al. Vascular perils during laparoscopic dissection of the oesophageal hiatus. Br J Surg 1997; 84:556–7.

137. Johansson B, Glise H, Hallerback B. Thoracic herniation and intrathoracic gastric perforation after laparoscopic fundoplication. Surg Endosc 1995; 9:917–18.

138. Watson DI, Jamieson GG, Mitchell PC et al. Stenosis of the esophageal hiatus following laparoscopic fundoplication. Arch Surg 1995; 130:1014–16.

139. Mitchell PC, Jamieson GG. Coeliac axis and mesenteric arterial thrombosis following laparoscopic Nissen fundoplication. Aust NZ J Surg 1994; 64:728–30.

140. Medina LT, Vientimilla R, Williams MD et al. Laparoscopic fundoplication. J Laparoendosc Surg 1996; 6:219–26.

141. Schauer PR, Meyers WC, Eubanks S et al. Mechanisms of gastric and esophageal perforations during laparoscopic Nissen fundoplication. Ann Surg 1996; 223:43–52.

142. Lowham AS, Filipi CJ, Hinder RA et al. Mechanisms of avoidance of esophageal perforation by anesthesia personnel during laparoscopic foregut surgery. Surg Endosc 1996; 10:979–82.

143. Swanstrom LL, Pennings JL. Safe laparoscopic dissection of the gastroesophageal junction. Am J Surg 1995; 169:507–11.

144. Collet D, Cadiere GB. Conversions and complications of laparoscopic treatment of gastroesophageal reflux disease. Am J Surg 1995; 169:622–6.

145. Hinder RA, Filipi CJ, Wetscher G et al. Laparoscopic Nissen fundoplication is an effective treatment for gastroesophageal reflux disease. Ann Surg 1994; 220:472–83.

146. Firoozmand E, Ritter M, Cohen R et al. Ventricular laceration and cardiac tamponade during laparoscopic Nissen fundoplication. Surg Laparosc Endosc 1996; 6:394–7.

147. Farlo J, Thawgathurai D, Mikhail M et al. Cardiac tamponade during laparoscopic Nissen fundoplication. Eur J Anaesthesiol 1998; 15:246–7.

148. Viste A, Horn A, Lund-Tonnessen S. Reactive pleuropericarditis following laparoscopic fundoplication. Surg Laparosc Endosc 1997; 7:206–8.

149. Viste A, Vindenes H, Gjerde S. Herniation of the stomach and necrotizing chest wall infection following laparoscopic Nissen fundoplication. Surg Endosc 1997; 11:1029–31.

150. Watson DI, Jamieson GG, Britten-Jones R et al. Pneumothorax during laparoscopic dissection of the diaphragmatic hiatus. Br J Surg 1993; 80:1353–4.

151. Wetscher GJ, Glaser K, Wieschemeyer T et al. Tailored antireflux surgery for gastroesophageal reflux disease: effectiveness and risk of post-operative dysphagia. World J Surg 1997; 21:605–10.

152. Collard JM, Romagnoli R, Kestens PJ. Reoperation for unsatisfactory outcome after laparoscopic antireflux surgery. Dis Esoph 1996; 9:56–62.

153. Watson DI, Jamieson GG, Game PA et al. Laparoscopic reoperation following failed antireflux surgery. Br J Surg 1999; 86:98–101.

154. McKenzie T, Esmore D, Tulloh B. Haemorrhage from aortic wall granuloma following laparoscopic Nissen fundoplication. Aust NZ J Surg 1997; 67:815–16.

155. Schorr RT. Laparoscopic upper abdominal operations and mesenteric infarction. J Laparoendosc Surg 1995; 5:389–91.

156. Janssen IM, Gouma DJ, Klementschitsch P et al. Prospective randomised comparison of teres cardiopexy and Nissen fundoplication in the surgical therapy of gastro-oesophageal reflux disease. Br J Surg 1993; 80:875–8.

157. Washer GF, Gear MWL, Dowling BL et al. Randomized prospective trial of Roux-en-Y duodenal diversion versus fundoplication for severe reflux oesophagitis. Br J Surg 1984; 71:181–4.

158. Torquati A, Houston HL, Kaiser J et al. Long-term follow-up study of the Stretta procedure for the treatment of gastroesophageal reflux disease. Surg Endosc 2004; 18:1475–9.

159. Tam WC, Holloway RH, Dent J et al. Impact of endoscopic suturing of the gastroesophageal junction on lower esophageal sphincter function and gastroesophageal reflux in patients with reflux disease. Am J Gastroenterol 2004; 99:195–202.

160. Hogan WJ. Clinical trials evaluating endoscopic GERD treatments: is it time for a moratorium on the clinical use of these procedures? Am J Gastroenterol 2006; 101:437–9.

161. Watson DI, Roy-Shapira A, Sonnenchein M et al. Transoral endoscopic anterior partial fundoplication without surgical incisions. Aust NZ J Surg 2006; 76(Suppl 1):A37–8 (Abstract).

162. Cadière GB, Rajan A, Rqibate M et al. Endoluminal fundoplication (ELF) – evolution of EsophyX, a new surgical device for transoral surgery. Minim Invasive Ther Allied Technol 2006; 15:348–55.

163. Triadafilopoulos G, DiBaise JK, Nostrant TT et al. The Stretta procedure for the treatment of GERD: 6 and 12 month follow-up of the U.S. open label trial. Gastrointest Endosc 2002; 55:149–56.

164. Corley DA, Katz P, Wo JM et al. Improvement of gastresophageal reflux symptoms after radiofrequency energy: a randomized, sham-controlled trial. Gastroentrology 2003; 125:668–76.
    A randomised trial of sham endoscopy vs. endoscopic application of radiofrequency energy to the gastro-oesophageal junction.

165. Devière J, Costamagna G, Neuhaus H et al. Nonresorbable copolymer implantation for gastroesophageal reflux disease: a randomized sham-controlled multicenter trial. Gastroenterology 2005; 128:532–40.

166. Noh KW, Loeb DS, Stockland A et al. Pneumomediastinum following Enteryx injection for the treatment of gastroesophageal reflux disease. Am J Gastroenterol 2005; 100:723–6.

167. Tintillier M, Chaput A, Kirch L et al. Esophageal abscess complicating endoscopic treatment of refractory gastroesophageal reflux disease by Enteryx injection: a first case report. Am J Gastroenterol 2004; 99:1856–8.

168. Fockens P, Bruno MJ, Gabbrielli A et al. Endoscopic augmentation of the lower esophageal sphincter for the treatment of gastroesophageal reflux disease: multicenter study of the Gatekeeper Reflux Repair System. Endoscopy 2004; 36:682–9.

169. Abou-Rebyeh H, Hoepffner N, Rösch T et al. Long-term failure of endoscopic suturing in the treatment of gastroesophageal reflux: a prospective follow-up study. Endoscopy 2005; 37:213–16.

170. Schwartz MP, Wellink H, Gooszen HG et al. Endoscopic gastroplication for the treatment of gastro-oesophageal reflux disease: a randomised, sham-controlled trial. Gut 2007; 56:20–8.
    A randomised trial of sham endoscopy vs. endoscopic mucosal suturing at the gastro-oesophageal junction.

171. Rothstein R, Filipi C, Caca K et al. Endoscopic full-thickness plication for the treatment of gastroesophageal reflux disease: a randomized, sham-controlled trial. Gastroenterology 2006; 131:704–12.

A randomised trial of sham endoscopy vs. endoscopic full-thickness plication of the gastro-oesophageal junction.

172. http://www.endogastricsolutions.com/index. php?src=gendocs&link=EsophyX

173. Cadière GB, Rajan A, Germay O et al. Endoluminal fundoplication by a transoral device for the treatment of GERD: a feasibility study. Surg Endosc 2007 (online publication); DOI: 10.1007/s00464-007-9618-9.

174. http://www.medigus.com/endoscopy.html

Treatment of the complications of gastro-oesophageal reflux disease and failed gastro-oesophageal surgery

Farzaneh Banki
Tom R. DeMeester

Complications of gastro-oesophageal reflux disease

Gastro-oesophageal reflux disease (GORD) is a common problem accounting for 75% of oesophageal disease in the USA.[1] It is not an inconsequential disease in that patients with GORD have a quality of life similar to patients with angina or heart failure.[2] Further, complications of GORD such as Barrett's oesophagus, oesophagitis and stricture can occur in 50% of patients, and other oesophageal and gastric abnormalities such as a paraoesophageal hernia or intrathoracic stomach are commonly associated with the disease.[3,4]

The prevalence and severity of the complications of GORD are directly related to the presence of a mechanically defective lower oesophageal sphincter and an increased oesophageal exposure to both acid and bile.[3] Simultaneous oesophageal acid and bilirubin monitoring has shown that the combined reflux of gastric acid and duodenal bile into the distal esophagus causes severe mucosal injury and a 300% increase in the risk of Barrett's oesophagus.[5]

Medical therapy consists mainly of acid suppression and has little effect on the bilious component of the refluxed gastric juice. For this reason antireflux surgery is particularly effective in managing the complications of GORD, provided the proper procedure is chosen and correctly performed. The recognition of complications and their effect on oesophageal function is crucial for planning surgical therapy. A short oesophagus, poor oesophageal motility or a large paraoesophageal hiatal hernia can require more complex and challenging surgery. Such surgery needs to be carefully planned and precisely performed. Improper planning or a poorly performed procedure can result in failure. In this chapter we will review the surgical treatment of complicated GORD, provide surgical tips on how to reduce the risk of a failure, and how to manage a patient with a failed procedure when it occurs.

There are seven complications or abnormalities associated with GORD that, when present, have a profound effect on the complexity and outcome of an antireflux procedure. They are a short oesophagus, a wide oesophageal hiatus, a strictured oesophagus, a paraoesophageal hiatal hernia, an intrathoracic stomach, a previous failed antireflux procedure and the condition of end-stage reflux disease.

Short oesophagus

Oesophageal shortening occurs most commonly in patients with advanced reflux disease and is due to acid- and bile-induced inflammatory changes in the muscular wall of the oesophagus. Healing followed by repetitive injury results in a longitudinal contracture of the tubular oesophagus. Oesophageal shortening, when unrecognised, is a threat to the success of an antireflux procedure.

The diagnosis of a short oesophagus should be suspected when the patient has a non-reducing hiatal hernia of 5 cm or longer on an upright barium swallow (**Fig. 14.1**), when a stricture or long-segment Barrett's oesophagus is seen on endoscopy or the measurement of a short oesophageal length on manometry.[6] The latter is only suggestive of a short oesophagus in that progressive shortening of oesophageal length occurs with progressive mucosal disease, but the individual variation is considerable. Consequently, there is no threshold length below which oesophageal shortening can be readily identified.

When one of the above clinical indicators are present the positive predictive value for the diagnosis of a short oesophagus is 84% (Fig. 14.1) and the degree of shortening is sufficient to require a gastroplasty in more than 58% of such patients. The only absolute way to identify a clinically significant shortened oesophagus is the inability to surgically mobilise 2–3 cm of the distal oesophagus into the abdomen and perform a tension-free antireflux

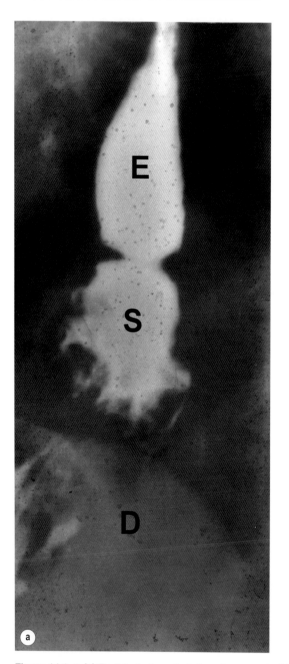

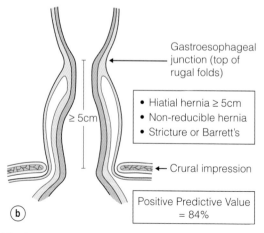

Gastroesophageal junction (top of rugal folds)

≥ 5cm

- Hiatial hernia ≥ 5cm
- Non-reducible hernia
- Stricture or Barrett's

Crural impression

Positive Predictive Value = 84%

Figure 14.1 • (a) Radiological manifestation of a non-reducible hiatal hernia in an upright position on an upper gastrointestinal study. D, diaphragm; E, oesophagus; S, stomach. **(b)** Suspicion of a short oesophagus.

repair. Less than 2 cm of abdominal oesophagus can place sufficient tension on a repair to cause it to herniate or disrupt over time. The diaphragm contracts 30 000 times a day with respiration and the oesophagus contracts 1000 times a day with swallowing. Consequently, unless the repair is free of tension, breakdown can be expected.

The best management of a short oesophagus is to recognise it prior to surgery, mobilise the lower half of the oesophagus to obtain 2–3 cm of tension-free abdominal length at the time of surgery and, if unable to do so, perform a Collis gastroplasty. In patients with a suspected short oesophagus, we prefer to perform the surgical procedure through an open transabdominal incision with transhiatal mobilisation of the distal half of the oesophagus. This approach also allows lengthening of the oesophagus with the Collis gastroplasty if necessary. A fundoplication done around a shortened oesophagus has a high failure rate due to herniation, disruption or slipping of the fundoplication. The latter is often confused with placement of a Nissen fundoplication too low because of the failure to recognise a short oesophagus. To perform a Collis gastroplasty a 48 French bougie is passed down the oesophagus. An EEA stapler is used to make a circular opening 5 cm from the gastro-oesophageal junction closely adjacent to the bougie. A GIA stapler is used to divide the stomach parallel and snuggly against the bougie. This provides 4–5 cm of additional oesophageal length (**Fig. 14.2**). A Nissen fundoplication is constructed around the neo-oesophagus. The procedure allows for a tension-free fundoplication and results in an effective antireflux mechanism. The procedure can leave a small segment of acid-secreting gastric mucosa proximal to the intact fundoplication. Complications of the procedure are persistent dysphagia from a too small gastroplasty tube or ischaemia of the gastroplasty tube, leading to ulceration, bleeding, necrosis and stricture.

Wide crura

A wide crural opening in patients with GORD requires particular attention since adequate and permanent crural closure is the 'Achilles heel' of an antireflux procedure. In a minority of patients with GORD the crura fail to develop properly and the distance between the right and the left crus is too wide to close effectively without tension. The abnormality is likely a congenital defect that deteriorates further with age. Usually the space between the crura is ovoid in shape, but in this condition the space is more circular (**Fig. 14.3**), and the distance between the right and left crus usually exceeds 4 cm. The right crus is often atrophic and holds sutures poorly, resulting in tearing of the muscle with separation of the crural closure and herniation of the

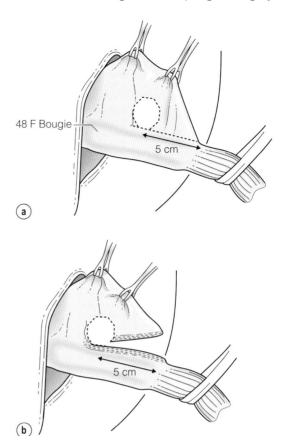

48 F Bougie

5 cm

(a)

5 cm

(b)

Figure 14.2 • Schematic presentation of an abdominal Collis gastroplasty using a 48 French bougie. **(a)** An EEA stapler is applied 5 cm from the gastro-oesophageal junction on the greater curvature. **(b)** The stomach is divided to create an extra 5 cm oesophageal length.

fundoplication. Strips of Surgisis® (Cook Biotech Inc., West Lafayette, IN) on each crus are used for reinforcement, and crural closure is done with 2-0 Ethibond figure-of-eight stitches. The stitches should incorporate large bites of crural muscle and the last crural stitches placed after the bougie used to size the fundoplication has been removed. The crural sutures are tied using the Ti-Knot® (LSi Solutions, Victor, NY) device, which approximates the crura gently with minimal tension. This method does not strangulate the crural muscle, thus reducing tissue necrosis and failure of the crural closure.

Strictured oesophagus

A peptic oesophageal stricture is a late complication of GORD and occurs in 1–5% of patients who develop oesophagitis. It is one of the most morbid and difficult complications to manage.[7] Aggressive acid suppression therapy with proton-pump inhibiters has reduced the incidence of strictures and lessened their recurrence after dilatation. Despite this

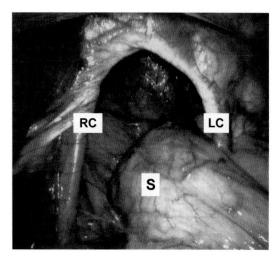

Figure 14.3 • Laparoscopic view of a wide crura. LC, left crus; RC, right crus; S, stomach.

advance in therapy, 30% of patients with strictures require a repeat dilatation within 1 year.[8] The presence of a stricture should suggest to the surgeon the possibility of a short oesophagus. The most efficient method of treating a reflux stricture has been dilatation followed by an antireflux procedure to obtain complete control of reflux. A stricture associated with severe oesophageal dysmotility is extremely difficult to manage. A stricture refractory to dilatation is likely due to a caustic pill-induced injury. In both situations oesophageal replacement is usually the best therapy.

Paraoesophageal hiatal hernia

Paraoesophageal hiatal hernias make up less than 5% of all hiatal hernias, but account for most of the hiatal hernia complications. They are unique in that the normal posterior phreno-oesophageal ligament that anchors the gastro-oesophageal junction within the abdomen is preserved and the body and fundus of the stomach herniate through a large anterior peritoneal lined opening in the oesophageal hiatus. Chest pain and dysphagia are the most common symptoms. The chest pain commonly occurs postprandially and is substernal in location, giving rise to concern that it is cardiac in origin. About 80% of patients with a paraoesophageal hiatal hernia complain of heartburn and have increased oesophageal acid exposure on pH monitoring.[9] The most common laboratory finding is chronic blood loss anaemia from erosions of the engorged gastric mucosa secondary to compression of the gastric veins at the hiatus.

The most common complication of a paraoesophageal hiatal hernia is an intermittent oesophageal obstruction from compression of the distal oesophagus by the distended, herniated stomach. Similarly, the

lung can be compressed by the distended stomach leading to episodes of shortness of breath. The stomach is unable to evacuate swallowed air due to the dependent position of the gastro-oesophageal junction. The repetitive episodes of distension lead to an increase in the size of the hernia over time. Some surgeons prefer to assess oesophageal motility prior to surgery, but passing a motility catheter can be challenging and at times impossible due to the altered anatomy.

Traditionally paraoesophageal hiatal hernias were repaired through a thoracotomy or laparotomy incision with a morbidity of 20% and a mortality of 2%.[10,11] The development of laparoscopic surgery has led to the repair of these complicated hernias by a minimally invasive approach. If the crural opening is >4 cm and primary closure of the diaphragmatic hiatus is under tension there is a significant risk of subsequent disruption of the crural closure and failure of the repair. To prevent this complication the use of a porcine biological mesh to reinforce the diaphragmatic closure has been advocated.[12]

Intrathoracic stomach

Patients with an intrathoracic stomach can present with chronic cough, repetitive pneumonia, chest pain, nausea, vomiting and anaemia. The symptoms are caused by aspiration and obstruction. The latter can lead to incarceration and strangulation of the stomach. A retrocardiac air–fluid level on a routine chest film is a common mode of discovery (**Fig. 14.4**). The obstruction is due to volvulus and distension of the herniated stomach. The upside-down stomach is unable to evacuate swallowed air and continues to distend, leading to obstruction at the level of the diaphragmatic hiatus. The condition is often associated with wide crura. Treatment requires surgery and is effective in relieving symptoms and preventing further episodes of obstruction, incarceration or strangulation. An oesophageal motility study is usually performed to assess the oesophageal body function as often this condition is associated with a history of chronic GORD. Placement of the motility catheter may be challenging and usually requires endoscopic guidance. All patients should have a video upper gastrointestinal barium study and an endoscopy prior to surgery so the surgeon can become familiar with the anatomy. We prefer to perform a transabdominal reduction of the intrathoracic stomach, excision of the hernia sac, partial or complete fundoplication and a crural closure with a biological mesh reinforcement. We use a transabdominal rather than a transthoracic approach as it provides similar results with less morbidity.

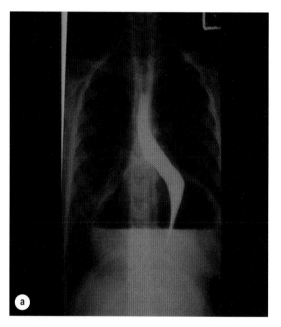
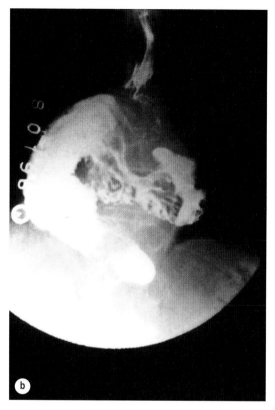

Figure 14.4 • Radiographic presentation of an intrathoracic stomach on a plain chest X-ray **(a)** and an upper gastrointestinal study **(b)** on two different patients.

Previous failed antireflux surgery

The majority of failed antireflux procedures are the result of inadequate patient selection, failure to recognise a short oesophagus or technical errors such as incomplete oesophageal mobilisation, failure to take down the short gastric vessels or inadequate closure of the oesophageal hiatus. These failures can be avoided if surgeons have a better understanding of the principles of antireflux surgery and take a diagnostic interest in the disease. Improving the diagnostic experience and technical know-how of the surgeon interested in performing antireflux procedures is one action that surgeons can take to decrease the rate of failed repairs.

Selection of patients for an initial antireflux procedure is of critical importance to avoid failure. Predictors of a successful antireflux procedure are the presence of the typical symptoms of heartburn and/or regurgitation, a symptomatic response to proton-pump inhibitor therapy that exceeds 50% improvement and a positive 24-hour oesophageal pH study off acid suppression therapy.[13] The latter is the most important predictor. Unfortunately,

often the initial surgery of a subsequent failed procedure was done without any preoperative objective evaluation.

The fundamental steps in the management of patients with a suspected failed antireflux procedure are: (1) confirm that the procedure has failed; (2) identify the cause of failure; and (3) select the correct surgical technique to construct a new antireflux barrier. Patients who suffer from a failed procedure complain of persistent, recurrent or new symptoms. They require a detailed analysis of their symptoms as the aetiology can be due to both natural disease and/or iatrogenic-induced disease. Further, their natural disease may not be GORD, but the consequence of their surgery may have produced GORD. In this situation their initial symptoms may not be relieved by a second antireflux operation.

To confirm that the previous antireflux procedure has failed, a 24-hour oesophageal pH study must be done with the patient off acid suppressive medication. It is not uncommon for the 24-hour pH study to be normal. In this situation the patient's symptoms are not due to reflux. It is likely they were caused by the surgery. If their symptoms are the same as before the surgery, it is likely they never had reflux disease.

To determine the cause of failure requires a video upper gastrointestinal barium study, endoscopy and a detailed analysis of the initial operative report. These studies may show evidence of a technical failure such as a slipped, twisted, herniated or tight fundoplication. An oesophageal motility study can often support a diagnosis of a tight fundoplication by a high lower oesophageal sphincter resting and residual pressure. Similarly, oesophageal motility is helpful in the diagnosis of a slipped fundoplication by showing interference with the manometric relaxation of the distal portion of the lower oesophageal sphincter on swallowing.

Most redo antireflux procedures are best done transabdominally through an open incision. The approach allows the greatest flexibility to deal with the unsuspected. It is the author's experience that, at this point in the disease, the patient is more interested in a fix than the approach used to do the fix.

Prior to performing a redo fundoplication, it is imperative to assess the integrity of the vagus nerves following failed antireflux surgery, especially if the patient presents with symptoms of delayed gastric emptying such as early satiety, nausea and vomiting. Vagal integrity can be assessed with a nuclear gastric-emptying scan where half of the emptying should occur within 90 minutes and 100% within 4 hours. In a patient with severe delayed gastric emptying, a subtotal gastrectomy and gastro-jejunostomy can be combined with an antireflux procedure. The fundoplication and the crural closure are done in the standard fashion, followed by a distal gastric resection with a Roux-en-Y gastro-jejunostomy. In selected cases a total gastrectomy and a Roux-en-Y oesophago-jejunostomy may be required.

An oesophageal fistula is an extremely rare complication of GORD but may develop following an antireflux procedure. The predisposing factor is the presence of a foreign body such as a plastic device or synthetic material. The most common presenting symptom is dysphagia and the most common endoscopic sign is a pinpoint oesophageal ulceration on top of a mound of oedematous mucosa. The use of Teflon pledgets on the diaphragmatic closure should be discouraged as contamination is not uncommon and usually leads to subsequent fistulisation into the oesophagus or stomach. Surgical treatment usually requires take-down of the previous repair, removal of all foreign material and a re-repair.

Evaluation of a failed antireflux procedure

The evaluation of a patient with a failed antireflux procedure can be done by an analysis of their symptoms and altered anatomy:

1. **Symptomatic analysis.** Patients with failed antireflux surgery can present with persistent symptoms (symptoms that were present prior to surgery and persist after surgery), recurrent symptoms (symptoms that initially resolved following surgery and reappeared after a period of time) and de novo symptoms (new symptoms that appeared following an antireflux procedure). A brief description of each category follows.

   a. **Persistent symptoms.** Persistent symptoms are more common in patients who initially present with atypical symptoms of GORD such as hoarseness, cough and adult-onset asthma. They are less common in patients with typical symptoms such as heartburn and regurgitation. Failure to relieve preoperative symptoms in a patient who otherwise meets the preoperative criteria is likely due to an initial misdiagnosis as to the cause of the symptoms. In particular, if the patient's initial preoperative symptoms were nausea or vomiting, it is more likely the patient had delayed gastric emptying rather than GORD.

   b. **Recurrence of preoperative symptoms.** Relief of symptoms following surgery that subsequently return should suggest the possibility of a disrupted, slipped or herniated fundoplication. In these patients a careful symptomatic evaluation is warranted. Commonly, the patient will also complain of chest pain and dysphagia as being new symptoms along with their recurrent symptoms.

   c. **New-onset symptoms.** Persistent dysphagia is the most common new symptom following Nissen fundoplication. In the early postoperative period it is due to mucosal oedema and eventually disappears within 3 months. Persistent dysphagia 6 months after a Nissen fundoplication is usually due to a too tight, misplaced or twisted fundoplication.

2. **Anatomical analysis.** To define the abnormal gastric anatomy requires familiarity with the endoscopic appearance of a normal intact Nissen fundoplication (**Fig. 14.5**). A well-reconstructed Nissen fundoplication has a triangular shape with depth of about 1–2 cm and is snug around the retroflexed endoscope. The squamocolumnar junction is usually visible within and near the base of the fundoplication. The three types of anatomical failures that can be discerned

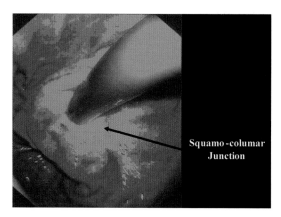

Figure 14.5 • Desired endoscopic appearance of a Nissen fundoplication. The fundoplication is triangular, has as adequate depth, is not twisted and the squamocolumnar junction is seen at the base of the fundoplication.

following a Nissen fundoplication are a slipped, herniated and twisted fundoplication. The endoscopic appearances of herniated and twisted fundoplications are shown in **Fig. 14.6**.

a. **Slipped fundoplication.** A slipped fundoplication is usually a misplaced fundoplication and is due to a failure to mobilise the oesophagus adequately and placing the fundoplication below the gastro-oesophageal junction around the upper stomach. This is likely to occur in patients with a short oesophagus or a

large hiatal hernia. Commonly, in patients with a slipped fundoplication there will be the inability of the distal portion of the lower oesophageal sphincter to relax on swallowing. When performing a Nissen fundoplication we routinely isolate the posterior vagus nerve (**Fig. 14.7**) and place the fundoplication between the posterior vagus nerve and the oesophagus (**Fig. 14.8**). This ensures that the fundoplication is placed around the oesophagus and not the stomach, since the posterior vagus nerve is loosely adherent to the oesophagus and dissects off easily, whereas its dissection off the stomach is difficult and causes bleeding. It is almost impossible to place the fundoplication around the stomach using this technique. We have not observed vagal nerve injury or evidence of postvagotomy symptoms following the technique. In fact, the nerve is protected since it is always identified.

b. **Herniated fundoplication.** Failure of adequate crural closure and incomplete mobilisation of the distal oesophagus are the main reasons for a herniated Nissen fundoplication. We place six to eight deep interrupted 2-0 Ethibond figure-of-eight stitches to close the crura. Stitches are tied loosely to achieve tissue approximation without strangulation. If the crural stitches are tied under tension, necrosis of the crura

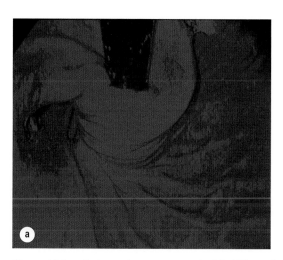

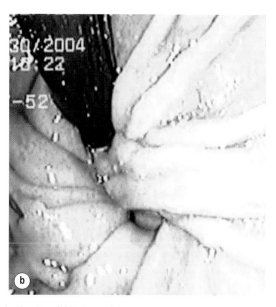

Figure 14.6 • Endoscopic appearance of a failed Nissen fundoplication. **(a)** Twisted. **(b)** Herniated wrap.

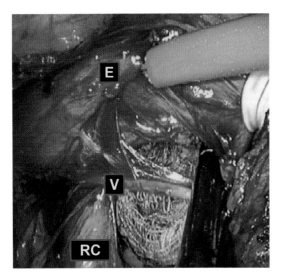

Figure 14.7 • Laparoscopic view of the isolated posterior (right) vagal trunk. E, oesophagus; RC, right crus; V, posterior (right) vagal trunk.

muscle can occur with disruption of the crural closure and subsequent herniation of the fundoplication. The crural closure should always be completed after the 60F bougie used to size the fundoplication has been removed. If the hiatal opening is large or the crura are atretic the closure is

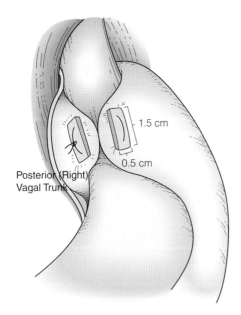

Figure 14.8 • Schematic presentation of the laparoscopic Nissen fundoplication.

reinforced using strips of Surgisis® on each crus.

c. **Twisted fundoplication.** If only the anterior gastric fundic wall is used to construct the fundoplication, twisting and tightening of the fundoplication with gastric distension can occur and cause dysphagia. This is usually reflected in an elevated sphincter pressure above normal levels, and poor anatomical and sometimes manometric relaxation. The fundoplication should be constructed using both the anterior and posterior gastric fundic walls to form a plication around the distal oesophagus, like putting a 'hot dog' bun around a 'hot dog'. The stomach should remain in its normal anatomical plane. The sutures that join the anterior and posterior fundic lips of the plication should lie on the right anterior lateral surface of the oesophagus.

The development of a fistula following antireflux surgery can also occur due to iatrogenic-induced ischaemia leading to necrosis of the oesophageal or gastric wall and subsequent fistulisation. The treatment may be medical or surgical depending on the patient's symptoms. A surgical repair is usually required if heartburn returns or episodes of bleeding occur.

Causes of a failed antireflux procedure

An error in the primary diagnosis is always a possible cause of failure of an antireflux procedure. The usual error is confusing achalasia for GORD. This occurs most commonly in patients with atypical symptoms of GORD such as asthma, cough and hoarseness. Patients with achalasia also commonly complain of respiratory symptoms, and distension of the oesophagus can produce a symptom similar to heartburn. A high degree of suspicion and a careful analysis of oesophageal motility are crucial to prevent this error. Other common causes of a poor outcome that are overlooked are:

1. failure to recognise gastric pathology causing delayed gastric emptying;
2. failure to recognise a short oesophagus or wide oesophageal hiatus;
3. failure to recognise global oesophageal dysmotility suggesting end-stage reflux disease;
4. failure to properly perform the surgical procedure.

It is important to remember that an antireflux operation differs from the simple surgical removal of a diseased organ. In the former the anatomy of an organ is rearranged to improve its function. In this situation surgical technique is paramount to a good outcome. Over time serious surgeons will perfect their antireflux procedure provided they follow their patients and tweak their technique based on analysis of their outcome. After 40 years of experience with antireflux procedures we have come to appreciate the following common errors in surgical technique that can lead to a failed repair:

1. Incomplete mobilisation of the oesophagus to obtain a 2–3 cm segment of abdominal oesophagus for a tension-free fundoplication.
2. Placing the fundoplication around the stomach instead of the oesophagus.
3. Incomplete mobilisation of the gastric fundus. Division of short gastric vessels has several advantages: first, it allows a complete mobilisation of the gastric fundus for construction of a fundoplication rather than performing a fundic wrap with only the anterior fundic wall; second, the stubs of the short gastric vessel provide a landmark for placing a stitch on the posterior fundic wall to draw it through a window between the posterior vagus nerve and the oesophagus to construct the fundoplication in the proper plane. At the completion of the fundoplication the greater curvature, identified by the location of the stubs of the short gastric vessels, remain on the left side of the abdomen in the same location they were prior to construction of the fundoplication. This approach prevents twisting of the fundoplication and stomach.
4. Incomplete crural closure or strangulation of the crural muscle by tight stitches leading to crural necrosis. Synthetic mesh used to reinforce the crural closure can become contaminated and erode into the stomach or oesophagus. If reinforcement is necessary use absorbable biological material.
5. Failure to use a bougie or using one with a diameter less than 60F to calibrate the fundoplication can result in a tight fundoplication and subsequent dysphagia.

The predominant factor in performing a redo operation once the cause of failure has been determined and a redo procedure is in order is to have a proven systematic operative approach so that the redo Nissen fundoplication will last a lifetime. The success of a third repair is less than 50% and the probability of an oesophagectomy to restore swallowing increases proportionally. The systematic steps we have perfected over 40 years of experience are as follows:

1. Mobilise the distal half of the oesophagus to obtain a comfortable abdominal oesophageal length of 2–3 cm in order to perform a tension-free fundoplication. If after mobilisation it is not possible to achieve a comfortable 2–3 cm of abdominal oesophagus a Collis gastroplasty should be performed provided there is adequate blood supply to the gastroplasty tube.
2. Partially close the diaphragmatic hiatus with 2-0 permanent sutures using figure-of-eight stitches. Make sure the crural stitches are not too tight. We prefer to tie the crural stitches to approximate the right and left crus without undue tension and place the knot squarely on the crural muscle. Complete the crural closure after removal of a 60F bougie used to size the fundoplication, since the passage of the bougie after crural closure may disrupt the stitches around the hiatal opening.
3. Divide and ligate the short gastric vessels along the upper third of the greater curvature to free the fundus. Place a draw stitch on the posterior wall of the stomach 6 cm down the greater curvature from the gastro-oesophageal junction and 2 cm in from the greater curvature on the posterior fundic wall.
4. Gently dissect and isolate the posterior vagus nerve from the oesophagus. Pull the tail of the draw stitch followed by the posterior lip of the fundoplication through the window between posterior vagus nerve and oesophagus. Grasp the anterior fundic wall and pull it to the right over the anterior surface of the oesophagus.
5. Pass a 60 French bougie to size the fundoplication.
6. Use 2-0 non-absorbable prolene suture with generous bites to construct the fundoplication. The prolene suture pulls smoothly through tissue and avoids forming a haematoma. Place the fundoplication in the right anterolateral position to keep the stomach in its normal plane. Use pledgetted stitches to avoid early disruption of the repair from unexpected gastric distension. Add well-oiled 2-0 silk stitches cranial and caudal to the fundoplication to give it a length of 1.5–2 cm.

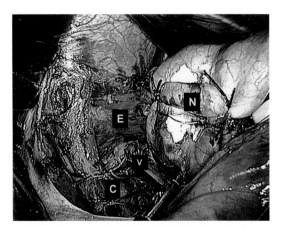

Figure 14.9 • C, crural closure; E, oesophagus;
N, Nissen fundoplication; v, posterior (right) vagus nerve.

7. Remove the 60 French bougie, retract the
complete fundoplication to the left and finish
the closure of the hiatus (**Fig. 14.9**). These
operative tips are summarised in Box 14.1.

End-stage gastro-oesophageal reflux disease

Chronic exposure of oesophageal mucosa to bile
and gastric juice produces irreversible damage
manifested by long segments of Barrett's oesophagus, global ineffective oesophageal motility and/or
strictures that gradually become refractory to therapy from repetitive dilatation. These patients have
end-stage reflux disease. They commonly have a
mechanically defective lower oesophageal sphincter, extensive injury to the oesophageal mucosa
and musculature, a long history of acid suppression therapy and/or multiple unsuccessful antireflux
operations. They are amongst the most challenging patients to manage and their treatment requires
careful and thoughtful assessment.

These patients often complain of dysphagia,
position-dependent regurgitation, and persistent bronchitis and/or repetitive pneumonia from
aspiration. A total fundoplication in the presence of global oesophageal dysmotility can stop
gastro-oesophageal reflux but may augment their
dysphagia, resulting in severe postoperative regurgitation and aspiration. A partial fundoplication
may not augment their dysphagia but provide
ineffective control of reflux with continued injury
to an already damaged oesophagus. Prior to surgical therapy oesophageal clearance should be
assessed with a video barium swallow and oesophageal motility. In patients with normal oesophageal motility, the surgeon should make efforts to

Box 14.1 • Summary of operative tips to perform a
Nissen fundoplication

1. **Oesophageal mobilisation**
   a. Mobilise the distal half of the oesophagus
   b. Ensure an intra-abdominal length of 2–3 cm
2. **Diaphragmatic closure**
   a. Close the diaphragmatic hiatus with deep 2-0
   permanent figure-of-eight stitches
   b. Do not make the crural stitches too tight
   c. Finish the crural closure after removal of
   the 60 French bougie used to size the
   fundoplication
   d. Reinforce the crural closure if the crura are
   separated by >4 cm or the crura sutures are
   under tension
3. **Construction of a window between the
   posterior vagal trunk and oesophagus**
   a. Separate the posterior vagus nerve with
   gentle dissection from the oesophagus. If the
   dissection is difficult or causes bleeding then
   the surgeon is dissecting too low and around
   the stomach
4. **Reconstruction of the fundoplication**
   a. Mobilise the gastric fundus by taking down of
   the short gastric vessels over the upper third of
   the greater curvature
   b. Place the posterior lip of the fundoplication
   between the oesophagus and the posterior
   vagus nerve
   c. Construct the fundoplication over a 60 French
   bougie
   d. Place the fundoplication in the right
   anterolateral position
   e. Use 2-0 non-absorbable pledgetted stitches
   with generous bites to construct the
   fundoplication
   f. Use 2-0 silk stitches caudal and cranial to the
   pledgets to give a fundoplication of 1.5–2 cm in
   length

preserve the oesophagus. Those with destroyed
oesophageal propulsive function are unlikely to have
a reasonable outcome from an additional attempt
at an antireflux procedure and an oesophagectomy
may be a better option. A global low contraction
amplitude throughout the distal half of the oesophageal body, i.e. all contractions in the distal half of
the oesophagus below 20 mmHg, is a sign of end-
stage disease. If >50% of oesophageal contractions
are above 20 mmHg and peristaltic and there is
adequate oesophageal barium clearance on the
contrast study, an attempt at a redo Nissen fundoplication can be considered. Below this threshold
it is likely the patient has end-stage reflux disease
with global oesophageal dysfunction.

Oesophagectomy is the best way to treat patients with end-stage reflux disease using, if possible, a vagal-sparing technique.[14,15] This procedure provides an effective oesophageal replacement without inducing the debilitating side-effects of vagotomy such as diarrhoea, dumping and early satiety. It has less overall complications compared to standard oesophagectomy and has an excellent functional outcome. The indications to perform a vagal-sparing oesophagectomy in patients with end-stage reflux disease are the symptoms of chronic dysphagia, regurgitation and aspiration. These patients commonly have either long-segment Barrett's oesophagus with severe oesophageal dysmotility, global ineffective oesophageal motility without Barrett's oesophagus or a refractory stricture. Oesophageal replacement is with a gastric tube of 2 cm diameter constructed along the greater curvature of the stomach. The left gastric artery is preserved to provide additional blood supply to the conduit. It is a simpler operation than a standard oesophagectomy, requires less dissection and provides a well-vascularised conduit for a reliable anastomosis to the cervical oesophagus. The technique of vagal-sparing oesophagectomy and the physiological results have been previously described.[14]

Summary

Antireflux surgery needs to be applied selectively and planned carefully. It is important to obtain a complete symptomatic assessment by reviewing in detail the patient's symptoms. A barium study is crucial to evaluate the reducibility of a hiatal hernia, oesophageal length and the clearance of swallowed barium. An oesophageal motility study is important to assess the oesophageal body function, rule out achalasia and determine the status of the lower oesophageal sphincter. Upper gastrointestinal endoscopy needs to be done by the operating surgeon to assess anatomical alteration of the oesophagus and cardia, and the degree of mucosal damage. A 24-hour oesophageal pH monitoring study is extremely important to confirm the diagnosis of GORD by the presence of increased oesophageal acid exposure. Laparoscopic Nissen fundoplication is a safe and effective operation provided it is applied selectively and correctly performed. The majority of failed antireflux surgeries are preventable by careful preoperative assessment and by performing an operation that incorporates techniques that are associated with lifelong effective repairs. Repair of a paraoesophageal hiatal hernia, an intrathoracic stomach or a redo antireflux procedure are more complicated. A redo operation should address the exact cause of failure and be performed in specialised, high-volume centres by experienced surgeons.

Key points

- The prevalence and severity of the complications of GORD are directly related to the presence of a mechanically defective lower oesophageal sphincter and an increased oesophageal exposure to both acid and bile.
- Antireflux surgery is particularly effective in managing the complications of GORD, provided the proper procedure is chosen and correctly performed.
- The only absolute way to identify a clinically significant shortened oesophagus is the inability to surgically mobilise 2–3 cm of the distal oesophagus and have it remain in the abdomen without the need for applied tension.
- A fundoplication done around a shortened oesophagus has a high failure rate due to herniation, disruption or slipping of the fundoplication.
- Paraoesophageal hiatal hernias make up less than 5% of all hiatal hernias, but account for most of the hiatal hernia complications.
- The majority of failed antireflux procedures are the result of inadequate patient selection, failure to recognise a short oesophagus or technical errors such as incomplete oesophageal mobilisation, failure to take down the short gastric vessels or inadequate closure of the oesophageal hiatus.
- Prior to performing a redo fundoplication, it is imperative to assess the integrity of the vagus nerves, especially if the patient presents with symptoms of delayed gastric emptying such as early satiety, nausea and vomiting.
- Oesophagectomy is the best way to treat patients with end-stage reflux disease using, if possible, a vagal-sparing technique.

References

1. DeMeester TR, Stein HJ. Surgical treatment of gastroesophageal reflux disease. In: Castell DO (ed.) The esophagus. Little, Brown & Co., Boston/Toronto/London. 1992; pp. 579–626.

2. Glise H, Hallerback B. Assessment of outcome after antireflux surgery. Semin Laparosc Surg 1995; 2:60–5.

3. Stein HJ, Barlow AP, DeMeester TR et al. Complications of gastroesophageal reflux disease. Role of the lower esophageal sphincter, esophageal acid and acid/alkaline exposure, and duodenogastric reflux. Ann Surg 1992; 216:35–43.

4. Spechler SJ. Complications of gastroesophageal reflux disease. In: Castell DO (ed.) The esophagus. Little, Brown & Co., Boston/Toronto/London. 1992; pp. 543–56.

5. Oh D, Hagen JA, Fein M et al. The impact of reflux composition on mucosal injury and esophageal function. J Gastrointest Surg 2006; 10(6):787–797.

6. Gastal OL, Hagen JA, Peters JH et al. Short esophagus: analysis of predictors and clinical implications. Arch Surg 1999; 134:633–6; discussion 637–8.

   This is one of the studies with the largest number of patients that has identified the predictors and the clinical implications of a short oesophagus. The study showed that the presence of a stricture was associated with oesophageal shortening sufficient to require gatroplasty.

7. Ferguson MK. Medical and surgical management of peptic esophageal strictures. Chest Surg Clin North Am 1994; 4:673–95.

8. Smith PM, Kerr GD, Cockel R et al. A comparison of omeprazole and ranitidine in the prevention of recurrence of benign esophageal stricture. Restore Investigator Group. Gastroenterology 1994; 107:1312–18.

9. Walther BS, DeMeester TR, Lafontaine E et al. Effect of paraesophageal hernia on sphincter function and its implication on surgical therapy. Am J Surg 1984; 147:111–16.

10. Ellis FH Jr., Crozier RE, Shea JA. Paraesophageal hiatus hernia. Arch Surg 1986; 121:416–20.

11. Pearson FG, Cooper JD, Ilves R et al. Massive hiatal hernia with incarceration: a report of 53 cases. Ann Thorac Surg 1983; 35:45–51.

12. Oelschlager BK, Pellegrini CA, Hunter J et al. Biologic prosthesis reduces recurrence after laparoscopic paraesophageal hernia repair: a multicenter, prospective, randomized trial. Ann Surg 2006; 244:481–90.

    This is a randomised trial designed to study the value of a biological prosthesis, small-intestinal submucosa (SIS), in laparoscopic paraesophageal hernia repair. The study concluded that buttressing the crural closure with SIS during laparoscopic paraoesophageal hernia repair reduces the likelihood of recurrence at 6 months, without mesh-related complications and side-effects.

13. Campos GMR, Peters JH, DeMeester TR et al. Multivariate analysis of the factors predicting outcome after laparoscopic Nissen fundoplication. J Gastrointest Surg 1999; 3:292–300.

14. Banki F, Mason RJ, DeMeester SR et al. Vagal-sparing esophagectomy: a more physiologic alternative. Ann Surg 2002; 236:324–35; discussion 335–6.

    This is the first study that has described the physiological result of the vagal-sparing oesophagectomy in comparison to standard gastric pull-up and colon interposition. The findings of this study make vagal-sparing oesophagectomy a particularly applicable surgical procedure for patients with end-stage benign and early-stage malignant diseases of the oesophagus. We further showed that this procedure is the ideal operation for intramucosal adenocarcinoma and Barrett's oesophagus with high-grade dysplasia (see Ref. 12).

15. Peyre CG, DeMeester SR, Rizzetto C et al. Vagal-sparing esophagectomy: the ideal operation for intramucosal adenocarcinoma and Barrett with high-grade dysplasia. Ann Surg 2007; 246:665–71; discussion 671–4.

15

Barrett's oesophagus

Richard Gillies
Ashref Tawil
Hugh Barr
Janusz Jankowski

Although columnar metaplasia of the oesophagus is commonly referred to as Barrett's oesophagus, the condition was first described by Tileston over 100 years ago.[1] In 1950, Barrett described the presence of gastric-type columnar mucosa in the distal oesophagus in combination with oesophagitis and an ulcer; however, he incorrectly believed this to be due to a congenitally short oesophagus.[2] Columnarisation of the lower oesophagus is believed to arise as a result of abnormal mucosal repair in response to chronic gastro-oesophageal reflux, and this has been demonstrated in an experimental model in dogs.[3] Three distinct types of columnar metaplasia have been identified: intestinal, cardiac and fundic. The most common type of metaplastic epithelium is intestinal and this has been identified as the precursor lesion of malignancy.

The importance of Barrett's oesophagus is clear: the incidence of adenocarcinoma of the oesophagus is increasing rapidly in the UK, especially for men, with a preponderance for tumours arising at the gastro-oesophageal junction. The UK incidence is currently 12.8 per 100 000, resulting in approximately 7600 new cases per year and making it the ninth most common cancer. The prognosis remains poor, with approximately 7400 deaths per year.[4] Barrett's oesophagus is accepted as a significant risk factor for adenocarcinoma of the oesophagus, with Barrett's patients having a 30–125-fold increased risk compared with the general population.[5] The UK has a particularly high incidence of Barrett's adenocarcinoma, two to three times that of other European countries or the USA.[6]

Definitions

It is important to clarify definitions used in describing Barrett's oesophagus as there remain differences in terminology. Barrett's oesophagus is defined as a metaplastic condition in which any portion of the normal squamous epithelium has been replaced by macroscopically visible columnar epithelium which is confirmed histologically. In the UK, the diagnosis does not require the histological identification of specialised intestinal metaplasia,[7] which is at odds with other countries, most notably the USA.[8] Although specialised intestinal metaplasia is recognised to be the malignant precursor lesion, it is not currently required for diagnosis at first endoscopy as missing this by sampling error might exclude patients from suitable surveillance programmes. It has recently been shown that a minimum of eight biopsies are required to confidently exclude intestinal metaplasia – if only four biopsies are taken the diagnostic yield is only 35%.[9]

It is important that both endoscopic and histological components of the diagnosis are met. During endoscopy vital landmarks must be identified. However, determining these measurements and the exact site of any biopsies can be difficult in a moving oesophagus, especially in the presence of a hiatus hernia. Studies have shown great inter- and intra-observer variation in the measured length of a Barrett's segment.[10] In an attempt to facilitate the diagnosis of Barrett's oesophagus and standardise the measurement of its extent, the Prague C & M criteria were developed.[11] The gastro-oesophageal junction is most practically defined as the proximal limit of the gastric mucosal folds: it is important that this is determined with minimal air insufflation as overinflation will flatten and obscure the gastric folds. The squamocolumnar junction is visible as the pale squamous epithelium merges into redder columnar mucosa. If the squamocolumnar junction is proximal to the gastro-oesophageal junction, biopsies should be taken from this area to confirm columnar metaplasia or Barrett's oesophagus. The circumferential extent (C value) and the maximum extent (M value) of columnar mucosa above the gastro-oesophageal junction should be recorded. These criteria have been shown to have a high degree of reliability between different endoscopists. The use of the terms long-segment Barrett's (>3 cm) and short-segment Barrett's (<3 cm) should now be discouraged.

Occasionally, biopsies will be histologically diagnostic for Barrett's oesophagus in that they contain a native oesophageal gland or, more usually, a duct from these glands in close juxtaposition to metaplastic mucosa. However, the superficial nature of most biopsies makes this unusual. More frequently, columnar epithelium is recognisable but must be correlated with confirmation of the biopsy location as intestinal-type mucosa may be found at the cardia or the stomach within a hiatus hernia and gastric- and fundic-type mucosa at the oesophagogastric junction or within the stomach. Histologically, these biopsies can only be said to be corroborative of an endoscopic diagnosis of Barrett's.

The development of adenocarcinoma in Barrett's oesophagus is thought to follow a progressive sequence from intestinal metaplasia to low-grade dysplasia (LGD) to high-grade dysplasia (HGD) and finally to cancer[12] (see **Fig. 15.1**). The presence of dysplasia is regarded as the best marker for malignant transformation in the epithelium. Dysplasia is classified histologically into low and high grade; when dysplasia cannot be clearly differentiated from the reactive or regenerative changes associated with inflammation, the term 'indefinite for dysplasia' should be used. This classification is a modification of histopathological classifications used in the rest of the gastrointestinal tract, most notably for colonic dysplasia associated with inflammatory bowel disease.[13] HGD is diagnosed when there are distinct cytological changes, particularly nuclear pleomorphism and loss of crypt architecture. LGD is more difficult to classify: there is loss of cellular differentiation and loss of goblet cells but with milder changes than those seen in HGD. Intramucosal cancer is said to have occurred when there is invasion through the basement membrane into the lamina propria. The term carcinoma in situ has been abandoned.

Pathophysiology

It is currently believed that Barrett's metaplasia develops as a mucosal 'adaptive' response to increased cell loss as a result of chronic inflammation, secondary to gastro-oesophageal reflux disease. Oesophageal squamous epithelium is highly sensitive to acid, alkaline and biliary reflux, which all cause inflammation, with cell loss, necrosis and ulceration. A recent study has provided strong evidence that the site of origin of Barrett's metaplasia is a progenitor stem cell located in the submucosal oesophageal gland

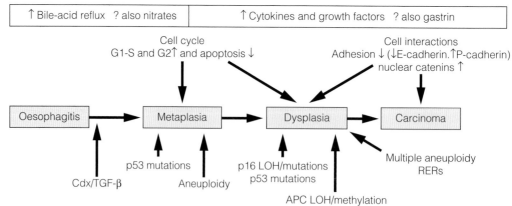

Figure 15.1 • The metaplasia–dysplasia–adenocarcinoma sequence. There are histological stages of progression (orange rectangles with coloured dots representing the clonal expansion of competing stem cells). In addition there are structural genetic changes in the form of mutations (vertical white arrows) and environmental changes (hollow white-edged rectangles) driving cell cycle and cell adhesion biological sequelae. Adapted from Jankowski J, Harrison RF, Perry I et al. Barrett's metaplasia. Lancet 2000; 356:2079–85.[15] With permission from Elsevier.
Cdx = CauDal protein gene; TGF-β = transforming growth factor-β; LOH = loss of heterozygosity; APC = adenomatous polyposis coli gene; RERs = random errors of replication.

ducts by demonstrating that a *p16* point mutation originating in microdissected squamous duct tissue was also present in adjoining metaplastic crypts.[14] Duodenal and gastric reflux-induced ulceration and inflammation is believed to induce tumour suppressor gene mutations, typically *p53* and *p16*, in some of the stem cell populations located in oesophageal gland squamous ducts which are present throughout the entire length of the oesophagus. Following this initiation phase multiple distinct clones of metaplastic tissue compete to colonise the oesophagus, creating a mosaic pattern of clones across the segment. Clonal expansion of populations with greater selective advantage, such as ability to survive in a markedly acid- or bile-rich environment, leads to dominant and widespread clones. Once initiated, the promotion and propagation of metaplastic clones is dependent on the surrounding microenvironment, particularly the presence of a chronic inflammatory cell infiltrate, characterised by T lymphocytes, and cytokines such as interleukin-1, tumour necrosis factor-α and transforming growth factor-β. These lead to an increase in cyclo-oxygenase-2, c-*myc* and cyclin D1, which increase proliferation and decrease apoptosis, and a reduction in E-cadherin, with resultant loss of cell adhesion and localisation of β-catenin to the nucleus[15] (see Fig. 15.1).

Although traditionally thought of as an acquired condition, genetic factors may play a part in a small proportion of Barrett's metaplasia as family and twin studies suggest a small subgroup of patients have a strong familial tendency to Barrett's oesophagus. However, no candidate genes have yet been definitely identified and inheritance is likely to be complex.[16]

Epidemiology

The exact prevalence of Barrett's oesophagus is unclear. Data obtained at post-mortem suggest it may be as high as 5%.[17] The incidence in unselected patients undergoing endoscopy is approximately 1%,[18] but in patients with symptoms of gastro-oesophageal reflux disease the incidence is much higher at 12%.[19] There is some evidence that the prevalence in the UK may be increasing[20] and a recent study in the Netherlands demonstrated an increase in the number of cases of Barrett's oesophagus despite a decrease in the number of endoscopies being performed over the same period, suggesting a true increase in incidence.[21] There is an increase in incidence with age, the mean age at diagnosis being approximately 62 years for men and 68 years for women, and it is more common in men than in women, with a ratio of approximately 1.7:1.[22] It predominantly affects Caucasians.[23] Early onset, increased frequency and long duration of reflux symptoms are associated with a higher risk of Barrett's oesophagus.[24]

This appears to correlate with the well-known association between increased frequency, duration and severity of reflux symptoms and increased risk of adenocarcinoma of the oesophagus.[25]

This has been clearly demonstrated in a Swedish case–control study. Patients with recurrent reflux symptoms when compared with asymptomatic patients had an odds ratio of 7.7 for oesophageal adenocarcinoma and 2 for adenocarcinoma of the gastric cardia. Patients with severe longstanding symptoms had an odds ratio of 43.5 and 4.4 for oesophageal and cardia adenocarcinoma respectively.[25]

Obesity and cigarette smoking have also been identified as risk factors.[26] The evidence regarding an association between mucosal damage such as ulceration or stricture formation and Barrett's oesophagus is conflicting.[24,27]

It is important to appreciate that a significant proportion of patients with Barrett's oesophagus are asymptomatic: the metaplastic columnar mucosa is less sensitive to further injury, resulting in patients with Barrett's being less aware of acid reflux than patients with uncomplicated reflux disease.[28] Gerson et al. attempted to determine the incidence of asymptomatic Barrett's in a population of patients attending for sigmoidoscopy to detect colorectal cancer: 110 patients with either no symptoms of reflux or infrequent symptoms underwent upper gastrointestinal endoscopy; patients with symptoms of gastro-oesophageal reflux disease occurring more than once a month, receiving therapy for the disease, or giving a history of previous endoscopy were excluded. Eight patients (7%) were found to have long-segment Barrett's oesophagus and 19 (17%) had short-segment disease, leading them to conclude that 25% of asymptomatic male veterans older than 50 had detectable Barrett's oesophagus.[29] This study has yet to be reproduced and most readers believe this to be related to a biased population attending the VA clinics. From the ProGERD study it is clear that progression to Barrett's oesophagus is very slow and few patients even with severe reflux do progress.[30]

Risk of cancer and mortality in Barrett's oesophagus

A large number of studies have estimated the risk of adenocarcinoma arising from Barrett's oesophagus, with variable results[31–40] (see Table 15.1). Concern has been expressed about the possibility of publication bias, with small studies only being published if they show a high incidence of cancer, leading to an overestimate of risk.[41] However, there appears

Table 15.1 • Studies reporting the incidence of adenocarcinoma in Barrett's oesophagus

Reference	Patients	Mean follow-up (years)	Total follow-up (patient years)	Risk (per patient year)
Robertson et al. (1988)[31]	56	2.9	168	1:56
Miros et al. (1991)[32]	81	3.6	289	1:96
Iftikhar et al. (1992)[33]	102	4.5	462	1:115
Wright et al. (1996)[34]	166	2.7	294 male	1:59
		2.9	167 female	1:167
Drewitz et al. (1997)[35]	177	4.8	834	1:208
Katz et al. (1998)[36]	102	5.0	563	1:188
Weston et al. (1999)[37]	108	3.3	362	1:72
Conio et al. (2003)[38]	166	5.5	1100	1:220
Hage et al. (2004)[39]	105	12.7	1329	1:221
Oberg et al. (2005)[40]	140	5.8	946	1:315

to be a real geographical variation in the incidence of carcinoma arising in Barrett's oesophagus in Western countries, with incidence rates in the UK and USA of approximately 1% and 0.5% per year respectively.[6]

It is important to appreciate that while patients with Barrett's oesophagus have an increased relative risk of adenocarcinoma, the majority of patients will die from other causes. A recent UK study demonstrated an increase in both overall mortality rate and oesophageal cancer mortality rate in Barrett's patients compared with the age- and sex-matched general population. However, only 10% of deaths were due to oesophageal cancer, while 49% were due to cardiorespiratory disease, especially ischaemic heart disease and bronchopneumonia, and 18% of deaths were due to other cancers.[42]

Natural history of dysplasia in Barrett's oesophagus

According to a recent systematic review involving a total of 1488 patients with Barrett's oesophagus, LGD was present at initial endoscopy in 169 patients (11%) and HGD in 18 patients (1.2%); 1301 (87%) had metaplasia with no dysplasia.[43]

The progression of Barrett's oesophagus from metaplasia to dysplasia has been reported to occur in 5–23% of patients undergoing surveillance. Miros et al. reported 10 out of 81 patients developing new LGD after mean follow-up of 3.6 years,[32] Katz et al. reported 19 new LGD and four new HGD cases out of 102 patients followed for 5 years,[36] and Weston et al. reported five new HGD cases out of 108 patients followed for a mean of 3.3 years.[37]

Low-grade dysplasia

A number of studies have reported on the natural history of LGD. Reid et al. followed 20 patients with LGD for a mean of 34 months and found that five patients developed either HGD or cancer, while 15 patients either regressed to Barrett's metaplasia without dysplasia (BM) or remained stable with LGD.[44] In a study of 25 patients with LGD, Skacel et al. reported that seven patients progressed to either HGD or cancer, while 18 patients either regressed to BM or remained stable after a mean follow-up of 26 months.[45] Weston et al. reported progression to HGD or cancer in 5 of 48 patients after a mean follow-up of 41 months, while 43 patients either regressed or remained stable.[46] More recently, Lim et al. reported progression to HGD or cancer in 9 of 34 patients after at least 8 years of follow-up, while three patients remained stable with LGD.[47] The largest study to date followed 156 patients for a mean of 4.1 years and reported progression to HGD or cancer in 13%, regression in 66% and stable LGD in 21%.[48]

While the natural history of LGD is still not fully understood, particularly in terms of time required to progress to HGD or cancer, it appears clear that the majority of patients with LGD will either remain stable or regress to BM. The risk of progression from LGD to HGD or cancer is between 10% and 28%.

High-grade dysplasia

Studies reporting the natural history of HGD have produced widely different results. Reid et al. followed 76 patients for 5 years and reported that

59% developed adenocarcinoma.[49] A study of 79 patients by Schnell et al. is particularly important because it reported that four patients had carcinoma detected during rigorous biopsies in the first year of surveillance, representing prevalent carcinoma: the subsequent incidence of carcinoma in the remaining 75 patients after a mean of 7 years was 15%.[50] In a study of 100 patients with HGD, 66 of whom underwent surveillance, 3 of 24 patients (13%) with focal HGD and 17 of 42 patients (40%) with diffuse HGD developed carcinoma after a mean follow-up of 41 and 23 months respectively.[51]

When considering the natural history of dysplasia in Barrett's oesophagus we must remember that in addition to potential problems with length of follow-up and sampling error at endoscopy, there is considerable inter- and intra-observer variation among experienced pathologists in the histological diagnosis of dysplastic Barrett's oesophagus. While pathologists can demonstrate acceptable levels of agreement in distinguishing HGD combined with carcinoma from no dysplasia combined with indefinite and low-grade dysplasia (kappa values of 0.8), there are much poorer levels of agreement in distinguishing between the four groups of no dysplasia, low-grade dysplasia combined with indefinite for dysplasia, high-grade dysplasia, and carcinoma (intra-observer kappa values of 0.64, inter-observer kappa values of 0.43).[52] It appears that pathologists find it difficult to separate inflammation in Barrett's oesophagus from LGD. In this situation pathologists should be encouraged to make use of the indefinite for dysplasia category: such a diagnosis does not mean that the pathologist is uncertain, but rather that it is not possible, with confidence, to exclude LGD in inflamed material. The diagnosis of HGD has serious implications for patient management and the diagnosis should be confirmed by two expert pathologists.

An important question to consider is what proportion of patients with a diagnosis of HGD who undergo oesophagectomy have an occult cancer detected in the resected specimen? Table 15.2 shows reported rates in the literature of 0–73%: overall the rate appears to be approximately 40%.[53-66] This emphasises the fact that patients thought to have HGD may in fact be harbouring an undetected cancer and confirms the importance of using strict biopsy protocols in patients with dysplasia. Levine et al. were able to correctly distinguish between HGD and carcinoma in 26 of 28 patients prior to surgery by using a rigorous biopsy protocol with a large channel endoscope and 9-mm open-span biopsy forceps (Olympus FB13K) used with a 'turn-and-suction' technique to maximise the mucosal biopsy size.[56] Samples must be taken from all areas of mucosal abnormality and any areas where HGD has been identified previously. All four quadrants of the oesophagus are also biopsied at 2-cm intervals. A large number of samples should be taken, up to 84 per patient in the study described above.

Table 15.2 • Studies reporting the incidence of adenocarcinoma in resected specimens following oesophagectomy for high-grade dysplasia

Reference	Patients with high-grade dysplasia	Invasive cancer at postoperative histology	Percentage
Altorki et al. (1991)[53]	8	4	50
Pera et al. (1992)[54]	18	9	50
Steitz et al. (1993)[55]	9	2	22
Levine et al. (1993)[56]	7	0	0
Peters et al. (1994)[57]	9	5	56
Edwards et al. (1996)[58]	11	8	73
Rice et al. (1997)[59]	16	6	38
Collard et al. (1997)[60]	12	4	33
Ferguson and Naunheim (1997)[61]	15	8	53
Cameron and Carpenter (1997)[62]	19	2	11
Falk et al. (1999)[63]	28	10	36
Headrick et al. (2002)[64]	54	19	35
Tseng et al. (2003)[65]	60	18	30
Sujendran et al. (2005)[66]	17	11	65
Total	**283**	**106**	**37**

Although some HGD may be stable or even regress, between 15% and 59% will progress to adenocarcinoma. If detailed biopsy mapping endoscopies showed no previous HGD (prevalent HGD), then the detection of new HGD (incident HGD) is associated with a risk of subsequent progression to cancer of only between 3% and 5% per year.[50,67]

Risk factors for progression to cancer

The length of the Barrett's segment has been shown to be a significant risk factor for progression to cancer, a doubling of length increasing the risk 1.7-fold.[68] Interestingly, while the extent of HGD appears to be a risk factor for progression to cancer,[51] it has not been shown to predict the presence of unsuspected carcinoma at oesophagectomy.[69] Recently, it has been suggested that the extent of LGD may also be a risk factor for progression to adenocarcinoma.[70]

Importantly, in a prospective longitudinal cohort study, individuals with Barrett's oesophagus who were regularly taking aspirin or other non-steroidal anti-inflammatory drugs (NSAIDs) were found to have a significantly lower 5-year cumulative incidence of adenocarcinoma compared with individuals not taking NSAIDs (6.6% and 14.3% respectively), suggesting that this may be an effective chemotherapeutic intervention.[71] To test this hypothesis, an ongoing large phase III multicentre randomised controlled trial has already recruited 1600 patients (aiming for 2500) – the AspECT trial (Aspirin and Esomeprazole Chemoprevention in Barrett's Metaplasia) is due to finish in 2016. The primary aim of this study is to determine whether acid suppression with proton-pump inhibition (high dose versus low dose) with or without aspirin can reduce mortality or the conversion from Barrett's metaplasia to HGD or adenocarcinoma. Both high- and low-dose acid suppression are being investigated as there remains doubt about the optimal dose of proton-pump inhibitor (PPI) to use, especially given the fact that Barrett's mucosa is relatively insensitive, thus rendering symptoms unreliable. There is an argument that incomplete acid suppression might increase the risk of cancer by exposing the mucosa to short pulses of acid, thus stimulating the proliferation of abnormal cells. In contrast, there is some epidemiological evidence that high-dose proton-pump inhibition might increase the risk of cancer as bile acid might become cytotoxic at neutral pH. Additionally, it is hoped that the trial may confirm whether aspirin is anticarcinogenic (oesophageal, gastric and colorectal) as well as cardioprotective, especially in patients with Barrett's who are at high risk of developing cardiac events. Early results from

this study, awaiting publication, confirm the previous observation that there is poor adherence to current guidelines among specialists (90%) in taking an appropriate amount of biopsies, mainly because of a perceived lack of strong evidence. Barrett's patients from centres involved in the AspECT trial have 37% more biopsies taken and adherence to guidelines is significantly greater.[72] Additionally, there is a trend to early referral of patients with HGD for surgical treatment (74%).[72]

 AspECT is the world's largest Barrett's randomised controlled trial and aims to decrease cancer conversion by 35% and cardiac deaths by 20%. The premise is that the shared cardiac and cancer comorbid factors mean that joint cardiac and chemoprevention is the best way to prevent premature death.

Molecular markers of increased risk

Due to the difficulties with the histological diagnosis of dysplasia and uncertainty about its natural history, attempts have been made to identify biological markers which signify increased cancer risk. Mutations in the *p53* tumour suppressor gene have been recognised in Barrett's oesophagus and oesophageal cancer. Younes et al. found *p53* mutation in 9% of Barrett's patients with LGD, 55% of patients with HGD and 87% of patients with carcinoma: no patients without dysplasia had a *p53* mutation.[73] Importantly, in a further study, 56% of patients with LGD and *p53* mutation progressed to HGD or carcinoma, whereas no patient with LGD without *p53* mutation progressed.[74] Similarly, Reid et al. demonstrated that loss of heterozygosity of gene 17 (*p53*) was found in 6% of patients without dysplasia, 20% of patients with LGD and 57% of patients with HGD.[75] Patients with loss of heterozygosity had a 16-fold increased risk of cancer after 3 years. These results have led to the suggestion that the subgroup of patients with low-grade or indefinite dysplasia and *p53* mutation should be subjected to more rigorous surveillance protocols. However, it is important to remember that not all oesophageal adenocarcinomas express *p53*, and patients without expression can progress to cancer.

Other markers which have been identified as conferring a high risk of progression are *p16* mutations,[76] cyclin D1 overexpression,[77] flow cytometry abnormalities such as aneuploidy and increase in the G2/tetraploidy fraction of DNA content,[78] and reduced expression of E-cadherin, with resultant loss of cell adhesion and localisation of β-catenin to the nucleus.[79] While these abnormalities may show some promise, the translation of potential biomarkers into useful predictive tools has been uncoordinated and not subject to large-scale clinical trials; therefore, they have no place in clinical practice at present.[80]

 There are currently no validated biomarkers of prognostic evaluation of Barrett's metaplasia ready for clinical use other than the presence or absence of dysplasia, especially HGD, as determined by histopathological assessment.

Effect of medical therapy and antireflux surgery

It has been shown that long-term acid suppression with PPIs can lead to an improvement in Barrett's metaplasia. A study of 23 patients following a regimen of omeprazole 40 mg daily for 2 years demonstrated a significant reduction in the length of columnar mucosa, an increase in squamous islands within the columnar epithelium and a reduction in the proportion of sulphomucin-rich intestinal metaplasia.[81] More recently a study of 188 patients followed for up to 13 years (mean 5 years) reported development of squamous islands in 48% of patients, although the mean length of Barrett's segment was not reduced and no patients regressed to squamous mucosa.[82]

 A randomised double-blind trial of omeprazole 80 mg daily versus ranitidine 300 mg daily in patients with proven Barrett's oesophagus and gastro-oesophageal reflux disease demonstrated a reduction in the length and surface area of columnar metaplasia in the omeprazole group but not in the ranitidine group, despite both treatments successfully controlling reflux symptoms.[83]

The effect of antireflux surgery on Barrett's metaplasia has proved a controversial subject. In a study of 56 patients, 9% underwent a complete regression to squamous mucosa and 34% a partial regression with a reduction in the length of Barrett's segment and the development of squamous islands; 16%, however, had an increase in the length of segment and 41% remained stable.[84] More recently, O'Riordan et al. demonstrated complete or partial regression of columnar metaplasia in 35% of patients 45 months after antireflux surgery, while 11% had an increase in the length of segment and 54% remained unchanged.[85] A randomised controlled trial of medical therapy versus antireflux surgery in 59 patients reported an increased length of

Barrett's segment in 40% of the medical group compared with 9% of the surgery group and a reduction in the length of segment in 7% of the medical group compared with 25% of the surgical group; 52% of the medical group and 66% of the surgical group remained unchanged.[86] Six patients (22%) in the medical group developed new dysplasia compared with just one in the surgery group (3%). It is important to note that not all patients in the medical group were treated with PPIs.

Perhaps the most important question is whether acid suppression with medical therapy or antireflux surgery can reduce the risk of progression to dysplasia and adenocarcinoma. In their study of Barrett's patients taking PPIs for a total of 966 treatment years, Cooper et al. reported 3% of patients developing new dysplasia and 1.6% developing adenocarcinoma after an interval of between 3 and 9 years of treatment: of the four patients who progressed to HGD or cancer, three were taking high-dose PPIs.[82] This equates to 1 case of cancer per 322 years of treatment or an incidence of 0.31%, significantly less than the incidence for the UK Barrett's population as a whole.[6]

In their study of 57 patients who underwent antireflux surgery, O'Riordan et al. reported that 6 of 8 patients with LGD prior to surgery regressed to BM with no dysplasia; however, two patients developed new LGD after surgery (4%) and two developed adenocarcinoma (4%) after an interval of 4 and 7 years.[85] Similarly, a study of 112 patients reported development of cancer in three patients (2.7%) at 13, 25 and 39 months after surgery.[87] Another large study of 161 patients reported the development of new dysplasia in 17 patients (10.5%) at a mean of 8 years after surgery and carcinoma in four patients (2.5%) 6 years after surgery.[88] It appears that the development of cancer in Barrett's patients after antireflux surgery is associated with failure of acid suppression but not necessarily development of symptoms.[85,87,88] It is important to remember that symptom relief is not a reliable indicator of acid suppression in Barrett's oesophagus.[89]

 A meta-analysis comparing the reported incidence of adenocarcinoma in Barrett's patients after antireflux surgery with patients treated medically found no statistically significant difference in the incidence rates of 3.8 and 5.3 per 1000 patient years respectively.[90] A recent systematic review reported a statistically significant lower incidence of adenocarcinoma after antireflux surgery compared with medical therapy (2.8 vs. 6.3 per 1000 patient years, $P = 0.03$); however, when uncontrolled case series were excluded and the analysis was confined to randomised trials and cohort studies there was no significant difference between the two treatments (4.4 vs. 6.5 per 1000 patient years, $P = 0.32$).[43] Accordingly, at present there is insufficient evidence to recommend antireflux surgery over proton-pump inhibition as a cancer-preventing procedure.

Screening for Barrett's oesophagus and adenocarcinoma

It is accepted that gastro-oesophageal reflux disease is a significant risk factor for the development of adenocarcinoma, with the well-known Swedish case–control study demonstrating a 44-fold increased relative risk in individuals with frequent heartburn of greater than 20 years duration.[25] This has led to the suggestion that screening individuals with chronic reflux symptoms to detect Barrett's oesophagus and cancer may be of benefit. However, it is important to appreciate two flaws in this concept: firstly, approximately 40% of individuals with cancer in the series mentioned above denied frequent heartburn; secondly, a significant proportion of individuals with Barrett's oesophagus are asymptomatic. In addition, Barrett's cases experience less symptoms of heartburn and use PPIs less frequently, compared with controls.[91,92]

The screening of individuals with chronic reflux symptoms to detect either Barrett's or cancer is not currently recommended in the UK.[93] This is because of the low absolute risk of developing adenocarcinoma in individuals with chronic reflux, combined with the knowledge that most individuals with Barrett's oesophagus die from causes other than oesophageal cancer. There are also concerns about the cost-effectiveness and invasiveness of endoscopy as a screening tool.

Surveillance and current guidelines for the management of dysplasia

The central concept of surveillance is that regular endoscopic examination and biopsy will allow the detection of cancer at an earlier stage than for symptomatic cancer, thereby resulting in better treatment outcomes. Several small series have shown better survival rates associated with surveillance-detected cancers than with non-surveillance-detected cancers.[54,55,57,94,95] However, it is possible that these non-randomised studies are affected by selection bias and length bias. In this regard the Barrett's Oesophagus

Surveillance Study (BOSS) will randomise patients with at least 1 cm Barrett's oesophagus to either surveillance ($n = 1250$) or telephone questionnaire only ($n = 1250$), the latter group being discharged unless they develop new symptoms or alarm symptoms. Clearly, surveillance is only appropriate for patients who are suitable for treatment of detected lesions, either HGD or cancer, and traditionally, as this was limited to oesophagectomy, this meant that individuals had to be of a relatively young age and lacking in any significant comorbidity. However, with the development of endoscopic techniques for mucosal ablation and resection the number of patients for whom surveillance is appropriate may increase.

There are a number of disadvantages and limitations to surveillance programmes. In addition to the physical and psychological burden imposed on patients, it must be remembered, and communicated to patients at enrolment, that surveillance does not guarantee to detect all cancers or to offer a cure for all detected cancers. The fundamental limitation of surveillance endoscopy to detect cancer is easy to appreciate when we consider that for a 2-cm-long segment of Barrett's, with a surface area of 13 cm², obtaining quadrantic biopsies results in only 3.5% of the surface area being sampled.[96] It is possible that, in the future, more advanced endoscopic imaging techniques may allow targeted biopsies from high-risk areas, thereby improving the yield over current random biopsies[97–101] (see Table 15.3).

 Current UK guidelines suggest that individuals with Barrett's oesophagus without dysplasia should undergo surveillance endoscopy every 2 years – this is based on a computer mathematical model and assumes the risk of developing adenocarcinoma in Barrett's oesophagus to be approximately 1% per annum.[93]

Biopsies should be taken from all four quadrants of the oesophagus at 2-cm intervals in addition to any areas of mucosal abnormality. As previously stated, at least eight biopsies are required to confidently diagnose Barrett's oesophagus.[9] Currently, the use of jumbo biopsy forceps is not recommended routinely.

The detection of LGD should lead to a course of high-dose acid suppression with a PPI for 8–12 weeks followed by repeat endoscopy with extensive biopsies. If LGD persists then surveillance endoscopy should be repeated at 6-monthly intervals and the patient should remain on a PPI. If regression to metaplasia without dysplasia occurs on two consecutive examinations then the surveillance interval may return to 2-yearly.

Individuals with biopsies reported as indefinite for dysplasia should also undergo extensive re-biopsy after an 8- to 12-week course of high-dose acid

Table 15.3 • Advanced endoscopic imaging modalities being investigated for use in Barrett's oesophagus surveillance programmes

Imaging modality	Concept	Reference
White light endoscopy		
High-resolution magnification endoscopy (HRME)	Greater magnification and resolution than normal endoscopy allowing more detailed visualisation of the mucosa	Sharma et al. (2003)[97]
Chromoendoscopy	Topical application of dyes improves visualisation of mucosal surfaces. Examples: methylene blue – absorbed with different patterns into different types of mucosa; indigo carmine – accumulates in mucosal fissures accentuating surface topography	Canto et al. (1996)[98]
Optical endoscopy		
Autofluorescence imaging (AFI)	Short-wavelength light causes excitation of endogenous biological tissues with subsequent release of longer wavelength fluorescent light	Kara et al. (2005)[99]
Narrow-band imaging (NBI)	Narrow-bandwidth green and blue light (with exclusion of red light) only superficially penetrates mucosa, improving visualisation of mucosal microvasculature and surface morphology	Gono et al. (2004)[100]
Trimodal imaging	Incorporates HRME, AFI and NBI in a single endoscope with ability to switch between modalities during procedure	Curvers et al. (2008)[101]

suppression. If this and a subsequent examination at 6 months fail to demonstrate dysplasia then surveillance may return to 2-yearly intervals.

The detection of HGD has serious implications for the patient. The diagnosis should always be confirmed by a second expert pathologist and if there is any doubt then a repeat examination with extensive re-biopsy should be undertaken without delay. The diagnosis of HGD is usually an indication to end surveillance and ideally all cases should be discussed in a multidisciplinary meeting with appropriate expertise in both surgical and endoscopic treatments, as well as histopathology. In a small minority of cases, some individuals may wish to continue with a 'watch-and-wait' policy until cancer is definitely detected, although the risk of this policy – namely the presence of undetected occult cancer – should be clearly communicated to the patient. In these circumstances, extensive biopsies should be obtained at 3-monthly intervals.

The management of HGD is a controversial subject in oesophageal surgery.[102] Traditionally, individuals who were fit enough were recommended to undergo oesophagectomy while endoscopic techniques were reserved for those unfit for resection. However, with increasing experience of endoscopic techniques many centres are now advocating their use as an alternative to oesophagectomy in patients who are fit enough for resection (see Chapter 6).

Endotherapy for Barrett's oesophagus

Endotherapy, including endoscopic mucosal resection (EMR) and ablative techniques, may be used alone or in combination with acid-reducing therapies.[103] These therapies potentially offer an attractive alternative to radical surgery in terms of reduced mortality and morbidity, but their long-term efficacy is unclear.[72] Of most concern, the subsequent development of cancer and cancer-related deaths have been reported in some series.

EMR techniques have been described which remove the entire circumference of Barrett's,[104,105] but there is a high rate of post-treatment stricture formation with this approach. In general, EMR appears to be a safe technique and most complications, including perforation, can be managed endoscopically.[105] It offers an advantage over ablative techniques in that removing an entire area of HGD and adjacent BM provides a histological specimen and eliminates some of the interpretive difficulties with conventional endoscopic biopsies, such as the inability to see mucularis mucosa.[105]

Endoscopic ablation techniques include thermal methods, such as argon-beam plasma photocoagulation (APC),[106] multipolar electrocautery (MPEC),[107] laser therapy and cryotherapy;[108] chemical methods, such as photodynamic therapy (PDT);[109] and radio-frequency (RF) ablation, such as the Barrx technique.[110] A randomised controlled trial comparing two thermal techniques, MPEC and APC, found no significant advantage with either technique over the other.[111] There are some concerns with these techniques, including stricture formation and incomplete ablation, and in particular 'buried' glandular mucosa beneath the neosquamous epithelium. The RF ablation technique may result in less 'buried glands' under the neosquamous epithelium as tissue is ablated to the level of the submucosa,[110] equivalent to the level of EMR – however, this is not as deep as PDT, which can reach as far as the muscularis propria. Recently there have been encouraging results from uncontrolled studies using the RF technique, with successful removal of over 90% of BM combined with minimal complications (<5%).[112]

It is unclear whether radical endotherapy that combines EMR with an ablative technique and is aimed at eradication of the entire Barrett's segment reduces the likelihood of either metachronous lesions or of recurrent dysplasia or cancer. Nevertheless, such an approach is advocated by some specialist centres.[72] Ultimately, these newer endoscopic therapies need to be tested against established surgery for HGD in randomised trials such as proposed by specialist centres in the UK.

Conclusion

In the last 5 years we have come a considerable way in the improved understanding and treatment of Barrett's oesophagus. We understand that histology when carried out correctly with intensive mapping, despite its obvious flaws, is a reasonable tool to detect premalignant cells in the majority of cases. Furthermore we have two strategies for the prevention of cancer, namely chemoprevention and surveillance, that are being tested in two of the world's largest randomised trials. Finally, we also now have excellent minimally invasive endoscopic therapies that need to be tested against the gold standard of oesophagectomy by surgical experts.

Key points

- The incidence of Barrett's adenocarcinoma is increasing and is especially high in the UK.
- The exact prevalence of Barrett's oesophagus is unclear – it may be present in up to 5% of the population. Most patients with Barrett's oesophagus are undetected in the community.
- Barrett's metaplasia develops as a mucosal 'adaptive' response as a result of chronic inflammation, secondary to gastro-oesophageal reflux disease. A recent study has provided strong evidence that the site of origin of Barrett's metaplasia is a progenitor stem cell located in the submucosal oesophageal gland ducts.
- The development of adenocarcinoma in Barrett's oesophagus is thought to follow a progressive sequence from intestinal metaplasia to low-grade dysplasia (LGD) to high-grade dysplasia (HGD) and finally to cancer. The presence of dysplasia is regarded as the best marker for malignant transformation in the epithelium.
- There is considerable inter- and intra-observer variation among experienced pathologists in the histological diagnosis of dysplastic Barrett's oesophagus.
- Most Barrett's epithelium is stable and will not undergo malignant transformation.
- The AspECT cancer prevention trial is the world's largest trial in this area and aims to decrease cancer by 35%.
- A randomised double-blind study has confirmed that acid suppression with a proton-pump inhibitor induces a partial regression of the columnar-lined segment.
- At present there is insufficient evidence to recommend antireflux surgery over proton-pump inhibition as a cancer-preventing procedure.
- Patients with intestinal metaplasia should have regular surveillance endoscopy and biopsy at 2-yearly intervals and should remain on a proton-pump inhibitor.
- Patients who have a surveillance-detected cancer survive longer following surgery than patients who develop symptomatic cancers.
- The detection of HGD is an indication to end surveillance.
- New endotherapies need to be tested in randomised trials to compare their efficacy with the gold standard surgery.

References

1. Tileston W. Peptic ulcer of the oesophagus. Am J Sci 1906; 132:240–2.

2. Barrett NR. Chronic peptic ulcer of the oesophagus and 'oesophagitis'. Br J Surg 1950; 38:175–82.

3. Bremner CG, Lynch VP, Ellis FH. Barrett's esophagus: congenital or acquired? An experimental study of esophageal mucosal regeneration in the dog. Surgery 1978; 68:209–16.

4. http://info.cancerresearchuk.org/cancerstats/types/oesophagus; accessed February 2008.

5. Wild CP, Hardie LJ. Reflux, Barrett's oesophagus and adenocarcinoma: burning questions. Natl Rev Cancer 2003; 3:676–84.

6. Jankowski J, Provenzale D, Moayyedi P. Oesophageal adenocarcinoma arising from Barrett's metaplasia has regional variations in the West. Gastroenterology 2002; 122:588–90.

7. Watson A, Shepherd NA. British Society of Gastroenterology guidelines for the diagnosis and management of Barrett's columnar-lined oesophagus: the definition of "Barrett's" columnar-lined oesophagus. http://www.bsg.org.uk/clinical-guidelines/oesophageal/index.html; 4–6.

8. Sampliner RE. The Practice Parameters Committee of the American College of Gastroenterology. Practice guidelines on the diagnosis, surveillance, and therapy of Barrett's esophagus. Am J Gastroenterol 1998; 93:1028–32.

9. Harrison R, Perry I, Haddadin W et al. Detection of intestinal metaplasia in Barrett's esophagus: an observational comparator study suggests the need for a minimum of eight biopsies. Am J Gastroenterol 2007; 102:1–8.

10. Dekel R, Wakelin DE, Wendel C et al. Progression or regression of Barrett's esophagus – is it all in the eye of the beholder? Am J Gastroenterol 2003; 98:2612–15.

11. Sharma P, Dent J, Armstrong D et al. The development and validation of an endoscopic grading system for Barrett's esophagus: the Prague C & M criteria. Gastroenterology 2006; 131:1392–9.

12. Jankowski JA, Wright NA, Meltzer SJ et al. Molecular evolution of the metaplasia–dysplasia–adenocarcinoma sequence in the esophagus. Am J Pathol 1999; 154:965–73.

13. Haggitt RC. Barrett's esophagus, dysplasia, and adenocarcinoma. Hum Pathol 1988; 25:982–93.

14. Leedham SJ, Preston SL, McDonald SA et al. Individual crypt genetic heterogeneity and the origin of metaplastic glandular epithelium in human Barrett's oesophagus. Gut 2008; 57(8):1041–8.

15. Jankowski J, Harrison RF, Perry I et al. Barrett's metaplasia. Lancet 2000; 356:2079–85.

16. Poynton AR, Walsh TN, O'Sullivan G et al. Carcinoma arising in familial Barrett's esophagus. Am J Gastroenterol 1996; 91:1855–6.

17. Cameron AJ, Zinsmeister AR, Ballard DJ et al. Prevalence of columnar-lined Barrett's esophagus. Comparison of population-based clinical and autopsy findings. Gastroenterology 1990; 99:918–22.

18. Cameron AJ, Lomboy CT. Barrett's esophagus: age, prevalence and extent of columnar epithelium. Gastroenterology 1992; 103:1241–5.

19. Winters C Jr, Spuring TJ, Chobanian SJ et al. Barrett's esophagus: a prevalent, occult complication of gastroesophageal reflux disease. Gastroenterology 1987; 92:118–24.

20. Prach AT, MacDonald TA, Hopwood DA et al. Increasing Barrett's oesophagus: education, enthusiasm or epidemiology? Lancet 1997; 350:933.

21. Van Soest EM, Dieleman JP, Siersema PD et al. Increasing incidence of Barrett's oesophagus in the general population. Gut 2005; 54:1062–6.

22. Caygill CP, Watson A, Reed PI et al. Characteristics and regional variations of patients with Barrett's oesophagus in the UK. Eur J Gastroenterol Hepatol 2003; 15:1217–22.

23. Spechler SJ, Zeroogian JM, Antonioli DA et al. Prevalence of metaplasia at the gastroesophageal junction. Lancet 1994; 344:1533–6.

24. Eisen GM, Sandler RS, Murray S et al. The relationship between gastroesophageal reflux disease and its complications with Barrett's esophagus. Am J Gastroenterol 1997; 92:27–31.

25. Lagergren J, Bergstrom R, Lindren A et al. Symptomatic gastroesophageal reflux as a risk factor for esophageal adenocarcinoma. Important confirmation in a case-controlled study that symptomatic reflux esophagitis leads to adenocarcinoma of the esophagus. N Engl J Med 1999; 340:825–31.

26. Smith KJ, O'Brien SM, Smithers BM et al. Interactions among smoking, obesity, and symptoms of acid reflux in Barrett's esophagus. Cancer Epidemiol Biomarkers Prev 2005; 14:2481–6.

27. Kim SL, Wo JM, Hunter JG et al. The prevalence of intestinal metaplasia in patients with and without peptic strictures. Am J Gastroenterol 1998; 93:53–5.

28. Trimble KC, Pryde A, Heading RC. Lowered oesophageal sensory thresholds in patients with symptomatic but not excessive gastro-oesophageal reflux: evidence for a spectrum of visceral sensitivity in GERD. Gut 1995; 37:7–12.

29. Gerson LB, Shetler K, Triadafilopoulos G. Prevalence of Barrett's esophagus in asymptomatic individuals. Gastroenterology 2002; 123:461–7.

30. Labenz J, Nocon M, Lind T et al. Prospective follow-up data from the ProGERD study suggest that GERD is not a categorial disease. Am J Gastroenterol 2006; 101:2457–62.

31. Robertson CS, Mayberry JF, Nicholson DA. Value of endoscopic surveillance in the detection of neoplastic change in Barrett's oesophagus. Br J Surg 1988; 75:760–3.

32. Miros M, Kerlin P, Walker N. Only patients with dysplasia progress to adenocarcinoma in Barrett's oesophagus. Gut 1991; 32:1441–6.

33. Iftikar SY, James PD, Steele R. Length of Barrett's oesophagus: an important factor in the development of dysplasia and adenocarcinoma. Gut 1992; 33:1155–8.

34. Wright TA, Gray MR, Morris AI et al. Cost effectiveness of detection of Barrett's cancer. Gut 1996; 39:574–9.

35. Drewitz DJ, Sampliner RE, Garewal HS. The incidence of adenocarcinoma in Barrett's esophagus: a prospective study of 170 patients followed for 4.8 years. Am J Gastroenterol 1997; 92:212–15.

36. Katz D, Rothstein R, Schned A et al. The development of dysplasia and adenocarcinoma during surveillance endoscopy of Barrett's esophagus. Am J Gastroenterol 1998; 93:536–41.

37. Weston AP, Badr AS, Hassanein RS. Prospective multivariate analysis of clinical, endoscopic and histological factors predictive of the development of Barrett's multifocal high-grade dysplasia or adenocarcinoma. Am J Gastroenterol 1999; 94:3413–19.

38. Conio M, Blanchi S, Lapertosa G et al. Long term endoscopic surveillance of patients with Barrett's oesophagus: incidence of dysplasia and adenocarcinoma: a prospective study. Am J Gastroenterol 2003; 98:1931–9.

39. Hage M, Siersema PD, van Dekken H et al. Oesophageal cancer incidence and mortality in patients with long-segment Barrett's oesophagus after a mean follow-up of 12.7 years. Scand J Gastroenterol 2004; 39:1175–9.

40. Oberg S, Wenner J, Johansson J et al. Barrett esophagus: risk factors for progression to dysplasia and adenocarcinoma. Ann Surg 2005; 242:49–54.

41. Shaheen NJ, Crosby MA, Bozymski EM et al. Is there publication bias in the reporting of cancer risk in Barrett's esophagus? Gastroenterology 2000; 119:333–8.

42. Moayyedi P, Burch N, Akhtar-Danesh N et al. Mortality rates in patients with Barrett's oesophagus. Aliment Pharmacol Ther 2008; 27:316–20.

43. Chang EY, Morris CD, Seltman AK et al. The effect of antireflux surgery on esophageal carcinogenesis in patients with Barrett's esophagus: a systematic review. Ann Surg 2007; 246:11–21.

A systematic review which failed to demonstrate a lower incidence of adenocarcinoma after antireflux surgery compared with medical therapy after excluding uncontrolled case series from analysis.

44. Reid BJ, Blount PL, Rubin CE et al. Flow-cytometric and histological progression to malignancy in

45. Skacel M, Petras RE, Gramlich TL et al. The diagnosis of low grade dysplasia in Barrett's esophagus and its implication for disease progression. Am J Gastroenterol 2000; 95:3383–7.

46. Weston AP, Banerjee SK, Sharma P et al. p53 overexpression in low grade dysplasia in Barrett's esophagus: immunohistochemical marker predictive of progression. Am J Gastroenterol 2001; 96:1355–62.

47. Lim CH, Treanor D, Dixon MF et al. Low-grade dysplasia in Barrett's esophagus has a high risk of progression. Endoscopy 2007; 39:581–7.

48. Sharma P, Falk GW, Weston AP et al. Dysplasia and cancer in a large multicenter cohort of patients with Barrett's esophagus. Clin Gastroenterol Hepatol 2006; 4:566–72.

49. Reid BJ, Levine DS, Longton G et al. Predictors of progression to cancer in Barrett's esophagus: baseline histology and flow cytometry identify low and high risk patient subsets. Am J Gastroenterol 2000; 95:1669–76.

50. Schnell TG, Sontag SJ, Chejfec G et al. Long-term non-surgical management of Barrett's esophagus with high-grade dysplasia. Gastroenterology 2001; 120:1607–19.

51. Buttar NS, Wang KK, Sebo TJ et al. Extent of high grade dysplasia in Barrett's esophagus correlates with risk of adenocarcinoma. Gastroenterology 2001; 120:1630–9.

52. Montgomery E, Bronner MP, Goldblum JR et al. Reproducibility of the diagnosis of dysplasia in Barrett's oesophagus: a reaffirmation. Hum Pathol 2001; 32:268–78.

53. Altorki NK, Sunagawa M, Little AG et al. High-grade dysplasia in the columnar-lined esophagus. Am J Surg 1991; 161:97–9.

54. Pera M, Trastek VF, Carpenter HA et al. Barrett's esophagus with high-grade dysplasia: an indication for esophagectomy? Ann Thorac Surg 1992; 54:199–204.

55. Steitz JM Jr, Andrews CW Jr, Ellis FH Jr. Endoscopic surveillance of Barrett's oesophagus. Does it help? J Thorac Cardiovasc Surg 1993; 105:383–8.

56. Levine DS, Haggitt RC, Blount PL et al. An endoscopic biopsy protocol can differentiate high-grade dysplasia from early adenocarcinoma in Barrett's esophagus. Gastroenterology 1993; 105:40–50.

57. Peters JH, Clark GW, Ireland AP et al. Outcome of adenocarcinoma in Barrett's esophagus in endoscopically surveyed and non-surveyed patients. J Thorac Cardiovasc Surg 1994; 108:813–21.

58. Edwards MJ, Gable DR, Lentsch AB et al. The rationale for esophagectomy as the optimal therapy for Barrett's esophagus with high-grade dysplasia. Ann Surg 1996; 223:585–9.

Barrett's esophagus: prospective endoscopic surveillance of a cohort. Gastroenterology 1992; 102:1212–19.

59. Rice TW, Falk GW, Achkar E. Surgical management of high-grade dysplasia in Barrett's esophagus. Am J Surg 1997; 174:1832–6.

60. Collard JM, Romagnoli R, Hermans BP et al. Radical esophageal resection for adenocarcinoma arising in Barrett's esophagus. Am J Surg 1997; 174:307–11.

61. Ferguson MK, Naunheim KS. Resection for Barrett's mucosa with high-grade dysplasia: implications for prophylactic photodynamic therapy. J Thorac Cardiovasc Surg 1997; 114:824–9.

62. Cameron AJ, Carpenter HA. Barrett's esophagus, high-grade dysplasia, and early adenocarcinoma: a pathological study. Am J Gastroenterol 1997; 92:586–91.

63. Falk GW, Rice TW, Goldblum JR et al. Jumbo biopsy forceps protocol still misses unsuspected cancer in Barrett's esophagus with high-grade dysplasia. Gastrointest Endosc 1999; 49:170–6.

64. Headrick JR, Nichols FC, Miller DL et al. High grade esophageal dysplasia: long-term survival and quality of life after esophagectomy. Ann Thorac Surg 2002; 73:1697–702.

65. Tseng EE, Wu TT, Yeo CJ et al. Barrett's esophagus with high grade dysplasia: surgical results and long term outcome – an update. J Gastrointest Surg 2003; 7:164–70.

66. Sujendran V, Sica G, Warren B et al. Oesophagectomy remains the gold standard for treatment of high grade dysplasia in Barrett's oesophagus. Eur J Cardiothorac Surg 2005; 28:763–6.

67. Konda VJ, Ross AS, Ferguson MK et al. Is the risk of concomitant invasive esophageal cancer in high-grade dysplasia in Barrett's esophagus overestimated? Clin Gastroenterol Hepatol 2008; 6(2):159–64.

68. Menke-Pluymers MBE, Hop WCJ, Dees J et al. Risk factors for development of an adenocarcinoma in columnar-lined (Barrett) esophagus. Gastroenterology 1993; 72:1155–8.

69. Dar MS, Goldblum JR, Rice TW et al. Can the extent of high grade dysplasia in Barrett's oesophagus predict the presence of adenocarcinoma at oesophagectomy. Gut 2003; 52:486–9.

70. Srivastava A, Hornick JL, Li X et al. Extent of low-grade dysplasia is a risk factor for the development of esophageal adenocarcinoma in Barrett's esophagus. Am J Gastroenterol 2007; 102:483–93.

71. Vaughan TL, Dong LM, Blount PL et al. Non-steroidal anti-inflammatory drugs and risk of neoplastic progression in Barrett's oesophagus: a prospective study. Lancet Oncol 2005; 6:945–52.

72. Das D, Ishaq S, Harrison R et al. Management of Barrett's oesophagus in the UK: overtreated, and underbiopsied but improved by the introduction of a national randomised trial. Am J Gastroenterol 2008; 103(5):1079–89.

73. Younes M, Lebovitz RM, Lechago LV et al. p53 protein accumulation in Barrett's metaplasia, dysplasia and carcinoma – follow-up study. Gastroenterology 1993; 105:1637–42.

74. Younes M, Ertan A, Lechago LV et al. p53 protein accumulation is a specific marker of malignant potential in Barrett's metaplasia. Dig Dis Sci 1997; 42:697–701.

75. Reid BJ, Prevo LJ, Galipeau PC et al. Predictors of progression in Barrett's esophagus II: baseline 17p (p53) loss of heterozygosity identifies a patient subset at increased risk for neoplastic progression. Am J Gastroenterol 2001; 96:2839–48.

76. Wong DJ, Paulson TG, Prevo LJ et al. p16 (INK4a) lesions are common, early abnormalities that undergo clonal expansion in Barrett's metaplastic epithelium. Cancer Res 2001; 61:8284–9.

77. Bani-Hani K, Martin IG, Hardie LJ et al. Prospective study of cyclin D1 overexpression in Barrett's esophagus: association with increased risk of adenocarcinoma. J Natl Cancer Inst 2000; 92:1316–21.

78. Menke-Pluymers MBE, Mulder AH, Hop WC et al. Dysplasia and aneuploidy as markers of malignant degeneration in Barrett's oesophagus. The Rotterdam Oesophageal Tumour Study Group. Gut 1994; 35:1348–51.

79. Bailey T, Biddlestone L, Shepherd N et al. Altered cadherin and catenin complexes in the Barrett's esophagus–dysplasia–adenocarcinoma sequence. Correlation with disease progression and dedifferentiation. Am J Pathol 1998; 152:1–10.

80. Preston SL, Jankowski JA. Drinking from the fountain of promise: biomarkers in the surveillance of Barrett's oesophagus – the glass is half full! Gut 2006; 55:1377–9.

81. Gore S, Healey CJ, Sutton R et al. Regression of columnar lined (Barrett's) oesophagus with continuous omeprazole therapy. Aliment Pharmacol Ther 1993; 7:623–8.

82. Cooper BT, Chapman W, Neumann CS et al. Continuous treatment of Barrett's oesophagus patients with proton pump inhibitors up to 13 years: observations on regression and cancer incidence. Aliment Pharmacol Ther 2006; 23:727–33.

83. Peters FTM, Ganesh S, Kuipers EJ et al. Endoscopic regression of Barrett's oesophagus during omeprazole treatment; a randomised double blind study. Gut 1994; 45:489–94.

A blinded randomised trial showing that acid suppression can result in alterations in Barrett's metaplasia.

84. Sagar PM, Ackroyd R, Hosie KB et al. Regression and progression of Barrett's oesophagus after anti-reflux surgery. Br J Surg 1995; 82:806–10.

85. O'Riordan JM et al. Long-term clinical and pathologic response of Barrett's esophagus after anti-reflux surgery. Am J Surg 2004; 188:27–33.

86. Ortiz A et al. Conservative treatment versus anti-reflux surgery in Barrett's oesophagus: long-term results of a prospective study. Br J Surg 1996; 83:274–8.

87. McDonald ML et al. Barrett's esophagus: does an antireflux procedure reduce the need for endoscopic surveillance? J Thorac Cardiovasc Surg 1996; 111:1135–40.

88. Csendes A et al. Dysplasia and adenocarcinoma after classic antireflux surgery in patients with Barrett's esophagus: the need for long-term subjective and objective follow-up. Ann Surg 2002; 235:178–85.

89. Ouatu-Lascar R, Triadafilopoulos G. Complete elimination of reflux symptoms does not guarantee normalization of acid reflux in patients with Barrett's esophagus. Am J Gastroenterol 1998; 93:711–16.

90. Corey KE et al. Does a surgical antireflux procedure decrease the incidence of esophageal adenocarcinoma in Barrett's esophagus? A meta-analysis. Am J Gastroenterol 2003; 98:2390–4.

    A meta-analysis demonstrating no difference between the incidence rates of adenocarcinoma in patients with Barrett's oesophagus treated medically or following antireflux surgery.

91. Wang KK, Sampliner R. Updated guidelines 2008 for the diagnosis, surveillance and therapy of Barrett's esophagus. Am J Gastroenterol 2008; 103(3):788–97.

92. De Jonge PJ et al. Risk factors for the development of esophageal adenocarcinoma in Barrett's esophagus. Am J Gastroenterol 2006; 101(7):1421–9.

93. Loft DE, Alderson D, Heading RC. British Society of Gastroenterology guidelines for the diagnosis and management of Barrett's columnar-lined oesophagus: screening and surveillance in columnar-lined oesophagus. http://www.bsg.org.uk/clinical-guidelines/oesophageal/index.html; 28–31.

94. Van Sandick JW et al. Impact of endoscopic biopsy surveillance of Barrett's oesophagus on pathological stage and clinical outcome of Barrett's carcinoma. Gut 1998; 43:216–22.

95. Fountoulakis A et al. Effect of surveillance of Barrett's oesophagus on the clinical outcome of oesophageal cancer. Br J Surg 2004; 91:997–1003.

96. Singh R et al. Barrett's esophagus: diagnosis, screening, surveillance and controversies. Gut and Liver 2007; 001(2):93–100.

97. Sharma P et al. Magnification chromoendoscopy for the detection of intestinal metaplasia and dysplasia in Barrett's oesophagus. Gut 2003; 52:24–7.

98. Canto MI et al. Methylene blue selectively stains intestinal metaplasia in Barrett's esophagus. Gastrointest Endosc 1996; 44:1–7.

99. Kara MA et al. Endoscopic video autofluorescence imaging may improve the detection of early neoplasia in patients with Barrett's esophagus. Gastrointest Endosc 2005; 61:679–85.

100. Gono K et al. Appearance of enhanced tissue features in narrow-band endoscopic imaging. J Biomed Opt 2004; 9:56.

101. Curvers WL et al. Endoscopic tri-modal imaging for detection of early neoplasia in Barrett's oesophagus: a multi-centre feasibility study using high-resolution endoscopy, autofluorescence imaging and narrow band imaging incorporated in one endoscopy system. Gut 2008; 57:167–72.

102. Barr H, Maynard ND. Controversial topics in surgery: high-grade dysplasia in Barrett's oesophagus. Ann R Coll Surg Engl 2006; 89:586–90.

103. Barr H, Stone N, Rembacken B. Endoscopic therapy for Barrett's oesophagus. Gut 2005; 54(6):875–84.

104. Seewald S et al. Endoscopic mucosal resection of Barrett's oesophagus containing dysplasia or intramucosal cancer. Postgrad Med J 2007; 83(980):367–72.

105. Peters FP et al. Multiband mucosectomy for endoscopic resection of Barrett's esophagus: feasibility study with matched historical controls. Eur J Gastroenterol Hepatol 2007; 19(4):311–15.

106. Attwood SE et al. Argon beam plasma coagulation as therapy for high-grade dysplasia in Barrett's esophagus. Clin Gastroenterol Hepatol 2003; 1(4):258–63.

107. Sampliner R et al. Reversal of Barrett's esophagus with acid suppression and multipolar electrocoagulation. Gastrointest Endosc 1996; 44:523–5.

108. Johnstone M et al. Endoscopic spray cryotherapy: a new technique for mucosal ablation in the esophagus. Gastrointest Endosc 1999; 1:86–92.

109. Overholt BF et al. International Photodynamic Group for High-Grade Dysplasia in Barrett's Esophagus. Five-year efficacy and safety of photodynamic therapy with Photofrin in Barrett's high-grade dysplasia. Gastrointest Endosc 2007; 66:460–8.

110. Hubbard N, Velanovich V. Endoscopic endoluminal radiofrequency ablation of Barrett's esophagus in patients with fundoplications. Surg Endosc 2007; 21(4):625–8.

111. Sharma P et al. A randomised controlled trial of ablation of Barrett's oesophagus with multipolar electrocoagulation versus argon plasma coagulation in combination with acid suppression: long term results. Gut 2006; 55:1233–9.

112. Dunkin BJ et al. Thin-layer ablation of human esophageal epithelium using a bipolar radiofrequency balloon device. Surg Endosc 2006; 20(1):125–30.

16

The management of achalasia and other motility disorders of the oesophagus

Derek Alderson

Introduction

Most patients who turn out to have oesophageal motor disorders undergo endoscopy and/or contrast radiology to make sure that their dysphagia is not due to cancer or their chest pain to gastro-oesophageal reflux disease. While these tests can provide the diagnosis, they are often normal leading to specific investigation of oesophageal motor function. Modified barium swallows to look at solid bolus transit using bread or marshmallow can provide added qualitative information. Radionuclide transit does much the same in a semiquantitative way, but the mainstay of specialised investigation is oesophageal manometry.

For many years oesophageal manometry was done using water-perfused systems that were difficult to set up and with many technical constraints. These were gradually replaced by solid-state pressure transducers and, with further miniaturisation and developments in computer software, it is now possible to construct thin catheters containing multiple pressure recording transducers (high-resolution manometry). Further details of manometry techniques are described in Chapter 12 and manometry of a normal swallow in Fig. 12.7.

Achalasia

Background

The term 'achalasia' comes from Greek, meaning 'failure to relax'. It was first used by Sir Arthur Hurst early in the twentieth century, although the clinical features were first described in 1697 by Thomas Willis. It is defined by the absence of peristalsis (this does not mean the absence of contractions) in association with a lower oesophageal sphincter (LOS) that fails to relax completely. Primary or idiopathic achalasia needs to be considered separately from secondary achalasia. While symptoms may be similar, the presence of a specific aetiology can influence management. These secondary causes are discussed later in this chapter.

Primary achalasia

This is an uncommon condition with an incidence in the Western world that is probably less than 1 case per 100 000 people per year.[1] It is due to progressive loss of ganglion cells in the myenteric plexus of unknown cause. The neural loss is somewhat selective as there is particularly severe loss of inhibitory nitrergic neurotransmission.[2,3] This process is often accompanied by an inflammatory infiltrate that has led to many theories regarding aetiology and while there is circumstantial evidence of viral exposure and autoimmune phenomena, neither provides a satisfactory explanation for all patients.[3]

Clinical features

The disease is most common in middle life, but can occur at any age. It typically presents with dysphagia and characteristically this affects fluids as well as solids. Symptom severity varies from day to day and patients often develop tricks to assist oesophageal emptying, such as Valsalva manoeuvres or air swallowing. Many admit to having been 'slow eaters' for many years. In patients who have remained untreated for many years, regurgitation is frequent and there may be overspill into the trachea, especially at night. In the early stages, achalasia may present with retrosternal discomfort and this may lead to a mistaken diagnosis of gastro-oesophageal reflux disease (GORD). Chest pain is common in achalasia and particularly so in those individuals said to have 'vigorous achalasia' (see below).

There are few physical signs that point specifically to any underlying motility disorder including achalasia. There are two important areas of physical examination that should be carefully evaluated as positive findings will play an important part in management. A careful examination of the respiratory system is essential. Recurrent chest infections due to episodes of aspiration from an oesophagus that is unable to clear itself may lead to acute and chronic signs as pulmonary performance deteriorates. It is not rare for these patients to be labelled as asthmatic. The other important area is to make a careful assessment of the patient's nutritional state. Insidious nutritional failure is easily missed in patients with a long history, although it is rare to see this in achalasia, where regular filling of the oesophagus with food and an upright posture eventually create a hydrostatic pressure that will overcome the LOS, causing the oesophagus to partially empty.

Investigations

Most patients with dysphagia are offered endoscopy as their first investigation. While achalasia may be suspected at endoscopy by finding a tight cardia and food residue in the oesophagus, early or vigorous achalasia is easily missed as the oesophagus is not dilated and still contracts.

Barium radiology may show hold-up in the distal oesophagus, dilatation of the oesophageal body, peristaltic dysfunction and a tapering stricture in the distal oesophagus, often described as a 'bird's beak'. The gastric gas bubble is usually absent, because most patients cannot swallow air through their non-relaxing LOS. It should, however, be emphasised that, like endoscopy, these typical features of well-developed achalasia are often absent and radiology is frequently passed as normal.

A firm diagnosis can only be made by oesophageal manometry. Classically, there is a hypertensive lower oesophageal sphincter that does not relax completely on swallowing, aperistalsis of the oesophageal body and a raised resting pressure in the oesophagus (**Fig. 16.1**). In practice, the LOS pressure is often normal. Once the oesophagus becomes dilated, contraction amplitudes become very low and may be non-existent. In vigorous achalasia, the non-dilated oesophagus exhibits obvious motor

activity with mainly simultaneous contractions, often of high amplitude.

Treatment

Achalasia responds well to treatment. There is no reliable drug therapy. Patients can be treated by endoscopic botulinum toxin injection into the LOS, but the two main methods are forceful (pneumatic) dilatation of the cardia and operative cardiomyotomy. Very rarely, patients require oesophagectomy.

Botulinum toxin injection

This involves the injection of 100 units of botulinum toxin into the LOS.

Whether a single treatment or multiple treatments is performed, only about a third of patients experience marked improvement in symptoms 1 year after the last treatment.[4–7]

When compared to pneumatic dilatation in a randomised trial, only 32% of patients who had received botulinum toxin were in symptomatic remission after a year compared to 70% after dilatation.[7] A Cochrane review published in 2006 came to the conclusion that botulinum toxin injection was inferior to pneumatic dilatation at 6 months.[8]

For this reason, botulinum toxin should be reserved for patients who are frail with major comorbidities.

Pneumatic dilatation

This involves stretching the cardia with a balloon to disrupt the muscle and render it less competent. The treatment was first described by Plummer in 1908. Many varieties of balloon have been described, but nowadays plastic balloons with a precisely controlled external diameter are used. If the pressure in the balloon is too high the balloon is designed to split along its length rather than expanding further. Balloons of 30–40 mm diameter are available and are inserted over a guidewire.

Perforation is the major complication. With a 30-mm balloon, the incidence of perforation should be <0.5%. The risk of perforation increases with the bigger balloons and they should be used cautiously for progressive dilatation over a period of weeks.

Forceful dilatation produces good to excellent relief of symptoms for more than a year in 70–90% of patients.[7,9,10]

There is wide variation in the incidence of GORD (between 4% and 40%) after successful dilatation, which reflects method of assessment (symptomatic

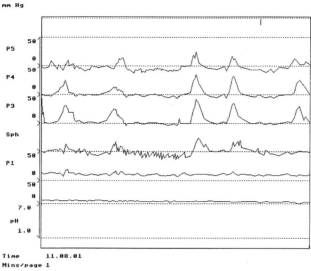

Figure 16.1 • Achalasia. High-resolution manometry from a patient presenting with dysphagia and regurgitation. The swallow is followed by a 'common cavity' rise in oesophageal pressure indicating filling. LOS relaxation is absent and there is a positive oesophagogastric pressure gradient. Upper oesophageal sphincter (UOS) relaxation shortly after the swallow was related to regurgitation of oesophageal contents.

versus endoscopic), the number of repeat dilatations and the length of follow-up.[11-13] In most patients, however, this can usually be controlled satisfactorily with a proton-pump inhibitor.

Cardiomyotomy

This operation is generally associated with Heller, who first carried it out in 1913. Heller's original description involved a double myotomy on the anterior and posterior walls at the cardia, but over the years a single anterior cardiomyotomy has become widely used, often in conjunction with an anterior partial fundoplication (Heller–Dor operation). Cardiomyotomy involves cutting the muscle of the lower oesophagus and cardia. The major complication is gastro-oesophageal reflux and this is less problematic by limiting the incision so that it does not extend for more than 1 cm on to the stomach and including a prophylactic antireflux operation.

In a small randomised trial, the addition of a Dor fundoplication reduced acid reflux documented by pH study from 48% to 9% at 6 months.[14]

It is customary to perform a partial rather than a total fundoplication in this situation because of the risk of causing dysphagia in the presence of an aperistaltic oesophagus. The proximal extent of the myotomy does not seem to matter provided that the obstructing segment is divided and this is easily determined by intraoperative endoscopy. Heller's myotomy is ideally suited to a minimal access approach and although it can be undertaken by thoracoscopy or laparoscopy, the latter approach seems far more popular.

There is some variation in success rates that mainly reflects the proportion of patients with marked oesophageal dilatation and the length of follow-up in different case series. In the normal-calibre oesophagus or where dilatation is minimal, cardiomyotomy is successful in more than 80% of patients.[11,15,16]

The impact of previous treatments on the safety and efficacy of subsequent surgery is unclear. Two large European case series involving nearly 350 patients (including more than 80 patients who had undergone previous botulinum toxin injection or pneumatic dilatation) came to different conclusions regarding the likelihood of perforation at laparoscopic surgery.[17,18]

Two randomised trials have compared balloon dilatation with surgical cardiomyotomy and found the surgical technique to be more effective in relieving dysphagia.[19,20]

Both are open to the major criticism of being statistically underpowered. In the trial published by Csendes et al. in 1981, a superior result in favour of surgery in terms of relieving dysphagia needs to be balanced against a higher rate of reflux. In addition, the pneumatic dilatation was of very short duration and there is no doubt that the results in that arm of the study were inferior to those achieved subsequently with more modern balloons. A more recent trial in Sweden that included a routine partial fundoplication as part of the surgery also identified more treatment failures in the dilatation arm.

A number of studies have used decision analysis (Markov modelling) techniques to identify optimal treatment strategies in the absence of good randomised trials.

When the outcome difference was expressed as quality-adjusted life years (QALYs), dilatation and surgery were equally effective.[21] Similar analyses examining cost-effectiveness tend to favour pneumatic dilatation.[22–24]

For these reasons, patient preference and levels of local expertise should be the main determinants in selecting treatment.

Revisional procedures and oesophagectomy

Failure to relieve dysphagia is usually because the myotomy is too short. The diagnosis is generally made on a contrast swallow but repeat manometry may be necessary. Balloon dilatation can be undertaken and there is no convincing evidence that this is more hazardous after a previous failed cardiomyotomy. The alternative is a redo operation conducted by thoracoscopy if the first attempt was laparoscopic or vice versa. Recurrent dysphagia is occasionally due to a slipped wrap and if symptoms are sufficiently troublesome, this should be surgically corrected.

Chest pain after surgery is more difficult to diagnose and manage. Some of these patients will have symptomatic gastro-oesophageal reflux, but chest pain related to swallowing and obstruction may not seem very different to heartburn for some patients. In vigorous achalasia, chest pain related to powerful simultaneous contractions can still persist after successful cardiomyotomy. Careful re-evaluation is necessary, potentially involving endoscopy, contrast radiology, manometry and 24-hour pH studies. A therapeutic trial of a proton-pump inhibitor may be worthwhile as well as being diagnostic. The addition of a fundoplication, where this was not done at the original operation, merits consideration in patients who are intolerant of proton-pump inhibitors. In other circumstances, unless a clear mechanical problem can be demonstrated (e.g. wrap disruption), revisional surgery is best avoided.

In a small proportion of patients, presentation is with a hugely dilated, flaccid oesophagus, and symptoms and signs of aspiration. Some patients also develop this as a late complication of previous treatment. While standard first-line treatments can be attempted, they often provide only very short-term relief of symptoms.

Oesophagectomy (ideally with vagal nerve preservation) may be the only solution.[25]

Primary achalasia is associated with a small increase in risk of developing squamous cell carcinoma of the oesophagus, presumably as a result of chronic inflammation related to food retention and fermentation. Most large studies estimate the increased risk to be about 30- to 40-fold.[26–29] A recent Swedish study has also highlighted a 10-fold increased risk of adenocarcinoma in men with achalasia.[30]

Secondary achalasia

In South America, chronic infection with the parasite *Trypanosoma cruzi* causes Chagas' disease, which has marked similarities to achalasia. The oesophagus becomes dilated ('megaoesophagus') and tortuous with a persistent retention oesophagitis due to fermentation of food residues. A severe cardiomyopathy is the main cause of death in these patients but some do require oesophagectomy.[31]

Pseudo-achalasia is an achalasia-like disorder that is usually produced by adenocarcinomas at the cardia or by any other tumour in the oesophageal wall at that level (e.g. gastrointestinal stromal tumours). While it seems attractive to suppose that the structural abnormalities related to these neoplasms must interfere with local neurotransmitters, pseudo-achalasia is sometimes also seen in patients with cancers outside the oesophagus (e.g. lung, pancreas), suggesting a paraneoplastic process.[32]

Secondary achalasia occasionally follows anti-reflux surgery. Provided there was preoperative evidence of peristalsis and this is not simply a case of misdiagnosis, the condition probably represents a wrap that is too tight for that patient. Interestingly, endoscopy is usually normal and manometry is required to establish that this is the problem. Truncal vagotomy is also recognised as a rare cause of secondary achalasia, but this can probably be condemned to history now.

Diffuse oesophageal spasm

This is also a rare condition of unknown cause characterised clinically by episodes of severe chest pain and/or dysphagia.[33] The upper oesophagus covered by striated muscle is usually unaffected in contrast to the lower two-thirds, where there is pronounced muscular thickening. Chest pain can be very severe and often occurs in isolation at night. Sometimes chest pain and dysphagia occur at the same time. Many patients undergo detailed assessment for cardiac causes of chest pain or reflux disease.

The diagnosis is rarely made by endoscopy or contrast radiology. Corkscrew oesophagus on a barium swallow is the exception rather than the rule. Diffuse oesophageal spasm is defined manometrically as the presence of two or more non-peristaltic sequences in a series of 10 wet swallows. These abnormal contractions are characterised by multipeaked waves of increased duration and amplitude[34] **(Fig. 16.2)**. They frequently exceed 300 mmHg. This definition, however, ignores a substantial group of patients who have a normal laboratory-based manometric study because they are not symptomatic when the test is done. Ambulatory manometry may be needed to clinch the diagnosis and has the advantage of correlating symptoms to the manometric abnormality.[35] It is evident that not all abnormal contractions produce a symptomatic event, but all symptomatic events are associated with abnormal manometric appearances.

These patients develop considerable thickening of the muscular wall of the oesophagus and treatment is usually directed towards this. Short-acting nitrates, calcium-channel blockers, phosphodiesterase inhibitors and botulinum injection have all been used to provide some patients with a degree of relief from mild symptoms, but there is no evidence that any specific drug treatment will reliably prevent attacks or provide sustained relief from symptoms. For patients with mild symptoms, a careful explanation of the cause of their symptoms and reassurance will often suffice, as there is no real evidence that this is a progressive condition in the majority of patients.

 A small number of patients have very severe symptoms and long oesophageal myotomy provides good symptomatic improvement in about 80% of patients.[36]

It seems important that the myotomy should encompass the entire length of the manometric abnormality so most surgeons advocate that this should be from the aortic arch down to within a few centimetres of the oesophagogastric junction. There is no consensus regarding the need to cross the cardia and incorporate an antireflux procedure. The operation is generally completed thoracoscopically.

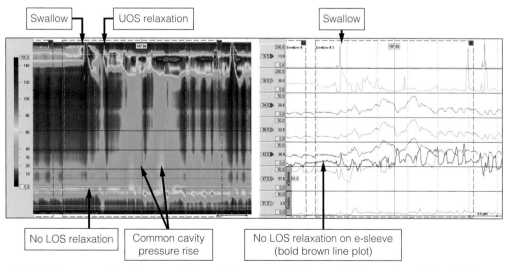

Figure 16.2 • Diffuse oesophageal spasm. High-resolution manometry from a patient presenting with dysphagia and chest pain. The swallow is followed by simultaneous, repetitive contractions in the mid-distal smooth muscle oesophagus. LOS relaxation is preserved. Note the sequential simultaneous contractions first in the middle and distal segments of the oesophagus and then LOS make it appear as if there is progressive peristalsis on the conventional line plots (dotted arrow). Repetitive contractions are seen clearly on both.

Nutcracker oesophagus, hypertensive lower oesophageal sphincter and non-specific oesophageal motor disorders

A number of 'conditions' can be identified by oesophageal manometry. In all cases, the correlation between manometric abnormalities and symptoms tends to be poor. Inevitably, patients undergoing the test have some oesophageal symptoms that have initiated the investigation in the first place, and it is tempting to imply a causal relationship.

Nutcracker oesophagus merely refers to high-amplitude contractions (>180 mmHg) with normal peristalsis during standard manometry. Hypertensive LOS (resting pressure >45 mmHg) is diagnosed when the sphincter still exhibits normal relaxation and there is normal peristalsis. Non-specific motor disorders cover a ragbag of manometric abnormalities that lie outside the normal range, such as low-amplitude peristalsis (<30 mmHg), non-transmitted or retrograde contractions and contractions of increased duration. Many patients with reflux disease will have one or more of these abnormalities and treatment should be directed towards their reflux disease. Inevitably, most patients with a non-specific manometric abnormality have oesophageal symptoms, but correlation with these manometric abnormalities is poor. Great care should be exercised in labelling patients with a manometric diagnosis.[37] There is virtually no evidence that any of these abnormalities responds to a specific treatment.

Oesophageal motor disturbances and autoimmune disease

Systemic sclerosis, polymyositis, dermatomyositis, systemic lupus erythematosus, polyarteritis nodosa and rheumatoid disease can all be associated with oesophageal dysmotility. The condition of most clinical relevance is systemic sclerosis. It is rare for the oesophageal involvement to occur as an early feature in any of these conditions.

Systemic sclerosis

This condition has characteristic cutaneous appearances with thickening, oedema and sclerosis of the skin associated with subcutaneous calcinosis. Unlike the other autoimmune collagen vascular disorders, visceral involvement is unusual except for the oesophagus, which is affected in up to 80% of patients. The striated muscle of the oesophagus is unaffected and there is smooth muscle atrophy involving the LOS. Peristalsis is weak and reflux common. The spectrum of oesophageal symptoms is wide from mild to severe dysphagia with regurgitation and aspiration, as well as reflux symptoms related to the LOS defect and poor clearance. Endoscopy, barium radiology and manometry are used as appropriate to understand the extent of disease in individual patients.

Treatment usually centres around reflux symptoms and the management of complications such as stricture development. Most patients are adequately managed by proton-pump inhibitors and antireflux surgery is only rarely required.

Polymyositis and dermatomyositis

Both of these conditions predominantly affect skeletal muscle and the most common clinical problems occur in the pharynx and at the level of the upper oesophageal sphincter. Up to 60% of patients have a swallowing problem and aspiration is a real concern. Dietary modification may be necessary to minimise this risk. Investigation is only needed to exclude other common causes of oropharyngeal dysphagia.

Systemic lupus erythematosus

Oesophageal involvement is rare, compared to the many other organs involved, including other parts of the gastrointestinal tract. The clinical spectrum is similar to that seen in systemic sclerosis and similar management approaches are therefore recommended.

Polyarteritis nodosa and rheumatoid disease

While many patients with these conditions have non-specific motor disorders on manometry, very few are symptomatic. Dysphagia in the rheumatoid patient may be related to arthritis in the cricoarytenoid joints and stricture in the upper third of the oesophagus has been reported.

Oesophageal diverticula

These can occur anywhere in the oesophagus. They are either congenital (rare) or acquired. In the case of the latter, they are described as traction (rare) or pulsion (common) diverticula.

Traction diverticula were said to arise from the effects of enlarged mediastinal lymph glands (particularly due to tuberculosis) and this was meant to account for the predominant location in the upper half of the oesophagus. Malignant mediastinal nodes, however, rarely cause these diverticula and with the reduction in tuberculosis, it is clear that most mid-oesophageal diverticula are of the pulsion type.

Pulsion diverticula therefore occur anywhere in the oesophagus but are most common in the lower half. Those that occur near the diaphragm are called epiphrenic diverticula. Most of these occur just above the diaphragm and for some reason tend to arise from the posterolateral wall of the oesophagus on the right.

 All pulsion diverticula represent the effects of an underlying motor disturbance where normally coordinated peristaltic activity is inconsistent and where a degree of functional distal obstruction is present.[38] Achalasia and diffuse oesophageal spasm can both lead to diverticulum formation and identifying the underlying motor abnormality may be important in management.[39]

Clinical features

Symptoms largely reflect the extent to which the diverticulum causes pressure effects and the disorder that gave rise to the diverticulum. Chest pain and/or dysphagia bring most diverticula to light, but large diverticula can be complicated by inflammation, fistula formation, perforation and neoplastic change.

Diagnosis

Most are discovered at endoscopy or during a barium swallow during investigation of the patient with chest pain or a swallowing problem. A large diverticulum containing food is sometimes picked up on a chest X-ray. Manometry may be necessary to characterise the motor abnormality, when symptoms are severe enough to warrant intervention.

Treatment

Small diverticula require no treatment in their own right and management should be directed towards the underlying motor disturbance. When the diverticulum itself is perceived to contribute to symptoms, surgery is aimed at correction of the motor disorder and excision of the diverticulum. There are three elements to consider: removal of the diverticulum with secure closure of the oesophagus, correction of distal obstruction by a myotomy of appropriate length and the need for an associated antireflux procedure. Good historical results with open surgery have largely been replicated by stapled excision and closure of the oesophagus with myotomy and a partial fundoplication using minimal access approaches.

Acknowledgements

All high resolution manometry figures were kindly supplied by Dr Mark Fox.

Key points

- Achalasia is an uncommon disorder that generally responds well to treatment by either pneumatic dilatation or surgery.
- Surgery is more effective than pneumatic dilatation in relieving dysphagia in achalasia but the techniques appear equally effective for outcome in terms of quality of life and dilatation has financial advantages.
- Botulinum toxin injection for achalasia should be reserved for patients with significant comorbidities.
- Diffuse oesophageal spasm usually presents with chest pain. It is difficult to diagnose because symptoms are intermittent. Ambulatory manometry is indicated in cases that are difficult to diagnose.
- A long myotomy may be indicated in patients with very severe diffuse oesophageal spasm but most patients should be treated non-surgically.
- Oesophageal involvement occurs in a variety of autoimmune disorders. It is particularly common in systemic sclerosis (affected in 80% of cases).
- The vast majority of oesophageal diverticula are of the pulsion type and arise within or proximal to an area of oesophageal motor disturbance.
- Treatment of an oesophageal diverticula is aimed at identifying and treating the underlying motility disorder. Additional diverticulectomy is only indicated when it contributes to symptoms.
- Non-specific manometric abnormalities are not diagnoses. The correlation with symptoms is poor. Patients should not be labelled with a manometric diagnosis. Many have underlying reflux and treatment of this is often effective.

References

1. Podas T, Eaden J, Mayberry M et al. Achalasia: a critical review of epidemiological studies. Am J Gastroenterol 1998; 93(12):2345–7.

2. Mearin F, Mourelle M, Guarner F et al. Patients with achalasia lack nitric oxide synthase in the gastro-oesophageal junction. Eur J Clin Invest 1993; 23: 724–8.

3. Kraichely RE, Farrugia G. Achalasia: physiology and etiopathogenesis. Dis Esophagus 2006; 19:213–23.

4. Pasricha PJ, Ravich WJ, Hendrix TR et al. Intrasphincteric botulinum toxin for the treatment of achalasia. N Engl J Med 1995; 322:774–8.

5. Fishman VM, Parkman HP, Schiano TD et al. Symptomatic improvement in achalasia after botulinum toxin injection into the lower oesophageal sphincter. Am J Gastroenterol 1996; 91:1724–30.

6. Gordon JM, Eaker EY. Prospective study of oesophageal botulinum toxin injection in high-risk achalasia patients. Am J Gastroenterol 1997; 92:1812–17.

7. Vaezi MF, Richter JE, Wilcox CM et al. Botulinum toxin versus pneumatic dilatation in the treatment of achalasia: a randomised trial. Gut 1999; 44:231–9.

   A small study, with no CONSORT diagram to explain recruitment and randomisation, and no power calculation.

8. Leyden JE, Moss AC, MacMathuna P. Endoscopic pneumatic dilatation versus botulinum toxin injection in the management of primary achalasia. Cochrane Database Syst Rev 2006; 18:CD005046.

   A careful overview of the relative merits of the two techniques. Nothing has changed in the last few years.

9. Kadakia SC, Wong RKH. Graded pneumatic dilatation using Rigiflex achalasia dilators in patients with primary oesophageal achalasia. Am J Gastroenterol 1993; 88:34–8.

10. Annese V, Basciani M, Perri F et al. Controlled trial of botulinum toxin injection versus placebo and pneumatic dilatation in achalasia. Gastroenterology 1996; 111:1418–24.

11. Vela MF, Richter JE, Khandwala F et al. The long-term efficacy of pneumatic dilatation and Heller myotomy for the treatment of achalasia. Clin Gastroenterol Hepatol 2006; 4:580–7.

12. Zerbib F, Thetiot V, Benajah DA et al. Repeated pneumatic dilatations as long-term maintenance therapy for esophageal achalasia. Am J Gastroenterol 2006; 101:692–7.

13. Leeuwenburgh I, Van Dekken H, Scholten P et al. Oesophagitis is common in patients with achalasia after pneumatic dilatation. Aliment Pharmacol Ther 2006; 23:1197–203.

14. Richards WO, Torquati A, Holzman MD et al. Heller myotomy versus Heller myotomy with Dor fundoplication for achalasia: a prospective randomized double-blind clinical trial. Ann Surg 2004; 240:405–12.

    A small study from a centre with a number of publications on achalasia. Compare this with their own results in earlier studies.

15. Sharp KW, Khaitan L, Scholz S et al. 100 consecutive minimally invasive Heller myotomies: lessons learned. Ann Surg 2002; 235:631–8.

16. Costantini M, Zaninotto G, Guirolli E et al. The laparoscopic Heller–Dor operation remains an effective treatment for esophageal achalasia at a minimum 6-year follow-up. Surg Endosc 2005; 19:345–51.

    The most useful recent article describing long-term outcomes, highlighting the paucity of data in relation to all achalasia treatments.

17. Bonavina L, Incarbone R, Reitano M et al. Does previous endoscopic treatment affect the outcome of laparoscopic Heller myotomy? Ann Chir 2000; 125:45–9.

18. Portale G, Costantini M, Rizzetto C et al. Long-term outcome of Heller–Dor surgery for esophageal achalasia: possible detrimental role of previous endoscopic treatment. J Gastrointest Surg 2005; 9:1332–9.

19. Csendes A, Velasco N, Braghetto J et al. A prospective randomized study comparing forceful dilatation and oesophagomyotomy in patients with achalasia of the oesophagus. Gastroenterology 1981; 80:789–95.

    An important study and clearly the first true comparison. It is inevitably open to criticism, mainly regarding the method of pneumatic dilatation. The late follow-up paper from the same group is worth reading.

20. Kostic S, Kjellin A, Ruth M et al. Pneumatic dilatation or laparoscopic cardiomyotomy in the management of newly diagnosed achalasia. Results of a randomised controlled trial. World J Surg 2007; 31:470–8.

    Another small and underpowered trial. Read in conjunction with Ref. 23 to see the effects of different endpoints.

21. Urbach DR, Hansen PD, Khajanchee YS et al. A decision analysis of the optimal initial approach to achalasia: laparoscopic Heller myotomy with partial fundoplication, thoracoscopic Heller myotomy, pneumatic dilatation or botulinum toxin injection. J Gastrointest Surg 2001; 5:192–205.

22. O'Connor JB, Singer ME, Imperiale TF et al. The cost-effectiveness of treatment strategies for achalasia. Dig Dis Sci 2002; 47:1516–25.

23. Kostic S, Johnsson E, Kjellin A et al. Health economic evaluation of therapeutic strategies in patients with idiopathic achalasia: results of a randomized trial comparing pneumatic dilatation with laparoscopic cardiomyotomy. Surg Endosc 2007; 21:1184–9.

24. Karanicolas PJ, Smith SE, Inculet RI et al. The cost of laparoscopic myotomy versus pneumatic dilatation for esophageal achalasia. Surg Endosc 2007; 21:1198–206.

25. Devaney EJ, Lannettoni MD, Orringer MB et al. Esophagectomy for achalasia: patient selection and clinical experience. Ann Thorac Surg 2001; 72:854–8.

    A highly informative case series that highlights the problems faced in dealing with end-stage disease.

26. Meijssen MA, Tilanus HW, van Blankenstein M et al. Achalasia complicated by oesophageal squamous cell carcinoma: a prospective study in 195 patients. Gut 1992; 33:155–8.

27. Aggestrup S, Holm JC, Sorensen HR. Does achalasia predispose to cancer of the esophagus? Chest 1992; 102:1013–16.

28. Streitz JM Jr, Ellis FH Jr, Gibb SP et al. Achalasia and squamous cell carcinoma of the eosophagus: analysis of 241 patients. Ann Thorac Surg 1995; 59:1604–9.

29. Sandler RS, Nyren O, Ekbom A et al. The risk of esophageal cancer in patients with achalasia. A population-based study. JAMA 1995; 274:1359–62.

30. Zendehdel K, Nyren O, Edberg A et al. Risk of esophageal adenocarcinoma in achalasia patients, a retrospective cohort study in Sweden. Am J Gastroenterol 2007 (Epub ahead of print).

31. Pinotti HW. A new approach to the thoracic esophagus by the abdominal trans-diaphragmatic route. Langenbeck's Arch Chir 1983; 359:229–35.

32. Portale G, Costantini M, Zaninotto G et al. Pseudoachalasia: not only esophago-gastric cancer. Dis Esophagus 2007; 20:168–72.

33. Osgood H. A peculiar form of oesophagismus. Boston Med Surg J 1889; 120:401–5.

34. Richter JE, Bradley LA, Castell DO. Esophageal chest pain: Current controversies in pathogenesis, diagnosis and therapy. Ann Intern Med 1989; 110:66–78.

35. Barham CP, Gotley DC, Fowler A. Diffuse oesophageal spasm: diagnosis by ambulatory 24 hour manometry. Gut 1997; 41:151–5.

    The first study to characterise diffuse oesophageal spasm in this way. It emphasises the importance of manometric abnormality and symptom correlation.

36. Leconte M, Douard R, Gaudric M et al. Functional results after extended myotomy for diffuse oesophageal spasm. Br J Surg 2007; 94:1113–18.

37. Hsi JJ, O'Connor MK, Kang YW et al. Nonspecific motor disorder of the esophagus: a real disorder or a manometric curiosity? Gastroenterology 1993; 104:1281–4.

38. Kaye MD. Oesophageal motor dysfunction in patients with diverticula of the mid-thoracic oesophagus. Thorax 1974; 29:666–72.

39. Di Marino AJ, Cohen S. Characteristics of lower esophageal sphincter function in symptomatic diffuse esophageal spasm. Gastroenterology 1974; 66:1–6.

17

Paraoesophageal hernia and gastric volvulus

Kyle A. Perry
John G. Hunter

Introduction

Paraoesophageal hiatal hernia is a relatively rare condition comprising approximately 10% of hiatal hernias. This condition was first identified on post-mortem examination in 1903,[1] and on upper gastrointestinal contrast radiography by Akerlund in 1926.[2] Since that time, the importance of these hernias has been recognised due to their propensity to develop potentially life-threatening complications including gastric volvulus with subsequent strangulation and perforation.[3] Management of para-oesophageal hernias has changed considerably since the development of laparoscopic repair and several areas of controversy remain as this technique continues to evolve.

Epidemiology

Hiatal hernias occur in approximately 10% of the population,[4] with approximately 15% of these being paraoesophageal hernias.[3,4] They typically present later in life with a 2:1 female preponderance, and are occasionally seen as a complication of antire-flux surgery. There is also a familial occurrence that confers a 20-fold increased risk in younger siblings of children with a hiatal hernia.[5]

Anatomy and natural history

The oesophagus enters the abdomen via the oesophageal hiatus of the diaphragm, which is comprised of the limbs of the right diaphragmatic crus,[6] although varying degrees of contribution of the left crus are often present. Although not anatomically correct, descriptions of hiatal dissection and repair, including those presented here, typically refer to these limbs simply as the right and left diaphragmatic crura. The intra-abdominal oesophagus is anchored to the diaphragm by the phreno-oesophageal ligament, which serves to maintain the position of the squamocolumnar junction within or slightly distal to the diaphragmatic hiatus and prevents displacement of the stomach through the diaphragm.[7]

Derangements in the normal anatomy of the gastro-oesophageal junction and oesophageal hiatus result in herniation of the stomach through this opening into the thoracic cavity. The aetiology of these hernias is often unclear. Hiatal hernias are rare in Asian and African populations, and are more common in conditions which create increased intra-abdominal pressure, such as obesity and pregnancy. Hiatal hernias are classified as types I–IV, with types II–IV representing forms of paraoesophageal hernia (**Fig. 17.1**). This nomenclature is slightly confusing, as giant hiatal hernias may appear to be a sliding or paraoesophageal hiatal hernia depending on the patient position. We prefer to use the term 'giant hiatal hernias' for the large hernias that are usually classified as type III and IV paraoesophageal hernia.

Most hiatal hernias (90%) are type I, or sliding, hernias in which the gastric cardia herniates upwards with proximal migration of the lower esophageal sphincter into the thorax. The phreno-oesophageal ligament is attenuated, but remains intact.[8] The term 'sliding hiatal hernia' is applied

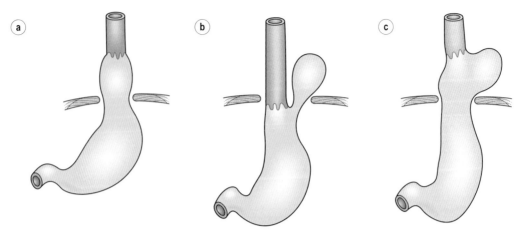

Figure 17.1 • Classification of hiatal hernias. **(a)** Type I (sliding). **(b)** Type II (true paraoesophageal). **(c)** Type III (combined).

here because the gastric wall comprises a portion of the hernia sac, analogous to retroperitoneal structures in sliding inguinal hernias.

Type II (true paraoesophageal) hiatal hernias are less common, constituting about 3% of hiatal hernias. In this type of hernia, the gastro-oesophageal junction remains anchored in its normal position, and the gastric fundus herniates through an enlarged hiatus. This defect is very rare because most paraoesophageal hernias evolve directly from type 1 (sliding hiatal hernia) to type III (mixed paraoesophageal hernia).

Type III (combined) hiatal hernias involve elements of both type I and II hernias, and represent the majority of paraoesophageal hernias presenting for surgical repair. These hernias result from enlargement of a type I hernia defect, to allow cephalad migration of the stomach in response to the transdiaphagmatic pressure gradient. There is a true hernia sac present with fundic herniation and proximal migration of the gastro-oesophageal junction into the thorax. This type of hernia is associated with laxity of the elements that retain normal gastric position, and the natural history is to progress to complete gastric herniation with the appearance of an upside-down intrathoracic stomach on contrast radiography.[9] This increased gastric mobility predisposes patients to gastric volvulus, which we will address in detail later in this chapter.

Type IV hiatal hernia refers to a large hernia defect with other viscera or abdominal organs contained within the hernia sac. The transverse colon is the most common other structure found in these hernias. Splenic herniation is extremely rare.

As with all hernias, the natural history of paraoesophageal hernia is progressive enlargement over time. Early in their course some are clinically silent, but most people have gastro-oesophageal reflux symptoms, which may have been treated with medical therapy or not at all. By the time the hernia grows large enough to allow a paraoesophageal hernia of the stomach, a cardio-oesophageal angle is recreated. Paradoxically, reflux symptoms may wane as the paraoesophageal herniation recreates a more competent antireflux valve.[10] The term 'giant paraoesophageal hiatal hernia' refers to defects in which at least half of the stomach is located within the thorax on contrast radiography, the hernia measures at least 6 cm in length on preoperative endoscopy, or a distance between the crura of at least 5 cm is noted on intraoperative inspection.[11,12] These hernias are repaired using the same principles required for all paraoesophageal hernias, but the large hernia sac and propensity for oesophageal shortening make these cases especially challenging.

Presentation and diagnosis

Approximately half of all paraoesophageal hernias are clinically silent and become apparent on imaging studies obtained for another reason. Symptomatic hernias may present with epigastric or chest pain, heartburn, postprandial fullness, regurgitation or dysphagia. Many of the signs and symptoms are non-specific and may mimic those of acute myocardial infarction, gastric ulcer or pneumonia. Type II hernias typically present without reflux symptoms, whereas type III hernias most typically present with postprandial chest pain with or without reflux symptoms (e.g. heartburn, dysphagia, regurgitation). Others present with iron deficiency anaemia secondary to chronic blood loss from erosions of the gastric mucosa caused by repeated movement across the hiatus, a phenomenon originally described by Collis in 1957,[13] or from an ulcer at the level of the diaphragm described by Cameron from the Mayo Clinic.[14,15]

In the acute setting of foregut obstruction, chest X-ray typically demonstrates a retrocardiac air–fluid level and often a second one below the diaphragm. A barium study will reveal obstruction at the level of the volvulus and can be used as a confirmatory study in this setting if the diagnosis remains uncertain. In the setting of ischaemia, the presentation is one of septic shock, with epigastric pain and resultant multiorgan system dysfunction. It should be emphasised that the catastrophic presentations of paraoesophageal hernia are quite rare.

Several tests may be used to classify the hernia, degree of gastro-oesophageal reflux and oesophageal motility prior to elective repair. Barium swallow may suggest the presence of a shortened oesophagus and classify the hernia to aid in decision-making, especially in frail patients with asymptomatic hernias. Manometry is useful in identifying oesophageal motility disorders, which may preclude the use of full fundoplication, but may not be technically possible due to difficulties positioning the catheter beyond the lower oesophageal sphincter. Upper gastrointestinal (GI) endoscopy is required to inspect for gastric ischaemia, ulceration or erosion. If a gastric ulcer is present, elective surgery should be delayed until after the ulcer is healed, or at least 6 weeks of proton-pump inhibitor treatment.

Operative indications

It has been generally accepted that reasonable surgical candidates should undergo repair regardless of symptoms. This recommendation is based on early series that showed an increased mortality after emergency surgery of 30% compared to 1% in elective cases. In 1967, Skinner and Belsey found that 6 of 21 patients with a known diagnosis of paraoesophageal hernia died from complications of their hernia when followed conservatively for 5 years.[11]

More recent studies have suggested differences in both the natural history of the disease and operative outcomes. Allen et al. followed 23 patients who refused operative repair of paraoesophageal hernias for a median follow-up of 78 months without development of any life-threatening complications.[16] Others have advocated that asymptomatic or minimally symptomatic paraoesophageal hernias may be managed by a strategy of 'watchful waiting', with emergency surgery required in only 1.2% of cases with an operative mortality of 5.4% in this setting.[17]

 The current recommendation is that all type II hernias should be repaired, and consideration should be given to type III hernias regardless of symptoms. However, in the case of an elderly, frail patient with significant comorbidities it may be appropriate to decide on a course of watchful waiting due to increased risks associated with surgical repair in these patients.

Operative approaches

Principles of paraoesophageal hernia repair

The repair of paraoesophageal hernias may be approached via thoracotomy, laparotomy or laparoscopy. The principles of proper surgical repair are the same with each approach:[18–20]

1. Complete excision of the hernia sac.
2. Reduction of the herniated stomach and 2–3 cm of distal oesophagus into the abdominal cavity.
3. Repair of the diaphragmatic hiatus.

Transthoracic repair

Traditionally, transthoracic repair of paraoesophageal hernias has been advocated. Approaching these via thoracotomy provides excellent visualisation of the hernia sac from within the mediastinum and allows extensive oesophageal mobilisation under direct vision. However, this approach has been associated with longer hospital stay and increased incisional discomfort. Blind reduction of the stomach also leaves the potential for recurrence of organo-axial rotation leading to postoperative intra-abdominal gastric volvulus.

Transabdominal repair

Paraoesophageal hernias may be approached via laparotomy, which provides most general surgeons with a familiar anatomical orientation, allows placement of the stomach in its proper orientation, and does not require single-lung ventilation or placement of an intercostal drain. Disadvantages include compromised ability to mobilise the oesophagus and perform oesophageal lengthening (Collis gastroplasty) when necessary.

Laparoscopic repair

Since its introduction by Cuschieri et al. in 1992,[21] laparoscopic paraoesophageal hernia repair has gained popularity and proven to be feasible, safe and effective.[22–29] Laparoscopy provides an attractive option because it appears to combine some of the advantages of both thoracotomy (access to the hiatus, ability to perform extensive mobilisation of the oesophagus under direct vision) and laparotomy (lower morbidity, no need for single-lung ventilation or postoperative chest tube). Further, this minimally invasive approach may be better suited for the elderly patients in which this disease most commonly occurs. However, this is a technically challenging operation that requires advanced laparoscopic skills, and questions remain about the recurrence rate.

Set-up and port placement

The patient is placed in the supine split-leg position under general anaesthesia. Intravenous antibiotics are given, and sequential compression devices and a Foley catheter are placed. The operating surgeon stands between the patient's legs, with the first assistant positioned on the patient's left side.

A total of five trocars are used (**Fig. 17.2**). Peritoneal access is gained using a Veress needle, and an 11-mm trocar is placed just left of the midline, 15 cm caudal to the xyphoid process. Two ports are placed in the left subcostal position, a 12-mm trocar 12 cm lateral to the xyphoid process, and a 5-mm trocar 8 cm further to the left. Finally, two 5-mm ports are placed along the right costal margin, one in the subxyphoid position and the second approximately 10 cm lateral. A Nathenson liver retractor is used to retract the left lobe of the liver and expose the oesophageal hiatus.

Reduction of hernia sac and fundic mobilisation

The stomach is gently reduced from the hernia sac (**Fig. 17.3**) and the left diaphragmatic crus is identified. The dissection is carried out along the left crus between the endothoracic fascia and the hernia sac. After the anterior phreno-oesophageal membrane is divided using ultrasonic dissection, the stomach is retracted to the left to expose the right crus. The pars flaccida of the lesser omentum is divided and the dissection continues along the right crus to the decussation of the crura. The gastrosplenic omentum is then divided using ultrasonic dissection, and the short gastric vessels are divided all the way up to the cephalad extent of the stomach. Division of the posterior gastric attachments creates a retro-oesophageal window through which a Penrose

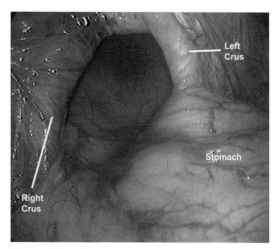

Figure 17.3 • A large paraoesophageal hernia with the stomach reduced into the abdomen prior to beginning the dissection.

drain is passed around the oesophagus to allow caudal retraction on the oesophagus and create exposure for the mediastinal dissection. Dissection proceeds from right to left, and the sac is opened to reveal a plane between the peritoneal sac and the mediastinum. Careful blunt and ultrasonic dissection develops this plane, with care taken to identify and preserve the vagal trunks and the scar tissue at the hiatus, which aids in the crural closure. With gentle retraction, the sac can be slowly mobilised out of the mediastinum and reduced into the abdominal cavity. Most individuals excise and remove the hernia sac, but excessive fastidiousness in this exercise risks injury to the vagi as they course in close apposition to the hernia sac in the epiphrenic fat. We usually remove the majority of the sac, including all sac and epiphrenic fat on the left side of the oesophagus, well away from the vagal trunks and the end branches of the left gastric artery.

Assessment of oesophageal length

When the hernia sac is completely reduced from the mediastinum, it is imperative to have at least 2.5 cm of tension-free intrabdominal oesophageal length. If a shortened oesophagus is identified an extensive circumferential mobilisation of the intrathoracic oesophagus is performed, which usually provides the desired oesophageal length. In cases of true shortened oesophagus, a wedge gastroplasty is performed over a large bougie. A point is marked 3 cm below the angle of His, and a transverse staple line is created with two or three applications of a linear endoscopic stapler inserted via

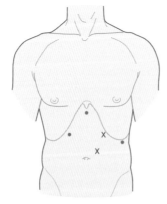

Figure 17.2 • Port placement for laparoscopic paraoesophageal hernia repair.

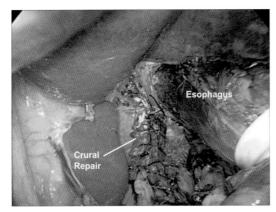

Figure 17.4 • Completed crural repair.

the left upper quadrant trocar. When the oesophageal dilator is reached, a vertical staple line created along the bougie creates a 3–4 cm neo-oesophagus, and the gastric wedge is removed from the abdomen.[30]

Crural dissection and repair

After complete reduction of the hernia sac and identification of an adequate length of intra-abdominal oesophagus, attention is turned to the crural closure. This is performed using interrupted, pledgetted, braided non-absorbable suture such as 0 silk (**Fig. 17.4**). It is frequently beneficial to reduce pneumoperitoneum pressure to 7 cm to close large diaphragmatic defects that are, in part, held open by the pneumoperitoneum. Once closed, the adequacy of closure may be tested by the passage of a 56–60 French Maloney dilator, which should completely fill the new hiatal aperture. If the diaphragmatic repair appears to be 'pinching' the oesophagus with dilator in place, a suture is removed. Conversely, if the closure is loose, the dilator is withdrawn into the upper oesophagus

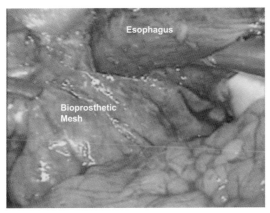

Figure 17.5 • Bioprosthetic mesh overlying the completed crural repair.

and another suture is added. In addition to suture repair, we have advocated the use of biological mesh for reinforcement of the crural repair. A 3 cm × 5 cm U-shaped piece of porcine small-intestinal submucosa mesh is fixed in place overlying the repair. Rather than struggle with difficult suture angles, or risking an intrathoracic injury by using hernia tacks to hold the mesh in place, we have been 'gluing' the mesh to the diaphragm with tissue sealant (**Fig. 17.5**).

Fundoplication

After the completion of the crural repair, we routinely perform an antireflux procedure because failure to do so has been associated with a 20–40% rate of postoperative reflux and preoperative testing cannot successfully predict postoperative reflux.[31–35] A Nissen fundoplication is performed unless the patient has a known history of severe oesophageal dysmotility, necessitating a partial fundoplication. A floppy Nissen is performed by passing the fundus of the stomach behind the oesophagus. When a wedge gastroplasty is performed, the staple line is opposed to the stomach wall and the most cephalad stitch of the fundoplication is placed on the true oesophagus above the neo-oesophagus, ensuring that no gastric mucosa lies above the wrap. The fundoplication is created using three 2-0 silk or braided nylon sutures incorporating the stomach and oesophagus with each 'bite'. An additional suture may be placed from the posterior portion of the wrap to the oesophagus.

Current controversies in paraoesophageal hernia management

Although many centres have adopted laparoscopic paraoesophageal hernia repair as their primary treatment approach, several technical considerations draw great debate. These include methods used to diminish hernia recurrence following laparoscopic para-oesophageal hernia repair, indications for adding an oesophageal lengthening procedure, and the need for prosthetic reinforcement of the crural repair.

Recurrence rate

As with any hernia repair, recurrence is a well-known complication of paraoesophageal hernia surgery, and the relatively high recurrence rate of 14–42% in several laparoscopic case series has been a criticism of this approach. However, only two studies have directly compared the open and laparoscopic approaches.

Hashemi et al. found that laparoscopic hernia repair had a higher recurrence rate compared to open repairs as detected by routine postoperative barium oesophagogram.[25] Conversely, another study found a higher incidence in open repairs; however, this study was based only on the recurrence of symptoms and did not employ routine postoperative imaging.[28]

One explanation for the high objective recurrence rate following laparoscopic repair is the decreased propensity to form adhesions that help prevent recurrent herniation after open repair. Most of these recurrences are small and asymptomatic, and they remain of questionable clinical significance without long-term studies examining their natural history. Two other factors that influence recurrence rates are recognition of shortened oesophagus and reinforcement of the crural closure.

Oesophageal lengthening procedures

Some oesophageal surgeons have argued against the existence of shortened oesophagus,[36] but most surgeons today agree that it is a real clinical entity that results from oesophageal inflammation in the setting of proximal migration of the gastro-oesophageal junction. Failure to recognise this condition during paraoesophageal hernia repair or fundoplication results in tension on the hiatal repair, which has been implicated in up to 33% of surgical failures after open and laparoscopic repairs.[37–39]

Short oesophagus has been recognised and studied for several decades, with the Collis gastroplasty described for its treatment in 1957.[40] Although preoperative testing can show the position of the gastro-oesophageal junction and suggest the presence of shortened oesophagus, these tests cannot reliably predict difficulty reducing the stomach to its anatomical position without tension intraoperatively.[41] Currently, shortened oesophagus is defined as the inability to gain 2.5–3 cm of tension-free intra-abdominal oesophagus following mediastinal dissection.

When adequate intra-abdominal length cannot be achieved via mediastinal mobilisation of the oesophagus, an oesophageal lengthening procedure can be performed to reduce tension, which favours a hernia recurrence by cephalad migration of the fundoplication through the crural repair. There are multiple laparoscopic approaches to oesophageal lengthening. The totally laparoscopic approach, favoured by the authors, has evolved from a method utilising circular and linear staplers[42] to the wedge gastroplasty previously

described.[30] Others have advocated a combined laparoscopic and thoracoscopic approach where by a linear stapler is passed through the hiatus via a thoracoscopic port to perform a stapled gastroplasty.[43,44]

Oesophageal lengthening procedures are required in up to 10% of paraoesophageal hernia repairs and their use is mandatory in cases when adequate tension-free oesophageal length cannot be obtained from mediastinal dissection alone.

Prosthetic crural reinforcement

The high recurrence rate documented in case series of laparoscopic paraoesophageal hernia repair has led to the development of several approaches to reinforcement of crural repair; however, a standardised approach to crural reinforcement has not been developed. The methods currently employed include pledgetted suture repairs and synthetic or bioprosthetic mesh repairs. Three prospective studies have shown decreased recurrence rates when prosthetic crural reinforcement is performed compared to primary repair.

Two prospective randomised trials have evaluated synthetic mesh reinforcement. One study showed a decreased recurrence rate with polytetrafluoroethylene reinforcement of the crural repair to a median follow-up of 78 months,[45] and another trial showed similar results with prolene mesh reinforcement of the hiatus.[46] These studies, however, did not carefully assess potential mesh-related complications, and the second series showed an increase in early postoperative dysphagia when mesh was used. Concern also exists about the use of synthetic mesh near the hiatus where movement of the mesh along the oesophagus with each respiration can cause complications including mesh erosion, ulceration, stricture and dysphagia.[31,47–49]

More recently, interest in bioprosthetic meshes has expanded to include crural repair. In 2006, a prospective randomised, multicentre trial examined the effect of bioprosthetic mesh on hernia recurrence.[50] This study showed a significant reduction in early recurrences (6-month follow-up) following bioprosthetic mesh repair, without increased dysphagia or impaired quality of life compared to those with primary crural repair. This repair appears to have potential, but no direct studies comparing it to synthetic mesh repair have been done, and long-term efficacy and complication rates of each approach need to be determined.

Acute gastric volvulus

Gastic volvulus, first described by Berti in 1896,[51] is defined as the rotation of the stomach greater than 180° around a fixed axis of rotation. Gastric strangulation from acute gastric volvulus is a dreaded complication of paraoesophageal hernia and it remains the driving force for recommending elective repair of asymptomatic hernias. Gastric strangulation occurs in up to 28% of cases of acute gastric volvulus,[52] and may progress to gastric necrosis, perforation and severe sepsis leading to cardiovascular collapse if it is not diagnosed quickly and aggressively managed.

Frequency and mechanism

The true incidence of gastric volvulus remains unknown, but it affects males and females equally. Approximately 20% of cases occur in infants and young children, with the remainder occurring in adults older than 50 years of age.

The anatomical classification of gastric volvulus is based on the axis of rotation (**Fig. 17.6**). **Organoaxial volvulus** is the most common type, and it accounts for almost all cases of acute gastric volvulus. This involves rotation of the stomach around the anatomical (longitudinal) axis, represented as a line drawn from the cardia to the pylorus,[9] frequently resulting in gastric strangulation. In **mesentericoaxial volvulus**, the antrum of the stomach rotates anteriorly and superiorly around a transverse axis that extends from the mid-lesser curvature to the mid-greater curvature.[9] The rotation is typically incomplete and results in intermittent gastric obstruction, rather than acute strangulation.

Presentation and diagnosis

Acute gastric volvulus typically presents with a history of dysphagia and high gastric obstruction. In 1904, Borchardt described the classic symptom triad of severe epigastric pain, retching and inability to vomit, and inability to pass a nasogastric tube.[53] Patients may also present with severe chest pain and minimal abdominal findings as the incarcerated segment is often located within the chest.[52]

The clinical history and a plain chest radiograph are usually sufficient for diagnosis. The X-ray shows a retrocardiac air–fluid level, often with a second air–fluid level present below the diaphragm. In cases where the diagnosis remains in question, barium swallow and meal is diagnostic and will show an obstruction at the level of the volvulus.

Management

Once the diagnosis has been made, intravenous fluid resuscitation should be initiated and an attempt made at gastric decompression with a nasogastric tube. If successful, this results in rapid symptom improvement, and allows time for intravenous fluid resuscitation prior to surgical repair. If nasogastric decompression is unsuccessful, the patient must be taken to the operating room immediately for emergency operative repair.

Surgical repair of gastric volvulus may be approached via thoracotomy, laparotomy or laparoscopy. The principles of repair include reduction of the hernia, release of the volvulus, debridement of all non-viable tissue, hiatal closure and anterior gastropexy or fundoplication to prevent recurrent volvulus. In cases where nasogastric decompression can be achieved preoperatively and adequate intravenous fluid resuscitation accomplished, most can be managed laparoscopically. Cases in the setting of acute peritonitis that cannot be relieved by gastric decompression are best approached via laparotomy or thoracotomy based on the preference of the operating surgeon.

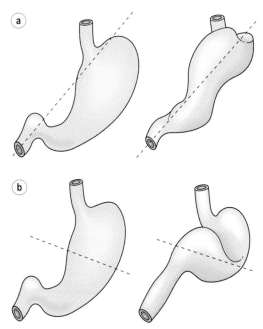

Figure 17.6 • Mechanisms of gastric volvulus.
(a) Organoaxial rotation. **(b)** Mesentericoaxial rotation.

Key points

- Paraoesophageal hernias comprise approximately 10% of hiatal hernias and, of these, type III hernias most commonly present for surgical repair.
- Paraoesophageal hernias should be repaired in symptomatic patients with reasonable surgical risk to prevent the development of potentially life-threatening complications.
- Watchful waiting is an acceptable management strategy in most asymptomatic individuals, especially the elderly or those with significant comorbidities.
- Laparoscopic paraoesophageal hernia repair is safe and effective in the management of paraoesophageal hernias and has become the operative approach of choice in many centres.
- Shortened oesophagus is defined as the inability to gain at least 2.5 cm of intra-abdominal oesophagus after standard mediastinal dissection. When encountered this can be managed by extensive mediastinal dissection and addition of an oesophageal lengthening procedure.
- Failure to recognise shortened oesophagus has been implicated in up to 33% of surgical failures in open and laparoscopic hiatal hernia repairs.
- Mesh reinforcement of the crural closure decreases the rate of early recurrence following laparoscopic paraoesophageal hernia repair, but data regarding the long-term efficacy and complication rates of these approaches are pending.
- Acute gastric volvulus is a serious complication of paraoesophageal hernias that requires aggressive management to avoid life-threatening complications of gastric strangulation, infarction and perforation.
- When gastric decompression of acute gastric volvulus can be obtained preoperatively, most operative repairs can be completed laparoscopically. However, in cases with acute peritonitis an open approach via laparotomy or thoracotomy should be utilised.

References

1. Andrew LT. The height of the diaphragm in relation to the position of certain abdominal viscera. Lancet 1903; 1:790.

2. Akerlund A, Onnell H, Key E. Hernia diaphragmatica hiatus oesophagi vom anatomischen unt rontgenologischen gesichtspunct. Acta Radiol 1926; 6:3–22.

3. Ellis FH Jr, Crozier RE, Shea JA. Paraesophageal hiatus hernia. Arch Surg 1986; 121:416–20.

4. Hill LD, Tobias JA. Paraesophageal hernia. Arch Surg 1968; 96:735–44.

5. Carre IJ, Johnston BT, Thomas PS et al. Familial hiatal hernia in a large five generation family confirming true autosomal dominant inheritance. Gut 1999; 45:649–52.

6. Marchand P. The anatomy of esophageal hiatus of the diaphragm and the pathogenesis of hiatus herniation. J Thorac Surg 1959; 37:81–92.

7. Kahrilas PJ, Wu S, Lin S et al. Attenuation of esophageal shortening during peristalsis with hiatus hernia. Gastroenterology 1995; 109:1818–25.

8. Skinner DB, Roth JLA, Sullivan BH et al. Reflux esophagitis. In: Berk JE (ed.) Gastroenterology, 4th edn. Philadelphia: WB Saunders, 1985; pp. 717–68.

9. Kahrilas PJ, Speiss AE. Hiatus hernia. In: Castell DO, Richter JE (eds) The esophagus, 3rd edn. Philadelphia: Lippincott, Williams & Wilkins, 1999; pp. 381–96.

10. Wo JM, Branum GD, Hunter JG et al. Clinical features of type III (mixed) paraesophageal hernia. Am J Gastroenterol 1996; 91:914–16.

11. Skinner DB, Belsey RH. Surgical management of esophageal reflux and hiatal hernia: long-term results of 1,030 patients. J Thorac Cardiovasc Surg 1967; 53:33–54.

12. Treacy PJ, Jamieson GG. An approach to the management of paraesophageal hiatus hernias. Aust NZ J Surg 1987; 57:813–17.

13. Collis JL. A review of surgical results in hiatus hernia. Thorax 1961; 16:1149.

14. Cameron AJ. Incidence of iron deficiency anemia in patients with large diaphragmatic hernia: a controlled study. Mayo Clin Proc 1976; 51:767–9.

15. Cameron AJ, Higgins JA. Linear gastric erosion: a lesion associated with large diaphragmatic hernia and chronic blood loss anemia. Gastroenterology 1986; 91:338–42.

16. Allen MS, Trastek VF, Deschamps C et al. Intrathoracic stomach: presentation and results of operation. J Thorac Cardiovasc Surg 1993; 105:253–8.

17. Stylopoulos N, Gazelle GS, Rattner DW. Paraesophageal hernias: operation or observation? Ann Surg 2002; 236:492–500.

18. Edye M, Salky B, Posner A et al. Sac excision is essential to adequate laparoscopic repair of paraesophageal hernia. Surg Endosc 1998; 12:1259–63.

19. Patel HJ, Tan BB, Yee J et al. A 25-year experience with open primary transthoracic repair of paraesophageal hiatus hernia. J Thorac Cardiovasc Surg 2004; 127:843–9.

20. Watson DI, Davies N, Devitt PG et al. Importance of dissection of the hernial sac in laparoscopic surgery for large hiatal hernias. Arch Surg 1999; 134:1069–73.

21. Cuschieri A, Shimi S, Nathenson LK. Laparoscopic reduction, crural repair, and fundoplication of large hiatal hernia. Am J Surg 1992; 163:425–30.

22. Diaz S, Brunt LM, Klingensmith ME et al. Laparoscopic paraesophageal hernia repair, a challenging operation: medium-term outcome of 116 patients. J Gastrointest Surg 2003; 7:59–66.

23. Edye MB, Canin-Endres J, Gattorno F et al. Durability of laparoscopic repair of paraesophageal hernia. Ann Surg 1998; 228:528–35.

24. Gantert WA, Patti MG, Arcerito M et al. Laparoscopic repair of paraesophageal hiatal hernias. J Am Coll Surg 1998; 186:428–32.

25. Hashemi M, Peters JH, DeMeester TR et al. Laparoscopic repair of large type III hiatal hernia: objective follow-up reveals high recurrence rate. J Am Coll Surg 2000; 190:553–60.

26. Horgan S, Eubanks TR, Jacobsen G et al. Repair of paraesophageal hernias. Am J Surg 1999; 177:354–8.

27. Mattar SG, Bowers SP, Galloway KD et al. Long-term outcome of laparoscopic repair of paraesophageal hernia. Surg Endosc 2002; 16:745–9.

28. Schauer PR, Ikramuddin S, McLaughlin MD et al. Comparison of laparoscopic versus open repair of paraesophageal hernia. Am J Surg 1998; 176:659–65.

29. Wiechmann RJ, Ferguson MK, Naunheim KS et al. Laparoscopic management of giant paraesophageal herniation. Ann Thorac Surg 2001; 71:1080–6.

30. Terry ML, Vernon A, Hunter JG. Stapled-wedge Collis gastroplasty for the shortened esophagus. Am J Surg 2004; 188:195–9.

31. Behrns KE, Schlinkert RT. Laparoscopic management of paraesophageal hernia: early results. J Laparoendosc Surg 1996; 6:311–17.

32. Trus TL, Bax T, Richardson WS et al. Complications of laparoscopic paraesophageal hernia repair. J Gastrointest Surg 1997; 1:221–7.

33. Casabella F, Sinanan M, Horgan S et al. Systematic use of gastric fundoplication in laparoscopic repair of paraesophageal hernias. Am J Surg 1996; 171:485–9.

34. Lal DR, Pellegrini CA, Oelschlager BK. Laparoscopic repair of paraesophageal hernia. Surg Clin North Am 2005; 85:105–18.

35. Swanstrom LL, Jobe BA, Kinzie LR et al. Esophageal motility and outcomes following laparoscopic paraesophageal hernia repair and fundoplication. Am J Surg 1999; 177:359–63.

36. Lam CR, Gahagan TH. The myths of the short esophagus. In: Nyhus LM, Harkins HN (eds.) Hernia. Philadelphia: JB Lippincott, 1964; p. 450.

37. DePaula AL, Hashiba K, Bajutto M et al. Laparoscopic reoperations after failed and complicated antireflux operations. Surg Endosc 1995; 9:681–6.

38. Ellis FH Jr, Gibb SP, Heatley GJ. Reoperation after failed antireflux surgery: review of 101 cases. Eur J Cardiothorac Surg 1996; 10:225–31.

39. Jobe BA, Horvath KD, Swanstrom LL. Postoperative function following laparoscopic Collis gastroplasty for shortened esophagus. Arch Surg 1998; 133:867–74.

40. Collis JL. An operation for hiatus hernia with short oesophagus. Thorax 1957; 12:181–8.

41. Gastal OL, Hagen JA, Peters JH et al. Short esophagus: analysis of predictors and clinical implications. Arch Surg 1999; 134:633–6.

42. Johnson AB, Oddsdottir M, Hunter JG. Laparoscopic Collis gastroplasty and Nissen fundoplication: a new technique for the management of esophageal foreshortening. Surg Endosc 1998; 12:1055–60.

43. Horvath KH, Swanstrom LL. Endoscopic esophageal lengthening procedures for the shortened esophagus: the combined laparoscopic/thoracoscopic Collis gastroplasty. In: Zucker CA (ed.) Surgical laparoscopy, 2nd edn. Baltimore: Williams & Wilkins, 2001; pp. 445–56.

44. Swanstrom LL, Marcus DR, Galloway GQ. Laparoscopic Collis gastroplasty is the treatment of choice for the shortened esophagus. Am J Surg 1996; 171:477–81.

45. Frantzides CT, Madan AK, Carlson MA et al. A prospective, randomized trial of laparoscopic polytetrafluoroethylene (PTFE) patch repair vs simple cruroplasty for large hiatal hernia. Arch Surg 2002; 137:649–52.

46. Kamolz T, Granderath FA, Bammer T et al. Dysphagia and quality of life after laparoscopic Nissen fundoplication in patients with and without

prosthetic reinforcement of the hiatal crura. Surg Endosc 2002; 16:572–7.

47. Granderath FA, Kamolz T, Schweiger UM et al. Impact of laparoscopic Nissen fundoplication with prosthetic hiatal closure on esophageal body motility: results of a prospective randomized trial. Arch Surg 2006; 141:625–32.

48. Paul MG, DeRosa RP, Petrucci PE et al. Laparoscopic tension-free repair of large paraesophageal hernias. Surg Endosc 1997; 11:303–7.

49. Tatum RP, Shalhub S, Oelschlager BK et al. Complications of PTFE mesh at the diaphragmatic hiatus. J Gastrointest Surg 2008; 12(5):953–7.

50. Oelschlager BK, Pellegrini CA, Hunter JG et al. Biologic prosthesis reduces recurrence after laparoscopic paraesophageal hernia repair: a multicenter, prospective, randomized trial. Ann Surg 2006; 244:481–90.

51. Berti A. Singulare attortigliamento dele' esofago col duodeno seguita da rapida morte. Gazz Med Ital 1896; 9:139.

52. Carter R, Brewer LA 3rd, Hinshaw DB. Acute gastric volvulus: a study of 25 cases. Am J Surg 1980; 140:99–106.

53. Borchardt M. Aus Pathologie und therapie des magenvolvulus. Arch Klin Chir 1904; 74:243.

18

Benign ulceration of the stomach and duodenum and the complications of previous ulcer surgery

John Wayman

Introduction

The role of the surgeon in the management of peptic ulcer disease has changed in the last few decades. Since the introduction of effective acid antisecretories and greater understanding of *Helicobacter pylori*, the role of the surgeon has become limited to the management of occasional resistant ulcers, emergency management of complicated ulcer disease and management of the side-effects of ulcer surgery.

Management of refractory peptic ulceration

Endoscopic confirmation

Gastric and duodenal ulcers may be considered 'refractory' to medical treatment if there is no sign of significant healing by 12 and 8 weeks respectively. Gastric ulcers must be carefully re-biopsied as there is a risk that an apparently benign gastric ulcer is in fact an early malignancy. Direct endoscopic inspection, adequate tissue biopsy and expert histological interpretation are essential to identify dysplasia, neoplasia or other more uncommon mucosal disease. Repeat endoscopy to confirm healing and re-biopsy are mandatory for all gastric ulcers but probably unnecessary for duodenal ulcers if symptoms have resolved. Persistent duodenal ulceration should be re-biopsied for similar, albeit less likely, reasons given above to identify the several neoplastic, infectious and inflammatory conditions that can mimic peptic ulcer disease.

Confirmation of persistent *Helicobacter* infection

Multiple diagnostic tests are available for determining the presence of *Helicobacter pylori* (HP) infection. Most tests have been evaluated in untreated individuals, while few studies have investigated their performance post-treatment when bacterial counts might be low. HP infection can be determined non-invasively by carbon isotope (^{13}C or ^{14}C) urea breath test, serologically by enzyme-linked immunosorbent assay or using endoscopic biopsy material by functional assay of urease activity and histological analysis. Which technique should be regarded as the 'gold standard' is uncertain. Several drugs, including proton-pump inhibitors, bismuth and antibiotics, temporarily suppress HP and render functional assays falsely negative. The sensitivity may be less following treatment, although using more than one biopsy may improve sensitivity.[1] Histological diagnosis is most sensitive using either the Warthin–Starry stain or the modified Giemsa stain, the latter being the simpler and cheaper and hence the most commonly used. Although frequently used as the reference method for other studies, this method is prone to inter-observer variability. False-negative diagnosis occurs in about 5–15% of cases, depending on the laboratory experience. Since the inoculum in the post-treatment case may be low and there may be proximal migration of the infection, diagnosis in this circumstance can be enhanced by analysis of biopsies from both the antrum and body of the stomach.[2] Immunohistochemistry using polyclonal antisera to HP can improve sensitivity and reduce inter-observer variation.[3] Use of the polymerase chain reaction allows detection of the presence of HP DNA in the absence of viable bacteria. Although this test may have the highest sensitivity, there are frequent false-positive results and the test adds little to existing diagnostic techniques. The urea breath test is particularly well suited to assessing HP status post-treatment.[4] The faecal antigen detection kit is a quick, technically simple non-invasive test and reports suggest a high degree of accuracy and good prediction of successful eradication.[5] Possible causes of failure of HP eradication are antibiotic resistance or if the patient has failed to comply with the prescribed regimen. The former may be overcome by appropriate modification of the antibiotic regime occasionally even using bacteriological culture to help direct treatment.

Idiopathic refractory ulceration

Ingestion of non-steroidal anti-inflammatory drugs (NSAIDs) should be re-evaluated. Surreptitious aspirin ingestion has been observed and if suspected can be established by assay of plasma salicylate levels. Any other factor that may be facilitating ulceration, such as smoking or intercurrent disease, should be sought and eliminated where possible. Diseases associated with peptic ulceration are chronic liver disease, hyperparathyroidism and chronic renal failure, particularly during dialysis and after successful transplantation. Those who smoke are more likely to fail both medical and, indeed, surgical ulcer treatment. Smoking impairs the therapeutic effects of antisecretories, may stimulate pepsin secretion and promote reflux of duodenal contents into the stomach. Smoking also increases the harmful effects of HP, and increases the production of free radicals, endothelin and platelet-activating factor. Smoking also affects the mucosal protective mechanisms by decreasing gastric mucosal blood flow and inhibiting gastric prostaglandin generation and the secretion of gastric mucous, salivary epidermal growth factor, duodenal mucosal bicarbonate and pancreatic bicarbonate.[6] Stopping smoking is an important first step to allow effective ulcer treatment.

A diagnosis of Zollinger–Ellison should be suspected in cases of *Helicobacter*-negative, non-NSAID-induced refractory ulceration and especially where there is ulceration of the second part of the duodenum or large confluent ulcers in the duodenum (see below). Hypergastrinaemia should be excluded prior to a decision to treat a refractory ulcer.

Where no cause for persistent ulceration can be found it may be necessary for the patient to take long-term antisecretory drugs. Alternatively, elective surgery may be considered in this group of patients. Inherent in this decision is a careful calculation of the relative risks and benefits of surgery against the potential risks and costs of continued medical treatment. The risks of complications of persistent ulcer disease, the degree of disability experienced by patients and their fitness for surgery should all be considered in the decision of whether or not to operate.

Elective surgery for resistant peptic ulceration

Definitive surgery for duodenal ulcer evolved around the concept of acid reduction either by resection of most of the parietal cell mass, vagal denervation of the parietal cells or resection of the antral gastrin-producing cells. The balance lay in minimising the chance of ulcer recurrence while at the same time trying to avoid the symptomatic side-effects and metabolic sequelae of the procedure that would affect the patient for the rest of their life.

The trend by the mid-1970s was towards highly selective vagotomy (HSV) or proximal gastric vagotomy, which denervated the parietal cell mass but left the antrum and pylorus innervated and so allowed a gastric emptying pattern that, while not completely normal, did not require a drainage procedure. This was the first ulcer procedure that did not involve bypass, destruction or removal of the pylorus and as a result has significantly fewer side-effects than other ulcer operations. The main concern with this operation, whether for duodenal or gastric ulcer, has been the recurrence rate. In the best hands recurrence rates of 5–10% have been achieved.[7]

Anterior seromyotomy with posterior truncal vagotomy probably denervates the proximal stomach more consistently.[8] It has proved that the posterior vagal trunk can be divided and the patient not experience significant diarrhoea, provided the pylorus is intact and innervated. There is now really no place for truncal vagotomy with either destruction, bypass or excision of the pylorus because of the lifelong risk of diarrhoea, which in a significant proportion of patients is socially disabling.[9]

Some surgeons advocated the use of truncal vagotomy and antrectomy, suggesting that this operation is the most effective for reducing acid secretion and has a very low recurrence rate of about 1%. The procedure was subsequently modified to a selective vagotomy and antrectomy, leaving the hepatic and coeliac fibres of the vagi intact. This did reduce the incidence of side-effects, especially diarrhoea, though dumping was still a problem. Bile gastritis and oesophagitis were also troublesome side-effects unless a Roux-en-Y reconstruction was used, though recurrent stomal ulceration was then more frequent unless a more extensive gastric resection was performed. The perfect ulcer operation has remained elusive and indeed there is none that has no side-effects or risks.

Operations for refractory duodenal ulcers

There is no good evidence on which to base the decision of operation in cases of resistant ulceration in the modern era. Intuitively, one might predict a poor result with HSV alone since its success rate historically was less than that of modern medical treatment. It seems likely that resection of the antral gastrin-producing mucosa and either resection or vagal denervation of the parietal cell mass is necessary. The operations that could be considered include the following:

- **Selective vagotomy and antrectomy.** Selective denervation is preferred because of a lower incidence of side-effects. It is not an easy procedure; in particular the dissection around the lower oesophagus and cardia has to be done very carefully. The vagotomy should be performed before the resection and tested intraoperatively. The reconstruction should either be a gastroduodenal (Billroth I) anastomosis or a Roux-en-Y gastro-jejunostomy. The latter is associated with fewer problems with bile reflux into the gastric remnant and oesophagus, but a higher risk of stomal ulceration and so at least a two-thirds gastrectomy is advised.
- **Subtotal gastrectomy.** Removal of a large part of the parietal cell mass is sound in theory and indeed ulcer recurrence after this operation is unusual. However, there is an incidence of postprandial symptoms and in particular epigastric discomfort and fullness that can limit calorie intake. Importantly, there is a high incidence of long-term nutritional and metabolic sequelae that require lifelong surveillance and can be difficult to prevent, although this is mainly in women.
- **Pylorus-preserving gastrectomy.** This operation involves highly selective vagotomy with resection of about 50% of the parietal cell mass and the antral mucosa, but preserving the pyloric mechanism and the vagus nerves to the distal antrum and pylorus. There is some evidence that this may be a superior technique with fewer sequelae compared to the traditional approaches.[10,11] Comparable results of the technique used in the context of treatment of early gastric cancer confirm a good long-term functional result.[12]

Operations for refractory gastric ulcers

There are no reliable data on which to base a recommendation for surgical treatment of refractory gastric ulcers. HSV is not recommended for pre-pyloric ulcers since they follow the same pattern as described for duodenal ulceration. The choice of operation for a more proximal ulcer, often along the lesser curve and often associated with atrophic gastritis, is between excision of the ulcer with HSV or partial gastrectomy. The recurrence rate is higher after HSV/excision, but the operative mortality is lower and side-effects fewer after this procedure.

Laparoscopic peptic ulcer surgery

Interest in minimally invasive procedures has led to many publications proving the feasibility of laparoscopic definitive ulcer operations. The indications and considerations for elective laparoscopic peptic ulcer surgery should be exactly the same as for open procedures.

Zollinger–Ellison syndrome (ZES)

Refractory peptic ulceration should raise the suspicion of ZES. Alternatively the syndrome may present with diarrhoea and weight loss and a third present with oesophagitis only. The disease may present more dramatically with perforation, haemorrhage, oesophageal stricture, jejunal or anastomotic ulceration. The condition should be suspected particularly when a duodenal ulcer coexists with primary hyperparathyroidism or metastatic adenocarcinoma of unknown origin. The aims of treatment are control of gastric acid hypersecretion most commonly by high-dose proton-pump inhibitors with, where possible, removal of the underlying tumour itself.

Pathology

Although originally described as a pancreatic endocrine tumour, the definition has also come to include extrapancreatic gastrin-secreting tumours. Where the condition is due to a pancreatic tumour, in two-thirds of cases the tumour will be multifocal within the pancreas.[13] At least two-thirds will be histologically malignant. One-third will already have demonstrable metastases by the time of diagnosis.[14] The most common extrapancreatic site is in the wall of the duodenum. Less frequently (6–11% of cases) ectopic gastrinoma tissue has been identified in the liver, common bile duct, jejunum, omentum, pylorus, ovary and heart.[15] These extrapancreatic tumours rarely metastasise to the liver and, even though they do metastasise just as frequently to regional lymph nodes, they tend to have a better prognosis than primary pancreatic tumours.

One-quarter of patients with ZES have other endocrine tumours as part of a familial multiple endocrine neoplasia (MEN-1) syndrome, particularly hyperparathyroidism.[14] This group of patients have a much worse prognosis than sporadic ZES, in part due to the multifocal nature of the tumour within the pancreas.

The majority of cases of ZES arise sporadically. Such tumours are more likely to occur in extrapancreatic sites than familial types. Prognosis is better in this group of patients.

Diagnosis

Diagnosis may be confirmed by the finding of fasting hypergastrinaemia associated with gastric acid hypersecretion. Hypergastrinaemia may occur in cases of achlorhydria such as ingestion of antisecretory drugs, postvagotomy, pernicious anaemia, atrophic gastritis, antral G-cell hyperplasia or gastric outlet obstruction. Hypergastrinaemia is also associated with a retained antrum after a Billroth II/Pólya-type gastrectomy where a small cuff of antrum has been included in the 'duodenal' closure: if a retained antrum is suspected, technetium pertechnetate scan may be useful in identifying the antral mucosa. If there is diagnostic uncertainty or the basal serum gastrin level is marginal, dynamic assay of serum gastrin following secretin (or alternatively calcium or glucagon) provocation may be required. Gastrin response to a standard meal helps to differentiate between hypergastrinaemia due to antral G-cell hyperplasia, which will result in an increase in serum gastrin levels, while no response would be expected in cases of gastrinoma.

Surgery for ZES

How aggressively surgery should be pursued in cases of gastrinoma is controversial. A prospective audit of outcome of cases treated surgically between 1981 and 1998 has shown that surgical exploration and resection resulted in excellent long-term results, with a 10-year survival rate of 94%.[16] If resectable solitary or multiple gastrinomas can be identified, surgical management should be considered in view of the high risk of malignancy. Whether that should be local enucleation or a wider resection is also controversial. In the past many would say that patients with MEN-1 and those with diffuse liver metastases should not be treated surgically. Nevertheless, impressive results from more than one centre have been reported even in the former group[15–17] and there is evidence that surgical resection of localised liver gastrinoma provides a cure rate similar to that of extrahepatic gastrinoma.[18]

Tumour localisation

A tumour may be localised initially by computed tomography. This may also identify metastatic disease. Endoscopic ultrasound (EUS) and intraoperative ultrasound have proved useful additional modalities. EUS is highly accurate in the localisation of pancreatic tumours and gastrinomas in the duodenal wall as small as 4 mm. Somatostatin receptor scintigraphy with [111In-DTPA (diethylenetriaminepenta-acetic acid)-DPhe1]octreotide (SRS) and selective arterial secretagogue injection (SASI) testing are the most reliable approaches to localising gastrinomas. SRS can identify 30% of gastrinomas ≥1.1 cm, 64% of those 1.1–2 cm and 96% of those >2 cm.[19] The test involves whole-body imaging, which is advantageous for the detection of extrapancreatic sites. Liver metastases can frequently be detected by conventional imaging, but SRS has proved a more sensitive investigation that may prevent unnecessary surgical exploration. SASI involves selective catheterisation of the feeding arteries of the duodenum and pancreas and the hepatic veins. Secretin is injected in turn into the splenic, gastroduodenal (GDA) and superior mesenteric (SMA) arteries. Corresponding hepatic venous gastrin levels are measured and allow identification of the main feeding vessel. More precise localisation can be achieved by more peripheral cannulation of the SMA and GDA or different points along the splenic artery. The test has greater than 90% sensitivity and specificity for preoperative tumour localisation.[17]

Surgical strategy

Exploration of the pancreas when preoperative investigations have failed to precisely localise a tumour is now a less frequent problem, particularly in specialist centres with access to SASI and SRS. Nevertheless, a laparotomy will detect a third more gastrinomas than even SRS.[19] If surgical exploration is performed then the pancreas must be mobilised along its entire length, inspected, palpated and if the facilities are available re-scanned intraoperatively by endoluminal or standard ultrasound. Palpation of the duodenal wall will identify 61% of duodenal gastrinomas. Intraoperative ultrasound does not detect any duodenal tumour that was not palpable, but duodenal transillumination by endoscopy will improve detection to 84% and duodenotomy identifies the remaining cases.[20] If no gastrinoma is found in the usual locations, other ectopic sites should be examined carefully.[15,16] Resection of these primary ectopic tumours can sometimes lead to durable biochemical cures.[15] Gastrinomas may be identified in 96% of surgical explorations if these approaches are adopted.[16] If no tumour is identified some would advocate that at most an acid-reducing operation should be considered. With the use of SASI in particular, though a tumour cannot be precisely localised, it may be sufficiently 'narrowed down' to allow a limited pancreatic and/or duodenal resection.[17] The intraoperative secretin test in which gastrin levels in response to secretin are measured before and after resection can be useful in assessing the effectiveness of resection.

Emergency management of complicated peptic ulcer disease

Although very few patients now require elective surgery, the number who require surgery for the complications of peptic ulcer disease has remained constant for many years.

Perforation

A number of factors associated with poor outcome in perforated peptic ulcer have been identified: delay in diagnosis, coexistent medical illness, shock on admission, leucocytosis and age over 75. A delay in treatment of greater than 24 hours is associated with a sevenfold increase in mortality, threefold risk of morbidity and a twofold increase in hospital stay. The elderly are particularly vulnerable and often more difficult to diagnose because of poorly localised symptoms and signs and fewer preceding symptoms. The principles of treatment of peptic ulcer perforation involve resuscitation, control of contamination and prevention of recurrence.

Conservative management

Study of the natural history of perforated peptic ulcers suggests that they frequently seal spontaneously by omentum or adjacent organs and that, particularly when this occurs rapidly, contamination can be minimal. Taylor showed that the mortality in his series of patients with peptic ulcer disease was half that of the contemporary reported mortality for perforation treated surgically.[21] In a recent small series, mortality by the conservative approach was 3% with conversion to operation in 6 of 34 because of progressive deterioration: five for unsealed gastric or duodenal ulceration and one for gangrenous cholecystitis.[22] A small, randomised controlled trial comparing conservative treatment with surgical treatment showed no difference in morbidity or mortality.[23] Eleven of 40 patients treated conservatively ultimately required surgical treatment; these cases were more often over 70 years of age. Hence some authors advocate an initial, closely monitored trial of conservative therapy of parenteral broad-spectrum antibiotics, intravenous acid antisecretories, intravenous fluid resuscitation and nasogastric aspiration in patients under the age of 70. Another adjunct suggested by some is the gastrograffin swallow; if the perforation is sealed, the patient can be treated non-surgically.[24] Such a policy requires careful interval assessment by an experienced surgeon with a low threshold for performing laparotomy if clinical improvement is not apparent both to confirm the diagnosis and oversew an unsealed perforation.

Surgery

In most cases the treatment of choice for patients with perforation of the duodenum is still laparotomy, peritoneal lavage and simple closure of perforation, usually by omental patch repair. The routine use of drains is unnecessary and may in fact increase morbidity. Additional biopsy of perforated gastric ulcers is mandatory. This simple treatment is safe and effective in the long term, when combined with pharmacological acid suppression. Ninety percent of perforations are associated with HP infection,[25] and HP eradication further significantly reduces the ulcer recurrence.[26]

In cases of 'giant' perforation, where the defect measures 2.5 cm or more, partial gastrectomy with closure of the duodenal stump should be considered (see also management of bleeding from giant duodenal ulcer below). Alternatively, in situations where the clinical situation or expertise dictates more expeditious surgery, the duodenal perforation should be closed as well as possible around a large Foley or T-tube catheter to create a controlled fistula. Other methods described include a free omental and jejunal serosal 'plug'.

Traditionally there has been a school of thought that, at the time of emergency laparotomy, definitive ulcer surgery should be performed. In particular, HSV has been strongly advocated to reduce the risk of recurrent ulceration and its complications. **The advances in understanding of the treatment of ulcers together with the decrease in experience of elective anti-ulcer surgery have made this argument no longer tenable.** The indications for emergency definitive surgery are exactly the same as the criteria for elective surgery and should now be extremely rare in the patient presenting with an acute perforation. There is no justification for performing vagotomy for complicated duodenal ulcer disease.[27,28]

Laparoscopic treatment of peptic ulcer perforation was first reported in 1990.[29]

A meta-analysis of 13 publications involving 658 patients has demonstrated 84.7% success rate by the laparoscopic approach with reduction of postoperative pain and wound infection but an increase in the rate of re-operation.[30]

A systematic review of 96 publications including 13 prospective and 12 retrospective studies identified shock, delayed presentation (>24 hours), confounding medical condition, age >70 years, poor laparoscopic expertise and American Society of Anesthesiologists (ASA) III–IV as risk factors for conversion to open and postoperative morbidity.[31] Statistically significant findings in favour of laparoscopic repair were less analgesic use, shorter hospital stay, less wound infection and lower mortality rate. Shorter operating time and less suture-site leakage were advantages of open repair.

 In 'low-risk' patients the laparoscopic approach has significant advantages. For higher risk patients (prolonged perforation for >24 h, shock on admission and confounding medical conditions) there is no evidence that the laparoscopic approach is advantageous. Some would interpret this to mean that in this group, until such evidence is available, the surgical approach should remain the more familiar open approach.

Bleeding

Management of acute haemorrhage from peptic ulceration of the stomach and duodenum has been revolutionised by rapidly developing endoscopic technology and expertise. The principle of successful management is by meticulous resuscitation, accurate endoscopic diagnosis and the timely application of appropriate therapy.

Medical therapy

 Although there is some evidence that proton-pump inhibitors given pre-endoscopy reduce the incidence of endoscopic findings of stigmata of recent haemorrhage, there is no evidence that this or any other any specific pre-endoscopy medical intervention has any effect on overall morbidity, mortality nor specifically the risk of re-bleeding or need for surgery.[32]

 There is compelling evidence that proton-pump inhibitors given after endoscopic control of bleeding are beneficial. A randomised controlled study (n = 240) from Hong Kong has demonstrated a significant reduction in re-bleeding following endoscopic treatment with a protocol of intravenous omeprazole (omeprazole 80 mg i.v. bolus followed by 8 mg/h infusion for 72 hours).[33]

 Meta-analysis of randomised, double-blinded trials with tranexamic acid reveal no significant difference in the incidence of re-bleeding but an increase in complications related to therapy such as stroke, myocardial infarction, deep vein thrombosis and pulmonary embolism.[34]

Somatostatin decreases gastric acid and pepsin secretion. Nevertheless, there is no proven benefit of somatostatin or its analogue (octreotide) in the management of active non-variceal upper gastrointestinal bleeding. Prostaglandin E_2 and its analogue (misoprostal) inhibits gastric acid production, stimulates mucosal perfusion and promotes bicarbonate and mucus secretion. Small studies to date have demonstrated no benefit of stopping acute bleeding or preventing re-bleeding.

Endoscopic therapy

The various techniques of endoscopic haemostasis have dramatically reduced the need for emergency surgery for bleeding due to peptic ulceration.

 Meta-analysis suggests that endoscopic therapy reduces the mortality of acute upper gastrointestinal bleed in patients' active bleeding or non-bleeding visible vessel by avoiding the often considerable morbidity or mortality of emergency surgery.[35]

Ulcers with a clean base or non-protuberant pigmented dot in an ulcer bed, which are at low risk of re-bleeding, do not require endoscopic treatment. For all others, including those who have active bleeding or non-bleeding visible vessels or have adherent blood clot, endoscopic treatment should be given.[36,37]

Injection with 4–16 mL 1:10 000 adrenaline around the bleeding point and then into the bleeding vessel achieves haemostasis in up to 95% of cases. Additional injection with sclerosants (sodium tetradecyl sulphate, polidoconal, ethanolamine) or absolute alcohol do not confer additional benefit and may cause perforation. Fibrin glue and thrombin may be more effective, but they are not widely available.

Techniques used commonly are the heater probe, multipolar coagulation (BICAP) and argon plasma coagulation. There is no strong evidence to recommend one thermal haemostasis technique over another.

Mechanical clips have had variable success reported when compared with other techniques. This may reflect the technical difficulties with their placement. In certain situations, such as active bleeding from a large vessel, they may be particularly useful.

 There is some evidence that for patients at higher risk of re-bleeding, treatment by a combination of two different modalities may be more beneficial than relying on one modality alone:[36,37] the commonest combination is likely to be adrenaline injection and heater probe application.

There is no evidence to support a repeat endoscopy unless there is a suggestion of further active bleeding or it is felt that the initial endoscopic treatment was suboptimal. Nevertheless, some clinicians do choose to re-evaluate higher risk cases after 24–48 hours and consider further endoscopic treatment.

Some recommend a second attempt at endoscopic treatment for re-bleeding before considering surgery.

 A prospective randomised study from Hong Kong looking at 92 patients who re-bled found that retreatment with adrenaline injection and heater probe led to a 73% control.[38] Overall, morbidity and mortality were greater in the group randomised to surgery; the complications of those re-endoscoped related to those of salvage surgery. Of those patients who failed to respond to second injection therapy, hypotension at randomisation and ulcer size >2 cm were significant risk factors.

Surgery

Operative intervention is mandatory if initial control of bleeding is not possible endoscopically. Surgery should also be considered if re-bleeding occurs following initially successful endoscopic treatment. Re-bleeding may be observed directly endoscopically or indirectly by continuing haematemesis, or the continuing need for transfusion. If there is doubt as to whether re-bleeding has occurred a check endoscopy should be performed before subjecting a patient to surgery.

Surgical intervention should be anticipated where there is a significant risk of re-bleeding. Various scoring criteria have been suggested to predict risk of significant re-bleeding and death; one commonly used is the Rockall system (Table 18.1). In addition,

the size of the ulcer (particularly >2 cm), its proximity to major vessels, such as the gastroduodenal ulcer on the posterior inferior wall of the duodenal bulb and the left gastric artery high on the lesser curve of the stomach, suggests a high risk of massive bleeding.

Bleeding duodenal ulcer

The first step is to make a longitudinal duodenotomy immediately distal to the pyloric ring. Haemostasis can be initially achieved by digital pressure. While it may be necessary to extend the duodenotomy through the pyloric ring, the pylorus should be preserved if at all possible. Older texts frequently assume that vagotomy is an integral part of ulcer surgery and recommend a larger pyloroduodenotomy, but this is usually not necessary. The stomach and duodenum should be cleared of blood and clots using suction to obtain optimal view of the bleeding site. If access is still difficult, kocherisation of the duodenum may help along with drawing up of the posterior duodenal mucosa using Babcocks' forceps.

The actively bleeding or exposed vessel should be secured. Points of note in securing the vessel are the limited access, the proximity of underlying structures such as the common bile duct and the tough fibrous nature of the base of a chronic ulcer. In view of these problems, a small, heavy, round-bodied or taper-cut semicircular needle with 0 or No. 1 suture material should be used. The argument of absorbable vs. non-absorbable suture is irrelevant: the sutures probably slough off as the ulcer heals.

The duodenotomy may be closed longitudinally. If vagotomy has been performed the pyloric ring should be divided and the duodenotomy closed transversely to create a Heinke–Mickulicz pyloroplasty

Table 18.1 • Rockall scoring system for risk of re-bleeding and death after admission to hospital for acute gastrointestinal bleeding

Variable	Score			
	0	**1**	**2**	**3**
Age	<60	60–79	>80	
Shock	No shock	Pulse >100 BP >100	Pulse >100 BP <100	
Comorbidity	None		Cardiac failure, IHD, major comorbidity	Renal failure, liver failure, disseminated malignancy
Diagnosis	Mallory–Weiss tear, no lesion, no SRH	All other diagnoses	Malignancy of upper GI tract	
Major SRH	None or dark spot		Blood in upper GI tract, adherent clot, visible or spurting vessel	

A total score of >3 is associated with good prognosis; <8 is associated with high risk of death.
BP, blood pressure; GI, gastrointestinal; IHD, ischaemic heart disease; SRH, stigmata of recent haemorrhage.

(Fig. 18.1a). If transverse closure is difficult because of the length of the duodenotomy, longitudinal closure may be performed and a gastro-jejunostomy fashioned. Alternatively, a Finney pyloroplasty may be fashioned (Fig. 18.1b).

In a giant ulcer, the first part of the duodenum may be virtually destroyed and, once opened, impossible to close. In this situation it is necessary to proceed to partial gastrectomy. The right gastric and right gastroepiploic arteries are divided. The stomach is disconnected from the duodenum by a combination of blunt and sharp dissection. Antrectomy is perfomed and continuity restored by a gastro-jejunostomy. The duodenal stump can then be closed. Although this can be achieved by pinching the second part of the duodenum away from the ulcer to allow conventional closure, this is probably more safely achieved by the technique of Nissen (Fig. 18.2). The duodenal stump is drained by either a tube or Foley catheter either through the duodenal suture line or more securely though the healthy side-wall of the second part of the duodenum (Fig. 18.3).

Long-term acid suppression is required postoperatively. With the advent of proton-pump inhibitors and the recognition of the role of HP, vagotomy should have no part of surgery for bleeding duodenal ulceration.

Bleeding gastric ulcer

The precise site of bleeding should already have been identified endoscopically. If not, intraoperative endoscopy and careful palpation of the stomach for induration should identify the site of the bleeding ulcer. If there is still doubt a generous incision should be made across the pylorus and duodenum followed by a more proximal gastrotomy if the source of bleeding is still not clear. Most chronic gastric ulcers are at the incisura or in the antrum. The traditional treatment for such ulcers that fail endoscopic therapy is partial gastrectomy. Some groups have advocated simple under-running of bleeding gastric ulcers. While this may be appropriate in selected cases with small bleeding gastric ulcers such as the Dieulafoy lesion, the only randomised trial

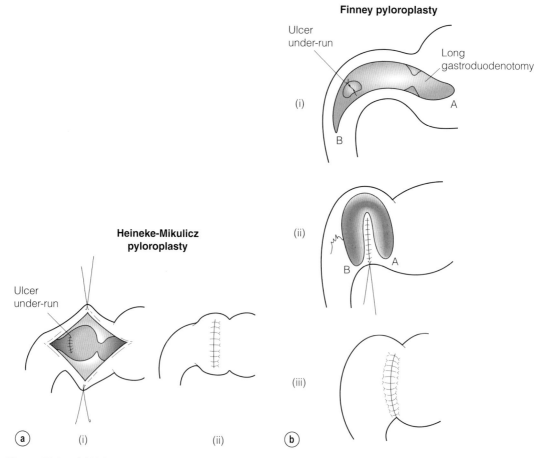

Figure 18.1 • **(a)** Heineke–Mikulicz pyloroplasty. **(b)** Finney pyloroplasty.

Nissen technique

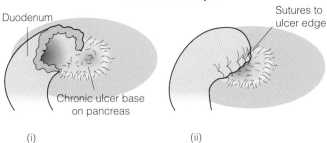

Figure 18.2 • Nissen technique.

Tube drainage

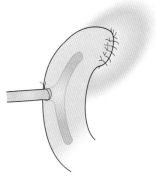

Figure 18.3 • Duodenal drainage following partial gastrectomy for duodenal ulcer.

to date ($n = 129$) suggests that this 'conservative' approach has a higher mortality and is more likely to result in re-bleeding if used unselectively.[39]

For proximal gastric ulcers, typically those high on the lesser curve eroding through into the left gastric artery, the choice of operation lies between total gastrectomy or local excision of the lesser curve (Pauchet's manoeuvre). Frequently such limited procedures involve as much mobilisation of the stomach as total gastrectomy. There is no evidence to recommend one approach over another, though the experience of the surgeon is a major factor in the decision-making process.

Pyloric stenosis

Gastric outlet obstruction can result from peptic ulcer disease of the duodenum or pre-pyloric region. It is a condition usually associated with chronic relapsing ulceration and is now fairly uncommon in the Western world.

Resuscitation and medical therapy

Initial management should consist of aggressive parenteral fluid and biochemical restoration with nutritional and vitamin supplementation as necessary. Nasogastric intubation with a wide-bore tube allows gastric washout of undigested food and so reduces antral stimulation. Aggressive parenteral antisecretory therapy and *Helicobacter* eradication, if appropriate, are used. In cases where the obstruction has been due to oedema and spasm, the situation can be expected to resolve once medical treatment has healed the ulcer.[40] Dietary changes to decrease the fibre content while providing a high calorie and protein intake are important until ulcer healing has occurred. In cases where the obstruction is due to fibrosis and cicatrisation of a pyloric ulcer, some form of intervention will be necessary.

Endoscopic treatment

The group of patients who develop gastric outflow obstruction are generally elderly and often with concomitant disease who tolerate poorly major surgery. Minimally invasive approaches are often appropriate in the first instance. Initial reports of successful resolution of pyloric stenosis following endoscopic balloon dilatation were challenged due to the relatively high number of cases that ultimately required open surgery (50% within 2 years).[41,42] Nevertheless, this remains a useful first-line endoscopic procedure that can be repeated on several occasions with good long-term results in up to 80% of patients.[42] The main risk of endoscopic dilatation is perforation and the procedure should only be performed on patients who have been appropriately worked up for surgical intervention if needed. Only if a combination of intensive medical treatment and dilatation fails to reopen the gastric outlet is surgery indicated.

Surgery

There are no published series that prove which procedure achieves the best results in this situation. Initial fears about the capacity of a large atonic stomach to resume function have not been realised. The operation with least complications is simple pyloroplasty (or gastroenterostomy where the inflammation around the pylorus is particularly intense), with the use of long-term medical acid suppression. Antrectomy and selective vagotomy or subtotal gastrectomy are more aggressive alternatives less likely to result in re-stenosis, but with a higher mortality and incidence of both short- and long-term side-effects.

Laparoscopic highly selective vagotomy with balloon dilatation has been attempted with some success in cases of pyloric stenosis. This has not been proven to be superior to dilatation and long-term acid suppression. Laparoscopic truncal vagotomy and gastroenterostomy has proven to be a technically feasible solution with good symptomatic, sustained response. The published series are small in numbers and the additional morbidity associated with the surgery suggest that balloon dilatation with acid suppression should still be the preferred first-line treatment in cases of pyloric stenosis.[43]

Complications of previous ulcer surgery

Although elective surgery for benign ulcer disease is now rare, there remains a large cohort of patients operated on prior to the mid-1980s with a variety of surgical procedures, of whom a small percentage will develop further symptoms, some of which may be severely disabling. Although numerous clinical syndromes have been well described (Box 18.1) patients presenting with pure syndromes are uncommon. The majority present with a mixed picture, but usually have a dominant symptom complex suggesting one main problem. This needs to be elucidated by a careful and detailed history of the clinical events occurring during a bad attack.

Preoperative evaluation

Endoscopy
Endoscopic examination is essential, and as with patients after previous antireflux surgery, it should be carried out by the surgeon considering any

Box 18.1 • Post-peptic ulcer surgery sequelae

Pathophysiological problems
- Gastro-oesophageal reflux
- Recurrent ulcer
- Enterogastric reflux
- Dumping
- Reactive hypoglycaemia
- Diarrhoea
- Malabsorption

Mechanical problems
- Loop obstruction
- Small stomach syndrome
- Bezoars

Other sequelae
- Cholelithiasis
- Carcinoma

revisional procedure. The exact anatomy, size of the gastric remnant, size and position of any drainage procedure, the presence of enterogastric reflux of bile, recurrent ulceration, the general state of the gastric mucosa and the presence of a hiatus hernia and/or reflux oesophagitis can be assessed. All abnormalities should be biopsied. All patients should be assessed for the presence of HP.

Radiology
Barium meal examination of the stomach is a useful adjunct where the anatomy remains unclear.

Gastric-emptying studies
Gastric-emptying studies may occasionally be useful. Barium meal examination may show rapid emptying of the contrast from the stomach and may demonstrate gross intestinal hurry with the meal reaching the caecum within a short time of leaving the stomach. Gastric emptying is, however, best studied using a radioactively labelled meal, either liquid or solid. In general, the radioactive liquid meals are easier to interpret than solid meals. The normal measured indices such as 10-minute emptying, the $T_{1/2}$ and the percentage retention after 60 minutes are often used in assessment. However, after gastric surgery these indices can be misleading as the patients often show a fast initial emptying component followed by a slower component.

Other tests
Congo red for the evaluation of the completeness of vagotomy and dumping provocation tests are now seldom performed. Oesophageal function tests will be required in those patients suspected of having gastro-oesophageal reflux. Enterogastric reflux can be assessed using the hepatobiliary dimethylacetanilideiminodiacetic acid (HIDA) scan. Bacterial overgrowth can be diagnosed by aspiration and culture of jejunal contents or by the [^{14}C]glycocholate breath test.

Various nutritional indices, including weight, serum albumin, transferase and corrected serum calcium concentration, should be measured in all patients. In selected patients full assessment for metabolic bone disease should be undertaken, especially in postmenopausal women. A full haematological survey should be carried out including measurement of serum iron, iron-binding capacity, folate and vitamin B_{12} levels.

Enterogastric reflux

Reflux of alkaline duodenal content into the stomach occurs following surgery that damages, bypasses or removes the pylorus. Enterogastric reflux is more common after gastrectomy, where reconstruction as a Billroth II gastro-jejunostomy has been carried out, but can largely be prevented by Roux-en-Y reconstruction.

The symptoms consist of persistent epigastric discomfort, sometimes made worse by eating and frequently associated with intermittent vomiting of bile-stained fluid or food mixed with bile, usually occurring within 90 minutes of a meal. Some patients become malnourished because of inadequate food intake, and anaemia develops in about a quarter of the patients as a result of chronic blood loss from the associated gastritis. Gastro-oesophageal reflux disease may also develop.

Endoscopy shows a diffuse gastritis with an oedematous hyperaemic friable mucosa and frequently superficial erosions. Endoscopic biopsy shows typical histological features including foveolar hyperplasia, glandular cystification, oedema of the lamina propria and vasocongestion of the mucosal capillaries, all in association with inflammatory cell infiltration.

Medical treatment

Cholestyramine has been shown to be an effective bile-acid-binding agent in vitro, although the results of several therapeutic trials have been disappointing. Antacids containing aluminium hydroxide have also been studied because of their bile-acid-binding capacity but the results have been equally unimpressive. In clinical trials sucralfate has been shown to reduce the inflammation within the gastric mucosa but this has not been associated with any improvement in symptoms. Prokinetic agents have also been used to improve clearance of the refluxate from the stomach, and the occasional patient may respond. These agents may, however, worsen dumping and diarrhoea. Ursodeoxycholic acid has been shown in one study to almost abolish the nausea and vomiting associated with enterogastric reflux and to significantly decrease the intensity and frequency of pain.

Surgical treatment

In patients with a previous truncal vagotomy and drainage, reversal of the drainage procedure can be undertaken provided at least 1 year has elapsed from the original operation. This is based on the premise that the stomach will regain some of its lost motility during this time. In fact, more than half of the patients with truncal vagotomy probably did not require a drainage procedure in the first place. Closure of gastro-jejunostomy for enterogastric reflux and bile vomiting is usually followed by improvement or complete relief in the vast majority of patients.[44] The risks of gastric stasis are minimal and conversion to a pyloroplasty should be avoided.

Reconstruction of the pylorus after pyloroplasty is a relatively straightforward operation. Having cleared the anteropyloroduodenal segment of all adhesions, the scar of the previous pyloroplasty is accurately opened. The pyloric ring is palpated and the scarred ends freshened if necessary. One approach is to make a small antral gastrotomy to allow the insertion of a size 12 or 14 Hegar dilator through the area of the pyloric reconstruction into the duodenum. Using a double-ended monofilament suture the pyloric ring is accurately opposed around the Hegar dilator before reapproximating the duodenum and antrum using a continuous serosubmucosal technique. Withdrawal of the Hegar dilator allows fingertip palpation of the reconstructed pylorus prior to closure of the antral gastrotomy. The overall results of pyloric reconstruction show that 80% of patients gain a satisfactory or good result,[45] although in one study only half of the patients with enterogastric reflux had a satisfactory or good response.[46]

If enterogastric reflux is not relieved, then the duodenal switch operation[47] would seem an appropriate further remedial procedure for patients whose symptoms necessitate further surgery (**Fig. 18.4**).

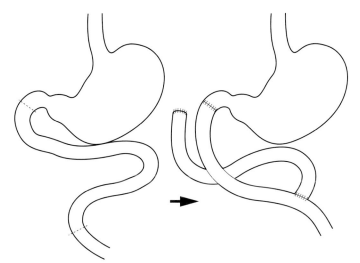

Figure 18.4 • Pylorus-preserving Roux loop – the duodenal switch operation.

Chapter 18

Recent experience with this has shown good results, although acid suppression is needed to prevent jejunal ulceration.[48]

In patients who have had a gastric resection or in those with a gastro-jejunostomy with pyloric stenosis, a Roux limb (approximately 45 cm in length) would seem an appropriate revisional procedure (with antrectomy in patients with pyloric stenosis). The procedure, however, does carry risks, as it is ulcerogenic because it diverts the buffering effect of upper gastrointestinal contents away from the gastroenteric anastomosis. The second problem is the development of delayed gastric emptying of solid food, producing a symptom complex of satiety, epigastric pain and non-bilious vomiting that has been termed the 'Roux syndrome'. Although many patients will demonstrate objective evidence of delayed gastric emptying of solids, this is usually of little or no clinical consequence except in a minority. The Roux syndrome is more likely to develop in patients who demonstrate delay in gastric emptying of solids prior to construction of the Roux limb and those who have a large residual gastric pouch. The syndrome may also be more likely to develop in those patients who require a completion vagotomy. Where these conditions exist, the operative procedure required is a more extensive gastric resection. The entire anastomosis should be resected to leave a small gastric pouch, and the Roux limb should be anastomosed to the stomach as an end-to-side Pólya-type gastro-jejunostomy. In those patients who develop severe symptoms from the Roux syndrome postoperatively, then the treatment is near-total resection of the gastric remnant with a Pólya-type gastro-jejunostomy.

Roux diversion will control enterogastric reflux in over 70% of patients, and recurrent jejunal ulcers can be avoided by checking and if necessary completing the truncal vagotomy as part of the operative procedure or, more commonly, relying on long-term treatment with proton-pump inhibitors.

Chronic afferent loop syndrome

The afferent loop syndrome can only occur after gastro-jejunostomy or a Billroth II-type reconstruction after partial gastrectomy. The condition is caused by intermittent postprandial obstruction of the afferent limb of the gastro-jejunostomy. The clinical picture is very similar to that produced by enterogastric reflux (Table 18.2). The problem is rarely encountered if surgeons use a short afferent jejunal loop. The cause of the obstruction may be due to anastomotic kinking, adhesions, internal herniation, volvulus of the afferent limb or obstruction of the gastro-jejunal stoma itself. Once diagnosed the treatment is always surgical. Conversion to a Billroth I anastomosis or a Roux-en-Y reconstruction of the afferent limb have both produced good results.

Dumping

The literature shows a considerable variability in the incidence of dumping after each procedure due at least partly to variations in definitions of the syndrome. A significant number of patients will develop dumping-type symptoms in the early period after their initial gastric operation but the majority have sufficient reserve to adjust to the changes without developing severe sequelae.

The symptoms of early dumping can be divided into vasomotor and gastrointestinal, as shown in Box 18.2. In a severe attack, the vasomotor symptoms are usually experienced by the patient towards the end of a meal or within 15 minutes of finishing, and the gastrointestinal symptoms develop a little later, but usually within 30 minutes after eating.

There is now clear evidence that dumping is associated with rapid gastric emptying leading to hyperosmolar jejunal content causing massive fluid shifts from the extracellular space into the lumen. This is associated with a significant fall in plasma volume. It is also known that plasma concentrations of several gut regulatory peptides are elevated in patients with the dumping syndrome, but it is not clear whether this is coincidental or causative.

Taking a careful history, delineating the vasomotor and gastrointestinal components usually makes the diagnosis of the dumping syndrome. Where there is any doubt, the patient should be encouraged to keep a diary card recording the foods eaten and the symptoms that develop thereafter. Rarely will the dumping provocation test be required; this should be carried out in hospital because of the severe and potentially life-threatening symptoms that can occur as a result of the test.

Table 18.2 • Differentiation between the chronic afferent loop syndrome and enterogastric reflux

Chronic afferent loop syndrome	Enterogastric reflux
Meal-related pain – relieved by vomiting	Constant pain (worsened by eating) – not relieved by vomiting
Vomitus contains bile	Vomitus contains bile and food
Vomiting projectile	Vomiting non-projectile
Rarely associated with bleeding/anaemia	Bleeding/anaemia found in 25% of patients

Vasomotor

- Palpitations
- Flushings
- Sweating
- Headache
- Weakness
- Faintness
- Anxiety

Gastrointestinal

- Vomiting
- Belching
- Fullness
- Colic
- Borborygmi
- Diarrhoea

Medical treatment

The majority of patients displaying the dumping syndrome can be managed satisfactorily by dietary manipulation. Reducing the carbohydrate content and restricting fluid intake with meals will help many of these patients. Avoiding extra salt and eating more frequent small meals may also be required. Assuming the supine posture after eating helps to slow gastric emptying and may minimise symptoms. Guar gum, a vegetable fibre, is known to reduce postprandial hyperglycaemia in both normal and diabetic patients. In a small study of postgastric surgery patients it has been shown to prevent the dumping syndrome and increase food tolerance in the majority of patients.[49] Pectin also delays gastric emptying but may precipitate attacks of diarrhoea. Somatostatin, and more recently its analogue octreotide, given subcutaneously prior to eating has been shown to significantly reduce or abolish the symptoms of dumping.[50] There is evidence that this is very effective for many patients in the short term but probably only works for around half of patients in the longer term.[51]

Surgical treatment

For patients with truncal vagotomy and drainage procedures, taking down the gastro-jejunostomy[52] should cure or improve dumping in over 80% of patients. Reconstruction of the pylorus produces similar results.[53] After gastrectomy, a number of procedures have been advocated for dumping. The simplest and probably the best is to convert the drainage procedure to a 45-cm Roux-en-Y gastro-jejunostomy. The delay in liquid emptying after this procedure is thought to be due to myoelectrical abnormalities within the Roux limb itself causing a degree of retrograde contraction. The delay in emptying of solids is probably a result of the vagotomy leading to a degree of gastric atony and loss of the antral prepulsive force to propel solid food into the small intestine. Reversal of the proximal 10 cm of the jejunal limb to create an antiperistaltic interposition is unnecessary and may lead to further stasis and dilatation of the interposed segment. This will worsen any symptoms of gastric retention. The interposition of a segment of upper jejunum between the gastric remnant and the duodenum has been advocated. Both isoperistaltic and antiperistaltic interpositions have been used, but these procedures can be associated with serious complications, and the long-term success rate is variable.[54]

Diarrhoea

Alteration in bowel habit occurs in the majority of patients who undergo truncal vagotomy and in most this is a change from constipation to a more regular habit with one or two motions per day. However, 11% of patients following truncal vagotomy and pyloroplasty had continuous diarrhoea that significantly interfered with their lifestyle.[55] A further 20% of patients will have episodic attacks of diarrhoea more than once a week.

The aetiology of postvagotomy diarrhoea remains poorly understood. Gastric stasis, abnormal small-bowel motility, and impaired biliary and pancreatic function have all been incriminated. Malabsorption, bacterial colonisation of the proximal small bowel and increased faecal excretion of bile salts and acid may all be contributing factors. Patients who have had a cholecystectomy are more likely to develop postvagotomy diarrhoea and have a particularly severe form.

Diarrhoea may be a component of the dumping syndrome, especially in patients after gastrectomy, but in many postvagotomy patients it is unassociated with dumping. The stool consistency varies from watery to soft, and in its severe form may be explosive in onset without warning, thus leading to incontinence. Patients may be unable to distinguish between the urge to pass flatus and a bowel motion. Occasionally symptoms will be so pronounced that weight loss and malnutrition become apparent.

Investigation of these patients includes the measurement of faecal fats, faecal elastase and vitamin B_{12} level. A barium enema should be carried out to rule out disorders of the colon, and if bacterial overgrowth is suspected the diagnosis may be confirmed by bacteriological examination of jejunal aspirates or by using the ^{14}C glycocholate breath test.

Medical treatment

The treatment of postvagotomy diarrhoea begins with dietary manipulation, and in particular the avoidance of refined carbohydrates and foods with a high fluid content. Restriction of fluid intake with meals is occasionally of benefit. Cholestyramine taken morning and evening may be of benefit, especially in patients who have also had a cholecystectomy. There are, however, long-term complications such as mega-loblastic anaemia due to folate deficiency in patients on long-term cholestyramine therapy. Codeine and loperamide may also be useful.

Surgical treatment

Closure of a gastro-jejunostomy will improve or cure diarrhoea in 80% of patients. A similar improvement is seen with reconstruction of the pylorus.[46,53] Various intestinal interpositions to act as an intestinal brake have been advocated. The use of a 10-cm antiperistaltic jejunal segment placed 100 cm distal to the duodenojejunal junction has been described.[56] The reversed segment produces a delay in the passage of contents through the small bowel. Many report poor results with these types of operation. The operation that has proved effective is the reverse distal ileal onlay graft, which creates a passive non-propulsive segment.[57]

Small stomach syndrome

This only occurs only after a high subtotal gastrectomy in which 80–90% of the stomach is removed and is very rare in the author's experience. Non-operative treatment consists of frequent small meals, antispasmodics, and mineral and vitamin replacement. Patients may also require fine-bore nasoenteric nutritional supplementation. In a small number of patients with uncontrollable symptoms, surgery may have to be considered. The reservoir jejunal interposition described by Cuschieri, a modification of the Hunt–Lawrence, is probably the procedure of choice.[58] Long-term follow-up of these patients is required as there is a tendency for the jejunal limb to elongate over several years and this can lead to stasis and ulceration.

Key points

- *Helocobacter pylori* infection and NSAID use are the primary risk factors for peptic ulcer disease.
- Smoking significantly increases the risk of complication from peptic ulcer disease and prevents effective healing.
- Gastric and duodenal ulcers may be considered 'refractory' to medical treatment if there is no sign of significant healing by 12 and 8 weeks respectively.
- Refractory ulceration should prompt biopsy from the ulcer margin and serum gastrin levels should be determined.
- A diagnosis of Zollinger–Ellison should be suspected in cases of *Helicobacter*-negative, non-NSAID-induced refractory ulceration and especially where there is ulceration of the second part of the duodenum or large confluent ulcers in the duodenum.
- There is no good evidence on which to base the decision of operation in cases of resistant ulceration in the modern era.
- Where ZES is due to a pancreatic tumour, in two-thirds of cases the tumour will be multifocal within the pancreas. At least two-thirds will be histologically malignant. One-third will already have demonstrable metastases by the time of diagnosis.
- The most common extrapancreatic site of gastrinomas is in the wall of the duodenum. Ectopic gastrinoma tissue has been identified in the liver, common bile duct, jejunum, omentum, pylorus, ovary and heart.
- One-quarter of patients with ZES have other endocrine tumours as part of a familial multiple endocrine neoplasia (MEN-1) syndrome, particularly hyperparathyroidism. This group has a much worse prognosis than sporadic ZES, in part due to the multifocal nature of the tumour within the pancreas.
- Somatostatin receptor scintigraphy with [^{111}In-DTPA-DPhe1]octreotide (SRS) and selective arterial secretagogue injection (SASI) tests are the most reliable approaches to localising gastrinomas.
- Delay in diagnosis, coexistent medical illness, shock on admission, leucocytosis and age over 75 are associated with poor outcome in perforated peptic ulcer disease.
- In 'low-risk' patients with perforated peptic ulcer, the laparoscopic approach has significant advantages but for those with prolonged perforation for more than 24 h, shock on admission and confounding medical conditions there is no evidence that the laparoscopic approach is advantageous.
- Endoscopic therapy reduces the mortality of acute upper gastrointestinal bleed in patients with active bleeding or non-bleeding visible vessel.

- Treatment of peptic ulcer bleeding by a combination of two different endoscopic modalities may be more beneficial than relying on one modality alone.
- Proton-pump inhibitors given after endoscopic control of peptic ulcer bleeding improve outcome.
- Only if a combination of intensive medical treatment and dilatation fails to reopen the gastric outlet is surgery indicated for benign pyloric stenosis.
- Although the spectrum of postgastric surgery syndromes is well described, the majority of patients will present with a mixed clinical picture. Careful appraisal will reveal a dominant problem.
- After antrectomy or other forms of partial gastrectomy, diversion of bile and pancreatic secretion is best carried out with a 45-cm Roux loop.
- Closure of a gastro-jejunostomy or reconstruction of the pylorus after pyloroplasty for enterogastric reflux and bile vomiting is usually followed by improvement or complete relief in the vast majority of patients. The risks of gastric stasis are minimal.

References

1. De Boer WA. Diagnosis of *Helicobacter pylori* infection. Review of diagnostic techniques and recommendations for their use in different clinical settings. Scand J Gastroenterol Suppl 1997; 223:35–42.

2. Boixeda D, Gisbet JP, de Raffael L et al. The importance of obtaining biopsies of the gastric body in the follow-up after treatment of HP infection. Med Clin (Barc) 1995; 105:566–9.

3. Vaira D, Holton J, Menegatti M et al. New immunological assays for the diagnosis of HP infection. Gut 1999; 45(Suppl 1):123–7.

4. Savarino V, Vigneri S, Celle G. The 13C urea breath test in the diagnosis of HP infection. Gut 1999; 45(Suppl 1): 118–22.

5. Odaka T, Yamaguchi T, Koyama H et al. Evaluation of the *Helicobacter pylori* stool antigen test for monitoring eradication therapy. Am J Gastroenterol 2002; 97:594–9.

6. Eastwood GL. Is smoking still important in the pathogenesis of peptic ulcer disease? J Clin Gastroenterol 1997; 25(Suppl 1):S1–7.

7. Johnston D, Axon ATR. Highly selective vagotomy for duodenal ulcer – the clinical results after 10 years. Br J Surg 1979; 66:874–8.

8. Taylor TV, Gunn AA, Macleod DAD et al. Anterior lesser curve seromyotomy with posterior truncal vagotomy for duodenal ulcer. Br J Surg 1985; 72:950–1.

9. Raimes SA, Smirniotis V, Wheldon EJ et al. Postvagotomy diarrhoea put into perspective. Lancet 1987; 2:851–3.

10. Yunfu L, Oinghua Z, Yongjia W. Pylorus and pyloric vagus preserving gastrectomy treating 125 cases of peptic ulcer. Minerva Chirugia 1998; 53:889–93.

11. Lu YF, Zhang XX, Zhao G et al. Gastroduodenal ulcer treated by pylorus and pyloric vagus-preserving gastrectomy. World J Gastroenterol 1999; 5(2):156–9.

12. Park do J, Lee HJ, Jung HC et al. Clinical outcome of pylorus-preserving gastrectomy in gastric cancer in comparison with conventional distal gastrectomy with Billroth I anastomosis. World J Surg 2008; 32(6):1029–36.

13. Ellison EH, Wilson SD. The Zollinger–Ellison syndrome: re-appraisal and evaluation of 260 registered cases. Ann Surg 1964; 160:512–20.

14. Zollinger RM, Ellison EC, O'Darisio TM et al. Thirty years of experience with gastrinoma. World J Surg 1984; 8:427–35.

15. Wu PC, Alexander HR, Bartlett DL et al. A prospective analysis of the frequency, location, and curability of ectopic (nonpancreaticoduodenal, nonnodal) gastrinoma. Surgery 1997; 122(6):1176–82.

16. Norton JA, Fraker DL, Alexander HR et al. Surgery to cure the Zollinger–Ellison syndrome. N Engl J Med 1999; 341(9):635–44.

17. Imamura M, Komoto I, Ota S. Changing treatment strategy for gastrinoma in patients with Zollinger–Ellison syndrome. World J Surg 2006; 30:1–11.

18. Norton JA, Doherty GM, Fraker DL et al. Surgical treatment of localized gastrinoma within the liver: a prospective study. Surgery 1998; 124(6):1145–52.

19. Alexander HR, Fraker DL, Norton JA et al. Prospective study of somatostatin receptor scintigraphy and its effect on operative outcome in patients with Zollinger–Ellison syndrome. Ann Surg 1998; 228(2):228–38.

20. Norton JA. Intraoperative methods to stage and localize pancreatic and duodenal tumors. Ann Oncol 1999; 10(Suppl 4):182–4.

21. Taylor H. Aspiration treatment of perforated ulcers. Lancet 1951; 1:7–12.

22. Gul YA, Shine MF, Lennon F. Non-operative management of perforated duodenal ulcer. Irish J Med Sci 1999; 168(4):254–6.

23. Crofts TJ, Park KGM, Steele RJC et al. A randomised trial of nonoperative treatment for perforated peptic ulcer. N Engl J Med 1989; 320(15):970–3.

24. Donovan AJ, Berne TV, Donovan JA. Perforated duodenal ulcer: an alternative therapeutic plan. Arch Surg 1998; 133(11):1166–71.

25. Mihmanli M, Isgor A, Kabukcuoglu F et al. The effect of *H. pylori* in perforation of duodenal ulcer. Hepato-Gastroenterology 1998; 45(23):1610–12.

26. Ng EKW, Lam YH, Sung JJY et al. Eradication of HP prevents recurrence of ulcer after simple closure of DU perf: randomised controlled trial. Ann Surg 2000; 231:153–8.

27. Gilliam AD, Speake WJ, Lobo DN et al. Current practice of emergency vagotomy and *Helicobacter* eradication for complicated peptic ulcer disease in the UK. Br J Surg 2003; 90:88–90.

28. Reuben BC, Stoddard G, Glasgow R et al. Trends and predictors for vagotomy when performing over-sew of acute bleeding duodenal ulcer in the United States. J Gastrointest Surg 2007; 11(1):22–8.

29. Mouret P, Francois Y, Vagnal J et al. Laparoscopic treatment of perforated peptic ulcer. Br J Surg 1990; 77:1006.

30. Lau H. Laparoscopic repair of perforated peptic ulcer: a meta-analysis. Surg Endosc 2004; 18(7):1013–21.

31. Lunevicius R, Morkevicius M. Systematic review comparing laparoscopic and open repair for perforated peptic ulcer. Br J Surg 2005; 92(10):1195–207.

32. Leontiadis GI, Sreedharan A, Dorward S et al. Systematic reviews of the clinical effectiveness and cost-effectiveness of proton pump inhibitors in acute upper gastrointestinal bleeding. Health Technol Assess 2007; 11(51):iii–iv, 1–164.

33. Lau JYW, Sung JJY, Lee KKC et al. Effect of intravenous omeprazole on recurrent bleeding after endoscopic treatment of bleeding peptic ulcers. N Engl J Med 2000; 343:310–16.

34. Henry D, O'Connel D. Effects of fibrinolytic inhibitors on mortality from upper gastrointestinal haemorrhage. Br Med J 1989; 298:1142–6.

35. Cook DJ, Guyatt GH, Salena BJ et al. Endoscopic therapy for acute non-variceal upper gastrointestinal hemorrhage: A meta-analysis. Gastroenterol 1992; 102:139–48.

36. British Society of Gastroenterolgy Endoscopy Committee. Non-variceal upper gastrointestinal haemorrhage: guidelines. Gut 2002; 51(Suppl IV):iv1–6.

37. Barkun A, Bardou M, Marshall JK et al. Consensus recommendations for managing patients with non-variceal upper gastrointestinal bleeding. Ann Intern Med 2003; 139:843–57.

38. Lau JYW, Sung JJY, Lam YH et al. Endoscopic re-treatment compared with surgery in patients with recurrent bleeding after initial endoscopic control of bleeding ulcers. N Engl J Med 1999; 340:751–6.

39. Poxon VA, Keighley MR, Dykes PW et al. Comparison of minimal and conventional surgery in patients with bleeding peptic ulcer: a multicentre trial. Br J Surg 1991; 78(11):1344–5.

40. Brandimarte G, Tursi A, di Cesare L et al. Antimicrobial treatment for peptic stenosis: a prospective study. Eur J Gastroenterol Hepatol 1999; 11(7):731–4.

41. Griffin SM, Chung SCS, Leung JWC et al. Peptic pyloric stenosis treated by endoscopic balloon dilatation. Br J Surg 1989; 76:1147–8.

42. Chisholm EM, Chung SCS, Leung JWC. Peptic pyloric stenosis – after the balloon goes up! Gastrointest Endosc 1993; 37:240.

43. Siu WT, Tang CN, Law BK et al. Vagotomy and gastrojejunostomy for benign gastric outlet obstruction. J Laparoendosc Adv Surg Tech A 2004; 14:266–9.

44. Green R, Spencer A, Kennedy T. Closure of gastro-jejunostomy for the relief of post-vagotomy symptoms. Br J Surg 1978; 65:161–3.

45. Koruth NM, Krukowski ZH, Matheson N. Pyloric reconstruction. Br J Surg 1985; 72:808–10.

46. Martin CJ, Kennedy T. Reconstruction of the pylorus. World J Surg 1985; 6:221–5.

47. DeMeester TR, Fuchs KH, Ball CS et al. Experimental and clinical results with proximal end-to-end duodenojejunostomy for pathological duodenogastric reflux. Ann Surg 1987; 206:414–26.

48. Strignano P, Collard JM, Michel JM et al. Duodenal switch operation for pathologic transpyloric duodenogastric reflux. Ann Surg 2007; 245(2):247–53.

49. Harju E, Larmi TKI. Efficacy of guar gum in preventing the dumping syndrome. J Parent Enter Nutr 1983; 7:470–2.

50. Primrose JN, Johnston D. Somatostatin analogue SMS 201-995 (octreotide) as a possible solution to the dumping syndrome after gastrectomy or vagotomy. Br J Surg 1989; 76:140–4.

51. Didden P, Penning C, Masclee AA. Octreotide therapy in dumping syndrome: analysis of long-term results. Aliment Pharmacol Ther 2006; 24(9):1367–75.

52. McMahon MJ, Johnston D, Hill GT et al. Treatment of severe side effects after vagotomy and gastroenterostomy by closure of gastroenterostomy without pyloroplasty. Br Med J 1978; 1:7–8.

53. Cheadle WG, Baker PR, Cuschieri A. Pyloric reconstruction for severe vasomotor dumping after vagotomy and pyloroplasty. Ann Surg 1985; 202:568–72.

54. Cuschieri A. Isoperistaltic and antiperistaltic jejunal interposition for the dumping syndrome. A comparative study. J R Coll Surg Edinb 1977; 22:319–42.

55. Raimes SA, Smirniotis V, Wheldon EJ et al. Post vagotomy diarrhoea put into perspective. Lancet 1986; 2:851–3.

56. Sawyers JL, Herrington JL Jr. Treatment of postgastrectomy syndromes. Am Surg 1980; 46:201–7.

57. Cuschieri A. Surgical management of severe intractable postvagotomy diarrhoea. Br J Surg 1986; 73:981–4.

58. Cuschieri A. Long term evaluation of a reservoir jejunal interposition with an isoperistaltic conduit in the management of patients with a small stomach syndrome. Br J Surg 1982; 69:386–8.

19

Oesophageal emergencies

Jon Shenfine
S. Michael Griffin

Introduction

The availability of upper gastrointestinal endoscopy and associated instrumentation has resulted in an increase in iatrogenic trauma, which now accounts for the majority of oesophageal injuries, although trauma can occur from a variety of insults from within or without, resulting in a spectrum of oesophageal damage. Unfortunately, most clinicians gain limited exposure to patients with oesophageal trauma due to its rarity and, as a result, misdiagnosis, incorrect investigations and inappropriate management are all too common. Lack of clinical experience is compounded by the lack of a management evidence base, with research limited to observational studies. Despite this, the management of such injuries is actually straightforward to a clinician familiar with the basic principles developed by oesophageal surgeons of the past to minimise morbidity and mortality. Hopefully the outcomes from these injuries will continue to improve with the changes in the structure of the service for patients with upper gastrointestinal disease and the provision of dedicated multidisciplinary specialist units with the inherent knowledge and skills to deal with them.

This chapter focuses on the diagnosis and management of injuries to the oesophagus from a number of different insults. In order, these are spontaneous and iatrogenic perforation, traumatic injuries, caustic injuries, and the management of foreign body and food bolus impaction.

Spontaneous perforation of the oesophagus

Definition and natural history

Boerhaave's syndrome is characterised by barogenic oesophageal injury leading to immediate and gross gastric content contamination of the pleural cavity. However, various degrees of damage and contamination are possible.[1,2] A number of clinical terms are used to describe this event: this text will only use the term 'spontaneous perforation of the oesophagus'; 'disruption' will also be used to describe the 'process' of perforation.

Aetiology and pathophysiology

Spontaneous perforation of the oesophagus is defined as complete disruption of the oesophageal wall occurring in the absence of pre-existing pathology. Since the oesophagus possesses no serosa, transgression of oesophagogastric contents rapidly leads to chemical and septic mediastinitis. A sudden rise in intra-abdominal pressure is present in 80–90% of cases, usually as a result of retching or vomiting, but cases have resulted from blunt trauma, weightlifting, parturition, defecation, the Heimlich manoeuvre or status epilepticus.[3] Vomiting is commonplace but spontaneous oesophageal perforation is rare, which suggests that other as yet unidentified factors may be important, such as pre-existing abnormalities of anatomy or pathology. In 10–20% of cases an underlying oesophageal pathology is identified, such as malignancy, peptic ulceration or infection, and as such do not truly represent spontaneous perforation. Mallory–Weiss tears are assumed to represent part of the spectrum of spontaneous perforation but it is likely that these mucosal injuries reflect 'shearing' rather than 'barogenic' trauma.[4]

Spontaneous perforations are usually single, longitudinal, 1–8 cm long with the mucosal injury being longer than the muscular tear, and occur most commonly in the left posterolateral position above the oesophagogastric junction. Pleural disruption occurs barogenically or from rapid gastric acid erosion and is exacerbated by the negative intrathoracic pressure. Caucasian males are predominantly affected, in a ratio of 4:1, which probably reflects a predisposition to alcohol ingestion, overindulgence and vomiting rather than a true gender variation.

Clinical presentation

The classical presentation is of severe chest pain following vomiting and the rapid development of subcutaneous emphysema. In a large case series this triad was only present in 7 of 51 patients (14%).[5] As such, the classical presentation is not necessarily the common presentation, which may account for misdiagnosis and treatment delay.

The most important feature is sudden, 'dramatic' chest pain following an episode of raised intra-abdominal pressure, most commonly vomiting. This pain is severe, constant, retrosternal or epigastric, exacerbated by movement and poorly relieved by narcotics. Patients are tachypnoeic and may sit up to splint their diaphragm and reduce excess movement. Abdominal pain and tenderness is common; in the same large case series 22 of 51 patients (43%) complained of abdominal pain leading to a negative laparotomy in three patients.[5] Although subcutaneous emphysema is pathognomonic it takes time to develop; mediastinal emphysema precedes this and may be visible on a plain chest radiograph. Due to a sympathetic nervous system response, patients appear pale and sweaty and are tachycardic with cool peripheries. With time the negative intrathoracic pressure draws air, food and fluids into the mediastinum and pleural cavities and a chemical pleuromediastinitis develops. A low-grade pyrexia ensues, which worsens as the systemic inflammatory response gives way to sepsis, and within 24–48 hours cardiopulmonary embarrassment and collapse develop as a consequence of overwhelming bacterial mediastinitis and septic shock. Survival is highly dependent on the evacuation of the contamination from the mediastinal and pleural cavities at the earliest possible opportunity.[6]

Diagnosis

A classical history is a reliable diagnostic aid but a high index of suspicion is essential as atypical symptoms, the similarity to more common cardiorespiratory disorders, and a shocked, confused and distressed patient may misdirect the clinician (Box 19.1). As a result, the diagnostic error is over 50%, with a diagnostic delay of more than 12 hours in the majority of cases and only 5% of cases diagnosed at presentation.[7] It may be that less than 35% of cases are correctly diagnosed pre-mortem.[8] Unfortunately, as time passes, the critical condition of the patient obscures relevant clinical features and the pursuit of incorrect investigations makes the diagnosis even more elusive.

Investigations

Plain radiography

The typical findings on plain chest radiography are subtle and are dependent on the site and the time interval following the insult. These are documented in Box 19.2 and **Fig. 19.1**. However, plain abdominal radiographs are helpful to exclude a perforated intra-abdominal viscus since an associated pneumoperitoneum is rare.[7]

Contrast radiography

Oral water-soluble contrast radiography is the investigation of choice for diagnosis and to ascertain the site, degree of containment and degree of drainage of the disruption (**Fig. 19.2**). Aqueous agents are rapidly absorbed, do not exacerbate inflammation and have minimal tissue effects, but may be associated with false-negative results in 27–66%.[9] Dilute barium may be used should an initial water-soluble study prove negative.

Box 19.1 • Common misdiagnoses for spontaneous perforation of the oesophagus

Medical
- Myocardial infarction
- Pericarditis
- Spontaneous pneumothorax
- Pneumonia
- Oesophageal varices/Mallory–Weiss tear
- Mesenteric ischaemia

Surgical
- Peritonitis
- Acute pancreatitis
- Perforated peptic ulcer
- Renal colic
- Aortic aneurysm (dissection/leak)
- Biliary colic
- Mesenteric ischaemia

Box 19.2 • Typical chest radiograph findings in spontaneous perforation of the oesophagus

- Pleural effusion
- Pneumomediastinum
- Subcutaneous emphysema
- Hydropneumothorax
- Pneumothorax
- Collapse/consolidation

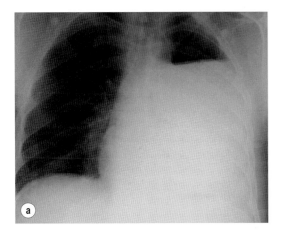

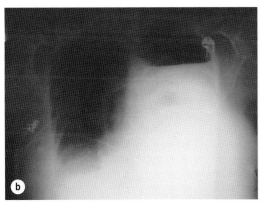

Figure 19.1 • (a,b) Typical chest radiograph findings of spontaneous oesophageal perforation.

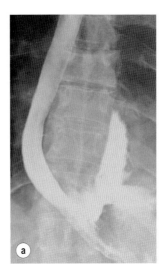

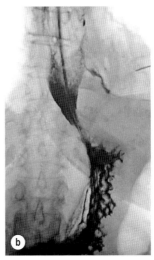

Figure 19.2 • (a,b) Contrast swallows demonstrating free extravasation of contrast media following spontaneous oesophageal perforation.

Upper gastrointestinal endoscopy

The risks of endoscopic assessment are minimised using modern, flexible videoscopes together with fluoroscopic guidance, but this should only be performed by a highly experienced endoscopist conversant with the consequences of their actions (**Fig. 19.3**).

 Video endoscopy has been used to examine the oesophagus in penetrating thoracic trauma and following oesophageal cancer surgery to examine the oesophagogastric anastomosis without additional morbidity.[10–12]

Endoscopic assessment excludes the diagnosis if normal, influences management if underlying pathology is discovered and facilitates placement of a nasojejunal tube to allow safe enteral feeding. In cases of contained 'intramural' oesophageal perforation, which are likely to be missed by traditional contrast radiography, endoscopic assessment is essential to avoid an unnecessary thoracotomy.

Computed tomography (CT)

Although CT is not a first-line investigation it is frequently performed in critically ill patients with an atypical presentation and is useful when contrast radiology or endoscopy are not available or possible.

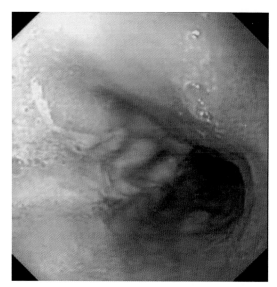

Figure 19.3 • Endoscopic appearance of spontaneous oesophageal perforation with full-thickness longitudinal disruption.

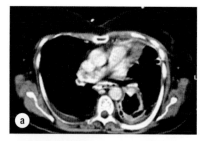

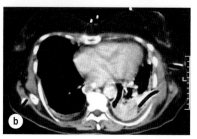

Figure 19.4 • CT appearances of spontaneous oesophageal perforation. **(a)** Left pleural hydropneumothorax. **(b)** Left basal intercostal chest drain in the same patient as in (a).

 In an intubated patient, the sensitivity of CT for spontaneous perforation is increased by placing a nasogastric tube just past cricopharyngeus to run in a small amount of contrast media[13] **(Fig. 19.4)**.

CT plays a significant role postoperatively and in assessing the adequacy of non-operative management, and the combination of CT with complex interventional radiological techniques has revolutionised the management of intrathoracic collections.

Other investigations

Aspiration of frank gastric contents on thoracocentesis is diagnostic – a pH of less than 6.0, a high amylase or microscopic squamous cells in the fluid can confirm disruption in difficult cases. Swallowed oral dyes, such as methylene blue, may also be diagnostically useful if a communicating drain is in situ.

Management

The rarity, the spectrum of damage and the consequences of inappropriate treatment have limited the ability to evaluate different management options. Published, observational case series often span many years, many centres, many surgeons and many techniques. Non-operative treatment is now standard for iatrogenic trauma, but surgery remains the mainstay of treatment for spontaneous perforation, and non-operative treatment should be viewed as 'radical'. The consequences of aggressive oesophageal surgery are well appreciated and patients require a multidisciplinary approach with input from intensive care, radiology, physiotherapy and rehabilitation services. Where possible these patients should be managed in specialist oesophageal surgery units. Hospitals lacking these facilities or the versatile surgical cover necessary to deal with the oesophagus by abdominal or left or right thoracic operative approaches should transfer the patients at the earliest opportunity after stabilisation.

Preoperative resuscitation

All patients require urgent respiratory and cardiovascular support and opiate-based analgesia whether or not shock, respiratory distress or organ dysfunction is present. An early anaesthetic review is recommended as many patients will develop respiratory failure requiring intubation and ventilation. Box 19.3 documents the initial resuscitation.

Non-operative treatment

Surgery is mandatory to remove gross contamination and limit further damage. However, non-operative management may be appropriate and successful in a small minority of patients who have either been diagnosed rapidly with minimal contamination and no mediastinitis or a contained perforation. It may also be considered in those with a delayed diagnosis who have demonstrated tolerance, especially with advances in radiological intervention, antibiotics and enteral nutritional supplementation.[6] Any demonstrable mortality or morbidity advantages with non-operative treatment are secondary to selection bias. Criteria to guide the selection of patients for non-operative treatment are documented in Box 19.4.

Box 19.3 • Initial resuscitation in spontaneous oesophageal perforation

- Control of airway and administration of supplementary oxygen
- Early anaesthetic involvement
- Large-bore intravenous access and intravenous fluid resuscitation
- Central venous access and arterial line monitoring ± inotropic support
- Urethral catheterisation and close monitoring of fluid balance
- Broad-spectrum antibiotic and antifungal agents
- Intravenous antisecretory agents (H$_2$-receptor antagonists or proton-pump inhibitors)
- Strictly nil by mouth
- Large-bore intercostal chest drainage – possibly bilaterally
- Nasogastric tube (only to be placed under endoscopic vision or radiological guidance)

Box 19.4 • Criteria for non-operative management of oesophageal perforation

- Perforation contained within the mediastinum
- Free drainage of contrast back into oesophagus
- No symptoms or signs of mediastinitis
- No evidence of solid food contamination of pleural or mediastinal cavities

Other factors to consider

- Perforation is controlled
- No underlying oesophageal disease
- No septic shock
- Availability for intensive observation and access to multidisciplinary care
- Low threshold for aggressive intervention
- Long delay in diagnosis such that the patient has already demonstrated tolerance
- Enteral feeding

Non-operative treatment comprises observation in intensive care or ward-based high-dependency units with patients kept strictly nil orally and fed enterally, if necessary via a feeding jejunostomy. A nasogastric tube should be placed under endoscopic and/or radiological assistance past the perforation to decompress the stomach. Where pleural perforation has occurred, chest drainage should be instituted and repeated contrast radiology, endoscopy and CT performed to monitor the status of the perforation. All patients should be given broad-spectrum intravenous antibiotics, antifungal and antisecretory agents, and a low threshold for surgical intervention should be maintained. Non-operative treatment should not be regarded as being 'conservative' and should be undertaken in the realisation that a change in plan with rapid surgical intervention may still be required.

The authors suggest that the temporary use of covered, self-expanding metal or plastic stents as a primary treatment to seal a spontaneous perforation is limited but that they may have a place to control a postoperative leak.[14-16] Transoesophageal debridement and mediastinal irrigation should be viewed as experimental.[17]

Surgery

The primary objective of surgical intervention is to restore oesophageal integrity and prevent further soiling. Thorough debridement, drainage, lavage and irrigation are more important for survival than the type of repair.[6] The authors advocate the formation of a feeding jejunostomy as a routine during surgery to facilitate enteral feeding. Management of the patients by a multidisciplinary team is again emphasised. Based on the site, a posterolateral thoracotomy is used to approach the oesophagus, most commonly on the left in the seventh or eighth intercostal space. Solid debris is removed and the pleural cavity thoroughly cleaned. The mediastinal pleura is widely incised to expose the injury, and necrotic, devitalised tissue debrided. A longitudinal myotomy is made as the mucosal injury is usually longer than the muscular one and the oesophagus repaired or closed over a T-tube.[18]

Success with one surgical technique over another probably reflects the expertise and experience of the individual centre rather than a true outcome difference.

Primary repair with or without reinforcement

A simple, primary suture repair is the most common surgical procedure used since Barrett first employed it successfully in 1947.[2] A single- or two-layered anastomosis is fashioned using 2/0 or 3/0 interrupted absorbable sutures (**Fig. 19.5**). A useful adjunct is to perform this repair over a small diameter bougie (40–46F).[19] However, primary repair is associated with a leak rate of at least 20% and if treatment is delayed past 24 hours this rises to over 50%.[20] Therefore, primary repair alone should be reserved for those operated on within 24 hours of the injury with demonstrably healthy tissue and limited soiling. Reinforcing the suture line with an onlay patch of nearby tissues (such as omentum, pleura, lung, pedicled intercostal muscle grafts, gastric fundus, pericardium or diaphragm) reduces the leak rate in experimental studies but this is difficult to confirm in vivo.[21,22]

T-tube repair

T-tube intubation was developed in the 1970s for late presenting patients who had tolerated perforation but had developed oesophagopleural fistulas

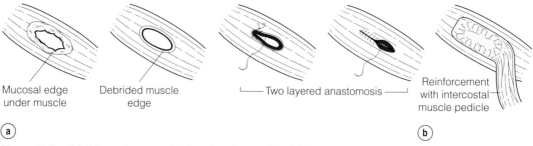

Mucosal edge under muscle

Debrided muscle edge

Two layered anastomosis

Reinforcement with intercostal muscle pedicle

(a)

(b)

Figure 19.5 • **(a)** Primary closure and buttressing of suture line. **(b)** Intercostal muscle flap.

since the oedematous tissues and localised sepsis excluded a primary repair.[23] The concept is of a controlled oesophagocutaneous fistula to divert secretions and facilitate healing without ongoing contamination. A large-diameter (6–10 mm) T-tube is placed through the tear with the limbs lying beyond the boundaries of the perforation and the oesophageal wall is closed loosely around the tube with fine interrupted, absorbable sutures (**Fig. 19.6**). The authors have not found it necessary to anchor the tube to the diaphragm as originally described.[7] The tube is externalised and secured at the skin, a further drain is placed down to the repair, and apical and basal intercostal chest drains are sited. Healing is monitored by contrast radiology and CT scans. The T-tube is left until a defined tract is established, with the majority removed between 3 and 6 weeks.

In view of the high leak rate for primary repairs, the T-tube technique is a recommended option for all patients.[24]

Resection

Oesophageal resection is a major undertaking with a high mortality, reserved for damage to a diseased oesophagus or in cases of extensive oesophageal trauma. The oesophagus can be immediately reconstructed if contamination is minimal or a delayed approach may be taken with limited demonstrable differences in outcome.[25] Techniques of exclusion and diversion are now historical.

Management algorithm

Diagnostic delay beyond 24 hours is classically associated with a poor outcome, but even when managed promptly and aggressively, spontaneous perforation of the oesophagus carries a significant mortality rate and reports to the contrary reflect selection bias. A management algorithm based on the therapeutic strategies outlined by the literature is demonstrated in **Fig. 19.7**. This is for guidance only and cases should be dealt with individually.

Personal experience and expertise may well determine the best management.

Perforation of the oesophagus secondary to underlying disease

Many conditions or their treatments predispose to perforation of the oesophagus, such as infections, malignancy, radiotherapy or chemotherapy.

In the presence of oesophageal cancer, the priority is to determine if the lesion was operable before the perforation, as an emergency subtotal oesophagectomy may be performed, although evidence suggests that perforation renders these lesions incurable and the associated surgical mortality is high.[26–28]

Non-perforated spontaneous injuries of the oesophagus

Barrett described full-thickness oesophageal perforation contained by the mediastinal pleura in 1947; this has since been termed 'intramural rupture'.[2,29] This can occur spontaneously or secondary to instrumentation, food impaction or coagulopathy. Endoscopically, there is a submucosal oesophageal haematoma with or without mucosal disruption. Non-operative treatment is usually successful as the perforation is contained, but a minority may require surgical intervention and intraluminal drainage of the haematoma may be necessary if there is airway compromise.[29,30]

'Black oesophagus syndrome' or acute oesophageal necrosis is an uncommon condition of circumferential mucosal and submucosal necrosis that ends sharply at the oesophagogastric junction in the absence of a caustic injury, most commonly presenting with upper gastrointestinal bleeding.[31] The most likely cause is vascular insufficiency from venous thrombosis as part of a 'two-hit' traumatic phenomenon associated with systemic hypotension from another cause. It has also been associated with thrombotic disorders.[32] Diagnosis is endoscopic and

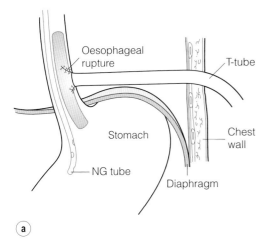

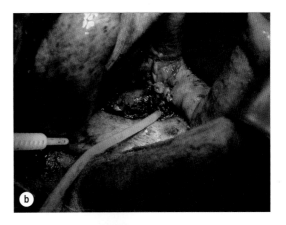

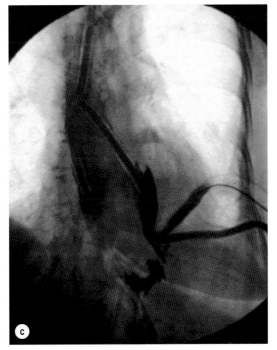

Figure 19.6 • (a) Diagrammatic representation of T-tube repair of spontaneous oesophageal perforation with T-tube in situ. **(b)** Operative photograph. **(c)** Contrast radiological image of the same patient as in (b); note additional intercostal chest drain.

treatment expectant with a low threshold for surgical resection as the condition can rapidly progress to perforation. Mortality is high, often secondary to the underlying cause.

Iatrogenic perforation of the oesophagus

Iatrogenic damage to the oesophagus leading to full-thickness disruption can occur from within, such as during endoscopic instrumentation, which accounts for 60–70% of such injuries, or from without, such as with paraoesophageal surgery.

Endoscopic injuries

Flexible video endoscopy has almost totally replaced rigid oesophagoscopy but despite the inherent safety of the procedure (0.03% perforation risk compared to 0.11% for rigid endoscopy), the dramatic increase in the number of examinations performed has led to an increase in the number of associated injuries.[33] Diagnostic endoscopic trauma is distal in

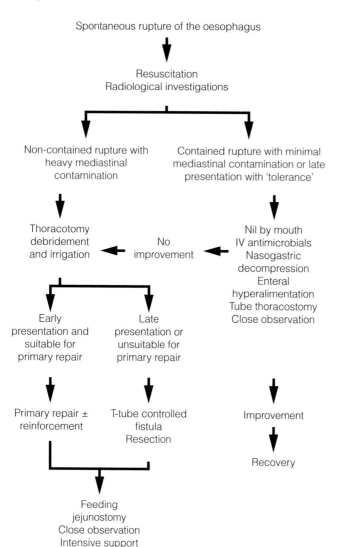

Figure 19.7 • Management algorithm for spontaneous oesophageal perforation.

75–90% of cases, usually just above an abnormality (Table 19.1). All therapeutic procedures carry a perforation risk of around 5%, which is increased in patients who have received prior radiotherapy or chemotherapy. Dilatation probably accounts for the majority of injuries and therefore the lower risk of perforation when placing self-expanding metal stents.[28] Benign pneumatic dilatation for achalasia carries a higher risk than graded dilatation, due to higher pressures and larger balloon size.[34] A recent development is transoesophageal echocardiography, which also carries a risk of pressure necrosis, especially when placed for perioperative monitoring.[35] A large case review of 75 patients with iatrogenic perforation of the oesophagus reported an overall mortality rate of 19%. Prevention is the real solution, and increasing awareness and training are likely to reduce the incidence.[36]

Clinical presentation and diagnosis

Most iatrogenic trauma is recognised immediately or there is at least a high index of suspicion. Clinical features depend on the cause, site and delay from injury but are similar to spontaneous perforation, with chest pain, dysphagia and odynophagia being most common. Patients can develop overt haemodynamic shock and a marked sympathetic nervous system response. Proximal cervical perforations are associated with neck pain, dysphonia, cervical dysphagia, hoarseness, torticollis and subcutaneous emphysema, but systemic symptoms are less common. The majority of the perforations have been visualised endoscopically or radiologically but plain radiography of the neck or chest may be useful, with contrast radiography or CT employed where necessary (**Fig. 19.8**).

Table 19.1 • Risk of iatrogenic oesophageal disruption through instrumentation

Medical instrumentation	Percentage risk of iatrogenic oesophageal disruption
Dilatation	0.5
Dilatation for achalasia	2
Endoscopic thermal therapy	1–2
Treatment of variceal bleeding	1–6
Endoscopic laser therapy	1–5
Photodynamic therapy	5
Stent placement	5–25

Management

In contrast to spontaneous perforations, which are associated with a 'full' stomach and gross mediastinal contamination, iatrogenic injuries usually occur in starved, hospitalised patients and are recognised early, hence contamination and treatment delay are markedly reduced. As such, there is considerable interest in non-operative, endoscopic and minimally invasive operative management options, all of which have been shown to be feasible. All patients require initial resuscitation and analgesia, and regular reassessment is mandatory as respiratory and cardiovascular support may become necessary.

Non-operative management

The basic principles of management of intrathoracic iatrogenic perforation are the same as those for

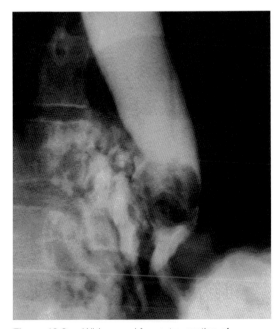

Figure 19.8 • Widespread free extravasation of contrast media as a result of iatrogenic rigid endoscopic perforation of distal oesophagus.

spontaneous perforation: a strict nil oral regimen, hyperalimentation (preferably enteral), broad-spectrum antimicrobial agents and drainage of collections. Criteria for selecting suitable patients for non-operative management are detailed in Box 19.4. Case series applying these criteria demonstrate a mortality rate between zero and 16%, but numbers are small and results are skewed by both selection and publication bias.[37–39] Non-operative management is not 'conservative'; patients require intensive observation and a low threshold for intervention, with up to 20% of patients requiring aggressive surgical salvage.[40] CT is the investigation of choice for assessment of collections and of progress, with contrast radiology still useful to assess leakage with a consequent lower radiation dose. The timing of investigations is best guided by the clinical condition of the patient but weekly serial contrast studies are not unreasonable. Iatrogenic cervical perforations are almost always contained and thus usually managed non-operatively with percutaneous drainage of collections where necessary. Any resulting oesophagocutaneous fistulas heal rapidly in the absence of distal obstruction. Occasionally, operative prevertebral lavage, primary closure and drainage using a left lateral incision anterior to the sternocleidomastoid is required, this being well tolerated by even critically ill patients.[41]

Endoscopic

The development of modern endoscopic technology means that an endoluminal approach is now possible that can replicate the principles of open surgery with minimal associated trauma. This is especially pertinent in patients where the benefits of surgical exploration are outweighed by the risk or by the ultimate outcome (advanced cancer) or in patients in whom the defect is small and clean and easily dealt with at the time of injury. However, all endoscopic approaches are technically difficult and should not be attempted by inexperienced operators unable to deal with the consequences of their actions. Two basic endoscopic treatments can be applied: closure and diversion.

Closure: clips and sealants

Endoclips are well established in closing small, clean defects after endoscopic mucosal resection or submucosal dissection for early cancer.[42] As such, in the absence of significant contamination, small perforations may be closed immediately using endoclips in addition to supportive non-operative treatment.[40] It is important to appreciate that endoclipping 'en face' in the oesophagus is challenging. Sealants such as fibrin glue have also been used successfully but this may require multiple endoscopic sessions and the authors do not believe that this significantly alters the clinical course from drainage alone.[36,43]

Diversion: stents

Many case reports describe the successful placement of self-expanding stents to seal oesophageal perforations, chronic fistulas and even postoperative anastomotic leaks.[16,44,45] Concerns have been raised regarding the extension of the defect through pressure necrosis and the trauma of ultimate stent removal.[42,46] Furthermore, stents were not designed for use in a normal oesophagus and migration rates approach 30%.[46] Publication bias means that failure rates, the consequences of failure or whether placement increases overall risk remain unknown. As such, stenting should be highly selective and always viewed as a temporary solution. However, in patients whose physical condition precludes more aggressive treatments and those in whom resection is not deemed suitable, stents do offer a serious alternative. The authors advise using a removable, softer material stent with planned removal within 3 months to avoid long-term complications.

Operative management

The indications for the operative management of iatrogenic perforations are identical to spontaneous perforation but underlying pathologies such as carcinoma, peptic stricture or achalasia are more common. As a result, specific operative intervention may be necessary and despite reduced contamination the associated surgical mortality is increased sixfold.[38] The indications for operative management are the corollary of those documented in Box 19.4.

Patients who sustain a perforation of a malignant stricture constitute a separate and difficult group to manage. Those who have known inoperable disease due to metastatic spread or who are unfit for surgery should be managed non-operatively, and in this situation the use of a sealing stent is appropriate. In patients with less clearly defined operability most authors recommend resection with a view to control of contamination and potential cure, but this strategy carries a considerable mortality rate of 11–75%.[25,27] There is evidence to suggest that despite resection, iatrogenic perforation of an operable carcinoma of the oesophagus compromises long-term survival such that these should be considered to have become palliation resections.[47] As such, every effort should be made to prevent perforation during staging endoscopic procedures.

Iatrogenic perforation of achalasia is uncommon (1–5%) and usually managed non-operatively or endoscopically as they are often small, recognised immediately and well contained. If thoracotomy and repair is required then it appears unnecessary to carry out a cardiomyotomy or antireflux procedure at the same time.

Laparoscopic approach

Since iatrogenic perforations are usually clean, circumscribed, recognised early and within a few centimetres of the oesophagogastric junction, it is reasonable for surgeons who are used to working at the hiatus to attempt repair and drainage laparoscopically by approaching the hiatus transperitoneally. This obviously requires advanced laparoscopic skills in specialist centres with appropriate facilities.[48]

Paraoesophageal surgery and procedural injuries

Direct oesophageal trauma is most commonly sustained during antireflux surgery, both open and laparoscopic, but the risk is low, of the order of 0–1.2%.[49] The risk increases with an intrathoracic approach, a previous hiatal operation and suturing of the wrap to the oesophagus. The majority of injuries are recognised and repaired immediately. The mortality of unrecognised and uncontained perforations approaches 20% and these require aggressive surgical intervention.

Trauma can also be sustained directly during thoracic and spinal surgery (<0.5% of procedures) or due to endotracheal intubation, nasogastric insertion and surgical tracheostomy. In ventilated patients, the clinical features of an injury may be concealed. Indirect trauma can occur through pressure necrosis or devascularisation, although the rich vascular supply of the thoracic oesophagus makes this extremely uncommmon.

Management algorithm

An algorithm for the management of iatrogenic injuries of the oesophagus is detailed in **Fig. 19.9**.

Traumatic injuries of the oesophagus

As a consequence of the protected posterior mediastinal position of the oesophagus, external trauma is rare, accounting for only 19% of all oesophageal injuries. Blunt trauma occurs in less than 1%.[50]

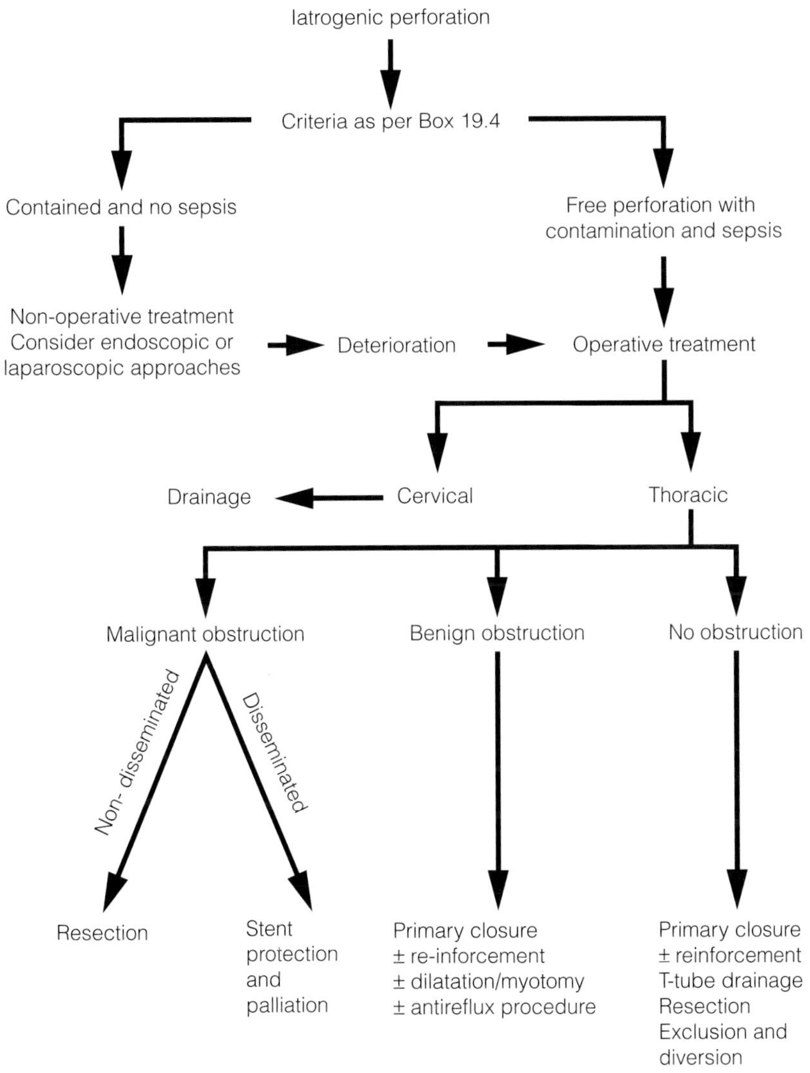

Figure 19.9 • Management algorithm for iatrogenic oesophageal perforation.

Iatrogenic perforation

Criteria as per Box 19.4

Contained and no sepsis

Free perforation with contamination and sepsis

Non-operative treatment Consider endoscopic or laparoscopic approaches → Deterioration → Operative treatment

Drainage ← Cervical

Thoracic

Malignant obstruction

Benign obstruction

No obstruction

Non-disseminated

Disseminated

Resection

Stent protection and palliation

Primary closure ± re-inforcement ± dilatation/myotomy ± antireflux procedure

Primary closure ± reinforcement T-tube drainage Resection Exclusion and diversion

Penetrating injuries

Penetrating injuries are easily missed since they usually occur in conjunction with serious injuries to surrounding viscera. Diagnostic delay and contamination greatly increase morbidity and mortality but any penetrating transcervical or transmediastinal wound, especially when gunshot derived, should raise suspicion of oesophageal injury. Damage may manifest as subcutaneous emphysema, cervical haematomas or on plain radiographic studies as a haemopneumothorax or soft tissue mediastinal or retropharyngeal oedema. Due to the limitations of performing contrast radiology in critically injured patients, direct visualisation with bronchoscopy and flexible oesophagoscopy is now preferred. If necessary these can be performed on table once stabilised from other more immediately life-threatening injuries.

 In a retrospective review of 55 trauma patients, Horwitz et al. demonstrated 100% sensitivity and 92.4% specificity for upper gastrointestinal endoscopy in confirming oesophageal perforation and although injuries were infrequent (prevalence 3.6%), no injuries were missed and the examination was safe.[11] In a similar study of 31 patients (24 of whom were intubated at the time of the examination), video endoscopy had a sensitivity of 100% and a specificity of 96% with no associated morbidity.[51]

Management

Some authors advocate mandatory surgery for penetrating cervical oesophageal injuries while others prefer a selective, non-operative approach. Contained perforations may be managed non-operatively irrespective of any delay, but repair should be undertaken when uncontained or in those requiring exploration for another reason, which is likely in any injury where the path traverses platysma or which passes through the mediastinum. Isolated cervical oesophageal injuries are best approached anterior to sternocleidomastoid via a left- or right-sided incision. Thoracic oesophageal trauma can be approached on the right side for the upper or mid-oesophageal thirds, and the left side for distal trauma, but other approaches may be required depending on the injury sustained. Virtually all transthoracic gun-shot wounds will require surgical exploration, and life-threatening cardiovascular, pulmonary and tracheobronchial injuries take precedence. Specialist advice and input should be sought but the majority of the oesophageal injuries will be able to be dealt with using the techniques described previously for spontaneous perforation of the oesophagus.

The overall mortality of penetrating thoracic oesophageal injuries is hard to ascertain but lies between 15% and 27% and is lower for cervical trauma at 1–16%.[52,53] The morbidity arises mostly from associated spinal and airway trauma for cervical injuries and from cardiorespiratory damage in thoracic trauma, and these injuries should be actively excluded.

Blunt trauma

Blunt cervical trauma usually results from impaction of the neck or upper chest on the steering wheel in high-velocity road traffic accidents, but may occur with extreme 'whiplash' flexion–extension. Similarly, thoracic oesophageal trauma can be sustained by rapid deceleration leading to traction laceration at fixed points such as the cricoid, carina or pharyngo-oesophageal junction, by barogenic damage after a sudden rise in intra-abdominal pressure from compression against a closed glottis or secondary to interruption of vascular supply. These are almost exclusively high-impact injuries so are often associated with more immediately life-threatening airway or cardiopulmonary damage and compromise. The diagnostic pathways and management strategies are similar to spontaneous and iatrogenic perforations, with an awareness of associated tracheobronchial and cardiopulmonary trauma, which is present in up to 56%.[50] It should be noted that even relatively minor thoracic blunt trauma can lead to late strictures from missed injuries, and oesophageal damage should be suspected and actively excluded.

Caustic injuries

Serious ingestion of a caustic substance is uncommon but devastating. The aetiology is distinct between the two age groups in which they occur. Ingestion by children is common and almost exclusively accidental whereas, in contrast, ingestion by adults is more often deliberate. Most caustic substances can be grouped into acids or alkalis. Dangerous acids are available as toilet cleaners (hydrochloric acid), battery fluid (sulphuric acid) and in metal working (phosphoric and hydrofluoric acids). Hydrofluoric acid is particularly dangerous, leading to dramatic, systemic fluctuations in metabolic calcium that can rapidly progress to refractory cardiac dysrhythmias; specialist poisons advice is recommended in these cases and emergency personnel should take care not to become contaminated themselves as even dermal exposure is hazardous. Strong alkalis are also readily available as cleaners and bleaches although, thankfully, most household agents are only mild caustic agents. Some button batteries contain powerful alkalis and ingestion of these is dealt with elsewhere in this chapter.

Misconception 1: tissue penetration by acids is minimised by coagulative necrosis whereas alkalis more rapidly penetrate transmurally through liquefactive necrosis. Although pathologically correct, this is clinically irrelevant as the ingestion of any strong caustic agent in sufficient quantity will inflict a potentially fatal oesophageal injury. Furthermore there is evidence to suggest that strong acid ingestion is associated with greater systemic effects, a higher perforation rate and a higher mortality than alkali ingestion.[54]

Misconception 2: acid ingestion causes gastric damage whereas alkali ingestion causes oesophageal injury. This is commonly cited but there is no evidence to support this.[55,56]

In summary, the severity of any injury is related to the corrosive properties, concentration, amount, viscosity and duration of contact between the particular caustic agent and the oesophageal mucosa. Intentional caustic ingestions are associated with larger ingested quantities of agent and so tend to lead to more severe injuries. In contrast, fortunately, the amount ingested accidentally by children is usually small.

Clinical presentation

Most patients survive to reach the hospital unless aspiration has occurred. In accidental ingestion, presentation is usually rapid and symptoms and signs may not yet be present. The clinical features are dependent on the substance and the time since ingestion, but the absence of oral burns or pharyngo-oesophageal symptoms does not exclude injury as the caustic agent may have passed rapidly through the mouth and the location of the most severe injury is not predicted by symptoms alone. Furthermore, in deliberate ingestion clinical features may be 'underplayed'. The clinical features of a caustic injury of the oesophagus are documented in Box 19.5.

Box 19.5 • Acute symptoms and signs of caustic injury of the oesophagus

- Refusal to eat or drink in children
- Facial oedema/burns
- Oropharyngeal pain
- Hypersalivation/drooling
- Stridor/hoarse voice
- Dyspnoea
- Chest pain
- Nausea and vomiting
- Epigastric pain/tenderness
- Haematemesis

Glossopharyngeal burns cause oedema that may threaten the airway and prevent clearance of secretions with drooling and hypersalivation, and injury to the epiglottis and larynx leads to stridor and a hoarse voice. Dyspnoea is uncommon unless aspiration has occurred. On inspection, oropharyngeal burns can range from mild oedema and superficial erosions to extensive mucosal sloughing and necrosis. Acid burns form a black eschar whereas alkali burns look grey and dull. Oesophageal injury is suggested by dysphagia and odynophagia, and gastric injury by epigastric pain, nausea, anorexia, retching, vomiting and haematemesis. Patients may present shocked or in respiratory distress.

Investigation and management

The immediate priorities are the establishment of a secure airway, the stabilisation of cardiovascular status and the relief of pain. Concurrent facial or eye burns should be irrigated and ophthalmology and plastic surgery specialist involvement should be sought. Oral intake is prohibited. Gastric lavage, induced emesis, nasogastric aspiration and the use of neutralising chemicals are currently contraindicated. Where possible the ingested agent and amount swallowed should be identified and regional poison centres can provide information regarding caustic properties.

Unintentional ingestion in asymptomatic patients with no oropharyngeal burns and normal or minor oesophageal findings may be discharged once they are able to take oral fluids.

All others require admission and flexible video endoscopy of the upper gastrointestinal tract by a skilled practitioner as soon as the patient is stabilised, preferably within 24 hours of ingestion, to assess the stage of the oesophageal injury and place a nasoenteral tube for early nutritional support – this may also act as a partial stent in preventing strictures.[55,57]

In cases with severe laryngopharyngeal burns or respiratory compromise, general anaesthesia may be required. Staging of the burn determines the optimum management, likelihood of subsequent stricture formation and is the only accurate predictor of systemic complications and death.[54] The severity of the injury is graded using a system similar to that for skin burns (Table 19.2) but differentiation between grades may be difficult, especially between second- and third-degree burns, with implications for management; consequently some patients will benefit from repeated evaluation (Table 19.3).[58,59] There has been recent interest in the use of oesophageal endosonography to assess the depth of necrosis, specifically damage to the muscle layers, as this would influence future stricture formation, but this currently offers no advantage over conventional endoscopic assessment.[60]

Most caustic injuries are managed non-operatively. The use of steroids and antibiotics during the acute phase remains controversial, with conflicting evidence regarding their benefits.[61]

Steroids form part of the treatment protocol of many units and research continues into their use for the prevention of strictures despite a prospective randomised, controlled trial that clearly demonstrated no benefit from steroids, with the development of oesophageal strictures related only to the severity of the corrosive injury.[62]

Patients with severe burns who are most at risk of stricture formation also represent the highest perforation risk and steroids may mask clinical

Table 19.2 • Depth of oesophageal burn

Depth of burn	Degree of burn	Endoscopic findings
Superficial	1	Mucosal oedema and hyperaemia
Transmucosal ± involvement of the muscularis	2a	Superficial ulcers, bleeding, exudates
	2b	Deep ulcers – focal or circumferential
Full thickness ± adjacent organ involvement	3a	Full-thickness focal necrosis
	3b	Extensive necrosis

Table 19.3 • Endoscopic staging of oesophageal caustic injury

Finding	First-degree	Second-degree	Third-degree
Bleeding	Hyperaemia only	Mild/moderate bleeding	Moderate/severe bleeding
Oedema	Mild	Moderate	Severe
Mucosal loss	None	Mucosal ulceration or blistering	Deep ulcers
Exudate	None	Present ± pseudomembrane	Present ± pseudomembrane
Appearance if endoscopy delayed	None	Granulation tissue	Eschar

symptoms.[63] As such, the authors believe there is no place for steroids in the initial management of a caustic injury.

 Similarly antibiotics should be reserved for those with proven infection, perforation or aspiration, and in these cases the authors suggest the additional use of antifungal agents.[64]

Intravenous fluids, analgesia, nutritional support and antisecretory agents should be given. Patients with grade 1 and 2a burns should be admitted and observed for 5–7 days with diet reintroduced gradually over 24–48 hours, and endoscopy or contrast radiology studies should be arranged for 6–8 weeks after discharge to assess for strictures. Patients who intentionally swallowed a caustic substance will require psychiatric assessment prior to discharge. It is reasonable to observe patients with grade 2b and 3 burns, continuing nasojejunal feeding and if there is no evidence of progression to perforation then clear fluids can be introduced from 48 hours, but be aware that the perforation risk is present for at least 7 days. Those who present with a perforation or deteriorate will require an emergency oesophagogastrectomy as the stomach is almost always injured. The authors do not believe that laparoscopy has a role. Immediate reconstruction with a substernal colonic interposition graft can be performed if there is minimal local contamina-

tion but more commonly reconstruction is delayed for 6–8 weeks. Resection should also be considered in patients with extensive circumferential mucosal injuries as problematic strictures and a cancer risk exist. The mortality for these injuries is 13–40%, with the majority of deaths occurring in the adult suicidal group.[56] Mortality mainly stems from respiratory complications and delay in the aggressive surgical treatment of transmural necrosis. There is no place for 'conservative' treatment in a severe caustic injury.

Long-term complications and outcomes

Strictures develop in 5–50% of patients, 95% of which are distal and can be graded according to the Marchand classification (Table 19.4).[65]

 Most strictures can be managed by Savary–Gilliard bougie dilatation.[66]

The procedure-related perforation incidence is less than 1%, but for safety the authors advise allowing approximately 6 weeks after injury before attempting dilatation. Antisecretory medication or even surgery may be required if reflux occurs after dilatation. Young patients with long, grade 3 or 4 strictures are likely to require a lifetime of repeated dilatations with a cumulative risk of iatrogenic perforation and

Table 19.4 • The Marchand classification of oesophageal strictures

Circumferential	Length	Consistency	Grade
Incomplete	Short	Fibrotic	1
String-like circumferential	Short	Elastic	2
Complete	≤1 cm	Fibrotic	3
Complete	>1 cm	Superficial fibrosis, easily dilated, non-progressive	4a
Compete	>1 cm	Deep fibrosis, tubular, progressive, not easily dilated	4b

ultimately of cancer, and in these patients surgery should be considered. Surgical options are to bypass or resect the obstructive segment or to perform a stricturoplasty. Bypass avoids dissection through mediastinal fibrosis, and using the retrosternal or subcutaneous route for the neo-oesophagus may avoid a thoracotomy. However, retaining the damaged oesophagus retains the long-term cancer risk and can lead to problems related to secretions and bacterial overgrowth. Thoracotomy, resection and colonic reconstruction (due to concurrent gastric damage) is therefore preferable. An alternative is an oesophageal stricturoplasty using a vascularised graft of colon, but again this retains the cancer risk. Many would advocate one definitive operation as the better option. An alternative is to use a temporary self-expanding stent for problematic strictures but experience is limited by numbers.[14]

Cancer risk

Up to 16% of caustic injuries are associated with squamous malignant transformation of the damaged oesophagus, a risk 1000 times that of the general population.[67] The severity of the injury is not proportional to the risk. Management options are early resection, since this is associated with low mortality rates, or surveillance. However, surveillance may be impractical as the latent period for the malignant change is 15–40 years. As such, simply an awareness of the risk by clinicians and patients should lead to earlier diagnosis and an increase in the number of curative resections.

Management algorithm

An algorithm for the management of caustic injuries of the oesophagus is detailed in **Fig. 19.10**.

Ingestion of foreign bodies

The oesophagus is the most common site for impaction of ingested foreign bodies within the gastrointestinal tract, accounting for 75% of cases.[68] The majority occur in children between the ages of 6 months and 6 years, with coins, toys, crayons and batteries being the commonest objects swallowed. In adults food boluses (predominantly meat) or impaction of bone fragments are more common. This is especially the case in edentulous patients due to decreased palatal sensation. Cases also occur in people with mental or psychiatric difficulties, or related to drug and alcohol abuse, and in those seeking secondary gain such as prisoners, and most upper gastrointestinal units are aware of a number of recurrent offenders.

Most foreign bodies impact in the cervical oesophagus, but impaction can occur at any of the physiological narrowings: cricopharyngeus, the aortic arch,

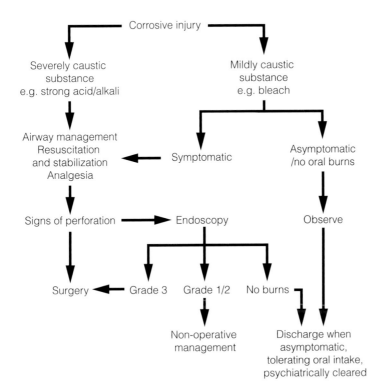

Figure 19.10 • Management algorithm for caustic oesophageal injuries.

the left main bronchus and the gastro-oesophageal junction. Benign pathology accounts for some cases (e.g. Schatzki rings, peptic strictures and eosinophilic oesophagitis); in contrast malignant strictures are uncommonly associated with impaction due to the long development phase, but there are significant food bolus impaction rates associated with palliative treatments of malignant oesophageal lesions such as plastic and self-expanding metal stents.[69]

Clinical presentation

In over 90% there is a clear history of ingestion associated with acute dysphagia at the level of the impaction and thus a rapid diagnosis.[70] However, in young children and uncooperative adults the diagnosis may not be so clear-cut. Suspicious symptoms in children are refusal of feeds, gagging and choking, but some cases may remain concealed for months or even years and chronic aspiration or reflux may represent long-standing impaction. A high index of suspicion is also required for psychiatric patients with features suggestive of foreign body ingestion. Respiratory symptoms occur in 5–15%, especially in children and in cervical impaction, leading to coughing, wheezing, stridor and dyspnoea. In adults, impaction in the cervical oesophagus can cause tracheal obstruction leading to the so-called 'café coronary' or 'steakhouse syndrome'. Typically sharp object ingestion (e.g. fish bones) can cause a persistent foreign body sensation despite easy passage through the oesophagus without impaction.

Physical signs are usually limited unless impaction causes obstruction leading to drooling or perforation leading to neck swelling, erythema, tenderness, subcutaneous emphysema or systemic effects. Long-standing impaction may lead to recurrent aspiration, empyema of the lung, perioesophagitis, oesophageal stenosis or fistulation into the airways or major vessels.

Diagnosis

Plain radiographs may localise both radio-opaque and non-radio-opaque objects and are useful if perforation is suspected (**Fig. 19.11**). Both anteroposterior and lateral projections should be obtained as objects may not be visible if overlying the vertebrae, and this also helps to distinguish whether objects are in the digestive or tracheobronchial tract. In young children and infants, extensive plain radiography may be required to confirm or refute the diagnosis of a swallowed radio-opaque foreign body. Even in the absence of symptoms or physical signs a potential history of ingestion should prompt the use of radiography, as in one study 17% of asymptomatic children with a history of coin ingestion had an impacted oesophageal coin.[71]

 Flexible video endoscopy is the investigation of choice. It has been used safely for over 30 years, is associated with a diagnostic sensitivity of 86% and specificity of 63%, and is therapeutic in 95%.[72,73]

Water-soluble contrast studies or CT scans may occasionally be required in cases of non-radio-opaque objects such as wood, aluminium, glass and

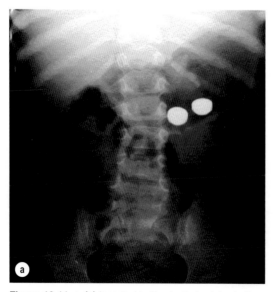
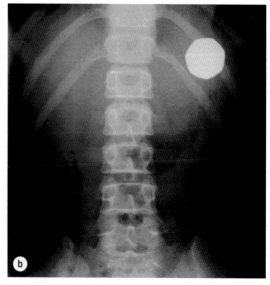

Figure 19.11 • (a) Ingested button batteries lying in the gastric antrum. **(b)** Ingested 50-pence coin.

plastics, but the use of hypertonic contrast media and barium should be avoided.

Management

In a Western population, the majority of ingested foreign bodies will pass through the gastrointestinal tract uneventfully, with 10–20% requiring endoscopic removal due to impaction and 1% requiring surgical removal.[73,74]

The indications for urgent intervention are:

1. Airway compromise.
2. Absolute dysphagia with aspiration risk.
3. Oesophageal impaction of sharp object or button battery.
4. Oesophageal impaction of greater than 24 hours duration.

The passage of a foreign body through the oesophagus does not always indicate success as objects over 5–6 cm long or 2 cm in diameter are unlikely to pass through the gastric pylorus or around the duodenal curves and, once impacted, endoscopic removal may be difficult and so expeditious retrieval while in the oesophagus is advised. Similarly, although the majority of ingested sharp objects entering the stomach will traverse the gastrointestinal tract without incident, the perforation risk of up to 35% suggests that retrieval if safe should be attempted.[75]

In all other situations, individual management strategies depend on the symptoms, objects and expertise of the receiving speciality, which includes paediatricians, surgeons and psychiatrists.

Observation of up to 24 hours is reasonable in asymptomatic patients with oesophageal coins or similar round, smooth objects as many of these will pass spontaneously.[76]

Failure to progress through the gastrointestinal tract or symptomatic deterioration should prompt surgical review. Therapeutic video endoscopy is as successful in object removal as rigid endoscopy but with a significantly lower complication rate (5% vs. 10%) and avoids general anaesthesia in the majority of cases. However, in a minority, the type of object, number of objects or the inability of the patient to cooperate (i.e. young children) may dictate that general anaesthesia is required. Rigid endoscopy is still useful for impaction in the pharynx as the view and access are superior, but it should be abandoned for distal obstructions. Patience is an important virtue in endoscopic removal but is rewarded with a success rate of around 95%.[73]

Failure is most likely to occur with long (>10 cm) or complex objects such as dental prostheses.

Smooth objects may be difficult to retrieve; a variety of graspers, snares, magnets and baskets may be required and it is useful to practise with the proposed grasper on a duplicate foreign body prior to the actual procedure. Coins should be orientated sideways to aid passage through cricopharyngeus and sharp or pointed objects may require an overtube or endoscopic hood for safe removal or manipulation to allow removal 'blunt end first'.

Food impactions tend to occur in the distal oesophagus and are usually accompanied by underlying pathology. Eosinophilic oesophagitis is of recent interest in this regard as a predisposing factor to acute dysphagia and food impaction. This is especially relevant as the oesophageal mucosa is thin, friable and easily traumatised by instrumentation and as such dilatation should be avoided. Mucosal biopsies are therefore a necessity in all cases. A number of techniques to dislodge food boluses without recourse to endoscopy have been reported. Proteolytic agents (e.g. papain) that dissolve the food bolus may cause oesophageal trauma and are dangerous if aspirated and they are not recommended. Effervescent agents, such as carbonated drinks and intravenous glucagon, which causes smooth muscle relaxation, were thought to help disimpact the food bolus but there is no good evidence to support their use.[77]

As such, the safest recourse is again video endoscopy, which allows relief of the impaction and diagnosis of any underlying pathology. In these situations, definitive treatment such as dilatation could be performed at the same time. Endoscopic removal of the food bolus may again be achieved using a variety of techniques and tools. Larger boluses may require piecemeal removal, using an overtube if repeated intubation is required. Once the endoscope has been passed distal to the bolus then the bolus may be gently pushed into the stomach, but this technique should never be performed 'blindly'.

'Disc' or 'button' batteries are now readily available and easily ingested by curious children. The electrical discharge or release of the alkaline contents can rapidly lead to local damage, necrosis and perforation. As such, urgent extraction is required if lodged within the oesophagus, and plain radiographs are helpful for localisation. However, if the battery has passed on to the stomach and duodenum then 80–90% will pass without complication. As such, observation with serial radiography is used to monitor progression and reserving endoscopic or surgical intervention if the battery fails to progress out of the stomach within 48 hours, if the patient develops symptoms of intestinal injury or if the battery fragments and there is evidence of mercury toxicity.

Surgery may be necessary when endoscopy fails for large objects, for objects embedded in the oesophageal wall or when there has been an associated or iatrogenic perforation.[68] The surgical approach depends not only on the site and severity of the injury, but also associated inflammation and any underlying oesophageal pathology. Surgery is also indicated in cases of deliberate narcotic packet ingestion where there is failure to progress, obstruction or rupture – endoscopic removal should not be attempted because of the risk of rupture.[78]

Summary

Oesophageal emergencies represent a widely heterogeneous group of conditions from a wide variety of insults leading to a wide spectrum of injury. The potential for disaster is omnipresent given the fragility of the oesophageal wall, the lack of serosa, the proximity of vital organs, the inaccessibility and the lack of symptoms and signs; these factors in combination mean that even minor injuries can be ultimately fatal. Because of the rarity of these difficult cases, most surgeons will deal with only a handful in their career; consequently such cases are best managed by specialist units with ancillary staff who are trained, equipped and experienced to prevent potentially disastrous consequences of misdiagnosis and inappropriate management. However, the best way to improve outcomes is through prevention where possible, for example through safe and thorough training in therapeutic endoscopy, better labelling of caustic substances, and development of smaller button batteries.

Key points

Spontaneous oesophageal perforation
- Diagnostic error and diagnostic delay are high.
- Oral water-soluble contrast radiography is the diagnostic investigation of choice.
- Flexible video endoscopic assessment may play an increasing role.
- Surgery remains the mainstay of treatment.

Iatrogenic oesophageal perforation
- 75–90% of iatrogenic perforations occur distally.
- Underlying pathology is common.
- Perforation of an oesophageal cancer renders these lesions incurable.
- Non-operative management is often successful.

Oesophageal trauma
- Penetrating trauma is easily missed with serious injuries to surrounding viscera.
- Bronchoscopy and video endoscopy are the investigations of choice.

Caustic injuries
- Investigation is mandatory in suspected caustic ingestion.
- Flexible video endoscopy is essential to assess the oesophagus within 24 hours of injury.
- There is no proven role for steroids or antibiotics in initial management.
- Most strictures can be managed by Savary–Gilliard bougie dilatation.
- Reconstructive surgery should be considered in young patients with refractory strictures.

Ingestion of foreign bodies
- Flexible video endoscopy is both the investigation and treatment of choice.
- The majority of ingested foreign bodies will pass uneventfully.
- Observation of up to 24 hours is reasonable in asymptomatic patients with round, smooth objects.

References

1. Derbes VJ, Mitchell RE Jr. Hermann Boerhaave's Atrocis, nec descripti prius, morbi historia, the first translation of the classic case report of rupture of the esophagus, with annotations. Bull Med Libr Assoc 1955; 43(2):217–40.

2. Barrett N. Report of a case of spontaneous perforation of the oesophagus successfully treated by operation. Br J Surg 1947; 47:216–18.

3. Mackler S. Spontaneous rupture of the oesophagus; an experimental and clinical study. Surg Gynecol Obst 1952; 95:345–56.

4. Hayes N, Waterworth PD, Griffin SM. Avulsion of short gastric arteries caused by vomiting. Gut 1994; 35(8):1137–8.

5. Griffin SM, Lamb PJ, Shenfine J et al. Spontaneous rupture of the oesophagus. Br J Surg 2008; 95(9):1115–20.

6. Altorjay A, Kiss J, Voros A et al. The role of esophagectomy in the management of esophageal perforations. Ann Thorac Surg 1998; 65(5):1433–6.

7. Shenfine J, Dresner SM, Vishwanath Y et al. Management of spontaneous rupture of the oesophagus. Br J Surg 2000; 87(3):362–73.

8. Levine PH, Kelley ML Jr. Spontaneous perforation of esophagus simulating acute pancreatitis. JAMA 1965; 191(4):342–5.

9. Buecker A, Wein BB, Neuerburg JM et al. Esophageal perforation: comparison of use of aqueous and barium-containing contrast media. Radiology 1997; 202(3):683–6.

10. Griffin SM, Lamb PJ, Dresner SM et al. Diagnosis and management of a mediastinal leak following radical oesophagectomy. Br J Surg 2001; 88(10):1346–51.

11. Horwitz B, Krevsky B, Buckman RF Jr et al. Endoscopic evaluation of penetrating esophageal injuries. Am J Gastroenterol 1993; 88(8):1249–53.

12. Srinivasan R, Haywood T, Horwitz B et al. Role of flexible endoscopy in the evaluation of possible esophageal trauma after penetrating injuries. Am J Gastroenterol 2000; 95(7):1725–9.

13. White CS, Templeton PA, Attar S. Esophageal perforation: CT findings. Am J Roentgenol 1993; 160(4):767–70.

14. Evrard S, Le Moine O, Lazaraki G et al. Self-expanding plastic stents for benign esophageal lesions. Gastrointest Endosc 2004; 60(6):894–900.

15. Petruzziello L, Tringali A, Riccioni ME et al. Successful early treatment of Boerhaave's syndrome by endoscopic placement of a temporary self-expandable plastic stent without fluoroscopy. Gastrointest Endosc 2003; 58(4):608–12.

16. Kiev J, Amendola M, Bouhaidar D et al. A management algorithm for esophageal perforation. Am J Surg 2007; 194(1):103–6.

17. Wehrmann T, Stergiou N, Vogel B et al. Endoscopic debridement of paraesophageal, mediastinal abscesses: a prospective case series. Gastrointest Endosc 2005; 62(3):344–9.

18. Walker WS, Cameron EW, Walbaum PR. Diagnosis and management of spontaneous transmural rupture of the oesophagus (Boerhaave's syndrome). Br J Surg 1985; 72(3):204–7.

19. Whyte RI, Iannettoni MD, Orringer MB. Intrathoracic esophageal perforation. The merit of primary repair. J Thorac Cardiovasc Surg 1995; 109(1):140–4; discussion 144–6.

20. Lawrence DR, Ohri SK, Moxon RE et al. Primary esophageal repair for Boerhaave's syndrome. Ann Thorac Surg 1999; 67(3):818–20.

21. Richardson JD. Management of esophageal perforations: the value of aggressive surgical treatment. Am J Surg 2005; 190(2):161–5.

22. Wright CD, Mathisen DJ, Wain JC et al. Reinforced primary repair of thoracic esophageal perforation. Ann Thorac Surg 1995; 60(2):245–8; discussion 248–9.

23. Mansour KA, Wenger RK. T-tube management of late esophageal perforations. Surg Gynecol Obstet 1992; 175(6):571–2.

24. Naylor AR, Walker WS, Dark J et al. T tube intubation in the management of seriously ill patients with oesophagopleural fistulae. Br J Surg 1990; 77(1):40–2.

25. Orringer MB, Stirling MC. Esophagectomy for esophageal disruption. Ann Thorac Surg 1990; 49(1):35–42; discussion 42–3.

26. Gupta NM. Emergency transhiatal oesophagectomy for instrumental perforation of an obstructed thoracic oesophagus. Br J Surg 1996; 83(7):1007–9.

27. Adam DJ, Thompson AM, Walker WS et al. Oesophagogastrectomy for iatrogenic perforation of oesophageal and cardia carcinoma. Br J Surg 1996; 83(10):1429–32.

28. Jethwa P, Lala A, Powell J et al. A regional audit of iatrogenic perforation of tumours of the oesophagus and cardia. Aliment Pharmacol Ther 2005; 21(4):479–84.

29. Steadman C, Kerlin P, Crimmins F et al. Spontaneous intramural rupture of the oesophagus. Gut 1990; 31(8):845–9.

30. Yen HH, Soon MS, Chen YY. Esophageal intramural hematoma: an unusual complication of endoscopic biopsy. Gastrointest Endosc 2005; 62(1):161–3.

31. Moreto M, Ojembarrena E, Zaballa M et al. Idiopathic acute esophageal necrosis: not necessarily a terminal event. Endoscopy 1993; 25(8):534–8.

32. Cappell MS. Esophageal necrosis and perforation associated with the anticardiolipin antibody syndrome. Am J Gastroenterol 1994; 89(8):1241–5.

33. Pasricha PJ, Fleischer DE, Kalloo AN. Endoscopic perforations of the upper digestive tract: a review of their pathogenesis, prevention, and management. Gastroenterology 1994; 106(3):787–802.

34. Borotto E, Gaudric M, Danel B et al. Risk factors of oesophageal perforation during pneumatic dilatation for achalasia. Gut 1996; 39(1):9–12.

35. Lecharny JB, Philip I, Depoix JP. Oesophagotracheal perforation after intraoperative transoesophageal echocardiography in cardiac surgery. Br J Anaesth 2002; 88(4):592–4.

36. Fernandez FF, Richter A, Freudenberg S et al. Treatment of endoscopic esophageal perforation. Surg Endosc 1999; 13(10):962–6.

37. Bladergroen MR, Lowe JE, Postlethwait RW. Diagnosis and recommended management of esophageal perforation and rupture. Ann Thorac Surg 1986; 42(3):235–9.

38. Michel L, Grillo HC, Malt RA. Operative and non-operative management of esophageal perforations. Ann Surg 1981; 194(1):57–63.

39. Sarr MG, Pemberton JH, Payne WS. Management of instrumental perforations of the esophagus. J Thorac Cardiovasc Surg 1982; 84(2):211–18.

40. Raju GS, Thompson C, Zwischenberger JB. Emerging endoscopic options in the management of esophageal leaks (videos). Gastrointest Endosc 2005; 62(2):278–86.

41. Brewer LA3rd, Carter R, Mulder GA et al. Options in the management of perforations of the esophagus. Am J Surg 1986; 152(1):62–9.

42. Qadeer MA, Dumot JA, Vargo JJ et al. Endoscopic clips for closing esophageal perforations: case report and pooled analysis. Gastrointest Endosc 2007; 66(3):605–11.

43. Cipolletta L, Bianco MA, Rotondano G et al. Endoscopic clipping of perforation following pneumatic dilation of esophagojejunal anastomotic strictures. Endoscopy 2000; 32(9):720–2.

44. Adam A, Watkinson AF, Dussek J. Boerhaave syndrome: to treat or not to treat by means of insertion of a metallic stent. J Vasc Interv Radiol 1995; 6(5):741–3; discussion 744–6.

45. Doniec JM, Schniewind B, Kahlke V et al. Therapy of anastomotic leaks by means of covered self-expanding metallic stents after esophagogastrectomy. Endoscopy 2003; 35(8):652–8.

46. Radecke K, Gerken G, Treichel U. Impact of a self-expanding, plastic esophageal stent on various esophageal stenoses, fistulas, and leakages: a single-center experience in 39 patients. Gastrointest Endosc 2005; 61(7):812–18.

47. Dresner SM, Lamb PJ, Viswanath YKS et al. Oesophagectomy following iatrogenic perforation of operable oesophageal carcinoma. Br J Surg 2000; 87(S1):29.

48. Bell RC. Laparoscopic closure of esophageal perforation following pneumatic dilatation for achalasia. Report of two cases. Surg Endosc 1997; 11(5):476–8.

49. Pessaux P, Arnaud JP, Ghavami B et al. Morbidity of laparoscopic fundoplication for gastro-esophageal reflux: a retrospective study about 1470 patients. Hepatogastroenterology 2002; 49(44):447–50.

50. Vassiliu P, Baker J, Henderson S et al. Aerodigestive injuries of the neck. Am Surg 2001; 67(1):75–9.

51. Flowers JL, Graham SM, Ugarte MA et al. Flexible endoscopy for the diagnosis of esophageal trauma. J Trauma 1996; 40(2):261–5; discussion 265–6.

52. Pass LJ, LeNarz LA, Schreiber JT et al. Management of esophageal gunshot wounds. Ann Thorac Surg 1987; 44(3):253–6.

53. Symbas PN, Tyras DH, Hatcher CR Jr. et al. Penetrating wounds of the esophagus. Ann Thorac Surg 1972; 13(6):552–8.

54. Poley JW, Steyerberg EW, Kuipers EJ et al. Ingestion of acid and alkaline agents: outcome and prognostic value of early upper endoscopy. Gastrointest Endosc 2004; 60(3):372–7.

55. Zargar SA, Kochhar R, Nagi B et al. Ingestion of corrosive acids. Spectrum of injury to upper gastrointestinal tract and natural history. Gastroenterology 1989; 97(3):702–7.

56. Zargar SA, Kochhar R, Nagi B et al. Ingestion of strong corrosive alkalis: spectrum of injury to upper gastrointestinal tract and natural history. Am J Gastroenterol 1992; 87(3):337–41.

57. Wijburg FA, Heymans HS, Urbanus NA. Caustic esophageal lesions in childhood: prevention of stricture formation. J Pediatr Surg 1989; 24(2):171–3.

58. Zargar SA, Kochhar R, Mehta S et al. The role of fiberoptic endoscopy in the management of corrosive ingestion and modified endoscopic classification of burns. Gastrointest Endosc 1991; 37(2):165–9.

59. Di Costanzo J, Noirclerc M, Jouglard J et al. New therapeutic approach to corrosive burns of the upper gastrointestinal tract. Gut 1980; 21(5):370–5.

60. Kamijo Y, Kondo I, Kokuto M et al. Miniprobe ultrasonography for determining prognosis in corrosive esophagitis. Am J Gastroenterol 2004; 99(5):851–4.

61. Ramasamy K, Gumaste VV. Corrosive ingestion in adults. J Clin Gastroenterol 2003; 37(2):119–24.

62. Anderson KD, Rouse TM, Randolph JG. A controlled trial of corticosteroids in children with corrosive injury of the esophagus. N Engl J Med 1990; 323(10):637–40.

A prospective randomised, controlled trial in 60 children with caustic injuries with a follow-up of 18 years comparing a steroid and antibiotic regimen with best supportive care. No benefit was demonstrated in the steroid and antibiotic group; the development of oesophageal strictures related only to the severity of the corrosive injury.

63. Oakes DD. Reconsidering the diagnosis and treatment of patients following ingestion of liquid lye. J Clin Gastroenterol 1995; 21(2):85–6.

64. Bauer TM, Dupont V, Zimmerli W. Invasive candidiasis complicating spontaneous esophageal perforation (Boerhaave syndrome). Am J Gastroenterol 1996; 91(6):1248–50.

65. Marchand P. Caustic strictures of the oesophagus. Thorax 1955; 10(2):171–81.

66. Cox JG, Winter RK, Maslin SC et al. Balloon or bougie for dilatation of benign esophageal stricture? Dig Dis Sci 1994; 39(4):776–81.

   A randomised study in 93 adult patients demonstrating a better and longer-lasting symptomatic result for lower cost with Savary–Gilliard bougie dilatation than balloon dilatation.

67. Imre J, Kopp M. Arguments against long-term conservative treatment of oesophageal strictures due to corrosive burns. Thorax 1972; 27(5):594–8.

68. Webb WA. Management of foreign bodies of the upper gastrointestinal tract. Gastroenterology 1988; 94(1):204–16.

69. Nandi P, Ong GB. Foreign body in the oesophagus: review of 2394 cases. Br J Surg 1978; 65(1):5–9.

70. Ciriza C, Garcia L, Suarez P et al. What predictive parameters best indicate the need for emergent gastrointestinal endoscopy after foreign body ingestion? J Clin Gastroenterol 2000; 31(1):23–8.

71. Hodge D3rd, Tecklenburg F, Fleisher G. Coin ingestion: does every child need a radiograph? Ann Emerg Med 1985; 14(5):443–6.

72. McKechnie JC. Gastroscopic removal of a phytobezoar. Gastroenterology 1972; 62(5):1047–51.

73. Li ZS, Sun ZX, Zou DW et al. Endoscopic management of foreign bodies in the upper-GI tract: experience with 1088 cases in China. Gastrointest Endosc 2006; 64(4):485–92.

74. Eisen GM, Baron TH, Dominitz JA et al. Guideline for the management of ingested foreign bodies. Gastrointest Endosc 2002; 55(7):802–6.

75. Vizcarrondo FJ, Brady PG, Nord HJ. Foreign bodies of the upper gastrointestinal tract. Gastrointest Endosc 1983; 29(3):208–10.

76. Waltzman ML, Baskin M, Wypij D et al. A randomized clinical trial of the management of esophageal coins in children. Pediatrics 2005; 116(3): 614–19.

   A prospective randomised controlled trial of 60 children with an asymptomatic oesophageal coin, comparing immediate endoscopic removal with observation, including radiography and endoscopic removal where deemed necessary. This demonstrated no benefit from immediate endoscopic removal and 25–30% of coins passed spontaneously without complications. They conclude that treatment could reasonably include a short period of observation, particularly in older children with distally sited coins.

77. Tibbling L, Bjorkhoel A, Jansson E et al. Effect of spasmolytic drugs on esophageal foreign bodies. Dysphagia 1995; 10(2):126–7.

   A multicentre placebo-controlled trial, showing no benefit of glucagon and diazepam over a placebo treatment in the treatment of food bolus impaction.

78. Lancashire MJ, Legg PK, Lowe M et al. Surgical aspects of international drug smuggling. Br Med J (Clin Res Ed) 1988; 296(6628):1035–7.

20

Surgery for the obese

Simon Dexter

Introduction

The resurgence of morbid obesity surgery, or bariatric surgery, over recent years has become obvious, as manifest by increasing media coverage as well as a dramatic increase in the number of publications in the surgical literature. The term bariatric derives from the Greek *baros* (weight) and *iatrikos* (physician). Patients, primary care physicians and commissioning bodies have all become more aware of the benefits of bariatric surgery. Pressure to provide access for the seriously overweight to weight loss surgery is set to become a major challenge in the next few years.

The increase in obesity surgery follows a worldwide epidemic in obesity. Procedures to counter morbid obesity were initially developed in the 1950s and 1960s but were either not regarded as mainstream surgery or fell within the practice of a few enthusiasts. The development and dissemination of laparoscopic bariatric surgery in the last 10 years, together with the endless burden of eligible patients, has brought it to the forefront of general surgery once more. Indeed, there are now more gastric bypasses performed in the USA per year than there are cholecystectomies.

The trend towards surgery seems set to continue as knowledge increases about the additional benefits of surgery over and above weight loss. The remarkable impact of surgery on comorbidities, especially diabetes mellitus, appears to be partly related to weight loss but also due to the type of surgical reconstruction used, and more detailed understanding of the effects of obesity surgery on diabetes has lead to the development of new procedures with primarily metabolic intent.[1]

Obesity

Obesity is defined as a body mass index (BMI) >30. Different classes of obesity are defined by the level of BMI (Table 20.1). Morbid obesity, or clinically severe obesity, is defined by a BMI of 40 or more. Another measure of obesity is waist circumference, as central obesity has a more direct relationship with health risk than BMI alone. In men risks increase with a circumference over 94 cm and intervention is suggested over 102 cm. In women the equivalent measurements are 80 and 88 cm respectively.[2]

Obesity has grown in epidemic proportions in Western countries such as the USA, Australia and the UK, and is even starting to become a significant problem in the Far East because of increasing affluence and the introduction of a Western diet.

In the UK the prevalence of obesity has tripled in women between 1980 and 2004 (from 8% to 23%) and quadrupled in men (from 6% to 23%). Currently nearly 2.5% of the adult population are morbidly obese, with a BMI >40.[3]

The aetiology of obesity is complex and has much to do with the free availability of high-calorie and fat-rich foodstuffs, combined with the sedentary lifestyle of the late 20th and 21st centuries. These very recent changes overwhelm body weight regulatory mechanisms, which have evolved over thousands of years of relative food scarcity.

Numerous genetic abnormalities have been linked to obesity but are not solely responsible for the obese phenotype. Twin studies confirm a strong

Table 20.1 • Definition of obesity according to BMI

BMI (kg/m²)	Description
20 or less	Underweight
20–25	Desirable
25–30	Overweight
Over 30	Obese
Over 40	Morbid (clinically severe) obesity
Over 50	Super-obesity

Box 20.1 • Comorbidity associated with morbid obesity

- Diabetes mellitus
  - Risk increases 4.5% per kg gained
- Arterial hypertension
- Coronary heart disease
  - Myocardial infarction
  - Heart failure
  - Cardiomyopathy
- Obstructive sleep apnoea
- Gallstones
- Liver steatosis
  - Non-alcoholic steatohepatitis
  - Cirrhosis
- High cholesterol/lipids
- Menstrual/reproductive disorders
  - Polycystic ovary syndrome
  - Infertility
  - Obstetric complications
- Stress incontinence
- Gastro-oesophageal reflux
- Stroke
- Cancer
- Arthritis
- Psychological disorders

genetic predisposition to obesity, but individual gene abnormalities are rarely implicated.[4]

The most common and best-known obesity syndrome is Prader–Willi syndrome (1 in 25 000), characterised by short stature, mental retardation, hypogonadism, small hands and feet, and upper body obesity. The genetic abnormality is usually a deletion on the long arm of chromosome 15.

Metabolic causes of obesity are also rare. Hypothyroidism commonly coexists with obesity, but treatment only results in, at most, modest weight loss, which is rarely of any impact in the morbid obese population. Cushing's syndrome causes progressive central obesity and should be distinguished from simple obesity by the relatively short history together with the various symptoms and physical signs.

The impact of obesity on individuals, their carers and society as a whole is considerable. Obesity is associated with an elevated risk of mortality compared to normal matched controls as a consequence of obesity-related comorbidity (Box 20.1), particularly cardiovascular disease and cancer. The direct costs of obesity in England in 1998 were £480 million, or 1.5% of the NHS budget, with indirect costs estimated at £2.1 billion.[5]

Box 20.2 • Criteria for bariatric surgery

- BMI ≥40
- BMI 35–40 with obesity-related comorbidity
- Age between 18 and 65*
- Obesity for more than 5 years
- Failed non-surgical attempts at weight loss
- Fit enough for surgery
- No specific clinical or psychological contraindications
- Understand risks of surgery
- Be committed to long-term follow-up

*No longer applied in latest NICE guidance.

 The ability of surgery to reverse obesity, obesity-related comorbidities and mortality risk has been confirmed by a number of trials, most notably the Swedish Obese Subjects study.[6,7] These data make a compelling argument towards surgery for patients who are morbidly obese and unable to lose weight by other means.

Indications for obesity surgery

Criteria for obesity surgery have been proposed by bodies such as the National Institutes of Health (NIH) in the USA[8] and the National Institute for Clinical Excellence (NICE) in the UK[5,9] (Box 20.2). Patients should be morbidly obese and have a BMI of 40 or greater, or a BMI >35 with obesity-related comorbidity such as diabetes mellitus, obstructive sleep apnoea or hypertension.

As surgery is a scarce and expensive resource, patients should be expected to have some insight into their condition and be knowledgeable enough to apply some nutritional principles to their diet. Patients should therefore have undergone meaningful attempts at non-surgical weight reduction over an extended period (5 years or more) and, ideally, should have attended a hospital-based weight management programme. They should not be addicted to alcohol or recreational drugs. Patients should understand the risks and implications of weight loss surgery and be committed to long-term follow-up.

Psychiatric disease is not a contraindication to weight loss surgery, and indeed depression is common amongst the morbidly obese population. However, significant psychiatric disease should be assessed in the context of the ability to understand the surgery and maintain compliance for dietary measures and nutritional supplements.

Age limits have previously been applied and tend to range from 18 to 55 years. These limits have been lifted in the most recent NICE guidance, as patients at both ends of the age spectrum can benefit from surgery.[9] Elderly patients have a higher morbidity and mortality after bariatric surgery and can expect more modest weight loss, but still experience major reductions in comorbidity and some survival benefit.[10,11] Weight loss surgery on children remains controversial, but may be indicated in obese children, beyond skeletal maturity. Children require a higher level of assessment both from an individual and a family perspective, and should be treated by a specialist childhood obesity team before surgery is considered.[9,12]

General considerations

There are many unique elements to a bariatric service, in addition to the technical surgery. The patient population are often well researched and many will attend with detailed questions, will have watched weight loss procedures on the internet or on television, and may be members of patient support groups. Nonetheless, media reporting of bariatric surgery may provide an unrealistic view. Patients can have completely inappropriate expectations of surgery and a poor understanding of why they are overweight. Prejudice against obesity is common, not only from the public, but also, sadly, from many health professionals. As a result patients are usually defensive about eating habits and lifestyle, fearing judgement or even a refusal to consider them for surgery if they own up to anything but the healthiest of eating patterns. They are very sensitive to ill-judged remarks about their size, despite in many cases presenting a cheerful or self-deprecating façade. It is important to deal with bariatric patients in a straightforward and non-judgemental fashion.

A well-planned patient pathway can improve the relevance of the surgical referral. If patients are channelled through a supportive weight management programme prior to surgical referral, they are more likely to be well prepared by the time they see a surgeon.

Patients are generally relatively young, often have young families and may function well despite their obesity and regard surgery as a way of preventing future health problems. The wider consequences of serious complications or a fatal outcome from surgery cannot be overstated, and the surgeon and their team should make every effort to minimise adverse outcomes by ensuring they are well trained, and are able to recognise and deal with problems. This requires commitment, teamwork and appropriate facilities.

In the USA population studies using insurance data have highlighted the variability in outcomes between units, with low-volume units and inexperienced surgeons experiencing elevated levels of mortality.[13,14]

These data prompted the development of a 'centres of excellence' programme through the American Society for Metabolic and Bariatric Surgery (ASMBS). The programme is supported by commissioners of healthcare, such as Medicare and other health insurance companies, who will only pay for surgery to be performed in registered centres of excellence, where results are demonstrably better.[15]

Multidisciplinary team working

The causes of obesity are multifactorial and the consequences of obesity affect patients psychologically and physically. The assessment and successful treatment of obesity requires a multidisciplinary approach. The team should include a dietician, physician, surgeon, anaesthetist and preferably a specialist nurse. In addition, patients need access to a clinical psychologist/psychiatrist. Perioperative support is enhanced by access to a patient support group.[16]

As with cancer, input from different professionals contributes to tailored care along best practice guidelines. The multidisciplinary meeting brings these opinions together and is highly appropriate for bariatric patients.

Risk management in obese surgical patients

Morbidly obese patients are commonly at higher than average risk for anaesthesia and surgery because of systemic comorbidity as well as their obesity.[17]

Diabetes, hypertension and hypoventilation/obstructive sleep apnoea are common conditions in patients undergoing obesity surgery. Preoperative assessment and management should aim to optimise these before elective weight-reduction surgery.

Diabetes is prevalent in a quarter to a third of patients who present for bariatric surgery, many of whom are previously undiagnosed. Whilst the majority will not require any long-term treatment, as surgery usually resolves diabetes, good glucose control during the perioperative period has been shown to reduce complications. Patients should be monitored after discharge to confirm glycaemic control.

Hypertension is often overlooked but requires an appropriate sized cuff to measure blood pressure. Obstructive sleep apnoea (OSA) is common in the obese population. OSA causes venous shunting, ventilation/perfusion mismatch and right heart strain, predisposing to congestive cardiac failure. Opiates used for pain relief after surgery can exacerbate apnoea and stop patients rousing during an apnoeic episode. For these reasons apnoea should be identified preoperatively by sleep studies, or patients at risk monitored closely in a critical care environment during the immediate postoperative period. Continuous positive airway pressure reduces the impact of sleep apnoea on cardiorespiratory morbidity and should be instituted before surgery where possible, particularly in more severe cases.

Patients should be encouraged to take responsibility for reducing their own operative risks, as bariatric surgery should be regarded as a partnership between surgeon and patient in order to achieve the best long-term outcomes. Active smoking is a major risk factor for bariatric surgery and is regarded by many surgeons as a contraindication to surgery. Smokers can significantly improve their operative risks by stopping smoking for at least 6 weeks before surgery.[18] Moreover, they should be encouraged to maintain abstinence from smoking given the paradox of pursuing a major but health-giving operation with a view to gaining years of life, whilst continuing to smoke.

Physical activity should be encouraged and any weight loss before surgery should be seen as a bonus. A requirement by some surgeons for patients to lose a certain amount of weight before surgery is based on the notion that it demonstrates commitment from the patient and may predict a better outcome. There are also definite improvements in operative risk with significant preoperative weight loss. In addition, 7–10 days of low-fat, low-carbohydrate diet results in marked loss of liver volume in the typical steatotic liver.[19] This reduction in volume renders the liver more flexible and allows it to be retracted with ease, reducing the risk of bleeding and possibly conversion or abandonment in the case of laparoscopic surgery.

Thromboembolic disease is a major risk in massive obesity and pulmonary embolism contributes up to 38% of perioperative bariatric surgery deaths.[20] Low-molecular-weight heparin should be given before and following surgery, and may be given with some additional benefit for several days following discharge. It may be difficult to fit conventional antithrombosis stockings, but calf compression devices can be used in the operating theatre.

Finally the surgical approach appears to be important in reducing complications.

Laparoscopic surgery results in earlier discharge, more rapid recovery and fewer complications than open surgery, most notably a reduction in wound-related complications.[21]

Surgical operations for obesity

Operations for obesity emerged in the early 1950s. Weight loss was induced by malabsorption through operations such as the jejuno-ileal bypass. By anastomosing the proximal jejunum to the distal ileum, much of the small bowel was taken out of circuit, resulting in a very short length of bowel for nutrient absorption. It became apparent that the excluded jejunum became a site for bacterial overgrowth, resulting in numerous major nutritional deficiencies, oxalate renal stones and liver failure. There have also been deaths from the metabolic consequences of the operation. As a result large numbers of these procedures have been reversed.

Gastric bypass emerged because Mason appreciated that patients lost weight after partial gastrectomy for ulcer disease, and so devised an operation that partitioned rather than resected the stomach. This was drained by a loop gastro-jejunostomy and became the first gastric bypass. Numerous developments have since followed, resulting in the modern gastric bypass, which is the most common procedure employed worldwide for obesity.[22] In addition, Mason continued to develop various restrictive gastroplasties to try and avoid the use of a small-bowel anastomosis, most notable the vertical banded gastroplasty, which until recently was one of the most popular operations in Europe for obesity.

Current procedures are generally performed laparoscopically and have altered slightly from open surgical techniques. Purely restrictive procedures include adjustable gastric banding and sleeve gastrectomy, with a small diehard minority continuing to use vertical banded gastroplasty. Combined restrictive and malabsorptive operations are the Roux-en-Y gastric bypass, which is predominantly restrictive, and bilio-pancreatic diversion and duodenal switch procedures, which rely more on malabsorption with a lesser degree of restriction.

Surgical technique

It is important that surgery is performed on operating tables designed to take the weight of these patients in both flat and steep head-up positions. Most surgeons will perform laparoscopic procedures from between the legs and some means of splitting the legs safely with head-up tilt is very important. A splitting table with footplates is ideal, but if extending boots are used for the legs these should be in as flat a position as possible, with the knees extended, to avoid them buckling and allowing the patient to slide down, whilst in a head-up position.

Anaesthetic considerations

The specific difficulties associated with operating on very large patients necessitate an experienced anaesthetist as well as surgeon.

Non-invasive measurement of blood pressure may be unreliable and an arterial line is usually of value for perioperative monitoring of blood pressure and volaemic status. Opiate analgesia is undesirable, especially for patients with sleep apnoea who need to be monitored in a high-dependency unit environment. Epidural anaesthesia is ideal, but may be difficult in the context of extreme obesity. Difficulties with the airway may on rare occasions necessitate the use of awake fibre-optic intubation. Where such difficulties are likely to be encountered the presence of two experienced anaesthetists may be valuable. However, the mere presence of obesity does not predict anaesthetic difficulties.

Open surgery

From the surgical perspective males, patients with central obesity, older patients and patients with large fatty livers usually present the greatest difficulties. The surgery can be made easier by standardising the approach and using appropriate retraction and position to achieve maximum exposure. A steep head-up position allows the viscera to fall away from the hiatal area and facilitates access, provided the diaphragm is supported by sternal retraction. This can be achieved either by a central sternal hook, attached to a crossbar, or by the Omnitract system, designed for bariatric surgery. Deep-bladed retractors are required with either approach, to hold open the upper midline incision used for open bariatric surgery.

As there is a high incidence of incisional hernia after open bariatric surgery, close attention should be paid to wound closure. Reflecting the fat away from the rectus sheath allows more precise approximation of the fascial wound edges and reduces hernia rates. In addition, the wound closure can be reinforced by using interrupted sutures along the length of the wound in addition to the continuous midline closure.

Laparoscopic surgery

The view at laparoscopic surgery is usually excellent with liver retraction and marked head-up tilt affording access to the hiatus and proximal stomach.

Most bariatric operations focus on the proximal stomach and port positions similar to those of hiatal surgery will be most familiar. Additional attention is needed to set up the port positions for access to the small bowel for gastric bypass and bilio-pancreatic diversion.

Peritoneal access is difficult to achieve by a Hasson technique because of the thickness of the abdominal wall. A Verres needle can be used safely for insufflation. The author's preference is to guide the needle carefully through the abdominal wall away from the midline in the left upper quadrant. Alternatively an optical trocar can be used if the surgeon has experience with the device.

Port placement through the thick abdominal wall is critical. Ports should be long enough to remain well in place in supine and head-up position. Leakage of gas into the abdominal wall from short cannulae partly sliding out creates problems with access. The angle of insertion of the ports should be towards the working position. If they are placed in the wrong direction, the thickness of the abdominal wall creates extra work on the instruments, increases friction, and results in imprecise use of the instrument and often gas leakage.

Long instruments are essential as is a reliable system for liver retraction. Stapling devices also come in longer lengths and are designed to be airtight for use in laparoscopic surgery.

Different surgical procedures

Obesity surgery generally falls into two categories:

1. Purely restrictive procedures.
2. Bypass/malabsorptive procedures (include restrictive element).

Restrictive procedures act to limit the volume of food intake. Bypass procedures add a small bowel bypass, which separates food from bilio-pancreatic enzymes for a determined length of the bowel, potentially reducing absorption of nutrients.

Some surgeons prefer a single procedure, although ideally one should attempt to tailor the procedure to the individual patient. Laparoscopic surgery has rapidly become the gold standard for bariatric surgery, although in some instances such as re-operative surgery, an open approach may be more appropriate.

Purely restrictive operations

Vertical banded gastroplasty (VBG)

This involves the fashioning of a vertical gastric pouch of around 20 mL volume with a synthetic band or ring wrapped around the pouch outlet. The site of passage of the ring is created using a circular stapler through the stomach, and the pouch

Chapter 20

fashioned with a vertical staple line from this point to the angle of His. Trials have demonstrated inferior results of VBG compared with gastric bypass.[23,24] In addition, VBG is associated with complications including pouch dilatation, gastro-gastric fistula, mesh erosion, vomiting, reflux disease and mild vitamin deficiency. The procedure is rarely undertaken currently as it has been superseded by adjustable gastric banding. Despite the loss of popularity of VBG there has been one randomised study in which it fared better than laparoscopic gastric banding in terms of weight loss and re-operations.[25]

Laparoscopic gastric banding

The concept of external gastric banding was initially developed in the 1970s but only really became popular in the 1990s, when it became routine to perform the procedure laparoscopically. There are currently a number of adjustable gastric bands on the market. Although slight variations exist between bands, the principles of the device are similar. The device consists of a rigid band with an inflatable silicone ring on the inside, which is connected to a reservoir placed on the abdominal wall or sternum.

The band is either preformed into a circle or can be drawn into a circular shape before locking into position around the stomach. The band is applied to the upper part of the stomach, creating an hourglass deformity with a small gastric pouch of around 20 mL above an adjustable outlet, or 'stoma', into the distal stomach. The fundus of the stomach is sutured over the band to create an anterior tunnel, to reduce the risk of band slippage. The stoma is adjusted postoperatively by filling the reservoir to the point where food passage is restricted, and slows emptying of the pouch. The pouch fills rapidly during eating, resulting in a sense of fullness with very small meals. Adjustments may take place several times over the first few months, starting 6–8 weeks following surgery.

Complications are rare at the time of surgery, but late complications include slippage and erosion. Slippage is potentially dangerous as the stomach prolapses through the band, compromising its blood supply. This complication is now rare, since abandoning the perigastric placement of bands for the now-favoured pars flaccida approach. Erosion of the band into the stomach occurs in 1–2% of cases and may result from, or present with, sepsis around the injection port. Oesophageal dilatation is more common in patients with pre-existing reflux and may result from an over-tight or misplaced band around the gastro-oesophageal junction. Leaks from the band usually occur from the port or tubing as it passes through the abdominal wall.

Gastric banding is an increasingly common procedure in the UK as a consequence of increased patient awareness through the media, including endorse-ments by several high-profile celebrities. Patients therefore often have unrealistic expectations of gastric banding and need to be counselled carefully to ensure compliance and to balance expectations.

The results from banding are greatly influenced by the quality of follow-up and support.[26] This may account for the variability in outcomes, which can be excellent in centres with a strong focus on banding,[27] but are often less impressive in other studies.

The perceived advantages of banding over other procedures include adjustable restriction, reversibility and maintenance of normal anatomy. Operative mortality is extremely low and it can be regarded as the safest of operative procedures. However, the safety of banding needs to be considered in the context of 'intention to treat'. Surgery improves long-term mortality with a small risk related to the surgery itself. Surgery thus represents a balance of risk; a poor outcome in terms of weight loss from a low-risk procedure is likely to be more dangerous than a good outcome from a higher risk operation in the longer term. In addition there is a potentially high rate of revisional surgery for complications or weight loss failure from banding, which adds greatly to the overall risk of the original procedure.[28] It is therefore essential that units focusing on bands because of their low risk produce good outcomes in terms of weight loss and maintain a low rate of revision in order to justify the claim to low morbidity.

Surgical technique

- Head-up position, surgeon between the split legs, assistant to patient's right side.
- Optical trocar insertion, 12 mmHg pressure, standard hiatal port positions.
- Band inserted into peritoneal cavity via 15-mm cannula.
- Angle of His identified and peritoneum over left crus incised.
- Pars flaccida opened and fat overlying right crus reflected by assistant.
- Peritoneum overlying right crus incised 0.5 cm cranial and anterior to point of fat encroachment onto the base of the right crus.
- Goldfinger® or equivalent blunt grasping instrument passed from epigastric port through aperture in peritoneum. This should pass **without any resistance** behind the proximal stomach to emerge over left crus at site of previous left crural incision.
- The band is drawn back around the tunnel created by Goldfinger and locked in place using its locking mechanism.

- An oesophageal bougie with intrinsic 20-mL balloon is positioned with the balloon between the band and the gastro-oesophageal junction, and the balloon inflated.
- Fundus of stomach is sutured with non-absorbable sutures to the pouch created by the balloon, providing a tunnel for the band. The left crus may be included in the lateral-most suture.
- Tubing is brought out through the 15-mm cannula, which is withdrawn over the tubing. The injection port is fixed to the rectus sheath, or presternal fascia, and tubing tunnelled to the site of the port, to which it is attached. The band should remain empty until first inflation several weeks later.
- Postoperatively patients can be discharged home the following day and are placed on a liquid diet for 4 weeks. The first band inflation is performed 6–8 weeks following surgery.

Sleeve gastrectomy

Vertical gastric stapling without a band (the Magenstrasse and Mill operation) was developed by Johnston et al. in order to avoid the use and subsequent complications of the synthetic band of the VBG.[29] The upper part of the stomach is divided lengthwise with staplers, creating a narrow tube of stomach. This tube has a small volume and, as with other restrictive procedures, limits the volume of food that can be eaten. The excluded upper part of the stomach (fundus) was left alone because it is closely applied to the spleen, was often relatively inaccessible and attempting its removal risked damage to the spleen.

Initial attempts to perform the procedure laparoscopically soon yielded to the development of sleeve gastrectomy, in which the fundus and body of the stomach are resected to the left of the 'sleeve', defined by a bougie lying against the lesser curve. The fundus is much easier to access safely laparoscopically than at open surgery and can be removed with minimal danger to the spleen.

Sleeve gastrectomy creates a long, narrow and restrictive gastric tube and removes the gastric fundus, greatly diminishing ghrelin production.[30] Ghrelin is an orexigenic hormone, produced predominantly in the gastric fundus, and by removing its major source appetite is reduced. Although gastric emptying is accelerated after sleeve gastrectomy, preservation of the antrum and pylorus prevents dumping and maintains duodenal continuity. Micronutrient malabsorption from the proximal small bowel is rare, although anaemia may occur from iron or occasionally B_{12} deficiency.

Weight loss is usually dramatic, but dilatation of the gastric tube over time can lead to weight gain. This is less common with the use of a narrow tube of 32–34 Ch. Complications include staple line leakage (2%), stenosis of the tube and gastro-oesophageal reflux. Reflux symptoms tend to predominate in the first year after surgery but reduce thereafter.[31]

Sleeve gastrectomy can be used as a primary weight loss operation, but is also used as the first stage of a two-stage procedure for extremely obese patients. The sleeve gastrectomy is performed and after sufficient weight loss, or when the weight loss reaches a plateau, the second stage of the procedure, often a duodenal switch, is undertaken. This may be a year or so later. At the time of the second stage operation there has usually been substantial weight loss and the operation is technically less challenging than would have been the case originally. This approach was initially endorsed by Gagner et al., who showed a marked difference in mortality for patients with a very high BMI, who underwent single-stage versus two-stage duodenal switch, and subsequently applied this approach to gastric bypass.[32]

Surgical technique

- Head-up position, surgeon between legs, assistant to patient's right.
- Optical trocar insertion, 12 mmHg pressure, ports placed to allow antral dissection/stapling and access to fundus.
- Antrum assessed for size and nerve of Laterjet identified.
- Greater curve mobilised from point of transection of antrum, close to the stomach wall, taking gastric branches of gastroepiploic arcade. Complete greater curve mobilisation may be performed before or after stapling of the gastric tube. Lesser sac adhesions are freed prior to initial stapling.
- Initial firing of stapler (author preference for 60-mm green cartridge with staple line reinforcement) 5–7 cm from pylorus, staying close to bougie up against lesser curve, preserving nerve of Laterjet.
- Continued firings of stapler, pushing bougie onto lesser curve. The stomach is stretched laterally to maintain approximation of stapler to bougie and avoid posterior fundal pouch on sleeve.
- Angle of His is dissected and posterior gastric vessel divided prior to final stapling at top end of tube. Staple line should not run onto oesophagus, to reduce risk of leakage from upper end of staple line.

- Haemostasis checked whilst good blood pressure maintained.
- Postoperatively liquid diet on day 1 and discharge home usually day 2.

Combined restrictive/malabsorptive procedures

Roux-en-Y gastric bypass (RYGB)

The RYGB remains the commonest operation worldwide for morbid obesity. Since the inception of gastric bypass by Mason in the 1960s there have been numerous adaptations to the procedure, more recently involving laparoscopic techniques.[22] The principles of the operation are the creation of proximal gastric pouch of <30 mL, based on the higher lesser curve, which drains via a Roux limb at least 75 cm long through an anastomotic stoma 1 cm in diameter. Variations of the operation include the addition of a restrictive band around the stoma to reduce stomal dilatation,[22] and the use of a long gastric tube with a loop gastro-jejunostomy.[33] Other variations include transection or stapling in continuity of the pouch from the stomach remnant, and variable limb lengths, as patients with higher BMIs achieve better weight loss with longer bypass limbs.[34]

The reason for weight loss after gastric bypass is down to a combination of factors. There is no doubt that restriction of food volume reduces calorie intake. Nutrient malabsorption is variable but uncommon after a standard gastric bypass and cannot be responsible for the degree of weight loss.

The impact of gastric bypass on gut hormone profiles may have much to do with the typical loss of appetite experienced after bypass surgery. This prolonged alteration of appetite is associated with elevated anorexigenic gut hormones such as peptide YY from the small bowel, and a reduction in the orexigenic hormone, ghrelin, produced in the fundus of the stomach.[30,35,36]

Gastric bypass also predisposes to dumping syndrome. This is more common following ingestion of excessive simple carbohydrates, and may be of benefit in sweet eaters, who will be discouraged from habitual sweet eating as a result of the unpleasant nature of the dumping symptoms.

RYGB produces better weight loss than the purely restrictive operations but has a different profile of significant complications, including marginal ulcer, stomal stenosis, anaemia (iron deficiency, vitamin B_{12} deficiency and folic acid deficiency), trace element deficiency (magnesium, calcium, zinc, selenium) and occasionally fat-soluble vitamin deficiency. Most of these complications can be anticipated and prevented by regular follow-up and blood tests, and the lifelong use of vitamin and mineral supplements. In addition, ulcer prophylaxis should be routine, at least for the first few months after operation, and in any patients requiring regular non-steroidal analgesics.

Surgical technique

- Head-up position, surgeon right side (small-bowel anastomosis) then between legs (pouch and top anastomosis).
- Optical trocar insertion, 12 mmHg pressure, ports placed to allow hiatal/proximal stomach dissection. Adjustments to ports to allow small-bowel dissection.
- Numerous techniques exist for laparoscopic gastric bypass. The author will describe his own technique.
- Greater omentum split along full length, giving access to the intracolic compartment and providing short route for antecolic Roux limb.
- Duodeno-jejunal flexure identified at base of transverse mesocolon and small bowel divided 75–150 cm distal to ligament of Treitz, depending on size of patient. Small bowel followed for a further equivalent length, taking Roux limb to right of divided bilio-pancreatic limb.
- Jejuno-jejunal anastomosis completed using linear stapler. Stapler fired in both directions creating wide anastomosis, and bringing residual enterotomy to front for closure with third, transverse firing of linear stapler.
- Jejuno-jejunal mesenteric defect closed with prolene.
- Liver retractor placed to obtain access to the hiatus.
- Angle of His identified and pouch sized by experience or initially by 20–25 mL intragastric balloon. Transection point of stomach usually around level of second branch of left gastric vessels, which should be divided whilst creating small perigastric window.
- Stomach transection initiated by transverse stapling 5 cm distal to oesophagogastric junction. Anvil of 21-mm circular stapler introduced via service gastrotomy away from pouch. Shaft of anvil pushed out along staple line, using an anvil grasper through small hole created by harmonic scalpel. Service gastrotomy stapled or sutured closed and pouch completed,

using two or three blue 45-mm staple firings, aimed towards angle of His.

- Stapler passed via extended port site into the abdomen and into the open end of the Roux limb. Spike advanced through side of jejunum and end-to-side gastro-jejunostomy fashioned. Jejunum closed with linear stapler and anastomosis leak tested using methylene blue instillation.
- Petersen defect closed from below with 2/0 prolene, taking Roux limb mesentery onto transverse mesocolon to right of duodeno-jejunal flexure.
- Extended port-site wound sutured to avoid postoperative hernia.
- Postoperatively liquid diet on day 1 and discharge home usually day 2.

Technical variations

The commonest variations involve the routing of the Roux limb and the technique of anastomosis. The Roux limb can be passed retrocolically (then usually antegastrically) via a fenestration in the mesocolon. This reduces the size of the Petersen defect but creates a new mesocolic defect, which needs closure around the Roux limb to avoid internal herniation.

The gastro-jejunal anastomosis can be hand-sewn, which requires a high level of technical expertise and, in most surgeon's hands, takes longer than stapling, or can be constructed using a linear stapler. This produces a more uncertain anastomotic diameter, and leaves an awkward combined enterotomy to close at the site of entry of the stapler, but is relatively easy to construct and does not require extension of any of the port sites. Finally the head of a circular stapler can be passed into the pouch and drawn into position by mounting the head onto an orogastric tube, which is passed per oram and out through a small hole in the tip of the completed pouch. This is only possible with a 'flip-top' circular stapler head, which passes through the pharynx, and has been made easier by the development of a pre-mounted device (Orvil, Covidien).

The technique of open gastric bypass differs in some respects. The pouch is often stapled without division from the remnant stomach, a retrocolic route is more commonly used for the Roux limb, and hand-sewn anastomoses are also more prevalent.

Concurrent cholecystectomy has been advocated because of difficulty accessing the biliary system after gastric bypass, as well as the development of gallstones in 30% of patients after rapid weight loss. However, only half of these patients will develop symptoms and a laparoscopic cholecystectomy following weight loss is not prejudiced by adhesions from the bypass surgery when performed laparoscopically. The risk of gallstone formation can be reduced by the administration of ursodeoxycholic acid postoperatively, although patient compliance is usually poor.

Malabsorption-predominant operations

Bilio-pancreatic diversion (BPD) is a malabsorption-predominant procedure, which was first introduced by Scopinaro and often is referred to by his name.[37] The operation involves transection of the ileum 250 cm proximal to the ileo-caecal junction. The distal ileal limb is anastomosed to a proximal stomach pouch, created by subtotal gastrectomy. The volume of the stomach remnant is adjusted according to the size of the patient and varies between 200 and 400 mL. The rest of the proximal small bowel (bilio-pancreatic limb) is anastomosed to the distal ileum 50 cm proximal to the ileo-caecal junction. This short common channel can only adapt to a certain extent and is unable to absorb more than around 1500 calories per day, although simple carbohydrates and alcohol can be absorbed in the more proximal small bowel and stomach.

The operation causes fat malabsorption and results in malodorous and frequent stools when fat is ingested. Protein is also malabsorbed and patients need to maintain a high-protein diet, with vitamin and micronutrient supplementation, to avoid long-term nutritional complications. These include protein calorie malnutrition (requiring reversal in 4%), osteoporosis from calcium and vitamin D malabsorption, and the consequences of the fat-soluble vitamin deficiencies, such as night blindness (vitamin A) and prolonged prothrombin time (vitamin K).

Bilio-pancreatic diversion (BPD) with duodenal switch (DS) is a modified version of the former technique in which the gastric volume is reduced by sleeve gastrectomy, preserving the antrum and pylorus. The duodenum is then transected 5 cm distal to the pylorus. The distal ileum is divided 250 cm upstream from the ileo-caecal valve and the ileal limb is joined to the first part of the duodenum. Most surgeons use a longer common channel of 100 cm than with a classical BPD, as the sleeve gastrectomy is somewhat more restrictive than the distal gastric resection. This reconstruction reduces the incidence of stomal ulcer, reduces dumping and has a lower incidence of protein malnutrition than BPD.[38,39]

Laparoscopic DS is a long and technically difficult operation. In patients with extreme obesity (BMI >65) the mortality from the operation may be substantial and is potentially reduced by a two-stage approach.

Choice of procedure

There is no clear guidance as to which procedure is most appropriate for any particular patient. The decision as to which procedure is most suitable should be a joint decision between surgeon and patient after a full explanation of the appropriate procedures, their risks, complications and lifestyle impact.

Factors that influence the decision include the extent of obesity and level of comorbidity. Malabsorptive procedures result in the greatest weight loss and may be more appropriate in the super-obese. However, the operations are long and complex and may be inadvisable in highly comorbid patients, particularly those with significant cardiac disease. The nutritional dangers of malabsorptive procedures require a thorough understanding and a commitment by the patient to adhere to dietary rules. Dietary compliance is also very important for successful weight loss from gastric banding. Patients who are low-volume eaters, snackers and sweet eaters may not be suitable candidates. Sweet eaters may find that dumping from sweets after gastric bypass helps control this aspect of their diet, although dumping is not invariable. The presence of comorbidities such as diabetes and dyslipidaemia are more predictably controlled by gastric bypass or BPD and patients should be aware of this.

The potential morbidity of the procedures differs and gastric banding is generally perceived to be the least morbid operation. Patients should understand that each operation carries a risk–benefit ratio and that they will need to achieve a good outcome in order to benefit from a low-risk operation. Failure to control their obesity leaves them at risk, however safe the procedure.

An attempt to use some of these factors to produce an algorithm is useful if a variety of procedures is on offer,[40] although individual patient preference should play a large role in determining the procedure. Patients who are coerced into an operation they do not want will often blame the choice of procedure if they do not fare well.

Laparoscopic versus open surgery

In recent years laparoscopic approaches to bariatric surgery have predominated. Whilst patient and technology driven initially, the benefits of laparoscopic surgery have emerged as patients appear to have fewer complications and better early recovery. Randomised trials have shown that laparoscopic surgery is associated with less post-operative pain, shorter hospital stay, a lower incidence of wound infection and a similar incidence of anastomotic leak. The incidence of incisional hernia is much higher 3 years after open gastric bypass (39% vs. 5%) with similar weight loss to laparoscopic bypass.[41] Stomal stricture may be more prevalent following laparoscopic gastric bypass, perhaps because of an increased use of staplers. There may be a higher incidence of internal hernia following laparoscopic surgery because of a lack of adhesion formation. Overall 30-day morbidity is lower after laparoscopic surgery (7% vs. 14.5%).[21]

All procedures can be completed laparoscopically, but can be very technically demanding. As such it is preferable for surgical teams to be specifically trained and to carry out large volumes of cases to minimise complications.

Revisional bariatric surgery

Revisional surgery is an inevitable consequence of the increasing number of bariatric operations being undertaken. The most common reasons for revision are weight gain or failed weight loss and specific complications of the procedure. Occasionally patients become intolerant of their procedure and request reversal or conversion to an alternative operation.

In the case of failed weight loss or weight gain, a contrast study should be performed to identify a cause, such as erosion, disassembly or leakage of a band, or a staple line disruption after VBG or gastric bypass. Sleeve gastrectomy dilatation and widening of the gastro-jejunal anastomosis after bypass may also be demonstrated.

Gastric band erosion can usually be dealt with by removing the band endoscopically using a band cutter, although the tubing needs to be cut and the port removed surgically. Staple line disruption after VBG or gastric bypass can be re-stapled with best results from isolating the pouch using a linear cutting stapler. Alternatives include conversion from VBG to gastric bypass, or placing an adjustable gastric band around the pouch.

A dilated sleeve can be re-stapled and reduced for weight gain after either isolated sleeve or duodenal switch.[42] Excess weight loss following malabsorptive operations may require lengthening of the common channel.

There is an argument towards pursuing a malabsorptive procedure after a failed restrictive operation. Many patients with failed bands will go on to have a revisional gastric bypass, with variable outcomes, but conversion of standard gastric bypass to a distal gastric bypass carries a high risk of protein malnutrition.[43] Patients who fail to do well after surgery need to be carefully assessed as to why they have failed before undertaking potentially risky revisional surgery.

Each case that presents for revisional surgery requires careful consideration by the whole multidisciplinary team, needs to understand the elevated level of risk of redo surgery and should undergo any procedure by an experienced surgeon, as the procedures can be very taxing surgically.

Outcomes from surgery

Weight loss

Weight loss can be presented as actual weight loss, percentage weight loss or percentage of excess weight loss; this is the proportion of excess weight over and above the ideal body weight of the patient that is lost and is the commonest term used in surgical literature. Success from weight loss surgery is usually reported as an excess weight loss of 50% or more, and should be assessed more than 5 years from surgery to be truly meaningful.

Weight loss is a function of the effect of the operation combined with dietary and lifestyle change from the patient. Pure restrictive operations tend to have poorer weight loss than hybrid or malabsorptive operations.

A recent meta-analysis of 22 000 patients in 136 studies showed a mean percentage excess weight loss for BPD/DS of 70.1%, gastric bypass of 61.6% and gastric banding of 47.5%.[44]

Modest weight loss carries quite positive health benefits, but improvement in quality of life as assessed by patients is generally proportional to weight loss.[45]

Mortality

Mortality risk is increased in morbid obese patients compared with the non-obese population, and the risk increases with higher BMI.[46]

The mortality risk from surgery should be <1%. Gastric banding is the lowest risk procedure, and BPD/DS carries the highest mortality.[20,44]

The above meta-analysis gave a mortality of 0.1% for restrictive surgery, 0.5% for gastric bypass and 1.1% for BPD/DS.

Patient factors have a major impact on operative death and high BMI (>65) males with hypertension carry the highest operative risk.[47]

Surgically induced weight loss significantly reduces mortality in the morbidly obese population, and improves numerous obesity-related comorbidities, including diabetes, hypertension and obstructive sleep apnoea. A dramatic impact of surgery on mortality has been suggested by a number of restrospective cohort studies.[48,49]

The improvement in mortality after bariatric surgery has been shown unequivocally by the recent analysis of the Swedish Obese Subjects study.[7]

This prospective controlled intervention study involved 4047 patients, of whom 2010 underwent surgery. Follow-up was completed for an impressive 99.9% of patients at a mean of 10.9 years. The majority of patients underwent restrictive operations (gastric banding or VBG) and weight loss was relatively modest. Despite this the hazard ratio for mortality risk was 0.71 ($P < 0.01$) after adjustment for age, sex and risk factors.

The greatest relative improvement in cause of death after gastric bypass appears to be from a reduction in cancer-related deaths (60% reduction at 7 years).[48] However, despite an overall reduction in mortality, non-disease-related deaths such as accidents and suicide are higher after surgery, perhaps reflecting some of the characteristics of patients who seek surgery.

Provided operative mortality is kept at low levels, it is safer for most patients to have surgery than to maintain conservative treatment for morbid obesity.

Comorbidity resolution

Weight loss is usually regarded as the primary outcome for weight loss surgery. However, reduction in mortality is related to reversal of comorbidities, which is brought about by successful weight loss surgery.

Resolution or improvement of comorbidities is predominantly due to weight loss. However, the foregut reconstruction applied in gastric bypass and bilio-pancreatic diversion has an immediate effect on diabetic control, which is initially independent of weight loss.[50]

Other diseases that improve with surgically induced weight loss include obstructive sleep apnoea, arterial hypertension, dyslipidaemia, non-alcoholic steatohepatitis, pseudotumour cerebri, stress incontinence, venous stasis and gastro-oesophageal reflux disease. Subfertility and polycystic ovary syndrome respond well to weight loss and even patients with presumed infertility should be advised to take contraceptive precautions during the early rapid weight loss phase.

The impact of surgery on type 2 diabetes mellitus is very dramatic. The most profound effect occurs with bilio-pancreatic diversion and gastric bypass, which results in remission of diabetes in around 97% and 85% respectively.[51,52]

Many patients achieve euglycaemia and are discharged home off medication within a few days of surgery and prior to any significant weight loss. The amount of weight lost is nonetheless important in reversing diabetes and is its major determinant after gastric banding, in which there is no foregut bypass[53] and in which diabetes resolves in around one-half to two-thirds of patients.

> The effect of gastric banding is most profound in lighter patients and has been shown in a randomised trial of surgery versus control in patients with a BMI of 30–40, who experienced 73% remission of diabetes, compared with 13% in the conventional therapy control group.[54]

Various theories exist to account for the rapid and prolonged improvement in diabetes. Foregut bypass results in exclusion of the duodenum and alters the gut hormone profile after food. Duodenal exclusion results in improvement in diabetic control through mechanisms that are as yet unclear.[50]

> Studies initially in animals, and subsequently humans, confirmed the role of the duodenum in diabetic control, as duodeno-jejunal bypass without gastric reduction causes remission of diabetes.[1,55]

In addition to this 'foregut theory' the hindgut also plays a role as the delivery of nutrients into the distal small bowel results in an exaggerated response in the production of gut hormones such as glucagon-like peptide 1 (GLP1).[35] GLP1 is an incretin, which increases postprandial insulin production and improves pancreatic β-cell function.

Complications of obesity surgery

Morbidly obese patients should constitute some of the highest risk patients for surgery, given the surgical, anaesthetic and nursing difficulties in dealing with them, as well as the range of comorbidities that are prevalent. Reassuringly, in the context of the modern multidisciplinary team approach, complications are rare and mortality is consistently below 1%.

Generic complications include bleeding, thromboembolism, chest infection, wound sepsis, dehiscence and wound hernia. All of these risks are increased in the obese population. Thromboembolism is a dangerous complication and pulmonary embolism, the leading cause of death among bariatric surgical patients, occurs in 0.25% of cases.

Wound sepsis and fascial dehiscence are commoner with open surgery, and the incidence of ventral hernia is often as high as 20%.

Procedure-specific complications can be technical and usually relate to the stoma or the reconstruction. In addition, the operations can cause nutritional and metabolic disturbances.

Vomiting and solid food intolerance can be due to stomal stenosis. This is easily treatable in the context of an adjustable band, which can be partially deflated. If the stenosis is at an anastomosis, balloon dilatation is usually effective, although rarely indolent strictures will require surgical refashioning.

Marginal ulcers occur in up to 10% of gastro-jejunal or gastro-ileal anastomoses. The occurrence of ulcers is highest within the first year of surgery. Predisposing factors include an oversized pouch, use of non-steroidals, *Helicobacter pylori* infection, anastomotic tension, smoking and rarely a gastrico-to-pouch fistula. Prevention includes routine anti-ulcer prophylaxis for the first 3–6 months after surgery.

Small-bowel obstruction occurs in 2% of patients in the early postoperative phase, when it is of major concern because of the potential for anastomotic or gastric remnant dehiscence upstream of the obstruction. Following laparoscopic surgery, obstruction may be due to a port-site or umbilical hernia, which if found should be repaired or left full of omentum, if incarcerated, at the time of surgery. Internal hernia occurs in up to 5% of cases, predominantly after laparoscopic surgery and particularly if internal hernia defects are not closed. Diagnosis of internal hernia can be difficult, with only computed tomography (CT) and re-exploration providing a high degree of diagnostic accuracy. Internal herniae can develop through the mesenteric defect of the jejuno-jejunostomy/ileostomy, the mesocolic defect (retrocolic reconstruction) and the Petersen space below the Roux limb mesentery.

Anastomotic leak is a rare, but life-threatening, complication most commonly affecting the gastro-jejunal anastomosis. Leaks can also occur at the small-bowel anastomosis or the duodenal stump after BPD/DS.

Leaks are technical and should be identified by leak testing during surgery, or occur late, often a week or so after operation, due to poor anastomotic blood supply. Any onset of unexplained pain, tachycardia, pyrexia or general deterioration within the first week or so of surgery should be considered to be a leak. CT if possible may be helpful and a contrast study may show the leak, but early re-exploration should always be contemplated. Treatment is usually by drainage and establishment of nutrition via remnant gastrostomy or jejunostomy. On occasions it may be possible to close the leak, although attempts are usually futile.

Failure to lose weight occurs in 10–15%. Treatment failure varies in different procedures, but is a complex issue. Weight gain or poor loss can be due to technical failure, such as a pouch-to-remnant fistula, but is often due to patient compliance. Failure to embrace lifestyle changes, including physical activity, and an emphasis on snacking and inappropriate foodstuffs predisposes to weight gain. Good patient support and follow-up and in some cases psychological support can minimise the risk of failure.

Loss of restriction after gastric bypass, often associated with widening of the stoma, can be prevented by banded bypass.[22] When it occurs and weight starts to climb, the stoma can be refashioned or banded. Recently some success has been achieved by placing an adjustable band around the pouch in these patients.[56]

Micronutrient deficiency occurs because of poor intake, reduced gastric volume and acid production, duodenal and proximal jejunal diversion, and in some cases fat malabsorption (fat-soluble vitamins).

Vitamin B_{12} deficiency is common owing to failure to cleave food-bound vitamin B_{12}. This results from reduced availability of intrinsic factor after RYGB and occasionally sleeve gastrectomy.

Calcium deficiency is common but difficult to detect as serum calcium is maintained by secondary hyperparathyroidism when intake is poor with or without vitamin D deficiency. Osteoporosis remains a long-term complication of foregut bypass surgery.

Thiamine deficiency is rare but has serious neurological consequences (Wernicke's encephalopathy). It is associated with poor intake and frequent vomiting in the early postoperative phase.

Trace element deficiencies are common before surgery because of poor diet. Reduced intake and absorption of zinc may contribute to hair loss.

Fat-soluble vitamin deficiency (vitamins A, D, E and K) can occur in the context of fat malabsorption and is common after bilio-pancreatic diversion.

Protein deficiency occurs in 5–10% of patients after malabsorptive surgery. Extreme protein deficiency is a serious concern, which requires hospitalisation and can lead to hepatic failure and late death.[43] Most patients respond to a period of parenteral nutritional support, but occasionally surgical lengthening of the common channel or reversal is needed.

Patients should be given dietary support, micronutrient supplementation and undergo long-term follow-up in order to identify and treat these potential deficiencies.

Summary

Morbid obesity is a complex condition and is associated with comorbidities that affect all of the body's major organ systems. Management of obesity should be multidisciplinary and surgery for the obese requires a dedicated and well-trained team.

Numerous operations exist, each with its own profile of efficacy and complications. The choice of operation for any individual patient is controversial but should be guided by patient factors as well as the surgeon's expertise. Patients require long-term follow-up after obesity surgery in view of the potential metabolic disturbances. In addition the results of surgery are improved by postoperative patient support.

Key points

- Morbid obesity, or clinically severe obesity, is defined by a BMI of 40 or more.
- In the UK the prevalence of obesity has tripled in women between 1980 and 2004 (from 8% to 23%) and quadrupled in men (from 6% to 23%). Currently nearly 2.5% of the adult population are morbidly obese.
- The ability of surgery to reverse obesity, obesity-related comorbidities and mortality risk has been confirmed by a number of trials, most notably the Swedish Obese Subjects study.[6,7]
- Patients should be morbidly obese and have a BMI of 40 or greater, or a BMI >35 with obesity-related comorbidity such as diabetes mellitus, obstructive sleep apnoea or hypertension, to be considered for surgery.
- The assessment and successful treatment of obesity requires a multidisciplinary approach. The team should include a dietician, physician, surgeon, anaesthetist and preferably a specialist nurse.
- Morbidly obese patients are commonly at higher than average risk for anaesthesia and surgery because of systemic comorbidity as well as their obesity.[17] Diabetes, hypertension and hypoventilation/obstructive sleep apnoea are the most common problems.

- The specific difficulties associated with operating on very large patients necessitate an experienced anaesthetist as well as surgeon.
- Laparoscopic surgery results in earlier discharge, more rapid recovery and fewer complications than open surgery, most notably a reduction in wound-related complications.[21]
- Purely restrictive procedures include adjustable gastric banding, sleeve gastrectomy and vertical banded gastroplasty.
- Combined restrictive and malabsorptive operations are the Roux-en-Y gastric bypass (RYGB), which is predominantly restrictive, and bilio-pancreatic diversion and duodenal switch (BPD/DS) procedures, which rely more on malabsorption with a lesser degree of restriction.
- Gastric banding is increasingly used and has the lowest operative risk of the bariatric procedures, but results are variable.
- The RYGB remains the commonest operation worldwide for morbid obesity.
- The impact of gastric bypass on gut hormone profiles may have much to do with the typical loss of appetite experienced after bypass surgery.
- There is no clear guidance as to which procedure is most appropriate for any particular patient. Malabsorptive procedures result in the greatest weight loss and may be more appropriate in the super-obese. However, the operations are long and complex and may be inadvisable in highly comorbid patients.
- Success from weight loss surgery is usually reported as an excess weight loss of 50% or more, and should be assessed more than 5 years from surgery to be truly meaningful.
- A recent meta-analysis of 22 000 patients in 136 studies showed a mean percentage excess weight loss for BPD/DS of 70.1%, gastric bypass of 61.6% and gastric banding of 47.5%.[44]
- The above meta-analysis gave a mortality of 0.1% for restrictive surgery, 0.5% for gastric bypass and 1.1% for BPD/DS.
- The improvement in mortality after bariatric surgery has been shown unequivocally by the recent analysis of the Swedish Obese Subjects study.[50]
- Resolution or improvement of comorbidities is predominantly due to weight loss. However, the foregut reconstruction applied in gastric bypass and BPD has an immediate effect on diabetic control, which is initially independent of weight loss.
- The impact of surgery on type 2 diabetes mellitus is very dramatic, especially BPD and RYGB, but also for gastric banding in lighter patients (BMI 30–40).

References

1. Cohen RV, Schiavon CA, Pinheiro JS et al. Duodenal–jejunal bypass for the treatment of type-2 diabetes in patients with BMI 22–34: a report of 2 cases. Surg Obes Relat Dis 2007; 33:195–7.

2. Lean MEJ, Hans TS, Seidall JC. Impairment of health and quality of life in people with large waist circumference. Lancet 1998; 351:853–6.

3. Health Survey of England 2004. NHS Health and Social Care Information Centre, Public Health Statistics, 2005.

4. Allison DB, Kaprio J, Korkeila M et al. The heritability of body mass index among an international sample of monozygotic twins reared apart. Int J Obesity 1996; 20:501–6.

5. National Institute for Clinical Excellence. Guidance on the use of surgery to aid weight reduction for people with morbid obesity. Technology Appraisal Guidance No. 46, 2002.

6. Sjostrom L, Lindroos A-K, Peltonen M et al. Lifestyle, diabetes, and cardiovascular risk factors 10 years after bariatric surgery. N Engl J Med 2004; 351:2683–93.

7. Sjostrom L, Narbro K, Sjostrom C et al. Swedish Obese Subjects study. Effects of bariatric surgery on mortality in Swedish obese subjects. N Engl J Med 2007; 357:741–52.

8. Gastrointestinal Surgery for Severe Obesity. Reprinted from NIH Consens Dev Conf Consens Statement, 25–27 March 1991; 9(1).

9. National Institute for Clinical Excellence. Obesity: Guidance on the prevention, identification, assessment and management of overweight and obesity

in adults and children. NICE Clinical Guideline 43, 2006.

10. Perry CD, Hutter MM, Smith DB et al. Survival and changes in comorbidities after bariatric surgery. Ann Surg 2008; 247:21–7.

11. Dunkle-Blatter SE, St Jean MR, Whitehead C et al. Outcomes among elderly bariatric patients at a high-volume center. Surg Obes Relat Dis 2007; 3:163–9.

12. Inge TH, Zeller M, Garcia VF et al. Surgical approach to adolescent obesity. Adolesc Med Clin 2004; 15:429–53.

13. Flum DR, Salem L, Elrod JA et al. Early mortality among Medicare beneficiaries undergoing bariatric surgical procedures. JAMA 2005; 294:1903–8.

14. Flum DR, Dellinger EP. Impact of gastric bypass surgery on survival: a population based analysis. J Am Coll Surg 2004; 199:543–51.

15. Pratt GM, McLees B, Pories WJ. The ASBS Bariatric Surgery Centers of Excellence program: a blueprint for quality improvement. Surg Obes Relat Dis 2006; 2:497–503.

16. Hildebrandt SE. Effects of participation in bariatric support group after Roux-en-Y gastric bypass. Obesity Surg 1998; 8:535–42.

17. Adams JP, Murphy PG. Obesity in anaesthesia and intensive care. Br J Anaesth 2000; 85:91–108.

18. Moller A, Tonnesen H. Risk reduction: perioperative smoking intervention. Best Pract Res Clin Anaesthesiol 2006; 20:237–48.

19. Fris RJ. Preoperative low energy diet diminishes liver size. Obesity Surg 2004; 14:1165–70.

20. Morino M, Toppino M, Forestieri P. Mortality after bariatric surgery: analysis of 13,871 morbidly obese patients from a national registry. Ann Surg 2007; 246:1002–7.

21. Hutter MM, Randall S, Khuri SF et al. Laparoscopic versus open gastric bypass for morbid obesity: a multicenter, prospective, risk-adjusted analysis from the national surgical quality improvement program. Ann Surg 2006; 243:657–66.

22. Fobi MA, Lee H, Holness R et al. Gastric bypass operation for obesity. World J Surg 1998; 22:925–35.

23. MacLean LD, Rhode BM, Sampalis J et al. Results of the surgical treatment of obesity. Am J Surg 1993; 165:155–60.

24. Hall JC, Watts JM, O'Brien PE et al. Gastric surgery for morbid obesity. The Adelaide study. Ann Surg 1990; 211:419–27.

25. Morino M, Toppino M, Bonnet G et al. Laparoscopic adjustable silicone gastric banding versus vertical banded gastroplasty in morbidly obese patients: a prospective randomized controlled clinical trial. Ann Surg 2003; 238:835–41.

26. Shen R, Dugay G, Rajaram K et al. Impact of patient follow-up on weight loss after bariatric surgery. Obesity Surg 2004; 14:514–19.

27. O'Brien PE, Dixon JB, Brown W et al. The laparoscopic adjustable gastric band (Lap-Band): a prospective study of medium-term effects on weight, health and quality of life. Obesity Surg 2002; 12:652–60.

28. Suter M, Calmes JM, Paroz A et al. A 10-year experience with laparoscopic gastric banding for morbid obesity: high long-term complication and failure rates. Obesity Surg 2006; 16:829–35.

29. Johnston D, Dachtler J, Sue-Ling HM et al. The Magenstrasse and Mill operation for morbid obesity. Obesity Surg 2003; 13:10–16.

30. Karamanakos SN, Vagenas K, Kalfarentzos F et al. Weight loss, appetite suppression, and changes in fasting and postprandial ghrelin and peptide-YY levels after Roux-en-Y gastric bypass and sleeve gastrectomy: a prospective, double blind study. Ann Surg 2008; 247:401–7.

31. Himpens J, Dapri G, Cadiere GB. A prospective randomized study between laparoscopic gastric banding and laparoscopic isolated sleeve gastrectomy: results after 1 and 3 years. Obesity Surg 2006; 16:1450–6.

32. Regan JP, Inabnet WB, Gagner M et al. Early experience with two-stage laparoscopic Roux-en-Y gastric bypass as an alternative in the super-super obese patient. Obesity Surg 2003; 13:861–4.

33. Rutledge R. The mini-gastric bypass: experience with the first 1,274 cases. Obesity Surg 2001; 11:276–80.

34. MacLean LD, Rhode BM, Nohr CW et al. Long- or short-limb gastric bypass? J Gastrointestinal Surg 2001; 5:525–30.

35. Le Roux CW, Aylwin SJB, Batterham RL et al. Gut hormone profiles following bariatric surgery favor an anorectic state, facilitate weight loss, and improve metabolic parameters. Ann Surg 2006; 243:108–14.

36. Cummings DE, Weigle DS, Frayo RS et al. Plasma ghrelin levels after diet induced weight loss or gastric bypass surgery. N Engl J Med 2002; 346:1623–30.

37. Scopinaro N, Adami GF, Marinari GM et al. Biliopancreatic diversion. World J Surg 1998; 22:936–46.

38. Hess DS, Hess DW. Biliopancreatic diversion with a duodenal switch. Obesity Surg 1998; 8:267–82.

39. Marceau P, Hould FS, Lebel S et al. Biliopancreatic diversion with a duodenal switch. World J Surg 1998; 22:936–46.

40. Buchwald H. A bariatric surgery algorithm. Obesity Surg 2002; 12:733–46.

41. Puzziferri N, Austrheim-Smith IT, Wolfe BM et al. Three-year follow up of a prospective randomized trial comparing laparoscopic versus open gastric bypass. Ann Surg 2006; 243:181–8.

42. Gagner M, Rogula T. Laparoscopic reoperative sleeve gastrectomy for poor weight loss after

biliopancreatic diversion with duodenal switch. Obesity Surg 2003; 13:649–54.

43. Sugerman HJ, Kellum JM, DeMaria EJ. Conversion of proximal to distal gastric bypass for failed gastric bypass for superobesity. J Gastrointestinal Surg 1997; 1:517–24.

44. Buchwald H, Avidor Y, Braunwald E et al. Bariatric surgery: a systematic review and meta-analysis. JAMA 2004; 292:1724–37.

45. Karlsson J, Taft C, Ryden A et al. Ten-year trends in health-related quality of life after surgical and conventional treatment for severe obesity: the SOS intervention study. Int J Obesity 2007; 31:1248–61.

46. Lew EA, Garfinkel L. Variations in mortality by weight among 750 000 men and women. J Chronic Dis 1979; 32:563–76.

47. Fernandez AZ Jr, Demaria EJ, Tichansky DS et al. Multivariate analysis of risk factors for death following gastric bypass for treatment of morbid obesity. Ann Surg 2004; 239:698–703.

48. Adams TD, Gress RE, Smith SC et al. Long term mortality after gastric bypass surgery. N Engl J Med 2007; 357:753–61.

49. Christou NV, Sampalis JS, Liberman M et al. Surgery decreases long term mortality, morbidity and health care use in morbidly obese patients. Ann Surg 2004; 240:416–24.

50. Hickey M, Pories W, MacDonald K et al. A new paradigm for type 2 diabetes mellitus. Could it be a disease of the foregut? Ann Surg 1998; 227:637–44.

51. Pories WJ, Swanson MS, MacDonald KG et al. Who would have thought it? An operation proves to be the most effective therapy for adult-onset diabetes mellitus. Ann Surg 1995; 222:339–50.

52. Scopinaro N, Marinari GM, Camerini GB et al. Specific effects of bilio-pancreatic diversion on the major components of metabolic syndrome. Diabetes Care 2005; 28:2406–11.

53. Dolan K, Bryant R, Fielding G. Treating diabetes in the morbidly obese by laparoscopic gastric banding. Obesity Surg 2003; 13:439–43.

54. Dixon JB, O'Brien PE, Playfair J et al. Adjustable gastric banding and conventional therapy for type 2 diabetes. A randomized controlled trial. JAMA 2008; 299:316–23.

55. Rubino F, Forgione A, Cummings DE et al. The mechanism of diabetes control after gastrointestinal bypass surgery reveals a role of the proximal small intestine in the pathophysiology of type 2 diabetes. Ann Surg 2006; 244:741–9.

56. Gobble RM, Parikh MS, Greives MR et al. Gastric banding as a salvage procedure for patients with weight loss failure after Roux-en-Y gastric bypass. Surg Endosc 2008; 22:1019–22.

Index

Note: Page numbers in *italics* refer to figures.
Page numbers in **bold** refer to tables.

Index

H

I

J

P